Hyperactivity is common, indeed it may be the most common disorder of childhood for certain age-groups, with an incidence of up to 5%. This is the second in a new series in child and adolescent psychiatry which brings together developmental studies with the latest information on psychopathology and management. Drawing upon international expertise, this volume provides balanced and in-depth reviews of different aspects of empirical research in the area of childhood hyperactivity ranging from epidemiology to experimental psychology and molecular biology. Its strong developmental perspective also incorporates early attachment theory, detailed behavioural observation research and longitudinal outcome studies into adulthood. The reviews of clinical treatment approaches provide practical information, and chapters on sex differences and cross-national studies are new in books in this field. As with all volumes in this series, clinicians and researchers in the fields of psychiatry, psychology, development, paediatrics and neurology will welcome this as a valuable resource.

Hyperactivity Disorders of Childhood

MONOGRAPHS IN CHILD AND ADOLESCENT PSYCHIATRY

Child and adolescent psychiatry is an important and growing area of clinical psychiatry. The last decade has seen a rapid expansion of scientific knowledge in this field and has provided a new understanding of the underlying pathology of mental disorders in these age groups. This series is aimed at practitioners and researchers both in child and adolescent mental health services and developmental and clinical neuroscience. Focusing on psychopathology, it highlights those topics where the growth of knowledge has had the greatest impact on clinical practice and on the treatment and understanding of mental illness. Individual volumes benefit both from the international expertise of their contributors and a coherency generated through a uniform style and structure for the series. Each volume provides firstly an historical overview and a clear descriptive account of the psychopathology of a specific disorder or group of related disorders. These features then form the basis for a thorough critical review of the aetiology, natural history, management, prevention and impact on later adult adjustment. Whilst each volume is therefore complete in its own right, volumes also relate to each other to create a flexible and collectable series that should appeal to students as well as experienced scientists and practitioners.

Already published in this series:
The Depressed Child and Adolescent edited by Ian M. Goodyer
ISBN 0 521 43326 6

CAMBRIDGE MONOGRAPHS IN CHILD AND ADOLESCENT PSYCHIATRY

Hyperactivity Disorders of Childhood

Edited by

SEIJA SANDBERG

CAMBRIDGE
UNIVERSITY PRESS

Published by the Press Syndicate of the University of Cambridge
The Pitt Building, Trumpington Street, Cambridge CB2 1RP
40 West 20th Street, New York, NY 10011-4211, USA
10 Stamford Road, Oakleigh, Melbourne 3166, Australia

First published 1996

Printed in Great Britain at the University Press, Cambridge

A catalogue record for this book is available from the British Library

Library of Congress cataloguing in publication data available

ISBN 0 521 43250 2 hardback

TAG

For Catharina

Contents

Contributors

Joanne Barton
Department of Child and Adolescent Psychiatry,
University of Glasgow
Caledonia House
Royal Hospital for Sick Children
Yorkhill
Glasgow G3 8SJ, UK

J. K. Buitelaar
University Hospital Utrecht
Department of Child and Adolescent Psychiatry
PO Box 95500
3508 GA Utrecht
The Netherlands

Charles Cunningham
The Hospital for Sick Children
555 University Avenue
Toronto, Ontario
Canada MSG1X8

Ruth Day
Department of Child Neurology and Child Development
Royal Hospital for Sick Children
Yorkhill
Glasgow G3 8SJ, UK

M. Elena Garralda
St Mary's Hospital Medical School
Imperial College of Science, Technology and Medicine
London, UK

Christopher Gillberg
Section of Child and Adolescent Psychiatry
University of Göteborg
Box 17113, S-402 61
Göteborg
Sweden

Lars Hellgren
Child Neuropsychiatry Centre
Annedial Clinic
University of Göteborg
5-413 45 Göteborg
Sweden

Ellen Heptinstall
MRC Child Psychiatry Unit
Institute of Psychiatry
De Crespigny Park
London SE5 8AE, UK

Shinichiro Kado
Kyoto Child Welfare Centre
Takeyamachi-Sembon-Higashi
Kamigyo-ku
Kyoto 602
Japan
Siu-Luen Luk
Department of Psychiatry
University of Melbourne
Melbourne
Victoria 3031
Australia

Sheryl Olson
Department of Psychology
University of Michigan
580 Union Drive
Ann Arbor, Michigan 48109-1346
USA

Seija Sandberg
Department of Child Psychiatry
The Royal London Hospital
Whitechapel
London E1 1BB, UK

Russell J. Schachar
Department of Psychiatry
The Hospital for Sick Children
555 University Avenue
Toronto, Ontario
Canada M5G 1XB

Robert Soussignan
Département de Psychologie
Université de Reims Champagne
57 rue Peirre Taittinger
51096 Reims Cedex
France

Jim Stevenson
Department of Psychology
University of Southampton
Highfield
Southampton SO17 1BJ, UK

Ryuro Takagi
Takagi Psychiatric Clinic
Karasuma-Oike-Agaru
Nakagyo-ku
Kyoto 604
Japan

Rosemary Tannock
The Hospital for Sick Children
555 University Avenue
Toronto, Ontario, Canada M5G 1X8

Eric Taylor
MRC Child Psychiatry Unit
Institute of Psychiatry
De Crespigny Park
London SE5 8AF, UK

Richard Tremlay
Research Unit on Children
University of Montreal
Montreal, Quebec
Canada

Gotz-Eric Trott
Department of Child and Adolescent Psychiatry
University of Würtzburg
Würtzburg
Germany

Herman van Engeland
Department of Child and Adolescent Psychiatry
University Hospital Utrecht
PO Box 85500
3508 GA Utrecht
The Netherlands

Jaap Van der Meere
Laboratory of Experimental Clinical Psychology
University of Groningen
Grote Kruisstraat 2/1
9712 TS Groningen
The Netherlands

Monographs in child and adolescent psychiatry

The 20th century has witnessed substantial progress in the understanding of child and adolescent development. Psychologists have established that cognitive, emotional, and social development are active processes, arising in the context of diverse social experiences in the home, school and peer group. In addition, the unique individuality and rights of children and adolescents have been recognised increasingly, and despite growing dependence on the state and the intrusion of specialist agencies, parents have attained fuller acknowledgement that they have responsibilities towards, as well as expectations of, their offspring. These scientific and social advances have been associated with the emergence of more sophisticated services for children and adolescents with emotional and behavioural difficulties. During the last 30 years, academic and clinical child and adolescent psychiatry and psychology have become established specialities, with the recognition that treating and managing mental disorder in young people require expertise which is not available readily in general psychiatry or psychology, or in paediatrics. Similar professional advances have characterised other child-related health care professions. In particular, the expansion of academic centres to foster research and teaching in child development and in the psychiatric disorders of childhood and adolescence has had considerable impact on the training and education of scientists, social scientists and practitioners in the field of child and adolescent mental health. The predominant feature of theory and clinical practice has been to emphasise the role of the family and social factors in the causation and management of child and adolescent psychiatric disorder. Towards the close of the 20th century, however, there is a growing awareness that the nature of child and adolescent mental disorders is highly complex, involving brain function as well as social and psychological processes. Three new major areas of endeavour have emerged, complementing existing research strategies investigating the aetiology, nature and outcome of mental disorders in young people, namely the role of genetic factors, the importance of neurobiology and the effectiveness of existing services. Associations between brain, mind and the environment will become fully understood only through interdisciplinary collaboration, bridging the gap between basic and clinical science and clinical practice. Fundamental advances in the understanding of neural structure and function are being accompanied rapidly by fuller interplay between neurochemistry and human behaviour. Combining behavioural measurement with non-invasive neuro-imaging procedures will provide more detailed information about the integrity of brain function in health and disease. Innovative neuroscientific approaches, combined with new techniques of behavioural genetic research, will result in a clearer definition of the important psychosocial mechanisms in the onset and outcome of psychiatric disorders, as well as providing new insights into pathogenesis. In addition, the need to determine what service provisions are in the best interests of children and their families and which treatments are the most effective under different service delivery conditions, becomes an increasingly important topic in clinical and public health research. The search for new methods to evaluate treatment outcome and the need to equate costs with the benefits of child mental health care are emerging as basic elements in health service planning and provision. Such ideas, in combination with research, educational and clinical advances, are fostered through closer collaboration between basic and clinical neuroscience and clinical practice in only a few centres around the world and, therefore, require dissemination to reach a wider scientific and clinical audience. Textbooks are an essential medium for the diffusion of research and clinical information. In child and adolescent psychiatry, a few comprehensive, multi-author textbooks, designed for library reference and for experienced postgraduate use, have become well-established as standard texts. These have been augmented by in-depth volumes devoted to a single topic. Some of the latter incorporate valuable introductory overviews of major disorders, usually intended for undergraduate or postgraduate readership. Others have reviewed specific areas, relevant to both student and specialist. As the scientific basis of child and adolescent psychiatry and the methods of treatment have widened, in-depth coverage by single authors has become correspondingly difficult.

Over recent years, a number of key advances in developmental science and child and adolescent psychiatry research have provided the stimulus for the evolution of a new developmental approach to the study of psychopathology. Continuities and discontinuities between normative developmental processes and the onset of emotional and behavioural disorders have been a growing focus of research. The identification of social risk factors for mental disorder is being supplanted by the need to determine the mechanisms and processes that arise from such factors and which are responsible for the onset and maintenance of disorder. There has been a recognition that such mechanisms will not be fully elucidated without new interdisciplinary research collaboration. Thus, the close relationship fostered between social, psychological and psychiatric researchers in the behavioural sciences will be promoted by collaboration with neuroscientists in the laboratory, in the clinical settings and the neuro-imaging centres. Determining mechanisms, involving brain and mind as well as psychosocial processes, will then assume an increasing reality.

This book is the second volume in a new series entitled Monographs in Child and Adolescent Psychiatry. The series is aimed at practitioners in child and adolescent mental health services and researchers in development and clinical neuroscience. Each volume will be dedicated to a specific topic within the field of child and adolescent psychopathology. While the general aim is to provide comprehensive coverage of the major syndromes, it is intended that there should be detailed consideration of topics less commonly dealt with in standard texts. In order to provide coherence within the series, a uniform style and structure will be utilised throughout, with due recognition of specialised aspects of such topics as are essential for inclusion, but which do not readily fit the standard structure. Each volume will open with a historical account of the topic, providing a perspective on the evolution of concepts and practices in present day usage. Since child and adolescent psychiatry has experienced rapid growth during the latter part of the 20th century, there is a tendency for the pace of change to obscure the contributions from previous generations. The historical chapters focus mainly on 18th to 20th century developments. Following this, there is a thorough exposition of the normal and the developmental biology pertinent to each topic. This will provide the necessary framework for comparing normal and abnormal mechanisms and processes, as well as continuities and discontinuities of thoughts, feelings and behaviours over time. These chapters will discuss, where appropriate, physio-chemical and neural, as well as social and psychological, aspects of normal behaviour.

The clinical components will include detailed expositions on the prevalence, nature, characteristics, evolution and outcome of the disorder. A life-span approach will be adopted to trace the course of childhood disorders into adult life. Recent advances in the classification of disorders, including comorbidity and the influence of development on presenting signs and symptoms, together with syndrome definition and recognition, will receive close attention. The application of behavioural genetics and the importance of gene-environment interaction will be covered, as well as environmental contribution to psychiatric syndromes. Family and peer group influences on onset, recovery and relapse will be discussed. Pathophysiological and pathopsychological accounts of the topic will be highlighted and, wherever possible, allocated separate chapters. Clinical chapters will include accounts of treatment and current public health policies. The differential impact of single and recurrent episodes on subsequent child and adult adjustment will form an important component of these clinical sections. Although the chapters will be written by international experts from widely different backgrounds and areas of expertise, each volume will conform to the overall structure of the series, providing a coherent approach to each topic. While complete in its own right, each volume will relate to the others in style and structure, creating flexible and collectable series, which should appeal to students, as well as experienced scientists and practitioners.

Preface

Hyperactivity disorders are common at certain ages – perhaps the most common disorders of childhood. According to large surveys, up to one in six children may be affected, with half of them likely to benefit from a referral to a specialist service.

However, hyperactivity/hyperkinetic disorder is also a condition over which there has been much disagreement between researchers in terms of its definition, frequency and significance. The disagreement has, in turn, been reflected in the attitudes of clinicians to the extent that in some centres, and indeed in some countries, very few children acquire the diagnosis while many are perhaps deprived of the treatment they would probably benefit from. In contrast, others may well have been unnecessarily given the label and 'medicated' for a hyperactivity disorder that they do not suffer from.

In this volume, a group of internationally merited researchers representing the various fields of child psychology, neurology and psychiatry have reviewed and synthesised the latest knowledge of childhood hyperactivity. The individual authors have approached the topic from separate, but inter-related perspectives of developmental and experimental psychology, neurochemistry, genetics and clinical psychopathology. Whenever possible, they have done this by following the common underlined thread of continuity from the normal to abnormal and of examining the impact of hyperactivity on the child's development in its different facets of physical, cognitive, emotional and social functioning.

Although the history of hyperkinetic disorder has at times been marked by conceptual muddles, often giving rise to widely inconsistent findings, many of these controversies appear to have been solved by the recent advances in research carried out with improved methodological rigour. These advances have made it possible for the authors of this volume to put forward a coherent account of the condition that continues to compromise the development of large numbers of children.

In the light of the current knowledge, hyperactivity disorders represent an outcome of continuing mutual influences between the constitutionally predisposed child and environmental stressors. The biological vulnerability can be translated into neurochemical dysfunction, most likely involving a multitude of so-called transmitters. The basis for such dysfunction appears at least partly genetically determined and exerts its primary influence in the form of some cognitive defect, mediated in many cases via language disorder. Recent research carried out in the socially more protected and far less studied gender, the girls, has further strengthened the evidence for a biologically based aetiology of hyperactivity disorder.

The extent to which the biological vulnerability gives rise to clinically relevant hyperactivity is largely determined by the presence of environmental stressors which act as triggers for the behavioural expression. Factors in the child's immediate social environment constitute the most powerful triggers. Of these, the affective content of the primary care giver–child interactions, stemming for example from parental depression, is probably the most influential. Its effect on the child's ability to modulate his level of activity and attention is likely to be mediated by inconsistent emotional feedback, lack of mutual contingencies, low level of cognitive stimulation and absence of rewarding experiences. Hyperactivity may therefore be conceptualised as a developmental defect of motivation, arising from the foundation of learned ineffectiveness, and leading to less rewarding transactions with the environment, and to loss of motivation to try.

Indeed, one of the most persuasive recent theoretical explanations for the so-called attention deficit, frequently part of hyperactivity disorder, is that instead of involving a defect in the child's ability to sustain attention or process information, it constitutes an 'output' deficit stemming from a disorder of self-regulation.

The problems of personal maladjustment are further accentuated in children with the more difficult temperamental disposition and, in the context of sub-optimal parent–child relationship, proceeding to oppositional or antisocial conduct disorder, not uncommonly found adjacent to hyperactivity. Wider social and cultural nouns and expectations in turn determine which children are labelled as hyperactive. These factors also influence willingness for help seeking and compliance with treatment. Untreated hyperkinetic disorder carries considerable risk for educational failure and future social maladjustment.

The most common treatment for hyperactivity is the use of phychostimulant drugs. In many cases these drugs are dramatically effective in reducing restlessness, improving concentration and cognitive performance, and increasing academic productivity albeit with little effect on actual learning. However, many hyperactive children gain little benefit from pharmacological treatments and, in some, side effects necessitate withdrawal of the drug. However, the most disappointing fact is the reoccurrence of the symptoms on termination of treatment. For these reasons, much effort has been spent in developing and refining psychological therapies usually based on cognitive behaviours techniques aimed at directly influencing the child's ability for self-regulation and self-monitoring. Best results are often obtained by combining drug treatment with psychological approaches. However, even given years of sustained therapeutic effort, the long-term prognosis of hyperactive children remains problematic with a substantial minority being left to cope with poor concentration, suboptimal interpersonal skills and exposed to risks of illicit drug use, motor accidents and poor employment record.

Thus, given the considerable burden hyperactivity can create for individual children and their families, the painstaking search for its causes and for cure, as demonstrated by research carried out in different parts of the world, seems well warranted. Although the level of knowledge represented in this book reflects many advances made in the past decades, it is unlikely to be the final truth, but will hopefully stimulate new and better research in the years to come.

Seija Sandberg London

1

Historical development

Seija Sandberg and Joanne Barton

INTRODUCTION

The constellation of overactivity, poor impulse control and inattention has been given a variety of diagnostic labels over the years. Although at present hyperkinetic disorder is a popular diagnosis, it is a relative newcomer in the diagnostic classification of child psychiatry. For example, even the latest (1957) edition of the child psychiatry textbook by Kanner contained no reference to hyperactivity as a diagnostic entity. On the European side of the Atlantic the condition, however, was recognised and referred to as 'hyperkinetic disorder' in Hoff's (1956) major textbook of general psychiatry. So, although at present hyperactivity tends to be associated as a particularly 'American' phenomenon, the history of the use of the term tells us otherwise. Though new as a diagnostic entity, hyperactive behaviour in children has been recognised and treated for much longer. Indeed, the current conceptualisation of the disorder represents a stage in a complex and varying developmental history, and therefore in order to appreciate our present perspective it is important to consider the chronological course in the development of the concept itself. In this chapter, an overview of the history of hyperactivity disorders will be presented, especially as they have appeared in the Western texts of childhood's behaviour disorders.

The earliest descriptions of the disorder are those by Still and Tredgold in the early 1900s. Their work will be discussed and examined in the context of the prevailing social and scientific climate. Both authors presented their analysis of the behavioural characteristics of a relatively small group of children, some of whom bear close resemblance to the hyperactive children of today. Still (1902) attributed such behaviour to a 'defect of moral control', believing it to be a biological defect which was inherited or resulted from some pre- or postnatal injury. His ideas about causation are best understood in the context of the widespread support being given at that time to Social Darwinism.

The theory of damage occurring in the early stages of the individual's development, though often mild and undetected, was adopted by Tredgold (1908); and at a later stage by others, such as Pasamanick, Knobloch & Lilienfeld (1956), as an attempt to explain the behavioural problems seen in hyperkinetic children. The encephalitis epidemic in 1917–1918 played a significant part in the history of hyperactivity. Following the epidemic, clinicians were confronted with children suffering from behavioural and cognitive sequelae, many presenting with the core features of what today would be termed hyperactivity.

For the first half of the twentieth century, the predominant view regarding the causation of hyperactivity was that of an association with brain damage. A plethora of terms such as 'organic drivenness', and 'minimal brain damage' were used to describe the disorder. During this period, the similarity between the behaviour of hyperactive children and that of primates subjected to frontal lobe lesions was noted. This was used by several investigators to support the idea that hyperkinetic disorders were due to defects in forebrain structures, despite the lack of evidence of such lesions in many children.

During the fourth and the fifth decades of this century, series of papers were published which marked the beginnings of child psychopharmacology in general, and the pharmacotherapy of behaviourally disturbed children, in particular. By the end of the 1950s, the concept of brain damage as the single causative factor in the causation of hyperkinesis was challenged. 'Minimal brain dysfunction' was substituted for 'minimal brain damage'. A variety of hypotheses was put forward at the time regarding the causation of hyperactivity, including the psychoanalytic theory of poor parenting. With the decline of the concept of 'minimal brain dysfunction', the idea of the 'hyperactive child syndrome' was being developed, with Stella Chess (Chess, 1960) as one of its chief proponents. Chess differed from her predecessors in that she viewed the prognosis of hyperactive children as reasonably good, with the condition in most cases having resolved by puberty. By the end of the 1960s the prevailing view was that hyperkinesis represented a form of brain dysfunction, and presented with a variety of symptoms of which motor overactivity was the most predominant.

It was during the 1960s that the split developed between Europe and North America over the conceptualisation of hyperkinesis. Clinicians in Europe maintained a narrower view of the disorder, seeing it as a rare syndrome of excessive motor activity; usually occurring in conjunction with some signs of brain damage. In North America, on the other hand, hyperactivity was seen as being relatively common, and in most cases not necessarily associated with overt signs of brain damage. The differences became highlighted in the diagnostic classificatory systems used (ICD and DSM, respectively).

In the 1970s, the emphasis moved away from motor overactivity and began to focus on the attentional aspects of the disorder. A number of authors demonstrated that hyperactive children had great difficulty with tasks involving sustained attention. At the same time, there was also a growing belief that hyperkinetic behaviour was due to environmental causes. This coincided with a move towards a healthier lifestyle and disquiet about the 'drugging' of school children. The idea that hyperactivity was, at least in every other case, due to an allergic reaction to food substances, particularly food additives, became popular at this time. Technological advance and other cultural influences were also put forward as causative factors. An additional development of the decade was the increase in the number of studies investigating the psychophysiology of hyperactivity.

During the 1980s the explosion of research in the field continued. With this came the development of 'research criteria' and standardised assessment procedures. Advancements were also made in the area of treatment, with new methods involving cognitive–behavioural therapies. Hyperactivity came to be seen as a condition with a strong hereditary component, chronic in nature and causing significant handicap in the areas of academic achievement and socialisation; with treatment requiring the complementary skills of a variety of professionals.

EARLY MEDICAL EXPLANATIONS

The modern history of hyperkinetic disorder is traditionally seen to begin with the writings of Sir George Frederick Still (1902) and Alfred F. Tredgold (1908), with many authors acknowledging that our present concept of hyperactivity has its foundation in their work (Ross & Ross, 1982). Preceding the studies by Still and Tregold, extensive descriptions of hyperkinetic children, mostly in the form of individual case studies, had already appeared in the psychiatric literature of the nineteenth century (Bourneville, 1897; Clouston, 1899; Hoffmann, 1845; Ireland, 1877; Maudsley, 1867); and continued to be published in the early decades of this century (Boncour & Boncour, 1905; Heuyer, 1914; Pick, 1904; Scholz, 1911)

Overexcitability and mental explosiveness: forerunners of hyperactivity?

Clouston (1899) described a series of very difficult morbid conditions that 'occur in neurotic children, but lie on the borderland of psychiatry'. He hypothesised that the disorders were all due to some dysfunction in the 'brain cortex', and were pathogenically 'states of deranged reactiveness of the neurones of the higher regions of the brain'. The derangement had arisen because the higher centres of the brain, responsible for inhibiting activity, had in some way been weakened and therefore become unable to cope with the amount of 'energising they have to control'.

Clouston, however, emphasised that such disorders should not be classified as 'out and out mental disorders'. He believed that the conditions were ultimately caused by 'hereditary and congenital peculiarities', with defects in the 'subtle and obscure process of central nerve development in childhood' acting as predisposing agents. He further postulated that certain areas of the brain 'running ahead' in their development, compared to others, were causing the derangement of its function. This in turn caused 'explosions which spread into other centres'.

Clouston (1899) outlined a series of disorders, which he proposed, all resulted from the same pathology; one of these resembles the hyperkinetic disorder of today. He called it 'simple hyperexcitability', arguing that the disorder resulted from 'undue brain reactiveness to mental and emotional stimuli'. It affected children from the age of 3 years until puberty, with overactivity and restlessness being the main symptoms. The disorder came in bursts and lasted from a few months to years. During the bursts the child would grow thin, not sleep and deteriorate in educational performance. Such clinical signs were ascribed to the children showing a 'delirium of pleasure in response to nice things', and interpreted as an exaggeration of the response one would expect from a child of nervous temperament.

Clouston concluded that the common feature of such disorders was the 'explosive condition of the nerve cells in the higher cortex'. This in his view was comparable to the overactivity of the motor cortex seen in persons suffering from epilepsy. Referring to the by then well-established findings that the process of brain development in childhood comprises rapid cell multiplication accompanied by the cells gradually becoming more stable, he argued that in the children suffering from 'hyperexcitability' this process of nerve stability does not occur, resulting in the children growing up with 'irregular explosive tendencies'.

The treatment Clouston recommended for such conditions was the use of bromides, 'fearlessly in large doses up to the point when symptoms of bromism are beginning to show themselves'. He did, however, emphasise that the drugs should not be used in isolation. Instead, the children should at the same time be given a good diet, plenty of fresh air, 'suitable amusement, companionship and employment'. The aim of the treatment was to 'reduce the cell catabolism and the reactiveness of the cerebral cortex whilst not interfering with brain anabolism'. The treatment had to be carefully monitored in order to ensure that it did not 'go too far'.

Still and the defect of moral control

Sir George Frederick Still (1868–1941), a paediatrician and the first professor of children's diseases at King's College Hospital, London, is primarily known for his description of chronic rheumatoid arthritis in children – Still's disease. In a series of lectures given in 1902 to the Royal College of Physicians, Still analysed in detail the case histories of 20 children, some of whom showed features of what we at present would call hyperactivity. In his descriptions, features such as extreme restlessness and 'almost choreiform' movements were frequently mentioned. Another common characteristic of the children was their 'abnormal incapacity for sustained attention', causing school failure even in the absence of intellectual retardation. In their behaviour, many of the children were mischievous, destructive and violent, and appeared not to respond to punishment.

According to Still, this pattern occurred more often in boys than in girls, became frequently apparent by early school years, was sometimes accompanied by peculiarities of physical appearance (e.g. epicanthic folds and high-arched palates), appeared often to be a function of temperament, generally showed little relationship to the child's training and home environment, and commonly shared a poor prognosis. Still suggested that the children he was describing suffered from a 'defect of moral control', whereby they demonstrated 'the reckless disregard for command and authority in spite of such training and discipline as experience shows will render a healthy child law-abiding'. Instead, such children displayed 'immediate gratification of self without regard either to the good of others or to the larger and more remote good of self'. Still also noted that, although many of the children with this condition came from chaotic families, a substantial proportion of them lived in homes where they appeared to receive an adequate upbringing. In fact, when refining his criteria for children with the disease, Still decided to exclude those who had been exposed to poor child rearing. This led him to hypothesise that the 'defect of moral control' was due to some 'morbid physical condition', which was either inherited, or resulting from a perinatal or postnatal injury.

The degree of uncertainty about the causation of the condition provided a logical basis for separating the children with such problems into subgroups. Still proposed a distinction between children with demonstrable gross lesions of the brain; those with a variety of acute diseases, conditions and injuries that would be expected to result in brain damage, although none could be demonstrated; and those with hyperactive behaviours that could not be attributed to any known cause. Thereby, Still laid the groundwork for the historical equivalents of three major diagnostic categories of brain damage, minimal brain dysfunction, and hyperactivity. In doing this, he also sowed the seeds for a terminological confusion so prevalent in the literature of hyperactivity over decades to come, but confusion that also gave the impetus to much excellent research on the nature of hyperactivity and its treatment.

It is to be noted that the social conditions, and the trends in scientific thought prevailing in Britain at the time, provide the context for the work of scientists such as Still. Nineteenth century Britain was marked by powerful economic, political and social transformations with the economy shifting progressively to mass production of goods in factories. Society was characterised by class hierarchy with the lower classes frequently suffering the adverse consequences of the transformed economy (Rowntree, 1901). Such adverse effects took the form of rising infant mortality, poor physical health of the workforce, and learning difficulties and delinquency in children. However, the intellectual and moral deficiencies of the lower classes tended to be identified as the cause, rather than the consequence, of their circumstances.

Concurrent with these developments was the rise of positivism in contemporary science, with beliefs that the progress of society could be achieved through the development of objective science. It was especially the theories of Darwin that provided a scientific rationale for various kinds of social deviance, with hypotheses suggesting that the environment conferred a selective advantage to some types of biological variation (Darwin, 1859). Deduced from his theories, the notion for the 'survival of the fittest' became elevated to a status of a 'law', in an attempt to explain social phenomena. This 'social Darwinism' soon found wide support among intellectuals and social reformers.

In keeping with the prevailing trend of his day, Still was keen to adopt the principles of social Darwinism and set out to explain the 'defects of moral control' of the children he was asked to treat. He claimed that moral consciousness and moral control were essentially innate characteristics. They were also 'the highest and latest product of mental evolution'. However, because they constituted a relatively recent evolutionary advance, they were also fragile and showed 'a special liability to loss and failure in development'.

Hyperactivity due to neuropathic diathesis

To support Still's reports of hyperactive behaviour pattern occurring when brain damage was suspected, but could not be substantiated, Tredgold (1908) proposed that some forms of brain damage, such as birth injury or relatively mild anoxia, though undetected at the time, could express themselves as behaviour problems or learning difficulties when the child is faced with the demands of early school years. Alfred F. Tredgold was a member of the English Royal Commission on Mental Deficiency. His book, *Mental Deficiency (Amentia)*, was published in 1908, updated in 1914, and remained in publication until 1952. In the book, Tredgold described many children who exhibited features of hyperactivity, and he is attributed by a number of authors (e.g. Ross & Ross, 1982) as being the first to provide an account of 'minimal brain damage'.

Tredgold's descriptions of hyperactivity derived from his observations of a group of child patients whom he labelled as 'high-grade feeble minded'. Although incapable of making use of education as provided in school, such children would in his judgement nevertheless benefit from individual attention and instruction. He also noted that a number of the children exhibited a variety of physical anomalies, including abnormalities of the palate, soft neurological signs, abnormal head shape and size, and poor co-ordination.

Apart from being educationally inferior, the children were also prone to criminal behaviour, despite having been raised in an adequate environment. Like Still, Tredgold attributed such moral deficiency to the impact of some 'organic abnormality on the higher levels of the brain', and argued that the areas of the brain where 'sense of morality' was located, also were the product of the more recent development in the course of human evolution; and were therefore more susceptible to damage. Tredgold believed that such moral deficiency was caused by the inheritance of some brain defect that was being passed on from generation to generation, and being able to take various forms, resulting in hyperactivity, migraine, mild forms of epilepsy, hysteria and neurasthenia. He called the defect by various names, such as 'neuropathic diathesis', 'psychopathic diathesis' 'blastophoria' or 'germ corruption'. In his view, environmental circumstances played no significant role in the causation of mental or moral deficiency.

With regard to the influence of slum life and all its associated conditions in producing amentia, it is necessary to sound a note of warning. It does happen sometimes that the real mental defectives of our large towns hail from the slums, although I do not think such is disproportionately the case. Still, a sufficient number of defective children come from such areas to make the superficial enquirer, content with that which is apparent, jump on the conclusion that the pernicious environment is therefore the cause of their defect. My own enquiries have convinced me that in the great majority of these slums cases, there is pronounced morbid inheritance, and that their environment is not the cause, but the *result*, of that heredity (quoted in Schachar, 1986).

In the decades that followed, a wide range of deviance was attributed to the interaction of brain disorder and constitutional predisposition by leading medical authorities on both sides of the Atlantic. Such biological variation could in turn have several different outcomes, ranging from school failure (Cornell, 1912), to criminality (Healy, 1915). In contrast, psychological and social explanations for cognitive and behavioural deviations were explicitly rejected. The core debate revolved around the relative contributions of inheritance and birth injury as factors of prime importance in leading to disturbed adaptability towards one's surroundings (Henderson, 1913).

Sequelae of the encephalitis epidemic

The link between hyperactive behaviour and demonstrable brain damage was strengthened by the epidemic of encephalitis spreading across Europe and the United States of America in 1917–1918. In its aftermath, many clinicians encountered children, who though having survived the infection, subsequently presented with behaviour problems and cognitive deficits. Hyperactivity, catastrophic changes in personality and learning difficulties were among the predictable sequelae of the disease (Hohman, 1922; Ebaugh, 1923). The term 'postencephalitic behaviour disorder' was adopted to encompass the various consequences. Observations of the child victims of subsequent outbreaks of encephalitis confirmed the same pattern of symptoms (Bender, 1942; Gibbs *et al.*, 1964). Cantwell (1975) and many others date the development of the North America's interest in hyperactivity to the encephalitis epidemic.

Hohman (1922), Ebaugh (1923) and Strecker & Ebaugh (1924) argued that the children who showed persisting problems with behaviour following the epidemic were also the ones who had been most severely affected by the disease; and were in most cases left with severe brain dysfunction. As such, however, only the problems of few of the children described would fit the present-day criteria for hyperkinetic disorder. It is also to be acknowledged that the available evidence was for an association between severe damage and severe behavioural disturbance. For some reason, this was subsequently extrapolated to claim that a similar connection existed between minimal brain damage and lesser degrees of disordered conduct.

As was the case with Still's disease, the influences of social Darwinism were also brought to bear on the sequelae of encephalitis, with the assumption that there was some inherited predisposition to developing the disease. People who contracted illnesses, such as encephalitis, were believed to be in some way constitutionally inferior (Bassoe, 1922; Bond & Appel, 1931).

Hyperkinetic disease

In the early 1930s, Kramer & Polnow described a syndrome characterised by restlessness, distractibility and speech disorder, called it 'hyperkinetic disease' and classified it as a form of childhood psychosis, usually of unknown origin (Hoff, 1956, pp. 543–4). The extreme restlessness, commencing in the third or fourth year of life, often came on suddenly, 'after a period of quiet', and was frequently followed by an epileptic seizure. The restlessness reached its most severe form at the age of 6 years, and then gradually decreased with the majority of cases achieving an almost complete recovery. Disturbances of speech and general mental development were often noted before the onset of restlessness.

The children were also described as being easily distracted. Their excessive motor activity, chaotic and aimless in nature, appeared to occur as a succession of uncorrelated impulses with no aim other than to respond to a stimulus. Their play also seemed to lack purpose, with toys tending to be broken rather than played with. The 'lack of discrimination', as noted, bears a resemblance to the 'impulsivity' described in children suffering from hyperkinetic disorders of today. The paucity of the children's interpersonal relationships was also remarked upon. They tended to be aggressive towards other children rather than play with them. Any attempts to restrain the child would be met with opposition and struggling.

The speech disorders, as recorded, consisted of poor articulation and 'inarticulate labelling'; the children's vocabulary was thought not to increase until their recovery from the condition. However, their intelligence, when observed daily at home, appeared to be higher than that detected on formal cognitive testing. Kramer & Pollnow (1932) argued that the disorder could be differentiated from others such as schizophrenia, dementia infantilism, encephalitis and schizophrenia-like psychoses.

In total 15 children presenting with 'hyperkinetic disease' were described. Of these one died, three suffered from definite mental defect, three recovered from the restlessness but were left with permanently impaired intelligence, four recovered partially, whilst another two recovered completely. Four children were less than 7 years old and were therefore felt to be still within the 'hyperactive stage.'

Organic drivenness

In 1934, Kahn & Cohen described three patients whose clinical condition was marked by hyperkinesis, inability to remain quiet, abruptness, clumsiness and explosiveness of voluntary activity. The authors argued that all the symptoms were secondary to a central behaviour abnormality – hyperactivity. This hyperactivity was a result of 'organic drivenness, or a surplus of inner impulsion'. They suggested that the hyperactive behaviour stemmed from abnormality in the organisation of the brain stem and was often caused by trauma, or 'prenatal encephalopathy or birth injury'. Acknowledging that, in a number of such hyperactive children, no history of trauma could be confirmed, Kahn & Cohen (1934) postulated a congenital defect in the activity-modulating system of the brain stem as being the cause of the condition. In their view, both the over- as well as the under development of certain areas of the brain were capable of leading to the same end result. They also added that features such as soft neurological signs, e.g. twitching, and minor congenital dysmorphisms, were evidence of the constitutional nature of these deficits.

Further evidence of a causative link between brain damage and hyperactivity was provided by studies of epilepsy and other brain disorders (Clark, 1926; Lord, 1937; Preston, 1945). Also, children with confirmed lead poisoning were often found to sustain severe neurological and psychological sequelae, one of the latter being a behavioural expression of hyperkinesis, short attention span, and impulsivity (Byers & Lors, 1943). The characteristics of the children suffering from 'motor restlessness syndrome', as appearing in the first recorded descriptions in Soviet psychiatry (Sukhareva, 1940), were very similar.

Associations with primate research

Studies carried out in the latter half of the nineteenth century (Fernier, 1876) had shown that frontal lobe ablation in monkeys produced excessive restlessness and poor concentration. During the 1930s, several researchers noted that there was a similarity between the behaviour shown by primates who had undergone frontal lobe ablation and that of hyperactive children (Blau, 1936; Levin, 1938). This was taken as evidence in support of hyperkinetic behaviour in children being the result of some defect in forebrain structures, even though signs of such lesions could not always be demonstrated in all affected individuals.

Psychostimulant treatments, and their effect on theory of hyperkinesis

The efficacy of amphetamines in the treatment of hyperkinesis was discovered purely by accident in children undergoing pneumoencephalogram investigations for their disturbed behaviour. Charles Bradley, working at the Emma Pendleton Bradley Home in Providence, Rhode Island, USA prescribed Benzedrine to increase blood pressure in an attempt to alleviate headaches. Bradley and his colleagues, having been impressed by the ideas of Khan & Cohen (1934), also working at the centre, decided to join in the efforts to demonstrate the nature of structural abnormalities in the brain that they believed were the cause of disruptive behaviour in children. For this purpose, pneumoencephalograms were widely employed with the consequence that many of the children were left with severe headaches.

Most of the children given Benzedrine for their headaches also showed a clear improvement in their behaviour and school performance (Bradley, 1937); in some there was also a rise in intelligence test scores (Bradley & Green, 1940) attributed to the drug's favourable effect on the child's emotional attitude towards the test. Furthermore, it was noted that a wide range of children benefited from the medication, and that the therapeutic effect was not specific to any particular behaviour, although the children who improved least turned out to have a demonstrable structural neurological deficit (Bradley & Bowen, 1940; 1941).

The mechanism of the drug's action was at first attributed to its effect of stimulating higher inhibitory centres and thereby producing increased voluntary control. In addition, Bradley (1957) commented on the importance of the euphoriant effect of amphetamines. He believed that children with behaviour problems, many of whom showed marked overactivity and restlessness, were unhappy, and that their deviant behaviour was their way of conveying this. Therefore, giving them amphetamines made them less unhappy, and took away some of their need to behave badly.

Laufer (1975) later suggested that the reason the drug was not widely used until the mid 1950s was because of the prevailing psychoanalytic climate, which resisted the idea that hyperactive behaviour was due to an underlying organic cause. Laufer and his colleagues took up the cause of amphetamines and set out to investigate the neurological mechanism underlying the 'hyperkinetic impulse disorder', and the action of amphetamines (Laufer & Denhoff, 1957; Laufer, Denhoff & Solomons, 1957). Attempting to secure some sound evidence for the drug's effectiveness, in the face of strong competition from those who promoted the role of poor parenting as the cause for hyperactive-type behaviour problems, was an uphill struggle.

Laufer's research was heavily built on the work of two of his contemporaries, Gastaut (1950), and Magoun (1952). Gastaut had developed a photo-Metrozol stimulation test which involved administering the drug Metrozol whilst lights were flashed at the child. The resulting myoclonic jerks of the forearm and spike-wave patterns on the EEG were then carefully monitored. Magoun's work centred on the importance of the ascending reticular activating system in preserving alertness.

Hypothesising that abnormalities of the reticular activating system led children to be over alert and over active, Laufer, Denhoff & Solomons (1957) embarked on a study of children with 'emotional disturbance', dividing them into those who showed evidence of 'hyperkinetic impulse disorder', and those who did not. They found that the hyperkinetic group required less Metrozol to induce myoclonic jerks in response to the stroboscope compared with the non-hyperkinetic group. However, when the hyperkinetic children were given amphetamines, the amount of Metrozol required increased to the same level as in the non-hyperkinetic children. The authors postulated that the central nervous system deficit of overactive children was located in the area of the thalamus. As a result of this, excess stimulation was not filtered out, but instead passed through to the brain causing the child to behave in an overactive way.

It has later been pointed out that Laufer's research did suffer from certain methodological flaws; for example, there had been a failure to record the photo-Metrozol levels of the non-hyperkinetic children. However, even though the original study has never been replicated, Laufer's early work has definitely fuelled much interest in the study of biological treatments in childhood hyperactivity.

From minimal brain damage to minimal brain dysfunction

The belief that brain damage could be inferred laid the foundation for the concept of minimal brain damage (Doll, Phelps & Melcher, 1932; Ehrenfest, 1926; Ingalls & Gordon, 1947; Smith, 1926). The publications and 'minimal stimulation' classroom programmes by Strauss and his associates (Strauss, *et al.*, 1955; Strauss & Lehtinen, 1947; Strauss & Werner, 1942, 1943), helped further to promote the idea that hyperactive behaviour was caused by minimal brain damage. The group studied the psychopathology and educational needs of children residing in the Wayne County Training School, Michigan, USA. The school provided rehabilitation for children considered to be of borderline intelligence, or 'higher grade morons'. Strauss *et al.* (1955) suggested that the borderline children should be divided into two distinct groups, which they called 'exogenous' and 'endogenous'. The 'exogenous' children had histories of physical damage to the central nervous system, either due to trauma or inflammatory process, but no family history of mental retardation. The medical histories of the 'endogenous' children did not contain any evidence of physical damage to the brain, but the children came from families with a history of mental retardation. The two groups also differed with regard to their behaviour and current functioning: the 'exogenous' children responded poorly to teaching, and appeared to be overactive and easily distracted. Prompted by their observations, the group set out to determine the nature of the brain-injured child's deficit, and to develop appropriate educational programmes for such children.

As a result of their observations, Strauss & Werner (1943) concluded that the behaviour of the brain-injured children closely resembled that of brain-injured adults. This led them to postulate species-specific innate patterns of behaviour. When a child suffers a brain injury, these particular behavioural patterns are triggered by less intense stimuli, but produce more intense responses, than is the case with adults. Although their initial studies were based on intellectually impaired children, the authors argued that there was no reason why these same behaviour patterns should not indicate brain damage in children of normal intelligence.

Research findings like these were appealing at the time, because they provided a biological explanation for children's behaviour problems and educational failure. They also excited paediatricians and child psychiatrists, who, when trying to help such children, had grown disillusioned and dissatisfied with the lack of success of treatments based largely on psychoanalytic theories. Although welcomed by many, the conclusions by Strauss and his colleagues were also met with scepticism by a number of people. The main criticisms related to the lack of clarity of the criteria by which organic brain disorder was defined. Also, the educational programmes that had been guided by the research, frequently turned out to be ineffective (Cruikshank *et al.*, 1961), and the attempts to replicate the psychometric results in most instances proved unsuccessful (Weatherwax & Benoit, 1962).

At the same time as the theories put forward by Strauss and his co-workers were struggling to gain wider acceptance, the validity of the concept of minimal brain damage was strengthened by a substantial body of foetal and animal research. Epidemiological studies demonstrated a strong association between maternal and foetal factors and subsequent behaviour problems in the children (Lilienfeld, Pasamanick & Rogers, 1955; Pasamanick, Rogers & Lilienfeld, 1956), and results of animal studies supported a relationship between disordered behaviour and minor degrees of brain damage (Cromwell, Baumeister &

Hawkins, 1963). Empirical evidence for a significant link between histories of anoxia at birth and later disorders of development appeared particularly suggestive (Graham *et al.*, 1957), as did the systematic clinical observations of the behaviour of children suffering from epilepsy (Ounsted, 1955), and of other forms of organic brain disorder (Ingram, 1956).

The introduction of the concept of a continuum of damage, with a corresponding continuum of medical, behavioural and educational consequences by Pasamanick and his colleagues presented a theoretical step forward (Knobloch *et al.*, 1956; Pasamanick, Knobloch & Lilienfeld, 1956; Pasamanick, Rogers & Lilienfeld, 1956). The argument was based on the observation that the cause of perinatal death in babies whose mothers had had severe complications of pregnancy, and/or where the pregnancy ended prematurely, was usually due to brain injury. Therefore, amongst the group of infants who did not die, some would be severely injured and develop a variety of disorders. Depending on the severity and location of the injury, these disorders ranged from cerebral palsy, through conduct disorders and learning difficulties to mild behaviour problems (Pasamanick & Knobloch, 1961). These findings stemmed from a study of children referred to the Division of Special Services of the Baltimore Department of Education, with non-referred children from the same classrooms being used as controls. The referred children were found to be three times more likely than the controls to have a history of perinatal complications such as anoxia or premature birth. This was particularly true of those children who presented with hyperactive-type behaviours. In a subsequent prospective study, involving 500 children who had been born prematurely, the incidence of such developmental abnormalities was found to increase with decreasing birth weight (Knobloch & Pasamanick, 1966). Although these were mainly interpreted as lending support for the role of gestational and perinatal factors in the later development of hyperactivity, an association between socio-economic status, race and complications of pregnancy was also recorded. There was a higher incidence of perinatal events in lower socio-economic and non-white populations. This led the authors to conclude that the perinatal complications and adverse environmental factors most likely stemmed from the same social disadvantage.

While Pasamanick and his colleagues were promoting their research as providing evidence for a link between minimal brain damage and hyperactivity, several authors criticised the idea, increasingly doubting the concept of brain damage as the sole cause of hyperactive behaviour in children. Birch (1964), Rapin (1964), and Herbert (1964) all questioned the assumption that, if brain damage caused behaviour problems, then all children with behaviour problems must have brain damage, even though there might not be any physical evidence to support the presence of damage.

Coinciding with this, the Oxford International Study Group of Child Neurology (Bax & MacKeith, 1963) also contended that brain damage should not be inferred from behaviour alone, and recommended that the term 'minimal brain damage' be replaced by 'minimal brain dysfunction' (MBD). It also recommended that attempts be made to reclassify the heterogeneous group of children, subsumed under the this label, into a number of more homogeneous subgroups. In the USA, a national task force formulated an official definition of the disorder (Clements, 1966).

The term minimal brain dysfunction syndrome refers...to children of near average, average, or above average general intelligence with certain learning or behavioural disabilities ranging from mild to severe, which are associated with deviations of function of the central nervous system. These deviations may manifest themselves by various combinations of impairment in perception, conceptualization, language, memory, and control of attention, impulse, or motor function .... during the school years, a variety of learning disabilities is the most prominent manifestation (quotation by Ross & Ross, 1982).

The definition was welcomed by those who believed hyperactivity to be an unequivocal diagnostic sign of brain damage (e.g. Wender, 1971), but criticised by many (e.g. Routh & Roberts, 1972; Rutter, 1977). Although the term 'MBD' was useful in emphasising the role of organic factors in the causation of hyperactivity and thus providing something of a challenge to the psychoanalytic views of the time, which proposed that the disorder was due to poor parenting, it was eventually recognised as being over-inclusive. 'MBD' was subsequently replaced by more specific terms relating to particular behavioural and developmental disorders, such as dyslexia, learning disabilities and language disorders. These terms were based on observed disabilities rather than hypothesised underlying mechanisms.

EMERGENCE OF BEHAVIOURAL DEFINITIONS

Three decades elapsed between Still's (1902) description of children with hyperactive behaviour unrelated to either demonstratable brain damage, or a history of suggestive damage and the first comprehensive discussion of hyperactive children. In 1935 Childers noted that only a small proportion of cases with hyperactivity seemed aetiologically related to substantiated or inferred brain damage. His discussion of children with no evidence of brain damage is notable for the differentiation made between the hyperactive child and the brain-damaged child.

Hyperkinetic behaviour syndrome

During the late 1950s and early 1960s, dissatisfaction with the term 'MBD' was growing. The influential publications by Laufer and his associates (Laufer & Denhoff, 1957; Laufer, Denhoff & Solomons, 1957), which introduced the concepts and terms of 'hyperkinetic behaviour syndrome', and 'hyperkinetic impulse disorder', signalled the onset of final acceptance of the construct of hyperactivity as we know it now.

Chess (1960) also emphasised the importance of excessive motor activity as a defining feature of the disorder, and that this should be observed rather than taken on an anecdotal account from the parents. In addition, she moved away from attributing the disorder to poor parenting or brain damage. Her findings were based on a group of 36 children, termed hyperactive, in a whole sample of 881 children attending a private practice. The features, documented in detail, resemble the present criteria of hyperactivity disorder, including sex ratio and age of onset. Aggression and impulsivity were seen as associated characteristics. Chess (1960) proposed that the disorder, in most cases, was due to 'physiologic hyperactivity', but also noted that hyperactivity could be associated with mental retardation, schizophrenia or organic brain damage. A treatment approach which incorporated behaviour modification, medication, special educational provision and psychotherapy was recommended.

The change in the concept and terminology served as a stimulus for a series of important empirical investigations (Huessy, 1967; Smith, 1962; Werry, Weiss & Douglas, 1964), and descriptive clinical studies (Bakwin & Bakwin, 1966; Stewart *et al.*, 1966; Werry, 1968). By the late 1960s, the concept of hyperactivity was firmly established in the literature.

Tools for assessment

In the late 1960s, Conners and his team developed parent and teacher rating scales for the assessment of symptoms of hyperactivity (Conners, 1969; 1970). At that time, these questionnaire-based instruments presented an invaluable step forward in allowing for a standardised measurement of children's behaviour with a particular emphasis on hyperactivity. Although initially devised for the measurement of change in behaviour during drug treatment, the scales have also been successfully employed in epidemiological research.

Psychophysiology and the importance of arousal level

Several psychological models have atributed hyperactive behaviour to an abnormality in the level of arousal in the central nervous system (CNS). However, the direction of postulated abnormality has been a matter of considerable dispute. The models viewing the deficit as one of over arousal have interpreted hyperactivity as a behavioural manifestation of an over aroused, or highly aroused CNS (Freibergs & Douglas, 1969; Kahn & Cohen, 1934; Knobel, Wolman & Mason, 1959; Laufer, Denhoff & Solomons, 1957; Strauss & Lehtinen, 1947). The under arousal models, on the other hand, have conceptualised the condition as a compensatory response by a sub optimally aroused individual through increased sensory input (Bradley, 1937; Werry & Sprague, 1970).

The psychophysiology of hyperactivity was extensively investigated during the 1970s. Several studies were published during this time examining a variety of physiological aspects, such as EEG, galvanic skin response, averaged evoked responses, etc. (Satterfield, 1973; Satterfield *et al.*, 1972; Satterfield, Cantwell & Satterfield, 1974; Satterfield & Dawson, 1971). Many of these also had considerable methodological problems and were highly criticised (e.g. Hastings & Barkley, 1978). One of the weaknesses of the psychophysiological research was that the studies were often based on out dated theories of the 1950s suggesting, for example, that hyperactivity was due to cortical over arousal. If anything, the evidence produced suggested that hyperactive children had a slower than normal response to stimulation, thus detracting from theories of over stimulated cortices in these children.

Deficits of attention and motivation

The 1970s saw a proliferation of research into hyperactivity and a fast growing volume of literature on various aspects of the disorder. Particularly in the United States, features such as short attention span, impulsivity and distractibility, previously considered to be associated characteristics, were now included in the defining symptoms. At the same time, the popularity of the concept of MBD was declining due to the lack of scientific evidence in its favour.

One of the turning points in the history of hyperactivity was when in the early 1970s, Douglas and her team at McGill University suggested that motor overactivity was not the core symptom in the syndrome of hyperkinesis; but rather deficits in the ability to sustain attention and control impulsive responding were more important. Douglas also argued that these were the areas in which stimulant medication was most effective (Douglas, 1972).

Employing a series of measures to assess the behavioural and cognitive aspects of the disorder, the McGill team demonstrated that hyperactive children experienced more problems with sustained attention particularly in situations where there were distractions, but that they were not generally more learning or reading impaired, or more distractible than normal children. However, in situations where the children were given continuous and immediate reinforcement, the hyperactive ones could perform at near normal and even normal levels of attention (Freibergs & Douglas, 1969). Another important observation was that, while the excessive motor restlessness usually declined by early teens, the difficulties in sustained attention and impulse control often persisted into adolescence.

One of the doubtless merits of the systematic and detailed work of Douglas and her colleagues was that it helped to establish a tradition of high quality research in the study of cognitive aspects of hyperactivity. Another notable feature of her work has been the way it has been guided by theory, which can be tested and revised when necessary; these are features which have been so often found wanting in the mushrooming hyperactivity research.

The work of Douglas and her team has definitely been influential in shaping the study of hyperactivity. It was probably the main reason for the American Psychiatric Association (1980) altering the diagnostic terminology in DSM III to Attention Deficit Disorder, +/- hyperactivity, thus focusing on the attentional aspects of the disorder, rather than on the motor overactivity. Although the theory of Douglas has subsequently been questioned in part, it nevertheless has provided the impetus for a new generation of high-quality research in the various aspects of hyperactivity, including the individual processes of attention, motivation, inhibitory control, etc. It has undoubtedly facilitated the development of links between the study of attention as behavioural manifestation of central processing of information and the neuro-anatomical and neurotransmitter processes, providing the focus for the more recent research in the field of hyperactivity.

The role of the environment

In the 1970s the trend against drugging children with behaviour disorders was accompanied by a number of alternative theories explaining the causation of hyperactivity. One such explanation, gaining long-lasting popularity, was that of food allergy. Feingold (1975) suggested that children demonstrated hyperactive behaviour as a result of an allergic or toxic reaction to food substances, especially food additives. This theory caught the imagination of both professionals and lay people. Several studies were set up to investigate the concept; the more rigorous of these have found no or minimal effect of food substances on the behaviour of children.

Poor parenting as a causative factor in hyperactivity was put forward by both psychoanalysts (Bettelheim, 1973), and behaviourists (Willis & Lovaas, 1977). The former suggested that an excessively negative reaction from an intolerant mother to a child, who demonstrates a negative or hyperactive temperament, would lead to the clinical presentation of hyperactivity. According to the latter, non-compliant and hyperactive behaviour developed as a result of poor conditioning to stimulus control by parental commands and instructions. However, in the search for psychosocial causes, the finding of possibly greatest potential importance was that by Tizard & Hodges (1978), demonstrating an association between institutional up-bringing and hyperactive behaviour. It suggested that a lack of continuity in parenting may impair the development of the normal modulation of activity and attention. The importance of disrupted core relationships for the development of hyperactive behaviour pattern was also highlighted by the observational study of Routh (1980), and the theoretical model of 'learned ineffectiveness' by Glow & Glow (1979).

The 1970s also saw the beginning of a vigorous sociological and medicolegal debate about the implications of the increasingly popular diagnosis of hyperactivity. Block (1977), for example, suggested that technological development, leading to rapid cultural change, was responsible for children becoming hyperactive. The resulting increased excitation and environmental stimulation could in 'pre-disposed' children cause hyperactive behaviour of clinical severity. Conrad (1976), on the other hand, argued that the expansion of the clinical diagnosis stemmed at least partly from the existence of powerful drug treatments for children's disruptive behaviours. The drugs, of course, had existed long before then, but their availability was convenient when physicians became increasingly confronted with referrals of children with puzzling troublesome behaviours, especially from schools. The issue was also picked up by authors of more popular texts. In the USA, for example, journalists Schrag and Divoky (1975) published a book about the 'myth' of childhood hyperactivity and, in Britain Steven Box (1977), in a popular sociological journal, referred to the 'scandalous silence' surrounding the mass labelling and drugging of school children who failed to conform. Whalen & Henker (1980) also drew attention to the apparent increased tolerance for diagnostic ambiguity and for greater tendency to make the diagnosis of hyperactivity once there was evidence of the child's behaviour having improved by the drug treatment.

The issue of a syndrome

The question of whether hyperactivity constitutes a syndrome in the sense of sharing a unitary cluster of symptoms, a common cause in terms of major aetiological factors, a consistent response to treatment, a predictable natural course, and whether or not it differs from other disorders, especially conduct disorder, in terms of these factors, has been a difficult one to settle. At times, the argument has led to considerable polarisation of views with some seeing the whole issue as more of a hindrance to progress of research (e.g. Ross & Ross, 1982), while others have regarded it as an invaluable stimulus for good study (e.g. Rutter, 1982).

The interest generated by the syndrome issue has led a small, but determined group of investigators to search for empirical support for the disorder. This process has helped to sharpen both the theoretical reasoning behind it (Quay, 1979; Rie & Rie, 1980; Rutter, 1982; Sandberg, 1981; Shaffer & Greenhill, 1979), and most notably to improve the search for aetiological processes (Loney, Kramer & Milich, 1981; Loney, Langhorne & Paternite, 1978; Sandberg, Rutter & Taylor, 1978; Schachar, Rutter & Smith, 1981; Shaffer, McNamara & Pincus, 1974; Taylor, 1983). The net result has been a considerable scientific advancement starting from early the 1970s and likely to continue for some time. The scientific and clinical developments of the 1980s and 1990s are the subjects of the individual contributions of the book, and, therefore, outside the remit of this chapter.

REFERENCES

American Psychiatric Association (1980). *Diagnostic and Statistical Manual of Mental Disorders, 3rd edn.* Washington DC.

Bakwin, H. & Bakwin, R.M. (1966). *Clinical Management of Behavior Disorders in Children.* Philadelphia: Saunders.

Bassoe, P. (1922). Diagnosis of encephalitis. *Journal of American Medical Association,* **79**, 223–5.

Bax, M.C.O. & MacKeith, R.C. (1963). Minimal brain damage – a concept discarded. In *Minimal Cerebral Dysfuction*, eds. R.C. MacKeith & M.C.O. Bax. Little Club Clinics in Development Medicine, No. 10. London: Heinemann.

Bender, L. (1942). Postencephalitic behavior disorders in children. In *Encephalitis: A Clinical Study*, ed. J.B. Neal. New York: Grune and Stratton.

Bettelheim, B. (1973). Bringing up children. *Ladies Home Journal,* **90**, 28.

Birch, H.G. (1964). *Brain Damage in Children. The Biological and Social Aspects.* Baltimore: Williams and Wilkins.

Blau, A. (1936). Mental changes following head trauma in children. *Archives of Neurology and Psychiatry,* **35**, 722–69.

Block, G.H. (1977). Hyperactivity: a cultural perspective. *Journal of Learning Disabilities,* **110**, 236–40.

Boncour, P. & Boncour, G. (1905). *Les anomalies mentales chez les écoliers, étude medico-pedagogique.* Paris: Alcan.

Bond, E.D. & Appel, K.E. (1931). Treatment of post encephalitic children in hospital school. *American Journal of Psychiatry,* **10**, 815–28.

Bourneville, E. (1897). Le *traitement medico-pedagogique des differentes formes de l'idiotie.* Paris: Alcan.

Box, S. (1977). Hyperactivity: the scandalous silence. *New Society*, 1st December, 458–60.

Bradley, C. (1937). The behavior of children receiving Benzedrine. *American Journal of Psychiatry* **94**, 577–85.

Bradley, C. (1957). Characteristics and management of children with behavior problems associated with organic brain damage. *Pediatric Clinics of North America,* **4**, 1049–60.

Bradley, C. & Bowen M. (1940). School performance of children receiving amphetamine (Benzedrine) sulfate. *American Journal of Orthopsychiatry,* **10**, 782–8.

Bradley, C. & Bowen, M. (1941). Amphetamine (Benzedrine) therapy of children's behavior disorders. *American Journal of Orthopsychiatry,* **11**, 91–103.

Bradley, C. & Green, R. (1940). Psychometric performance of children receiving amphetamine (benzedrine) sulfate. *American Journal of Psychiatry,* **97**, 388–94.

Byers, R.K. & Lord, E.E. (1943). Late effects of lead poisoning on mental development. *American Journal of Diseases of Children*, **66**, 471–94.

Cantwell, D.P. (1975). *The Hyperactive Child.* New York: Spectrum.

Chess, S. (1960). Diagnosis and treatment of the hyperactive child. *New York State Journal of Medicine,* **60**, 2379–85.

Childers, A.T. (1935). Hyperactivity in children having behavior disorders. *American Journal of Psychiatry,* **120**, 142–8.

Clark, L.P. (1926). Psychology of essential epilepsy. *Journal of Nervous and Mental Disease,* **63**, 575–85.

Clements, S.D. (1966). *Task Force One: Minimal Brain Dysfunction in Children.* National Institute of Neurological Diseases and Blindness, Monograph No. 3. US Department of Health Education and Welfare.

Clouston, T.S. (1899). Stages of over-excitability, hypersensitiveness, and mental explosiveness in children and their treatment by the bromides. *The Scottish Medical and Surgical Journal,* IV, (6), 481–90.

Conners, C.K. (1969). A teacher rating scale for use in doing studies with children. *American Journal of Psychiatry,* **126**, 884–8.

Conners, C.K. (1970). Symptom patterns in hyperkinetic, neurotic and normal children. *Child Development,* **41**, 667–82.

Conrad, P (1976). *Identifying Hyperactive Children.* Massachusetts: Lexington Books.

Cornell, W.S. (1912). *Health and Medical Inspection of School Children.* Philadelphia: F.A. Davis.

Cromwell, R.L., Baumeister, A. & Hawkins, W.F. (1963). Research in activity level. In *Handbook of Mental Deficiency,* ed. NR. Ellis. New York: McGraw-Hill.

Cruickshank, W.M., Bentzen, F.A., Ratzeburgy, F.H. & Tannhauser, M.T. (1961). *A Teaching Method for Brain Injured and Hyperactive Children: A Demonstration Pilot Study.* Syracuse, New York: Syracuse University Press.

Darwin, C.R. (1859). *On the Origin of Species by Means of Natural Selection or the Preservation of the Favoured Races in the Struggles for Life*. London: John Murray.

Doll, E.A, Phelps, W.M. & Melcher, R.T. (1932). *Mental Deficiency due to Birth Injuries.* New York: Macmillan.

Douglas, V.I. (1972). Stop, look and listen: the problem of sustained attention and impulse control in hyperactive and normal children. *Canadian Journal of Behavioral Science,* **4**, 259–82.

Ebaugh, F.G. (1923). Neuropsychiatric sequelae of acute epidemic encephalitis in children. *American Journal of Diseases of Children,* **25**, 89–97.

Ehrenfest, H. (1926). Birth injuries of the child. *Gynecological and Obstetrical Monographs.* New York: Appleton.

Feingold, B. (1975). *Why Your Child is Hyperactive.* New York: Random House.

Fernier, D. (1876). *The Functions of the Brain.* New York: Putnam.

Freibergs, V. & Douglas, V.I. (1969). Concept learning in hyperactive and normal children. *Journal of Abnormal Psychology,* **74**, 388–95.

Gastaut, H. (1950). Combined photic and Metrazol activation of the brain. *Electroencephalography and Clinical Neurophysiology,* **2**, 249–61.

Gibbs, F., Gibbs, Spies, H. & Carpenter, P. (1964). Common types of childhood encephalitis. *Archives of Neurology*, **10**, 1–11.

Glow, P.H. & Glow, R.A. (1979). Hyperkinetic impulse disorder: a developmental defect of motivation. *Genetic Psychology Monographs,* **100**, 159–231.

Graham, F.K., Caldwell, B.M., Ernhart, C.B., Pennoyer, M.M. & Hartmann, A.F., Sr. (1957). Anoxia as a significant perinatal experience: a critique. *Journal of Pediatrics,* **50**, 556–69.

Hastings, J.E. & Barkley, R.A. (1978). A review of psychophysiological research with hyperactive children. *Journal of Abnormal Child Psychology,* **7**, 413–47.

Healy, W. (1915). *The Individual Delinquent.* Boston: Little Brown.

Henderson, L.J. (1913). *The Fitness of the Enviroment.* New York: Macmillan.

Herbert, (1964). The concept and testing of brain damage in children – A review. *Journal of Child Psychology and Psychiatry,* **5**, 197–217.

Heuyer, G. (1914). *Enfants anormaux et delinquants juveniles.* Paris. Thèse De Médicin.

Hoff, H. (1956). *Lehrbuch der Psychiatrie, Band II.* Basel: Benno Schwabe & Co.

Hoffmann, H. (1845). *Der Struwwelpeter.* Frankfurt: Literarische Anstalt.

Hohman, L.B. (1922). Post encephaltic behavior disorders in children. *Johns Hopkins Hospital Bulletin,* **33**, 372–5.

Huessy, H.R. (1967). Study of the prevalence and therapy of the choreatiform syndrome or hyperkinesis in rural Vermont. *Acta Paedopsychiatrica,* **34**, 130–5.

Ingalls, T.H. & Gordon, J.E. (1947). Epidemiologic implications of developmental arrests. *American Journal of Medical Science,* **241**, 322–8.

Ingram, T.T.S. (1956). A characteristic form of overactive behaviour in brain-damaged children. *Journal of Mental Science,* **102**, 550–8.

Ireland, W.E. (1877). *On Idiocy and Imbecility*. London: Churchill.

Kahn, E. & Cohen, L.H. (1934). Organic drivenness. A brain stem syndrome and an experience with case reports. *New England Journal of Medicine*, **210**, 748–56.

Kanner, L. (1957). *Child Psychiatry.* 3rd edn. Springfield. Ill: Charles C. Thomas.

Knobel, M., Wolman, M.B. & Mason, E. (1959). Hyperkinesis and organicity in children. *Archives of General Psychiatry,* **1**, 310–21.

Knobloch, H., Rider, R., Harper, P. & Pasamanick, B. (1956). Neuropsychiatric sequelae of prematurity: a longitudinal study. *Journal of the American Medical Association*, **161**, 581–5.

Knobloch, H. & Pasamanick, B. (1966). Prospective studies on the epidemiology of reproductive casualty. Methods, findings, and some implications. *Merrill-Palmer Quarterly,* **12**, 27–43.

Laehr, H. (1975). Uber den Einflub der Schule auf die Verhinderung von Geistesstorungen. *Allg. Ztschr Psychiatry,* **32**, 216.

Laufer, M.N. (1975). In Osler's day it was syphilis. In *Explorations in Child Psychiatry,* ed. E.J. Anthony, pp. 105–24. New York: Plenum Press.

Laufer, M. & Denhoff, E. (1957). Hyperkinetic behavior syndrome in children. *Journal of Pediatrics,* **50**, 463–74.

Laufer, M.W., Denhoff, E. & Solomons. (1957). Hyperkinetic impluse disorder in children's behavior problems. *Psychosomatic Medicine,* **19**, 38–49.

Levin, P.M. (1938). Restlessness in children. *Archives of Neurology and Psychiatry,* **39**, 764–70.

Lilienfeld, A.M., Pasamanick, B. & Rogers, M. (1955). Relationship between pregnancy experience and the development of certain neuropsychiatric disorders in childhood. *American Journal of Public Health,* **45**, 637–43.

Loney, J., Kramer, J. & Milich, R. (1981). The hyperkinetic child grows up: predictors of syptoms, delinquency and achievement at follow-up. In *Psychosocial Aspects of Drug Treatment for Hyperactivity*, eds. K.D. Gadow & J. Loney, pp. 381–415. Colorado: Westview Press.

Loney, J., Langhorne, J.E. & Paternite, C.E. (1978). An empirical basis for subgrouping the hyperkinetic/minimal brain syndrome. *Journal of Abnormal Psychology*, **87**, 431–41.

Lord, E.E. (1937). *Children Handicapped by Cerebal Palsy*. New York: Commonwealth Fund.

Magoun, H.W. (1952). An ascending reticular activating system in the brain stem. *Archives of Neurology and Psychiatry,* **67**, 145–54.

Maudsley (1867). *The Physiology and Pathology of the Mind.* London: Macmillan.

Ounsted, C. (1955). The hyperkinetic syndrome in epileptic children. *Lancet*, ii, 303–11.

Pasamanick, B. & Knobloch, H. (1961). Epidemiological studies on the complications of pregnancy and the birth process. In *Prevention of Mental Disorders in Children. Initial Explorations,* eds A. Caplan, pp. 74–94. New York: Basic Books.

Pasamanick, B., Knobloch, H. & Lilienfeld, A.M. (1956). Socio-economic status and some precursors of neuropsychiatric disorder. *American Journal of Orthopsychiatry,* **26**, 594–601.

Pasamanick, B., Rogers, M.E. & Lilienfeld, A.M. (1956). Pregnancy experience and the development of behavior disorder in children. *American Journal of Psychiatry,* **112**, 613–18.

Pick, A. (1904). Uber einige bedeutsame Psycho-Neurosen des Kindesalters. *Sammlung zwangsloser Abhandlungen aus dem Gebiete der Nerven- und der Geisteskrankheiten*, **5**, 1–28.

Preston, M.I. (1945). Late behavioural aspects found in cases of prenatal, natal, and postnatal anoxia. *Journal of Pediatrics,* **26**, 353–66.

Quay, H.C. (1979). Classification. In *Psychopathological Disorders of Childhood, 2nd edn.*, eds. H.C. Quay & J.S. Werry, pp. 1–42. New York: Wiley.

Rapin, I. (1964). Brain damage in children. In *Practice of Pediatrics*, ed. J. Brennemann, vol. 4. Hagerstown: M.D. Prior.

Rie, H.E. & Rie, E.D. (1980). *Handbook of Minimal Brain Dysfunctions: A Critical Review.* New York: Wiley.

Ross, D.M. & Ross, S.A. (1982). *Hyperactivity: Current Issues, Research and Theory*, 2nd edn. New York: Wiley.

Routh, D.K. (1980). Developmental and social aspects of hyperactivity. In *Hyperactive Children: The Social Ecology of Identification and Treatment*, eds. C.K. Whalen & B. Henker, pp. 55–73. New York: Academic Press.

Routh, D.K. & Roberts, R.D. (1972). Minimal brain dysfuction in children: Failure to find evidence for a behavioral syndrome. *Psychological Reports,* **31**, 307–14.

Rowntree, B.S. (1901). *Poverty: A Study of Town Life.* London: Macmillan.

Rutter, M. (1977). Brain damage syndromes in childhood: concepts and findings. *Journal of Child Psychology and Psychiatry,* **18**, 1–21.

Rutter, M. (1982). Syndromes attributed to 'minimal brain dysfunction' in childhood. *American Journal of Psychiatry,* **139**, 21–33.

Sandberg, S.T. (1981). The overinclusiveness of the diagnosis of hyperkinetic syndrome. In *Strategic Interventions for Hyperactive Children*, ed. M. Gittelman, pp. 8–38. New York: Sharpe Inc.

Sandberg, S.T., Rutter, M. & Taylor, E. (1978). Hyperkinetic disorder in clinic attenders. *Developmental Medicine and Child Neurology*, **20**, 279–99.

Satterfield, J.H. (1973). EEG issues in children with minimal brain dysfunction. *Seminars in Psychiatry*, **5**, 35–46.

Satterfield, J.H. & Dawson, M.E. (1971). Electrodermal correlates of hyperactivity in children. *Psychophysiology*, **8**, 191–7.

Satterfield, J.H., Cantwell, D.P., Lesser, L.I. & Podosin, R.L. (1972). Physiological studies of the hyperkinetic child. *American Journal of Psychiatry*, **128**, 1418–24.

Satterfield, J.H., Cantwell, D.P. & Satterfield, B.T. (1974). Pathophysiology of the hyperactive child syndrome. *Archives of General Psychiatry*, **31**, 839–44.

Scholz, F. (1911). *Die Charakterfehler des Kindes.* Leipzig: E.H. Mayer.

Schachar, R.J. (1986). Hyperkinetic syndrome: Historical development of the concept. In *The Overactive Child*, ed. E.A. Taylor, pp. 19–40, Clinics in Developmental Medicine, No. 97, Spastics International Publications. Oxford: Blackwell.

Schachar, R., Rutter, M. & Smith (1981). The characteristics of situationally and pervasively hyperactive children: implications for syndrome definition. *Journal of Child Psychology and Psychiatry*, **22**, 375–92.

Schrag, P. & Divoky, D. (1975). *The Myth of the Hyperactive Child.* New York: Pantheon.

Shaffer, D. & Greenhill, L. (1979). A critical note on the predictive validity of 'the hyperkinetic syndrome'. *Journal of Child Psychology and Psychiatry*, **20**, 61–72.

Shaffer, D., McNamara, N. & Pincus, J. (1974). Controlled observation on patterns of activity, attention, and impulsivity in brain-damage and psychiatrically disturbed boys. *Psychological Medicine*, **4**, 4–18.

Smith, G.B. (1926). Cerebral accidents of childhood and their relationships to mental deficiency. *Welfare Magazine,* **17**, 18–33.

Smith, A. (1962). Ambiguities in concepts and studies of 'brain-damaged' 'organicity'. *Journal of Nervous and Mental Disease,* **135**, 311–26.

Stewart, M.A., Pitts, F.N., Craig, A.G. & Dieruf, W. (1966). The hyperactive child syndrome. *American Journal of Orthopsychiatry,* **36**, 861–7.

Still, G.F. (1902). The Coulstonian Lectures on some abnormal physical conditions in children. *Lancet*, **1**, 1008–12; 1077–82; 1163–8.

Strauss, A.A., & Lehtinen, L.E. (1947). *Psychopathy and Education of the Brain-Injured Child.* New York: Grune and Stratton.

Strauss, A.A. & Werner, H. (1942). Disorders of conceptual thinking in the brain-injured child. *Journal of Nervous and Mental Disease,* **96**, 153–72.

Strauss, A.A. & Werner, H. (1943). Comparative psychopathology of the brain injured child and the traumatic brain injured adult. *American Journal of Psychiatry,* **99**, 835–8.

Strauss, A.A., Kephart, N.C., Lehtinen, L.E. & Goldenberg, S. (1955). *Psychopathology and Education of the Brain Injured Child. Vol. 2, Progress in Theory and Clinic.* New York: Grune and Stratton.

Strecker, E.A. & Ebaugh, F.G. (1924). Neuropsychiatric sequelae of cerebral trauma in children. *Archives of Neurology and Psychiatry,* **12**, 443–53.

Sukhareva, G.E. (1940). Neskolko polozhenyo printsipakh psikhiatricheskoi diagnostiki. *Voprossy Detskoi Psikhiatrii, Moscow*, pp. 1–38.

Taylor, E.A. (1983). Drug response and diagnostic variation. In *Developmental Neuropsychiatry,* ed. M. Rutter, pp. 348–68. New York: Guilford Press.

Tizard, B. & Hodges J. (1978). The effect of early institutional rearing in the development of eight-year-old children. *Journal of Child Psychology and Psychiatry*, **19**, 99–118.

Tredgold, C.H. (1908). *Mental Deficiency (Amentia).* New York: W. Wood.

Weatherwax, J. & Benoit, E.P. (1962). Concrete and abstract thinking in organic and non-organic mentally retarded children. In *Readings on the Exceptional Child: Research and Theory,* eds. E.P. Trapp & P. Himmelstein. New York: Appleton –Century – Crofts.

Wender, P.H. (1971). *Minimal Brain Dysfunction in Children.* New York: Wiley.
Werry, J.S. (1968). Developmental hyperactivity. *Paediatric Clinics of North America,* **15**, 581–99.
Werry, J.S. & Sprague, R.C. (1970). Hyperactivity. In *Symptoms of Psychopathology*, ed. C.G. Costello. New York: Wiley.
Werry, J.S., Weiss, G. & Douglas, V. (1964). Studies on the hyperactive child: I. some preliminary findings. *Canadian Psychiatric Association Journal*, **9**, 120–30.
Whalen, C.K. & Henker, B. (1980). The social ecology of psychostimulant treatment: a model for conceptual and empirical analysis. In *Hyperactive Children: The Social Ecology of Identification and Treatment*, eds. C.K. Whalen & B. Henker, pp. 3–54. New York: Academic Press.
Willis, T.J. & Lovaas, I. (1977). A behavioral approach to treating hyperactive children: the parent's role. In *Learning Disabilities and Related Disorders*, ed. J.B. Millichap, pp. 119–40. Chicago: Year Book Medical.

2

Epidemiological approaches

Jan K. Buitelaar and Herman van Engeland

INTRODUCTION

Hyperactivity has been recognised for a long time as a rather common problem of childhood. Many, if not all, children may manifest hyperactive behaviour for a short period of time, such as when they are excited, anxious or very tired, or in the prodromal or reconvalescence phase of a somatic illness. Hyperactive behaviour may further be a concomitant phenomenon in an array of child psychiatric disorders, ranging from pervasive developmental disorders and emotional disorders to conditions ascribed to psychosocial deprivation. But there are also children who are primarily characterised by a persistent pattern of overactive, restless and uncontrolled motor behaviour. In this chapter such a persistent pattern of overactive behaviour is entitled as hyperactivity. The disruptive behaviours of these children may be a burden for their surroundings, and consequently often constitute a reason for clinical referral. It is obvious, however, that referral is determined by a mixture of factors which in part are external to the symptomatology of the particular child, as the tolerance and management capacities of the caregivers, the availability of services, and mental health system politics. The study of hyperactivity in clinic cases may therefore lead to wrong conclusions which are based upon an unrepresentative selection of children with a specific disorder.

Epidemiology, in contrast, is the study of a disorder in the general population. Three closely related components characterise epidemiology (Verhulst & Koot, 1992). The first is the assessment of the prevalence rate of a disorder, which refers to the proportion of the population at risk that develops the disorder within a given time period. Because epidemiology is concerned with the individual case of a disorder, there is the problem of how a 'case' is to be defined in a categorical framework, outside the clinical setting. The second component is the assessment of the distribution of the disorder. Questions involved are who has the disorder, when and where (Costello, 1990). For example, what is the male–female ratio of hyperactivity, does there exists a relationship with age or developmental factors, or is the manifestation of hyperactivity bound to specific psychosocial environments, or is it differentially influenced by urban–rural status? Finally epidemiology is concerned with how a particular individual got the disorder. What are the mechanisms that explain the genesis of hyperactivity, and which factors are associated with the variation in prevalence and distribution of hyperactivity?

WHAT IS A CASE?

Assessment of psychopathology

In epidemiology there are basically two main approaches to the assessment of psychopathology. The first one is the psychometric approach. This approach derives from efforts in psychology to measure psychological traits or behavioural dimensions by means of standardised tests and instruments. Rating scales which are completed by parents, teachers or the children themselves may cover a variety of symptoms and problem behaviours. The application of (multivariate) statistical techniques permits the establishment of cut-off scores and allows the comparison of a child's score with those of normative sex- and age mates. The psychometric approach converges with the conceptualisation of hyperactivity as a behavioural dimension or as a temperamental variation. For example, analyses of rating scale data obtained from large populations of children show a continuous distribution of scores on the 'hyperactivity' factor (e.g. Taylor, 1986 *a, b*; Trites & Laprade, 1983). At the more extreme scores there are progressively a smaller number of subjects; by no means is there evidence for a bimodal distribution and for a discrete and discerned pathological group. As has been pointed out before (Rutter, 1989*a*; Taylor *et al.*, 1991) such a continuous distribution fitting a dimensional model of psychopathology does not exclude that at extreme scores different mechanisms may be operative, making subjects not only quantitatively but also qualitatively different from subjects scoring in the 'normal' range.

The second approach is the method of clinical assessment and the assignment of subjects to specific diagnostic categories. Rather confusingly, there are some alternative definitions of a category of hyperactivity. DSM-III comprised a category of attention deficit disorder characterised by its main features of inattention and impulsivity; a further subdivision was made according to the presence or absence of symptoms of motor hyperactivity (ADDH or ADD, APA, 1980). In DSM-III-R the category of ADD was dropped; on the other hand, hyperactivity was added as an essential symptom for the diagnosis of attention-deficit hyperactivity disorder (ADHD, APA, 1987). Another difference between DSM-III and DSM-III-R in the diagnostics of a category of hyperactivity concerns the weight that has to be attached to information gathered from informants. In DSM-III it is explicitly stated that priority should be given to the observations at school as reported by teachers, whereas in DSM-III no such diagnostic rule is included. A third and different diagnostic scheme for a category of hyperactivity is described in the ICD-9 and the ICD-10-draft under the heading if hyperkinetic disorder (World Health Organisation, 1978, 1988). The defining features of this category are extreme overactivity and inattention that are manifest across different situations (pervasiveness) and the absence of pervasive developmental disorders and affective disorders. ICD-10-draft includes as an additional requirement for the diagnosis that abnormalities of attention and of motor activities should be directly observed and not be based solely on reports of parents and/or teachers.

Both methods to assess hyperactivity in epidemiological studies have their pros and cons. Rating scale data are rather easy and cheap to gather, and constitute a cost-effective way of screening large populations for the presence of particular constellations of symptoms; as a drawback however, they lead to arbitrary cut-offs on a dimensional scoring system. As such, rating scale data are not well suited to draw a sharp line between cases and non-cases. Further, a problem of many rating scales is the large overlap between different factors. For example, 'hyperactivity' factors derived after multivariate analyses of rating scales usually contain other disruptive behaviour symptoms as well; further 'hyperactivity' and 'aggression' factors strongly correlated in many studies (Hinshaw, 1987). It is self-evident that the examination of associations between scores on 'hyperactivity' factors and developmental data or psychosocial adversity may be confounded by this loss of power to discriminate hyperactive behaviours from those of aggression. A final limitation of the use of rating scale data is that it is difficult to obtain reliable information relating to the period of time during which the symptoms were manifest, and of the onset of the symptoms. Knowledge of the duration and persistence of the symptoms may be gathered only by the repeated administration of rating scales at certain time intervals, or, of course, by interviews.

These limitations may be overcome to a considerable extent by the clinical assessment approach. The diagnosis-based assessment has yet its own drawbacks. Diagnostic interviewing puts high demands on budgets for personnel and time. Further, diagnostic criteria and decisions should be made as explicit as possible and also the same for each investigator. This allows one to make diagnosis assignments in a reliable way: a child should receive the same diagnosis no matter who conducts the assessment. The search for reliability has stimulated the development and use of structured and semi-structured interview schedules, some of which may be applied by both clinicians and lay-interviews (for review see Edelbrock & Costello, 1988). In practice, most epidemiological studies strive to cut down the amount of interviewing by using a combination of dimensional and clinical approaches in a two-stage design. Questionnaire ratings are used in a screening phase to select all high-scoring subjects and a randomly chosen subgroup of low-scoring children for more intensive investigations in the second stage of the study.

Further issues in the case definition

The establishment of a psychiatric diagnosis is a necessary but not sufficient condition for the definition of a case. Since the golden criterion of a referral to mental services is of no help, additional considerations should be given to estimates of the severity of the disorder, to the perceived need for treatment, and to the concordance of symptoms reported by multiple informants (Brandenburg, Friedman & Silver *et al.*, 1990). We shall return to severity estimates and the need for treatment when discussing individual studies in more detail. Introduced as a standard in the Isle of Wight studies conducted by Rutter and his colleagues (Rutter, Tizard & Whitmore *et al.*, 1970; Graham & Rutter, 1973), there is now general consensus that information gleaned from multiple informants (parents, teachers and the children themselves), facilitates the best estimate of diagnosis in an individual case. However, there is still considerable disagreement about how conflicting information from several sources should be weighted and collapsed into a final diagnosis. Concerning hyperactivity, for example, 'situational hyperactivity' limited to either home or school, and 'pervasive hyperactivity' which is present across all situations, can be discerned. We shall explore the validity and the usefulness of this distinction on the basis of epidemiological studies to be discussed further on.

Some other questions pertaining to the subdivision of hyperactivity disorders are of interest. Is there any evidence for an independent syndrome of attention-deficit disorder without hyperactivity (ADD), and can this be differentiated from attention-deficit disorder with hyperactivity (ADDH)? And if so, what is the relationship between these two disorders? What are the relationships between hyperactivity disorders and specific learning disorders? What is the diagnostic overlap between hyperactivity disorders and other disrupted behaviour disorders such as oppositional and antisocial conduct disorder? And, to what extent is there co-morbidity between hyperactivity and emotional disorders? Finally, is there a meaningful association between hyperactivity and minor neurological dysfunctions on the level of the general population?

We shall attempt to answer these questions by reviewing population-based studies of overall psychopathology, and of hyperactivity in particular, in children and adolescents, published in the last decade. This time period was selected because the comparison between studies over larger time spans would be of less value, in view of changes in society and, more importantly because of huge variance in methodologies applied in the different studies. Questionnaire-based surveys that reported on the frequency distribution of hyperactivity symptoms but did not provide information on hyperactivity factors derived from multivariate analyses were not included (Rahim & Cederblad, 1984; Wang fu-Yeng *et al.*, 1989; Matsuura *et al.*, 1989; Ekblad, 1990). The same applied to studies that failed to specify cut-off scores differentiating hyperactive and non-hyperactive children (Taylor & Sandberg, 1984; Luk, Leung & Lee, 1988). In the same way, interview-based surveys that did not explicitly report data on hyperactivity disorders (Connell, Irvine & Rodney 1982; Whitaker *et al.*, 1990), or were drawn from referred populations (Costello *et al.*, 1988), were excluded.

REVIEW OF QUESTIONNAIRE-BASED STUDIES

Methodology

Table 2.1 presents an overview of questionnaire-based studies on the epidemiology of hyperactivity, published in the last decade. The Table includes author and year of publication, sample size and sample frame, the ages of the children studied, the method of diagnosis, the prevalence of situational hyperactivity (SH) and pervasive hyperactivity (PH) when specified, and the male/female ration (M/F), age trends, and the cognitive, psychosocial and developmental correlates of the disturbances, when reported.

As is evident from Table 1 studies differ widely in sampling characteristics and in the measurement of hyperactivity. Concerning differences in sampling procedures, some studies were done on normal school samples (a, d, i, j, k, m, o), which would not include children who were absent from school for various reasons, or those who attended special schools or treatment facilities. These unsampled children may constitute a high risk group for hyperactivity. The Isle of Wight study (b) was a total population study, while the Trites and Laprade and the Goldstein studies (f,i) were based on stratified population samples. Three studies (c, e, h) were conducted on a birth cohort. Goodman & Stevenson (1989*a*,*b*) studied a representative sample of London twins. Samples differed also in size, the range being from 219 to 29 889, and in age of the subjects recruited, the range being from 3 to 15 years. The Sandberg *et al.*, and Pelham *et al.* studies (a, o) surveyed boys only. One study (b) drew its subjects from a rural area, three were conducted in explicit urban areas (a, c, n), while the remaining studies involved rather mixed rural–urban populations.

Variations in the measurement of hyperactivity include the constellation of symptoms chosen to define 'hyperactivity', the type of informant used, the threshold score to make a diagnosis, and whether the definition of hyperactivity accounts for co-morbidity with aggressive behaviours. Most questionnaires focus on the symptoms of hyperactivity (e.g. Rutter A and Rutter B scales), or on a combination of hyperactivity and inattention (Conners PTQ 'hyperactivity' and 'inattention' scores). Even when using the same instruments (*in casu* the Conners PTQ), studies may differ in the factor solution of the questionnaire data (Trites & Laprade, 1983; Taylor & Sandberg, 1984; Luk *et al.*, 1991; Hinshaw, 1987). Other questionnaires (used in interview-based surveys to be discussed below) include such symptoms as temper tantrums, irritability, moodiness, emotional lability, emotional immaturity, low frustration tolerance, speech problems, impulsivity and motor clumsiness in their construct of 'hyperactivity'. An illustration of discrepant findings that result from the use of different questionnaires may be found in the Sandberg *et al.*, and in Holborrow *et al.* studies (a, g). In the former study there was a modest, albeit significant correlation (pearson $r = 0.46$) between teachers' hyperactivity ratings on the Conners and Rutter scales. In the latter study, three teacher rating scales, the Conners abbreviated, the Queensland, and the Pittsberg ones, were compared and revealed an overlap of only 3.5% of the sample to be hyperactive on all three scales.

A second difference in measurement of hyperactivity relates to the type of informant used. Most studies used teachers' information, either alone (d, f, g, i, j, k, l, m, o,), or in combination with parents' reports (a, b, h, i, m), but in Nichols and Chen (c) study, a psychologist rated the child's behaviour during a psychological test. Chapel *et al.* (1982) (e) used a combination of parents' and psychologist's judgement. Thirdly, some studies simply required a cut-off score of 1.5 or 2.0 S.D above the mean to qualify as hyperactive (a, c, d, f, g, i, j, k, m), while other studies established a cut-off that was validated against clinical judgement (b, h, n). The Pelham *et al.* study (o) used the cut-off as pro-

Table 2.1.

Study	Size	Age	Frame	Assessment	Prevalence %	Other findings
a. Sandberg *et al.* (1980)	226	5–9	Boys from 19 primary schools in Inner London, UK	Conners TQ and Rutter B	SH school 13 SH home 8 PH 1.4	SH school high social disadvantage SH home: maternal distress perinat. –
b. Schachar *et al.* (1981)	1536	10–11; 14–15 (f.u.)	Total population on Isle of Wight	Rutter B (teachers) and Rutter A (parents); score > 3	SH school 8.3 SH home 9.9 PH 2.2	PH but not SH correlated with persistence, other disorders and cognitive deficits; M/F 2.9:1
c. Nichols & Chen (1981)	29 889	7	Birth, cohort, collaborative project USA	Questionnaire; 1.0 S.D.	SH during psychol. examin. 7.9	SES +; M/F 1.6:1 prenatal +
d. King & Young (1982)	219	7–9	Boys from elementary school, sample, Indiana, USA	Rating scale composed of DSM-III criteria for ADDH and ADD (teachers)	SH school: ADDH 12 ADD 4.1	
e. Chapel *et al.* (1982)**[a]**	1017	3	Birth cohort, Dunedin, New Zealand	Two-item questionnaire assessing hyperactivity and inattention (parents, psychologist)	SH home 7.0 (2.9) SH psychol. 6.0 (1.2) PH 5.5 (0.9) **b**	SES –; M/F 1.4:1 perinatal +; SH/PH behind in language and motor skills
f. Trites & Laprade (1983)	9229	4–12	Stratified random sample, Ottawa, Canada	Conners TQ (teachers); 2.0 S.D.	SH school 5.7	age n.a.: M/F n.a.

Table 2.1. (*cont.*)

Study	Size	Age	Frame	Assessment	Prevalence %	Other findings
g. Holborrow *et al.* (1984)	1908	6–12	School sample, Queensland, Australia	Conners Abbreviated Q (teachers); 2.0 S.D.	SH school 5.6	no age effect; M/F 2.4:1; SES +
h. McGee *et al.* (1984*a*,*b*,1985)[a]	949	7	Birth cohort, Dunedin, New Zealand	Rutter A (parents), Rutter B (teachers); score > 5 and 4 resp.	SH 13 either PH or persistent hyperactivity 7	M/F 1.6:1; in boys hyperactivity but not aggression correlated with general cognitive deficits; SES –; perinatal –
i. Kuijper & Hirasing (1986), Hirasing *et al.* (1988)	747	5	All children at school in Hoorn, Netherlands	Conners Abbreviated Q (teachers, parents); score > 15	SH school 7 SH home 11 PH 2	M/F 1.7:1; SES +; prenatal but not perinatal problems correlated with hyperactivity
j. Holborrow & Berry (1986)	1593	6–12	School sample, Queensland, Australia	Conners Abbreviated (teachers); Q 2.0 S.D.	SH school 7.7	M/F 2:1; SES +; 27% SH also learning disorder
k. Shapiro & Garfinkel (1986)	315	7–12	All children attending a rural public school	Conners TQ (teachers); I/O factor > 7[c]; attentional battery and DICA (child)	SH school 5.3	M.F n.a. SES +; attention and learning and tests: +
l. Goldstein (1987)	7119	6–11	Multistage probability sample of households	Three-item questionnaire assessing attentiveness, hyperactivity and aggressivity (teachers)	SH school 5.7 (hyperactivity+ inattentiveness)	M/F 4:1; age n.a.: inattentiveness, but not hyperactivity correlated with lower cognitive performance

Table 2.1. (*cont.*)

Study	Size	Age	Frame	Assessment	Prevalence %	Other findings
m. August & Garfinkel (1989)	1038 (50 index and 47 controls in extended study)	5–14	All children at two suburban schools, Minnesota, USA	Conners TQ, Inventory with DSM-III items for ADHD and CD (teachers); HI index <15; cognitive and attentional tests (child);	SH school 9.2	M/F 7:1; age n.a.; two subtypes of ADHD:1) behavioural, 2) cognitive with learning disorder and attention deficits
n. Goodman & Stevenson (1989*a*,*b*)	570	13	Representative sample of London twins	Rutter B (teachers) and Rutter A (parents); score > 3	SH home 12.7 SH school 7.2 PH 4.6	M>F on inattentiveness; PH (and SH school) more cognitively impaired; hereditary factors explained 30–40% variance
o. Pelham *et al.* (1992)	931	5–14	Boys from regular schools from around North America	Rating scale composed of DSM-III-R criteria for disruptive behaviour disorders (teachers)	ADHD (school) 6.6	No age effect; co-morbidity OD/CD 30%

a Dunedin population and follow-up project (Chapel *et al.*, 1982; McGee *et al.*, 1984*a*,*b*, 1985, 1990; Anderson *et al.*, 1987).
b between brackets rates for the combination of hyperactivity and inattentiveness
c according to Loney & Milich (1982).
SH=situational hyperactivity; PH=pervasive hyperactivity; M/F=male/female ratio.
ADDH=attention deficit disorder with hyperactivity (DSM-III).
ADD=attention deficit disorder without hyperactivity (DSM-III).
ADDH=attention deficit hyperactivity disorder (DSM-III-R)

posed in the DSM-III-R. Fourthly, several studies did not explicitly report on aggressive behaviours (d, e, g, i, j); from the studies that did take account of aggressive and oppositional behaviours as well as hyperactivity, some reported on the overlap between the domains of hyperactive and aggressive behaviours (a, h, k, m, n, i, o), but other studies did not (b, c).

PREVALENCE

The prevalence of questionnaire-based situational hyperactivity (SH) varies from 5.3% to 13% for SH-school and from 8% to 12.7% for SH-home. The prevalence of ADDH and ADD in boys (both DSM-III) was 12% and 4.1%; for ADHD (DSM-III-R) in boys 7.1%. With regard to pervasive hyperactivity (PH), prevalence rates were found to very from 1.4% to 4%. These rates for PH contrast somewhat with rates from PH from two large-scale epidemiological studies on hyperactivity which will be discussed in more detail in the next section. In the Ontario Child Health Study PH was estimated to be prevalent on 0.5% of the population (Szatmari, Offord & Boyle, 1989a), while in the study by Taylor and his colleagues in East London (Taylor *et al.*, 1991), PH was found to be prevalent in 8% of the boys aged 6–7 years, which would correspond with a rate for boys and girls together of approximately 4–6%. The prevalence rates for PH are hardly comparable with the prevalence rate of 7% reported by McGee *et al.* (h), because in this study cross-situational hyperactivity and hyperactivity that persisted from age 5 to 7 year were lumped together into one category. Separate mention deserved also the prevalence rates extracted from Chapel *et al.* (1982) study (e). When their figures are recalculated from the combination of hyperactivity and inattentiveness, lower rates (between brackets in Table 2.1) are found. Nonetheless, the variation in prevalence figures seems to be rather small, relative to the fluctuations in methodology as described above.

CORRELATES AND RISK FACTORS

Sex and age influences

The expected excess of hyperactive boys was found, with the male/female ratio varying from 1.6:1 to 7:1 (median ratio 2.4:1). Three studies (g, j, o) observed an about equal proportion of children to be hyperactive across the age range studies, while two other ones (f, i, m) did not report on age effects. Goodman and Stevenson (1989*a*) reported a systematic difference in attentiveness score between boys and girls to the advantage of girls.

Cognitive correlates

Cognitive correlates of hyperactivity were examined in six studies (b, h, i, k, m, n). Schachar *et al.* (b) explored the differences between SH and PH children and demonstrated that PH could be distinguished from SH and non-hyperactivity by significant cognitive impairments. PH children were found to be below the mean for non-verbal intelligence both at age 10–11 years and at age 14–15 years, in particular. The association between PH and cognitive impairment could not be attributed to social class. However, the study did not address the question of whether co-morbidity with aggressive behaviours confounded the association between hyperactivity and cognition. The same criticism applies to the deficits in attention and learning reported by Shapiro and Garfinkel (1986). This issue was addressed in the reports from the Dunedin follow-up project (h) and the London twin study (n).

McGee *et al.* (1984*a,b*), (h) selected four groups of children, pure hyperactive, pure aggressive, combined hyperactive–aggressive and controls. It was found that both hyperactive groups scored generally lower than the aggressive and control groups on measures of verbal and nonverbal intelligence. In addition, a significant specific reading retardation was revealed in the group characterised by both hyperactivity and aggression. These cognitive differences between the two hyperactive and the aggressive and control groups at the age of 7 could be traced back to a lower intelligence measured at 3 years of age. Furthermore, at follow-up at the age of 9 years, both of the hyperactive groups were still significantly behind the other two groups in spelling and reading scores.

In the London twin study (n) PH children had more attentional and educational problems than non-hyperactive children with pervasive antisocial behaviour, while situationally hyperactive children resembled situational antisocial children in their pattern of cognitive correlates (Goodman & Stevenson, 1989*a*).

Thus both the Dunedin study (h) and the London twin study (n) provided strong evidence that pervasive hyperactivity is associated with significant and persisting deficits in intelligence. The next question is whether it is hyperactive behaviour per se or inattentiveness that is associated with cognitive abilities.

An attempt to answer this is provided by Goldstein (1987). In this study, somewhat limited by a rather crude definition of hyperactivity, inattentiveness and aggression on the basis of teacher reports only, inattentiveness, but not hyperactivity, appeared to be associated with lower performance on tests of intelligence, reading and arithmetic achievement. More robust data to provide information on this issue is available from the follow-up of the Dunedin project when the children were 9 years old (McGee, Williams & Silva, 1985) (h). The parent and teacher ratings of inattention were predicted by both cognitive (performance IQ, reading, and spelling) and motor (speech articulation and tapping speed), ability. Family background measures, on the other hand, were associated with hyperactive and aggressive behaviours as rated by parents and teachers.

Finally, important suggestions for further differentiation of questionnaire-defined ADHD were provided by August & Garfinkel (1989) (m). They described two subtypes: a behavioural subtype (80% of their ADHD sample) which in its severe forms was indistinguishable from conduct disorder, and a cognitive subtype (20%) with information-processing defects and learning disorders. This converges with data from Holborrow and Berry (1986) who found an overlap of 27% between school based SH and learning disorders.

Psychosocial background factors

Although some studies (a, b, c, g, i, j, k) (Table 2.1) report a somewhat increased prevalence of hyperactivity in children of lower SES families, none of these associations was found to be specific for hyperactivity. A further problem inherent in the use of SES is that the mere association between SES and children's behaviour/problems does not tell anything about the mechanisms involved. This has inspired the study of more specific background factors such as parental psychopathology, family functioning and life events in relation to child psychopathology. In three studies (a, c, h) hyperactivity was found to be associated with social disadvantage and family problems, but these associations equally applied to aggressive behaviour without hyperactivity and to learning problems.

In the London twin study (n), adverse family factors were found to explain only 8% of the variance both on trait hyperactivity ratings and in composite inattentiveness scores, while 30–40% of the variance could be explained by hereditary factors.

Table 2.2.

Study	Location	Size	Age	Frame	Case definition
A. Gillberg *et al.* (1982,1983)	Göteborg, Sweden	3448 (141)[b]	6–7	All children attending public preschools in Göteborg	Pervasive hyperactivity (home, psychiatric and neurologic examination)
B. Taylor *et al.* (1991)	Newham, East London, UK	2462 (194)	6–7	All boys at school in Newham	Pervasive hyperactivity (home, school); DSM-III, ICD-10-draft
C. Satin *et al.* (1985)	Long Island, New York, USA	294 (92)	6–9	Selected school age sub-sample (boys) at highest risk, taken from census tract stratified sample	DSM-III
D. Esser, Schmidt & Woerner(1990)	Mannheim, FRG	1444 (356)[c]	8; 13 f.u.	All 8 yr old children living in Mannheim	ICD-9 and severity rating scale
E. Verhulst, Berden & Sanders-Woudstra (1985)	Zuid-Holland, Netherlands	334 (116)	8,11	Birth registries stratified by age and sex, restricted to Dutch nationality	DSM-III; Severity rating scale (moderate, severe)
F. Shekim *et al.* (1985) -	Missouri, Columbia USA	114 (114)	9	Sample of general population	DSM-III
G. Vikan (1985)	North Troendelag County, Norway	1510 (139)	10	All children born in North Troendelag County in 1969	Rutter classification; Rutter Severity criterion and need for treatment
H. Anderson *et al.* (1987)[a]	Dunedin, New Zealand	892 (792)	11	All surviving children born to mothers residing in Dunedin in 1971 and 1972	DSM-III op the basis of 3 sources of information: 'strong pervasive' if criteria met by more than one source; 'situational' if criteria met by only one source; 'weak pervasive' if criteria met only by combining all 3 sources.

Table 2.2 (*cont.*).

Study	Location	Size	Age	Frame	Case definition
I. Kashani et al. (1987)	Columbia, Missouri, USA	150 (150)	14–16	All adolescents at public schools in Columbia	DSM-III;Severity rating scale (moderate, severe)
J. McGee *et al.* (1990)[a]	Dunedin, New Zealand	943 (943)	15	Same as in Anderson et al. (1987)	DSM-III criteria met by abbreviated DISC responses
K. Bird *et al.* (1988)	Puerto Rico, USA	777 (386)	4–16	Multistage probability sample of households	DSM-III; CGAS Severity rating scale
L. L. Szatmari *et al.* (1989*a*,*b*)	Ontario, Canada	2679 (194)	4–16	Multistage probability sample of households	DSM-III; Rutter Severity criterion
M. M. Shen Yu-cun *et al.* (1985*a*,*b*)	Beijing, China	2770 (161)	7–14	Total population of six elementary schools	DSM-III criteria for ADDH (modified)
N. N. Cohen *et al.* (1987)	Albany and Saratoga counties, USA	775 (775)	9–19	Multistage probability sample of households	DSM-III-R;Severity rating scale composed of DISC symptom scales at least 2 SD above the mean

a Dunedin population and follow-up project (see also Chapel *et al.*, 1982; McGee *et al.*, 1984*a*,*b*, 1985, 1990; Anderson *et al.*, 1987).
b Between brackets the number of subjects interviewed or examined.
c Mannheim longitudinal study, 356 subjects were re-examined at age 13 yr.
CGAS children global assessment scale.
DISC diagnostic interview schedule for children.

Table 2.3.

Study	Assessment	Prevalence	Other findings
A. Gillberg *et al.* (1982, 1983)	First stage: questionnaire aimed at detecting MBD problems (teachers) second stage: psychiatric, neurological and psychological examinations (child), questionnaire and interview (parents)	Overall p.d. n.a. MBD 7.1% (1.2% 'severe') ADDH n.a. ADD n.a. PH n.a. HK n.a. OD/CD n.a. MBD + HK 2.2%	Co-morbidity n.a. male / female 2.6:1 SES increase in low SES age n.a. non-optimal rearing + familial-hereditary +
B. Taylor *et al.* (1991)	First stage: Rutter Scale A (parents), Rutter Scale B, supplemented with items from the Conners TQ (teachers) second stage: battery of attentional performance tests, behaviour observation and neurological examination (child), PACS (parents), standardised interview (teachers)	Overall p.d. n.a. ADDH 17% ADD 1.5% PH 9% HK 1.7% OD/CD 18.5%	Co-morbidity: CD 46%, ED 14% male/female n.a. age n.a. SES - (ADD +) cognitive impairments: lower IQ and attention deficits in ADD and HK; adverse family factors correlated with persistence of disorder; perinatal adversity and neurological abnormalities in HK
C. Satin *et al.* (1985)	First stage: Conners Abbr.Q (parents, teachers) second stage: psychiatric and psychological examinations (child), parent interview (parents)	Overall p.d. n.a. ADDH 24% ADD n.a. PH 8% HK n.a. OD/CD n.a.	Co-morbidity n.a. male / female n.a. age peak 6–9 years; SES increase in low SES attention and cognition
D. Esser, Schmidt & Werner (1990)	First stage: Conners Q. (parents, teachers); second stage: parent interview, (8,13 yr), child interview (13 yr)	Overall p.d. 16.2% ADDH n.a.ADD n.a. PH n.a. 8 yr: HK 4.2% OD/CD 1.8% 13 yr: HK 1.6% OD/CD 8.4%	Co-morbidity n.a. HK only in boys! longitudinal risk: learning disabilities and family adversity

Table 2.3. (*cont.*)

Study	Assessment	Prevalence	Other findings
E. Verhulst et al. (1985)	First stage: CBCL (parents), TRF (teachers) second stage: CAS (child), Graham/Rutter interview (parents)	Overall p.d. 26% (moderate and severe), 7% (severe) ADDH 7% (moderate and severe), 3% (severe) ADD n.a. PH n.a. HK n.a. OD/CD 5%	Co-morbidity: n.a. male/female 2.2:1 SES n.a. age 8 yr > 11 yr
F. Shekim et al. (1985)	DISC-C (child); DISC-P parents	Overall p.d. n.a. ADDH 14% (either DISC-C or DISC-P), 2% (both DISC-C and DISC-P) ADD 2% PH 2% HK n.a. OD/CD 20%	Co-morbidity OD/CD 69% ED 38% Male / female 2:1 SES no effect
G. Vikan (1985)	First stage: Rutter Scale A abridged (parents), Rutter Scale B abridged (teachers) second stage: Rutter/Graham interview (child, parents)	Overall p.d. 5% ADDH n.a. ADD n.a. PH n.a. HK 0.5% OD/CD n.a.	Co-morbidity: n.a. male / female n.a. SES n.a. age n.a.
H. Anderson *et al.* (1987, 1989)	DISC (child), Rutter Scale A, supplemented with items assessing ADD and depression (parents), Rutter Scale B with additional items relating to ADD (teachers)	Overall p.d. 17.6% ADDH 6.6% (4.4% 'strong pervasive') ADD 1% PH 4.4% HK n.a. OC/CD 9.1%	Co-morbidity OD/CD 47% ED 26% Male / female 5.1:1 SES n.a. age n.a. IQ in ADDH lower than OC/CD; co-morbid cases ADDH/CD and CD had marked family disadvantage

Table 2.3. (*cont.*)

Study	Assessment	Prevalence	Other findings
I. Kashani et al. (1987)	DICA-C (child), CBCL and DICA-P (parents)	Overall p.d. 18.7% ADDH 2% OD/CD 14.7% ADD n.a. PH n.a. HK n.a.	Co-morbidity n.a. Male / female M=F SES n.a. age n.a.
J. McGee *et al.* (1990)	DISC-C abbreviated and social competence measures (child), RBPC and questions concerning global functioning (teachers)	Overall p.d. 22% ADDH 2.1% ADD n.a. PH n.a. HK n.a. OD/CD 9%	Co-morbidity OD/CD 20% ED 20% Male / female 2.5:1 SES n.a. age n.a.
K. Bird *et al.* (1988)	First stage: CBCL (parents), TRF (teachers) second stage: DISC-C (child), DISC-P (parents)	Overall p.d.(CGAS <61) 16% ADDH (CGAS <61) 9.5% OD/CD (CGAS <61) 9.9%	Co-morbidity OD/CD 54% ED 39% male / female M > F SES increase in low SES
L. Szatmari *et al.* (1989*a*,*b*,*c*)	First stage: semistructured interview with subsample of parents, teachers and children to establish cutoffs onchecklist scores second stage:CBCL modified version (child 12–16 yrs, parents,teachers)	Overall p.d. n.a. ADDH 6.3% ADD 1.4% PH 0.5% HK n.a. OD/CD 3.1%	Co-morbidity OD/CD 58% ED 14% male / female 2.7 : 1 SES: CD more psychosocial disadvantage than ADDH; age 4–11 yrs > 12–16 yrs (age effect in boys only); ADDH younger, more developmental problems than CD
M. Shen Yu-cun *et al.* (1985)	First stage: 4-item questionnaire (teachers) second stage: psychiatric and physical examination (child)	Overall p.d. n.a. ADDH 5.8% ADD n.a. PH n.a. HK n.a. OD/CD n.a.	Co-morbidity n.a. male / female 7:1 SES increase in low SES age peak at age of 9 yr

Table 2.3. (*cont.*)

Study	Assessment	Prevalence	Other findings
N. Cohen *et al.* (1987); Velez, Johnson & Cohen (1989)	DISC-C (child), DISC-P (parents)	Overall p.d. 16.7% ADHD 4% ADD n.a. PH n.a. HK n.a. OD/CD 5.6%	Co-morbidity n.a. Male / female 1.7 : 1 SES increase in low SES age 9–12 yrs > 13–18 yrs

MBD =minimal brain dysfunction; Overall p.d. =Overall psychiatric disorder.
ADDH =attention deficit disorder with hyperactivity (DSM-III).
ADD = attention deficit disorder without hyperactivity (DSM-III).
PH =pervasive hyperactivity; HK =hyperkinetic disorder.
OD/CD =oppositional/conduct disorder; ED =emotional disorder.
n.a. =not assessed.
CBCL =child behaviour checklist; TRF =teacher report form.
DISC =diagnostic interview schedule for children.
CAS =child assessment schedule.
DICA = diagnostic interview for children and adolescents.

Developmental correlates

A further point of significance concerns he relationship between hyperactivity and development factors. Prenatal and perinatal complications and neurodevelopmental abnormalities were not correlated with hyperactivity or aggression in two studies (a, h). In the Dutch study (i) prenatal problems (such as hypertension and drug treatment), but not perinatal problems, were found to be associated with hyperactivity. This study did not, however, sufficiently differentiate hyperactive from aggressive behaviour. In the Dunedin project (e) perinatal factors were clearly linked with hyperactivity (not controlled, however, for other problems) at the age of 3 years. Moreover, at 3 years, hyperactive children also had significant language and motor delay. The Nichols and Chen prospective birth cohort study (c) provides a large data set on developmental variables and hyperactivity. Several statistically significant associations could be established between hyperactivity at the age of 7 and a number of antecedent variables, such as cigarette smoking by mother during the pregnancy, delayed motor development at age of 1 year, and small head circumference at birth and or at 1 year, and excessive motor activity at the age of 8 months and 4 years. It should, however, be noted that the predictive power of the identified antecedent variables proved to be rather modest. Furthermore, there was a substantial overlap in developmental correlates of hyperactivity and those of learning difficulties with or without neurological soft signs but in the absence of hyperactivity. For example, in the London twin study (n) perinatal adversity was not related to later hyperactivity.

INTERVIEW-BASED POPULATION SURVEYS

Methodology

Over the past decade, 14 epidemiological reports could be identified on childhood and adolescent psychopathology with prevalence estimates based upon direct interviews of the subjects. Table 2.2 presents an overview of the studies, including information on authors, location, sample characteristics and case definition. In Table 2.3 a synopsis is provided of assessment methods, prevalence estimates and findings on co-morbidity and other correlates, when available, from these studies. As is evident from Table 2.2 and 2.3, the studies again differ widely in a number of ways.

First, eight surveys were conducted with the principal aim to estimate the overall prevalence of psychiatric disorder in the population rather than to focus on the prevalence of hyperactivity disorders, in particular (studies D, E, G, H, I, J, K, N). As a spin-off, however, these surveys provided data on the prevalence of hyperactivity in proportion to the rate of overall psychiatric disturbance. The explicit purpose of the other six surveys (A, B, C, F, L, M) was to examine the distribution of hyperactivity disorder in the general population, but without taking account of overall psychiatric morbidity of children and adolescents. This latter group of studies, Gillberg *et al.* in Sweden (A), in fact, concentrated on the prevalence of the minimal brain dysfunction syndrome (MBD), defined as a combination of attentional deficits or hyperactivity together with either problems of motor control or perceptual difficulties. In the second phase of analysis the rate of generalised hyperkinesis among the MBD children was estimated and extrapolations were made to the general population. The Chinese study (M) had a rather narrow focus by examining DSM-III-defined ADDH only, whereas the other surveys were targeted to also examine adjacent diagnostic groups such as oppositional and antisocial conduct disorder (studies B, C, F, L), attention deficit disorder without hyperactivity (studies B, L), and anxiety disorders (study L).

Second, there are huge differences between the studies in sampling methodology. Sampling units have included, for example, the year of birth, the school, the household. In some studies where school was the sampling unit, children living in institutions and those attending special educational facilities were excluded from the sample (A, I, N). Such children were also excluded in the Ontario Child Health Study (L), in spite of the sample being based on household. Although all investigators have attempted to maximise the representativeness of the sample in terms of demographic and socio-economic distributions, it nevertheless remains a problem in two small-sized studies with a high non-response rate (C,F). Nine studies used the multi method–multistage approach to select potential cases (A, B, C, D, E, G, K, L, M). However, the Mannheim (D) study based its prevalence estimates solely on subjects selected at random from the general population, and not on the highest scoring children from the first stage. In five other studies (F, H, I, J, N) all subjects identified through the initial sampling procedure were eligible for further diagnostic examinations. Other differences between the individual interview-based surveys concerned sample size, sex and age distribution. In five studies, the initial sample was over 1,500 (A, B, G, L, M), which contrasts with the small sample sizes of 114 and 150 in two studies (F, I). There was also a considerable variation in the number of subjects actually examined, the range being from 92 (study C) to 943 (study J). The majority of surveys involved almost equal numbers of boys and girls, however, two studies (B, C) restricted participation to boys only. The ages covered were predominantly in the primary school age range (A, B, C, D,

F, G, H). Adolescents, in particular, were investigated in two studies (I, J), while four studies (K, L, M, N) opted for a very broad age range.

Thirdly, and most importantly, studies differed in their approach to the definition of 'caseness'. The majority of the studies applied diagnostic categories from the DSM-III classification, while one (N) used the DSM-III-R criteria. In four studies from Western Europe (A, B, D, G) categories chosen (hyperkinetic disorder) were derived from the ICD-9 system and/or Rutter classification. Of all the studies, the most stringent criterion for hyperkinetic disorder was set by Taylor *et al.* (B). These investigators stipulated hyperkinetic disorder to be a combination of pervasive hyperactivity and inattentiveness which persists for longer than 6 months; in addition, they argued that 'impulsivity' was a concept too ambiguous to serve as a diagnostic criterion and consequently removed it from the definition of hyperkinetic disorder.

Many studies defined caseness beyond the mere application of diagnostic criteria for a psychiatric disorder and required additional considerations regarding the severity of the disorder, the perceived need for treatment, and whether or not there was converging evidence from multiple informants across different situations. Concordance of diagnostic information was employed in the case definitions of three studies (A, B, H). All the remaining studies, except for (C, F, J, M), included a severity rating scale which synthesised information about the level of adaptive functioning in different domains of the child's life.

Fourthly, discrepancies in the assessment instruments were prominent among the surveys reviewed. Of the different rating scales employed, three had been used in previous epidemiological and clinic-based studies and had known psychometric properties: the Rutter A (parents), and B (teachers), scales (Rutter *et al.*, 1970); the Child Behaviour Checklist (CBCL), and the related Teacher Report Form (TRF) (Achenbach & Edelbrock, 1983, 1986); and the Conners Teacher Questionnaire and Conners Abbreviated Questionnaire (Barkley, 1988). Modified versions of these ratings scales were employed in four studies: Rutter scales (study G), the Conners Teacher (study B, D) and Parents Questionnaire (study D) and the CBCL (study L). In three other studies (A, L, M), purposefully developed questionnaires were used.

Ten surveys did use (semi) structured interview schedules in eliciting diagnostic information from children and/or parents. Schedules used were the Rutter/Graham interview for parents (D, E, F), and for children (D, G); the Child Assessment Schedule (CAS) (Hodges *et al.*, 1982) (E); the Diagnostic Interview for Child and Adolescents in parents and child version (DICA, Herjanic & Reich, 1982) (I); and the Diagnostic Interview Schedule for Children in parallel versions for children and parents (DISC, Costello *et al.*, 1984) (F, H, J, K, N). The DISC in a fully structured instrument designed for use by lay interviewers, while the Rutter/Graham interview and the CAS require considerable training, and the former, in particular, should preferably be used by a person with clinical experience.

The London study (B) deserves to be specially mentioned because it is the only one employing a standardised investigator-based interview, the Parental Account of Children's Symptoms (PACS, Taylor *et al.*, 1986*a*) targeted to collect diagnostic information on hyperactivity, defiance and emotional disorder symptoms. As a related instrument, a standardised teacher interview schedule was used. Both instruments are to be applied by experienced clinicians. From a methodological point of view the London survey (B) stands out among all other surveys for its detailed measures on attentional performance, social and family backgrounds, neurological aspects and developmental data.

PREVALENCE

Comparing like with like as much as possible, the prevalence of DSM-III defined in surveys primarily envisaging overall rates of disturbance (studies E, G, H, I, H, J, K, N) ranges from 2.0% to 9.5% for boys and girls together. The median prevalence rate is 4.2%. The lowest rates were found in the adolescent samples (I, J), whereas the highest rates were detected in Zuid-Holland, the Netherlands, and in Puerto Rico (studies E, K). The overall rates of psychiatric disturbance ranged from 17.9% to 26%. However, given the methodological discrepancies of these surveys, the variations in prevalence of ADDH and overall disorder are rather small. It is of interest, however, to also compare the studies on the proportional prevalence of ADDH, i.e. prevalence of ADDH divided by the overall prevalence of psychiatric disorder. In this respect, the fluctuations become much more impressive: in Puerto Rico (study K) 59% of the overall psychiatric disorder is to be ascribed to ADDH, in New Zealand 38% (study J), 11% and 10%. These latter two studies with the lowest proportional ADDH prevalence cover the adolescent age period; thus, there are indications that the highest proportional prevalence of ADDH is more likely to be found in children of the younger age group. There are in addition other valuable explanations for these discrepant findings of in particular the Bird *et al.* study. The population of Puerto Rico is characterised by strong indicators of social disadvantage, including high rates of unemployment and divorce, high consumption of alcohol and high indexes of criminality (Bird *et al.*, 1988). Furthermore, diagnostic decision procedures seem to have differed to a considerable extent. For example, CBCL total problem scores were much higher in the Puerto Rican sample compared with those from the USA and the Netherlands; however, in spite of almost identical diagnostic criteria being applied the prevalence rates for overall psychiatric disorder ranged from 16% to 26%.

Surveys conducted with the particular aim of yielding prevalence estimates for ADDH report higher rates than the more general surveys reviewed above. Estimates vary from 5.6% to 14% for boys and girls together; the two studies that restricted participation to boys only (B, C) reported rates of 17% and 24% respectively with regard to the male/female ratio (to be discussed below) these latter figures would presumably correspond to a combined boys–girls rates of 12% and 17%, respectively. Three factors appear among other things to be associated with the higher rates found in surveys with a narrower focus: first, the lack of use of a severity rating along with DSM-III criteria in diagnostic procedures in the surveys reporting the highest ADDH rates (B, C, F); secondly, the inclusion of children aged 6–9 years who generally are at a higher risk for hyperactivity disorder; and thirdly, it is not surprising that examining a population especially for hyperactivity disorder yields a higher prevalence, since in surveys with a broad aim and multistage design, subjects whose pathology is limited to a single disorder (such as hyperactivity) may more easily remain undetected by virtue of their lower total problem scores.

Turning now to the more restrictively defined variants of hyperactivity disorder, the prevalence of pervasive hyperactivity, PH (defined as diagnostic agreement across different sources), ranges from 0.5% to 9%, with reported intermediate rates of 2 %, 4.4% and 8%. The highest detected rates (8% and 9% in studies B, C) need to viewed in light of the considerations outlined above: these studies sampled only boys aged 6–9 years. For example, in the Ontario Child Health Study (L) the prevalence estimate for PH in boys aged 4–11 years was 1.5%, which is only a sixth of the prevalence for PH in the London study. This discrepancy between the two most recent and comprehensive surveys with a narrower focus is the more striking when looking at the rather similar rates for situational hyperactivity (defined as DSM-III ADHD): 17% in London (boys 6–7 years), and 10.1% in Ontario (boys 4–11 years). The message therefore is that, when school-aged boys are hyperactive, they have a 50% chance to be rated as pervasively hyperactive in London, but a 15% chance to be similarly rated in Ontario. Different factors may contribute to this discrepancy: first, the Ontario sample comprised a mixed urban–rural population, whereas the London sample was an urban, and hence high-risk, population; second threshold scores might have been relatively lower in the London than in the Ontario study. This is an important point to keep in mind when the correlates and background factors for hyperactivity derived from the two studies will be discussed (see below).

Prevalence rate for hyperkinetic disorder in boys aged 6–7 years was 1.7% in the London survey (B). This rate would correspond to an overall rate for boys and girls of 0.9%–1.4%. The closest study to the British one is the study by Gillberg *et al.* (A). The Swedish researchers report a combined rate of 2.2% for minor neurological dysfunction (MND) and hyperkinetic disorder; the prevalence of hyperkinetic disorder as such, defined most similarly to British study as a persisting disorder of cross-situational hyperactivity and inattentiveness, was estimated to be close to 1%. It is difficult to compare this with the rate of 0.5% reported by Vikan (G) since in the Norwegian study three cases could be identified; the same applied to the high rates (4.2% at age 8, and 1.6% at 13 years) in the Mannheim study (D) as it is not clear how far pervasiveness and persistence of disorder were included in the diagnostic definition of hyperkinetic disorder.

Finally, rates for attention-deficit disorder without hyperactivity (ADD) have been reported as 1.0%, and 1.4% for boys and girls together (studies H, L); and 1.5% and 2.0% for boys only (studies B, F). It can be added that fluctuations in the ADD rates across the various studies were remarkably small.

Of all the prevalence rates quoted above, only some have been corrected for co-morbidity with related disorders. For example, the 9% pervasive hyperactivity in the London study was composed of 4% 'pure' pervasive hyperactivity combined with conduct disorder. Co-morbidity of ADDH with oppositional and/or antisocial conduct disorder varied across different studies from 30% (study I) to 69% (study M); the median rate was 47%–54%. In the same way, co-morbidity of ADDH with emotional disorders varied from 14% (studies B, L), to 39% (study K); with median rates of 20%–26%. The overlap between hyperkinetic disorder and pervasive developmental disorders was reported by Gillberg and Gillberg (1988) in a follow-up to study A: of the 14 children with hyperkinetic disorder, 8 showed autistic-type traits.

CORRELATES AND RISK FACTORS

Sex differences

Data on the male/female ratio for interview based diagnosis of hyperactivity disorder have indicated a consistent overall excess of hyperactive boys. The comparable ratios reported for ADDH have varied from 1:1 in the small-scale adolescent study (I) conducted in Missouri, USA, to 7:1 in the Beijing study (M), with median male/female ratio of 2.5:1. The latter implies that hyperactivity in girls is perhaps more frequent than it was supposed to be, and therefore it is not exclusively a problem of the male gender.

Age influences

There is a consistent trend in all surveys to suggest that the prevalence rates for hyperactivity disorder peak in children aged 4–9 years. Two studies (C, L) reported the highest rates for 6–9 year-olds, one study (K) found an earlier age peak, around the age of 4–5 years. It cannot, however, by any means be stated that hyperactivity disorders are only confined to younger children. DSM-III-defined ADDH was found prevalent in adolescents in 2%–5% of the population (studies I, J, L, N), – and this indicates that the true adolescent rates were perhaps higher than was previously thought. Age influences have been shown to manifest interactions with the situation-pervasive distinction, with sex differences, and with the 'source' reporting in hyperactivity. First, pervasive hyperactivity, defined as presence of hyperactivity according to the information gathered from parents and child, was rarely reported in adolescents in one study (L), while in another two studies (I, J) it was non existent. Secondly, the peak prevalence, reported in children aged 6-9 years has been found in boys only, whereas the Ontario project (L) was unable to substantiate any age effects of hyperactivity in girls. Thirdly, in the same study the parents rated more children as ADDH in the 12–16 age group than in the 4–11 age group, while teachers rated both boys and girls aged 4-11 more hyperactive than adolescents (Szatmari *et al.*, 1989*a*).

Cognitive and attentional correlates

The study with the most extensive data on cognitive and attentional correlates of hyperactivity is reported by Taylor *et al.* (1991). In the second stage of the London survey, cognitive performance was examined in five carefully defined contrast groups of children, namely a pure hyperactive group (defined as pervasive ADDH), a pure conduct disorder group, a mixed hyperactive–conduct disorder group, a group of children with ADD without hyperactivity, and a normal control group. The battery of psychological tests administered included five subtests from the WISC-R (similarities, vocabulary, block design, object assembly, and digit span), reading tests, a continuous performance task (CPT), a central-incidental learning test, a matching familiar figures (MFF) test, and the paired associate learning test (PAL). As a result, the ADD group proved to be clearly different from the normals in revealing a lower IQ and more speech problems, and in having poorer reading skills. The mixed hyperactive–conduct disorder group was also delayed in their reading abilities, but did not score lower on IQ. The hyperactive and conduct disorder groups were neither different from one another, nor different from the normal controls on IQ, in speech, development, or in reading skills. On a composite score of attentional performance, the pure ADD and the mixed hyperactive conduct disorder groups were found to be significantly impaired by comparison with the normal children. Furthermore, the two hyperactive groups scored lower on attention tests compared with the pure conduct disorder group. All differences reported in speech and reading skills and in attention performance were found even when covarying for the IQ. The authors concluded that the children with pure ADD were characterised by marked general cognitive impairments, including deviations in IQ, speech and reading skills and attention performance. The children with pervasive ADDH in turn, manifested more subtle attention deficits compared with the conduct disordered children, but not such a general impairment. When the analysis was shifted to the even more restrictive definition of hyperkinetic disorder, the hyperkinetic boys revealed more generalised cognitive deficits compared with both the conduct disordered and pervasively ADDH boys. Such deficits included lower IQ scores, reading delay and deviations on digit span, MFF and PAL tests. Therefore to sum up, both the ADD and the hyperkinetic disorder were characterised by general cognitive and attentional problems, while pervasive ADDH was associated with more subtle attention impairments which, however, were not severe enough to manifest on IQ tests. The overall position of pervasive ADDH boys on cognitive tests was intermediate between that of boys with the hyperkinetic syndrome and that of normal boys.

On a much smaller data set, Satin *et al.* (1985) (C) did not find cognitive differences (Peabody Picture Vocabulary Test, Beery Visual Motor Integration, reading and mathematics achievement) between children with ADDH and their comparison groups.

Anderson *et al.* (1989) (H) reported on the cognitive correlates of pervasive hyperactivity from the Dunedin prospective follow-up project. Hyperactive children (probably ADDH or ADD), and children with multiple disorders one of which was hyperactivity, were consistently rated lower than children with other disorders on full-scale IQ, verbal IQ, reading and spelling achievement across the 5–11 year age range.

Psychosocial correlates

The findings on SES show a inconsistent picture: in some studies, hyperactivity disorder has appeared more prevalent in lower SES children (A, C, M). However, the same association was found for other disorders as well in the three studies which did address the issue (K, D, N). In one study no association between SES and hyperactivity was found (L). The most informative data on psychosocial correlates of hyperactivity disorders were collected by Taylor *et al.* (1991), (B), and Szatmari, Offord & Boyle (1989*b*,*c*)(L).

In the London survey (B) the ADD group appeared to be associated with low occupational status of the parents and generally with more social disadvantage. Furthermore, measures of family relationships did distinguish the mixed hyperactive conduct disorder group, or the children with the more restricted hyperkinetic disorder from the remaining groups. It also turned out that persistence of disorder at follow-up 9 months later was significantly associated with the presence of intrafamilial problems and maternal depression.

In the Ontario Child Health Study (Szatmari, Boyle & Offord 1989*c*)(L), children with 'pure' ADDH children were younger and had experiences less psychological disadvantage, but more developmental delays than 'pure' CD children. The differences between ADDH and CD appeared to be stronger in boys than in girls. These findings were confirmed in an identical analysis of the same Ontario data set in a comparison of ADDH children and children without any disorder (Szatmari *et al.*, 1989*b*). A number of psychosocial, demographic, family and child-centred factors indicating disadvantage were more common in children with ADDH children with than in normal children. However, when co-morbidity was controlled for child-centred variables, including problems in motor and speech development, emerged as the most important; the association between psychosocial factors and ADDH was not significant over and above that found for other disorders, conduct disorder, in particular.

Taken as a whole, the findings on psychosocial variables from the Canadian study were at variance with the results of the London survey. However, the methodological differences make it difficult to carry out the appropriate comparisons between the two: the Ontario study included mostly situationally hyperactive boys and girls of a broad age range; the London study was based on pervasively hyperactive 6–7 year-old boys. Furthermore, the Canadian researchers did not measure the quality of family relationships in the different groups of children.

Developmental correlates

In the London survey (B) there were no differences between pure hyperactive, pure aggressive, mixed hyperactive–aggressive, pure attention deficit and normal children in minor complications of delivery, or in adverse prenatal and perinatal events. Neither did the five contrast groups differ from one another in motor development or in motor coordination. As has already been noted above, pure inattentiveness (ADD without hyperactivity) correlated significantly with language delay. Perinatal problems, as well as language delay, were, however, far more common in children with more restrictively defined hyperkinetic disorder. The results of the Gillberg, Carlstrom & Rasmussen (1983) study (A) were less clear-cut: non-optimal prenatal and postnatal factors accounted for only 6% of the variance in hyperkinetic disorder.

By contrast, in the Ontario Study (L), as depicted above, situationally and/or pervasively hyperactive children were distinguished from the CD and normal children by increased problems in their motor and speech development .

Neurological correlates

Epidemiological studies offer an opportunity to investigate the possible associations between hyperactivity disorder, neurological abnormalities and physical anomalies in the general population. Such an association was found only for hyperkinetic disorder, but not for the more loosely defined pervasive hyperactivity, nor for the other four contrast groups in the London study (B). In the Swedish survey (A) the population was first screened for MBD features; the children with hyperkinetic disorder were from the 'screen positives'. When the parameters relating to minor neurological dysfunction (due to the initial design), were left out of the analysis, it was found that 12% of the variance of hyperkinetic disorder was explainable by the presence of minor physical anomalies and 14% by familial/hereditary factors.

SUMMARY AND CONCLUSIONS

In summary, as has been extensively discussed above, epidemiological studies of hyperactivity disorders, both those with broad and narrow focus, show substantial differences in methodology which makes adequate comparisons between studies a difficult task. As is bound to happen in such a situation, a number of contradictory results across different studies emerge. There is therefore an urgent need for the researchers in this field to combine efforts and to reach consensus in developing uniform, standardised assessment procedures in order to employ common methodologies. Furthermore, only a couple of studies have progressed into investigating the pathogenetic mechanisms leading to, or being associated with symptomatology (Rutter, 1988). Surprisingly few studies have, for example, managed to adequately address and measure the relationship between attention deficits and hyperactivity in groups of children selected from the general population. So far, the yield of epidemiological approaches to studying hyperactivity disorders, and especially in deepening our understanding of these intriguing psychopathological conditions of childhood, has been rather meagre. In this last section we summarise the patterns of findings and discuss unresolved questions.

PREVALENCE

Hyperactivity disorder is common, perhaps at certain ages the most common, disorder of childhood. The median prevalence rate for interview-based and DSM-III defined ADDH was 4.2% in surveys with a broad focus, but rates were substantially higher, up to 17% in surveys with a narrower focus. These figures, however, disregard estimates of the severity of illness. Taking these into account, it seems reasonable to put ADDH rates in the range of 2% (in adolescence), to 8% (in school-age children in high risk urban populations). Pervasive hyperactivity, defined as hyperactivity with cross-informant concordance of diagnostic criteria, showed a broad range, from 0.5 in the Ontario study to 4%–6% in the London study. The studies 'in the middle-range' report 2%–4% pervasive hyperactivity. The even more restrictively defined hyperkinetic disorder was found prevalent close to 1%.

Prevalence varies considerably across age and gender. Almost all studies reported a preponderance of hyperactive males, and median figures for the male–female ratio were 2.5:1. Gender influences were most apparent in younger school-aged children, and in fact, the excess of hyperactive males seemed to be largely ascribed to teacher ratings of the behaviour of boys aged 6–9 years. Overall, children aged 6–9 years seem to be at the highest risk for hyperactivity disorder. The available studies raise a number of outstanding issues concerning sex and age influences which remain to be pursued in future research. These involve, for example, the relative difficulty of identifying pervasively hyperactive females and the absence of age effects in females. Another important conclusion is that, even given the age and gender effects, hyperactivity disorders appear relatively common in adolescence and in girls, which should have both clinical and research implications concerning these populations. One task, among others, is to reconsider and refine the type and number of diagnostic criteria required for a diagnosis of hyperactivity disorder dependent on age and gender factors.

Rural–urban status seems to have some impact on the prevalence of hyperactivity. In general, there appears to be a trend for populations in urban areas to manifest higher prevalence rates, but rural–urban comparisons within the same study have proved to be of minor importance (e.g. Szatmari *et al.*, 1989*a*). Of course, the rural–urban dichotomy is usually a crude distinction and may obscure the effects of associated factors, such as poverty, and other indices of socio-economic disadvantage which may well exert a more direct influence on the prevalence of hyperactivity. For example, in the London twin study, prevalence rates were associated with urban adversity, but not with urban residence *per se* (Goodman & Stevenson, 1989*a*).

DIAGNOSTIC ISSUES

ADD

Rates for ADD have consistently been reported in the 1%–2% range. In the Ontario Child Health Study, the diagnosis of ADD was almost exclusively made in adolescent girls. The debate of whether ADD is a separate diagnostic entity, sufficiently distinct from ADDH, dates back a long time. The consistent reporting of its prevalence across different studies, as well as the distinct cognitive, attentional and developmental correlates described by Taylor *et al.* (1991), add proof to ADD as a useful and valid diagnostic concept. This agrees with a growing body of research literature, mostly based on clinical samples, indicating that children with ADDH and ADD differ in a number of ways (Bauermeister *et al.*, 1992; Cantwell & Baker, 1992; Carlson, 1986; Lahey & Carlson, 1991). For example, children with ADDH have been described as more impulsive, aggressive, distractible and socially uninhibited. By contrast, children with ADD have been reported to be sluggish and drowsy, socially withdrawn, and exhibiting few conduct problems, but more affective symptomatology. There are, however, some questions markes concerning the continuity between ADDH and ADD over time: follow-up data from a clinical sample indicated that in the course of time, children with ADD have a high risk to obtain the diagnosis of ADDH (Cantwell & Baker, 1989); which may suggest that ADD is a temporal carnation of ADDH. Such findings may well stimulate research into differential neurobiological, cognitive and social-behavioural characteristics of children with ADDH and ADD. Another important question indeed is whether the attention deficit in ADDH and ADD differs, when examined with the appropriate neuropsychological and/or psycho-physiological designs.

Co-morbidity

Rates for co-morbidity with oppositional and/or antisocial conduct disorders (median 47%–54%), agree with the data from clinical samples (for review, see Biederman, Newcorn & Sprich, 1991). Or to put it better in reversed terms: the co-morbidity of hyperactivity and conduct disorder in referred cases is not to be ascribed to referral bias. The association of these two disorders is much stronger than it to be expected on the basis of the prevalence of the individual disorders (Szatmari *et al.*, 1989*c*). Different supplementary hypotheses have been put forward to explain this association (Rutter, 1989*a*), and one mechanism seems very plausible in particular: hyperactivity constitutes a considerable risk for the development of antisocial conduct disorder. Arguments are mainly based on data from short-term and long-term follow-up studies (Klein & Mannuzza, 1991), and on findings from cross-sectional epidemiological studies indicating that children with ADDH are younger than children with conduct disorder (Szatmari *et al.*, 1989*c*). Admittedly, the expected increase in their percentage of co-morbidity in older children and adolescents, compared to younger school-age children, is not, however, found across all surveys reviewed in this chapter. Methodological variance may be responsible for this negative finding. Another possibility, of course, is that hyperactivity disorders change into conduct disorders with age.

The co-morbidity with emotional disorders is reported fairly consistently across different surveys. However, to complicate the matters further, this association may be partly due to the associated conduct symptoms. Other routes that have been proposed are; first, that symptoms of hyperactivity and inattention as such, induce anxiety symptoms at an early age (for example, performance anxiety and phobic mechanisms), or secondly, that hyperactivity may in some cases be a manifestation of 'nervous restlessness'.

Remarkably, only one survey has addressed the diagnostic relationship between hyperactivity disorders and pervasive developmental disorders. Many PDD cases present with overactive and uncontrolled motor behaviour and inattentiveness; this issue does merit further attention in forthcoming studies.

SITUATIONAL–PERVASIVE DISTINCTION

The epidemiological studies by Schachar, Rutter & Smith (1981), by Goodman & Stevenson (1989*a*), and Taylor *et al.* (1991) have all made a strong claim that pervasive hyperactivity is qualitatively different from situational hyperactivity in its associations with cognitive and attentional impairments. Earlier support for this distinction has been provided by follow-up studies of hyperactive preschoolers. Persistence of disorder tended to be much stronger in PH preschoolers than in those with SH (Schleifer *et al.*, 1975; Campbell, Endman & Bernfield, 1977; but see, Cohen & Minde, 1983, for a negative result). In a more recent follow-up study, Gillberg & Gillberg (1988) replicated and extended these findings: 50% of a sample of children diagnosed as PH at the age of 7 years were still pervasively hyperactive at the age of 15 years; their academic achievement was also significantly poorer than that of children with SH. Neither initial IQ nor social class were clear predictive factors for such outcome. All these follow-up studies are, however, limited by the fact that co-morbidity for aggressive behaviours has not been allowed for. The same limitation applies to a Canadian study in which small groups of children with pervasive ADDH, situational ADDH and those not sharing hyperactivity were sampled from a general school population; pervasive ADHD, but not situational ADHD, was found to be associated with lower scores on verbal IQ and reading achievement (Boudreault *et al.*, 1988). Other relevant data are provided by clinical studies. Using a multivariate cluster analysis in a sample of 60 referred boys, aged 6–10 years, with problems of disruptive behaviour, Taylor *et al.* (1986b) identified a robust cluster of cases with high scores on all measures of hyperactivity and inattention. Additional features of these boys with PH were a lower IQ, earlier age of onset of behaviour problems, a good response to methylphenidate medication, abnormal findings on neurological examination and a history of developmental delays (Taylor *et al.*, 1986*a*; 1987).

Despite this body of evidence, there are still unresolved questions concerning validity, reliability and utility of the situational–pervasive distinction. First, the suggestions from the Ontario Child Health Study that pervasive hyperactivity is strongly related to age and gender factors, should be pursued in future research. A crucial question therefore appears to be whether the main issue concerns pervasive hyperactivity as such, or is it hyperactivity as typically present in boys aged 6–10 years? Secondly, another lead from the Goodman & Stevenson study (1989*a*), as enumerated in their discussion, was that there was a degree of deviant behaviour which seemed to increase progressively from home hyperactivity to school hyperactivity to pervasive hyperactivity. Thus, school hyperactivity was more similar to pervasive hyperactivity than was home hyperactivity. Other studies have corroborated the findings that teacher ratings of hyperactivity, and of psychiatric symptoms in general, correlate better with cognitive and attentional impairments than parent ratings do (Szatmari *et al.*, 1990; McGee *et al.*, 1986). Perhaps the key issue is the situational specificity of hyperactive symptomatology in relation to cognitive impairment; and the key distinction that between home and school hyperactivity, rather than between situational and pervasive hyperactivity. Thirdly, some measurement problems still remain. The unresolved questions include: how to weigh the manifestation of hyperactive behaviour in contexts other than school or home; for example, during psychological testing or psychiatric interviewing? Furthermore, how are the children selected as pervasively hyperactive by different instruments, such as the Rutter questionnaires or the CBL/TRF scales, comparable? And, whether the definition of pervasiveness should not be based on exceeding cut-offs on questionnaires, but on endorsing a sufficient number of ADDH or ADHD criteria from each source? Fourthly, Szatmari *et al.* (1989*c*) described differential correlates in comparison to those of conduct disorder in a more leniently defined hyperactivity disorder, comprising only 15% pervasive hyperactivity. It is, however, possible that the Canadians by their definition of ADHD, and the item pool and cut-offs of their modified CBCL checklists, albeit mainly resulting in situational ADDH diagnoses, selected a group of hyperactive children that was robust enough to find differential correlates, in spite of mainly constituting of subjects with the diagnosis of situational ADDH. Fifthly, it is worthwhile to examine whether the situational–pervasive distinction coincides with the demarcation of neurobiological abnormalities, for example, in cerebral monoaminergic neurotransmission, or in patterns of cerebral perfusion and regional metabolic rate. Sixthly, is pervasive hyperactivity not synonymous with severe hyperactivity, and if so, what are the contributions of other potential aspects of severity such as early age of onset, persistence over time, concomitant oppositional and aggressive behaviour, familial–genetic loading, lower IQ, and also the degree of overall behavioural deviance in the case of situational hyperactivity, related to age and sex norms? Clearly, many of these aspects are interrelated, but which comes first? Is it pervasiveness of symptoms that causes persistence, or is it persistence that leads to pervasiveness, or is excessive school hyperactivity the core problem? In conclusion, an alternative approach would be to explore the usefulness of a severity scale of hyperactivity symptoms. This should comprise elements of pervasiveness, degree of situational deviance, persistence, age of onset, co-morbidity, IQ, attentional performance and biological loading.

DEVELOPMENTAL, PSYCHOSOCIAL AND NEUROLOGICAL CORRELATES

The epidemiological data reviewed above allow a few firmly based conclusions regarding the correlates of hyperactivity disorder to be drawn. In general, hyperactivity does not seem to be associated with psychosocial adversity, not at least when corrections are made for co-morbid aggressive behaviours, and when compared with psychiatric disorder in general. So far, little attention has, however, been paid to intrafamilial problems, and to patterns of family interaction. The cross-sectional data suggest at best weak links between intrafamilial problems and hyperactivity, although persistence of disorder seems to be determined by psychosocial disadvantage (McGee *et al.*, 1991; Taylor *et al.*, 1991). Two caveats, however, have to made here: first, perhaps it is not motor restlessness *per se*, but inattentiveness that is associated with low SES (Taylor *et al.*, 1991); unfortunately, most studies have not differentiated these two core symptoms in the study of parameters that are associated with hyperactivity disorders. Secondly, it should be stressed that the extraction of significant correlates of hyperactivity has been based on cross-sectional designs, with only a few exceptions (Anderson *et al.*, 1987; Cohen *et al.*, 1987; Velez, Johnson & Cohen, 1989; McGee *et al.*, 1991). Therefore, the direction of the effects found may not be inferred, and thus, knowledge of the correlates gives only limited insight into the pathogenetic mechanisms of hyperactivity.

Developmental deviations and retardation of language, speech and motor functions are reported in excess in hyperactive children compared with disorder in non-hyperactive children. This suggests that hyperactivity ought to be at least partly conceptualised within the framework of general developmental immaturity. Correlations between hyperactivity, perinatal adversity and neurological abnormalities have proved to be rather weak and non-specific. There are cues, however, that perinatal and neurological non-optimality are related to the degree of severity of the hyperactivity disorder: perinatal and neurological parameters did discriminate children with severe hyperkinetic disorder from children with milder degree of hyperactivity. The evidence reviewed does, however, refute the old concept of 'minimal brain dysfunction' in the sense that subtle or minimal brain damage gives rise to a uniform behavioural picture of hyperactivity. The same argument has been put forward previously by Rutter, 1989*a* and Schmidt *et al.*, 1987. As far as early prenatal and perinatal variables have been adequately charted in relation to the genesis of hyperactivity, prenatal factors operating during embryogenesis and cerebrogenesis, but not perinatal factors, appear to be particularly significant, in combination with genetic influences (Goodman & Stevenson, 1989*b*).

COGNITIVE IMPAIRMENTS

The majority of the few studies, which have investigated association between hyperactivity and cognitive impairments, establish meaningful links. The findings include lower IQs, reading impairments and worse scores on attention performance tests in hyperactive children, compared with non-hyperactive and aggressive children. Studies differ, however, regarding the type of hyperactivity disorder to which these findings apply; there are clear suggestions that the more severe and or pervasive the hyperactivity disorder, the stronger is the association in the cognitive impairments (Taylor *et al.*, 1991; Goodman & Stevenson, 1989*a*; Schachar *et al.*, 1981).

A few additional points regarding the relationship between cognitive factors and hyperactivity deserve to be briefly mentioned: First, the nature of the attention deficits has not been clarified. For example, in the London survey continuous performance test results did not differentiate the hyperactive group from the contrast groups, casting doubt on the existence of deficits in sustained attention. It therefore remains unclear whether the cognitive deficit associated with hyperactivity is of a specific or rather general nature. It may also be asked whether more detailed neuropsychological and psychophysiological examinations than those employed so far will be able to result in a whole variety of different cognitive deficits? At this stage of our knowledge there are no indications of one specific deficit, and cognitive and attentional heterogeneity seem likely. Further studies are needed into the characterisation of attention deficits, and also into the ecological validity of cognitive tests employed (Barkley, 1991). Secondly, few epidemiological studies have explicitly focused on the co-morbid association between hyperactivity and learning disorders. (For further discussion, see Semrud-Clikeman *et al.*, 1992; Cantwell & Baker, 1991.) Thirdly, at present there does not appear to be sufficient knowledge to determine what are the pathogenetic mechanisms behind the association between inattentiveness (and hyperactivity), and general cognitive impairments (lower IQ), or specific cognitive impairments (poor reading achievement). Of course, inattentive behaviour interferes with the orientation to, and processing of, important information, that are the bricks of cognitive constructs and operation. If inattentiveness causes a lower IQ, then it might be predicted that inattentiveness is not only associated with cognitive impairment, but this association will be relatively stronger, dependent on the age of onset of the disorder, and the age of child. For example, the IQ deviations between hyperactive and normal children should be larger in adolescence compared with earlier school-age years. Data from the Dunedin follow-up project, where no interaction effect of age was found (Anderson *et al.*, 1989), preclude such a straightforward explanation; more complex explanatory models are indeed needed. It is, of course, possible that both attention deficits and cognitive impairments derive from the same underlying neurobiological dysfunctions. Similar considerations apply to the relationship between inattentiveness and reading disorders; further insightful comments on this topic and examples of explanatory models can be found in Rowe & Rowe (1992*a*,*b*) and in McGee & Share (1988). The topic is also fully discussed in Chapter 11 of this volume.

BEHAVIOURAL PRECURSORS

A number of questions remain unanswered regarding the precursors of hyperactivity: For example, what are the psychopathological precursors of hyperactivity and inattentiveness diagnosed in school-age children? At how early an age does it make sense to diagnose a child as suffering from ADHD or from hyperkinetic disorder? Is it possible, at toddler-age, to identify hyperactive and/or inattentive children at high risk for ADHD, ADD or hyperkinetic disorder? To what extent do temperamental variations, or characteristics of the early child-caregiver interaction contribute meaningfully to such a prediction? Are hyperactive and inattentive behaviours clustering together at pre-school age? Can temperamental variations be differentiated from precursors of later psychiatric disorder (Rutter, 1989*b*)? Although studies have approached this area of research, one common problem is that attention has been focused on the occurrence of isolated symptoms such as motoric overactivity, restlessness and poor concentration in pre-schoolers (Earls, 1980; Richman, Stevenson & Graham, 1975), but not so much on the identification of clusters of behaviour, or disorders of behaviour (Luk *et al*., 1991; Koot & Verhulst, 1991).

A few studies deserve to be cited in this context. Richman, Stevenson & Graham (1982) extracted five clusters, two of which comprised rather broadly defined disturbances of conduct, including overactive and restless behaviour at the age of 3 years; the two clusters applied to 33% of the sample studies. Valuable suggestions of the influence of early caregiver–child interactions were provided in a prospective study on antecedents of hyperactivity (Jacobvitz & Sroufe, 1987). Intrusive or overstimulating maternal care and child distractibility as assessed at 42 months or earlier, were best predictors of hyperactivity at the age of 5–6 years. Results on early identification, at the age of 2–3 years, of children at risk for later hyperactivity disorder nonetheless remain conflicting. For example, Chapel *et al*. (1982) found a low degree of stability of problem behaviour in children identified as hyperactive and/or inattentive from the age of 3 to the age of 5. It may be, of course that the precursors only become manifest after the child has entered school and should be capable of task-oriented behaviour along with his group of peers.

RECOMMENDATIONS FOR FURTHER EPIDEMIOLOGICAL STUDIES

In order to enlarge our knowledge of hyperactivity disorders, it seems exigent, in future epidemiological studies, to follow the exemplary design of Taylor *et al.* (1991), and to move beyond the mere task of establishing prevalence rates and correlated parameters. Progress can only be made by carefully studying selected groups of children from the general population by using multi-stage designs. In such studies, the concurrent validity of different instruments (e.g. Rutter scales, CBCL/TRF, Conners scales) should be established in the initial screening stage. In the second stage it is essential to include first, direct measurement of information processing within neuropsychological or psychophysiological designs; secondly, familial–genetic assessments, following, for example, the methods used by Biederman *et al.* (1986; 1987*a,b*); thirdly, refined and reliable measurements of family-interaction patterns. Further gains may be obtained if neurobiological measures are also included. The association with pervasive and specific developmental disorders deserves special attention as does the validity of attention-deficit disorder without hyperactivity. Ideally, such an epidemiological study should be based on the design of a prospective follow-up study starting at pre-school age and including measures of temperament and of child–caregiver interaction. The strategies of data analyses should include techniques such as structural equation modelling in order to test predictive hypotheses and to progress to testing of confirmatory models (Rowe & Rowe, 1992a). This would allow the real pathogenetic mechanisms to be studied and the gap between large-scale epidemiological and detailed clinical approaches to hyperactivity to be bridged.

REFERENCES

Achenbach, T.M. & Edelbrock, C.S. (1983). *Manual for the Child Behaviour Checklist and Revised Profile*. Burlington, University of Vermont, Department of Psychology.

Achenbach, T.M. & Edelbrock, C.S. (1986). *Manual for the Teachers's Report Form and the Teachers' Version of the Child Behaviour Profile*. Burlington, University of Vermont, Department of Psychology.

American Psychiatric Association (1980). *Diagnostic and Statistical Manual of Mental Disorders*. Third Edition Washington, DC:APA.

American Psychiatric Association (1987). *Diagnostic and Statistical Manual of Mental Disorders*. Third Edition Revised. Washington, DC:APA.

Anderson, J.C., Williams, S., McGee, R. & Silva, P.A. (1987). DSM-III disorders in pre-adolescent children. *Archives of General Psychiatry*, **44**, 69–76.

Anderson, J.C., Williams, S., McGee, R. & Silva, P.A. (1989). Cognitive and social correlates of DSM-III disorders in pre-adolescent children. *Journal of the American Academy of Child and Adolescent Psychiatry,* **28**, 842–6.

August, C.J. & Garfinkel, B.D. (1989). Behavioural and cognitive subtypes of ADHD. *Journal of the American Academy of Child and Adolescent Psychiatry,* **28**, 739–48.

Barkley, R.A. (1988). Child behaviour rating scales and checklists. In *Assessment and Diagnosis in Child Psychopathology*, eds. M. Rutter, A.H. Tuma & I.S. Lann, pp. 113–55. New York: Guilford Press.

Barkley, R.A. (1991). The ecological validity of laboratory and analogue assessment methods of ADHD symptoms. *Journal of Abnormal Child Psychology* **19**, 149–78.

Bauermeister, J.J., Alegria, M., Bird, H., Rubio-Stipec, M. & Canino, G. (1992). Are attentional-hyperactivity deficits unidimensional or multidimensional syndromes? Empirical findings from a community survey. *Journal of the American Academy of Child Adolescent Psychiatry* **31**, 423–31.

Biederman, J., Munir, K., Knee, D., Habelow, W., Armentano, M., Autor, S., Hoge, S.K., & Waternaux, C. (1986). A family study of patients with attention deficit disorder and normal controls. *Journal of Psychiatry Research*, **20**, 263–74.

Biederman, J., Munir, K., Knee, D., Armentano, M., Autor, S., Hoge, S.K., Waternaux, C. & Tsuang, M. (1987*a*). High rate of affective disorders in probands with attention deficit disorders and in their relatives: a controlled family study. *American Journal of Psychiatry,* **144**, 330–3.

Biederman, J., Munir, K. & Knee, D. (1987*b*). Conduct and oppositional disorder in clinically referred children with attention deficit disorder: a controlled family study. *Journal of the American Academy of Child and Adolescent Psychiatry,* **26**, 724–7.

Biederman, J., Newcorn, J. & Sprich, S. (1991). Co-morbidity of attention deficit hyperactivity disorder with conduct, depressive, anxiety, and other disorders. *American Journal of Psychiatry,* **148**, 564–77.

Bird, H.R., Canino, G., Rubio-Stipec, M., Gould, M.S., Ribera, J., Sesman, M., Woodbury, M., Huertas-Goldman, S., Pagan, A., Sanchez-Lacay, A. & Moscoso, M. (1988). Estimates of the prevalence of childhood maladjustment in a community survey in Puerto Rico: the use of combined measures. *Archives of General Psychiatry,* **45**, 1120–6.

Boudreault, M., Thivierge, J., Cote, R., Boutin, P., Julien, Y. & Bergeron, S. (1988). Cognitive development and reading achievement in pervasive-ADD situational-ADD and control children. *Journal of Child Psychology and Psychiatry,* **29**, 611–19.

Brandenburg, N.A., Friedman, R.M. & Silver, S.E. (1990). The Epidemiology of childhood psychiatric disorders: Prevalence findings from recent studies. *Journal of the American Academy of Child and Adolescent Psychiatry,* **29**, 76–83.

Campbell, S.B., Endman, M.W. & Bernfield, G. (1977). A three-year follow-up of hyperactive pre-schoolers into elementary school. *Journal of Child Psychology and Psychiatry,* **18**, 239–49.

Cantwell, D.P. & Baker, L. (1989). Stability and natural history of DSM-III childhood diagnoses. *Journal of the American Academy of Child and Adolescent Psychiatry,* **28**, 691–700.

Cantwell, D.P. & Baker, L. (1991). Association between attention-deficit hyperactivity disorder and learning disorders. *Journal of Learning Disabilities,* **24,** 88–95.

Cantwell, D.P. & Baker, L. (1992). Attention deficit disorder with and without hyperactivity: a review and comparison of matched groups. *Journal of the American Acaemy of Child Adolescent Psychiatry*, **31**, 432–8.

Carlson, C.L. (1986). Attention deficit disorder without hyperactivity. *Advances in Clinical Child Psychology,* **9**, 153–75.

Chapel, J.A., Robins, A.J., McGee, R., Williams, S.M. & Silva P.A. (1982). A follow-up of inattentive and/or hyperactive children from birth to 7 years of age. *Journal of Operational Psychiatry,* **13**, 17–26.

Cohen, N.J. & Minde, K. (1983). The hyperactivity syndrome in Kindergarten children: comparison of children with pervasive and situational symptoms. *Journal of Child Psychology and Psychiatry,* **24**, 443–55.

Cohen, P., Velez, N., Kohn, M., Schwab-Stone, M., & Johnson, J. (1987). Child psychiatric diagnosis by computer algorithm: theoretical issues and empirical tests. *Journal of the American Academy of Child and Adolescent Psychiatry,* **26**, 631–8.

Connell, H.K., Irvine L. & Rodney, J. (1982). The prevalence of psychiatric disorders in rural school children. *Australian and New Zealand Journal of Psychiatry,* **16**, 43–6.

Costello, A.J., Edelbrock, C.S., Dulcan, M.K., Kalas, R. & Klaric, S.H. (1984). *Development and Testing of the NIMH Diagnostic Interview for Children in a Clinic Population: Final Report.* Rockville, MD. NIMH, Centre for Epidemiological Studies.

Costello, EJ. (1990). Child psychiatric epidemiology. *Advances in Clinical Child Psychology,* **13**, 53–90.

Costello, E.J., Costello, A.J., Edelbrock, C., Burns, B.J., Dulcan, M.K., Brent, D. & Janiszewski, S. (1988). Psychiatric disorders in paediatric primary care: Prevalence and risk factors. *Archives of General Psychiatry,* **45**, 1107–16.

Earls, F. (1980). Prevalence of behaviour problems in 3-year-old children: a cross-national replication. *Archives of General Psychiatry,* **37**, 1153–7.

Edelbrock, C. & Costello, A.J. (1988). Structured psychiatric interviews for children. In *Assessment and Diagnosis in Child Psychopathology,* eds. M. Rutter, A.H. Tuma & I.S. Lann, pp. 87–112. New York: Guilford Press.

Ekblad, S. (1990). The children's behaviour questionnaire for completion by parents and teachers in a Chinese sample. *Journal of Child Psychology and Psychiatry,* **31**, 775–91.

Esser, G., Schmidt, M.H., & Woerner, W. (1990). Epidemiology and course of psychiatric disorders in school-age children – results of a longitudinal study. *Journal of Child Psychology and Psychiatry,* **31**, 243–63.

Gillberg, I.C. & Gillberg, C. (1988). Generalized hyperkinesis: follow-up study from age 7 to 13 years. *Journal of the American Academy of Child and Adolescent Psychiatry,* **27**, 55–9.

Gillberg, C., Rasmussen, P., Carlström, G., Svenson, B. & Waldenström, E. (1982). Perceptual, motor and attentional deficits in six-year-old children. Epidemiological aspects. *Journal of Child Psychology and Psychiatry,* **23**, 131–44.

Gillberg, C., Carlström, G. & Rasmussen, P. (1983). Hyperkinetic disorders in seven-year-old children with perceptual, motor and attentional deficits. *Journal of Child Psychology and Psychiatry,* **24**, 233–46.

Goldstein, H.S. (1987). Cognitive development in low attentive, hyperative, and aggressive 6- through 11-year-old children. *Journal of the American Academy of Child and Adolescent Psychiatry*, **26**, 214–18

Goodman, R. & Stevenson, J. (1989*a*). A twin-study of hyperactivity – I. An examination of hyperactivity scores and categories derived from Rutter Teacher and Parent Questionnaires. *Journal of Child Psychology and Psychiatry,* **30**, 671–89.

Goodman, R. & Stevenson, J. (1989b). A twin study of hyperactivity – II. The aetiological roles of genes, family relationships and perinatal adversity. *Journal of Child Psychology and Psychiatry,* **30**, 691–709.

Graham, P. & Rutter, M. (1973). Psychiatric disorders in the young adolescent: a follow-up study. *Proceedings of the Royal Society of Medicine,* **66**, 1226–9.

Hirasing, R.A., Kuijper, A. & Stolk, H.J.J. (1988). Ontwikkelingsverloop van het kind en hyperactiviteit (Course of children's development and hyperactivity). *Nederlands Tijdschrift voor Geneeskunde,* **132**, 1688–92.

Hinshaw, S.P. (1987). On the distinction between attentional deficits/hyperactivity and conduct problems/aggression in child psychopathology. *Psychological Bulletin,* **101**, 443–63.

Herjanic, B. & Reich, W. (1982). Development of a structured psychiatric interview for children: agreement between child and parent on individual symptoms. *Journal of Abnormal Child Psychology,* **10**, 307–24.

Hodges, K., Mknew, D., Cytryn, L., Stern, L. & Kline, J. (1982). The Child Assessment Schedule (CAS) diagnostic interview: a report on reliability and validity. *Journal of the American Academy of Child and Adolescent Psychiatry* **21**, 468–73.

Holborrow, P., Berry, P. & Elkins, J. (1984). Prevalence of hyperkinesis: a comparison of 3 rating scales. *Journal of Learning Disabilities.* **17**, 411–15.

Holborrow, P.L. & Berry, P.S. (1986). Hyperactivity and learning difficulties. *Journal of Learning Disabilities,* **19**, 426–31.

Jacobvitz, D. & Sroufe, L.A. (1987). The early caregiver–child relationship and attention-deficit disorder with hyperactivity in kindergarten: a prospective study. *Child Development,* **58**, 1488–95.

Kashani, J.H., Beck, N.C., Hoeper, E.W., Fallahi, C., Corcoran, C.M., McAllister, J.A., Rosenberg, T.K. & Reid, J.C. (1987). Psychiatric disorders in a community sample of adolescents. *American Journal of Psychiatry*, **144**, 584–9.

Klein, R.G. & Mannuzza, S. (1991). Long-term outcome of hyperactive children: a review. *Journal of the American Academy of Child and Adolescent Psychiatry,* **30**, 383–7.

King, C. & Young, R.D. (1982). Attentional deficits with and without hyperactivity. *Journal of Abnormal Child Psychology*, **10**, 483–95.

Koot, H.M. & Verhulst, F.C. (1991). Prevalence of problem behaviour in Dutch children aged 2–3. *Acta Psychiatrica Scandinavica,* **83**, *Suppl 367.*

Kuijper, A. & Hirasing, R.A. (1986). Prevalentie van hyper actief gedrag bij vijf-jarigen (Prevalence of hyperactivity in five-year old children). *Tijdschrift voor Orthopedagiek, Kinderpsychiatrie en Kinderpsychologie,* **11**, 120–30.

Lahey, B.B. & Carlson, C.L. (1991). Validity of the diagnostic category of attention deficit disorder without hyperactivity. *Journal of Learning Disabilities*, **24**, 110–20.

Loney, J. & Milich, M. (1982). Hyperactivity, inattention and aggression in clinical practice. In *Advances in Developmental and Behavioral Pediatrics*, eds. M. Wolraich & D.K. Routh, pp. 113–147. Greenwich, Conn: JAI Press Inc.

Luk, S.L., Leung, P.W.L. & Lee, P.L.M. (1988). Conner's Teacher Rating Scale in Chinese children in Hong Kong. *Journal of Child Psychology and Psychiatry,* **29**, 165–74.

Luk, S.L., Leung, P.W.L., Bacon-Shone, J. & Lieh-Mak, F. (1991). The structure and prevalence of behavioural problems in Hong Kong preschool children. *Journal of Abnormal Child Psychology,* **19**, 219–32.

Matsuura, M., Okubo, Y, Kato, M., Kojima, T., Takahashi, R., Asai, K., Endo, T., Yamada, S., Kimura, K. & Suzuki, M. (1989). An epidemiological investigation of emotional and behavioural problems in primary school children in Japan. *Social Psychiatry and Epidemiology,* **24**, 17–22.

McGee, R.& Share, D.L. (1988). Attention deficit disorder-hyperactivity and academic failure: which comes first and what should be treated? *Journal of the American Academy of Child and Adolescent and Psychiatry,* **27**, 318–25.

McGee, R., Williams, S. & Silva, P.A. (1984*a*). Behavioural and developmental characteristics of aggressive, hyperactive and aggressive hyperactive boys. *Journal of the American Academy of Child Psychiatry,* **23**, 270–9.

McGee, R., Williams, S. & Silva, P.A. (1984*b*). Background characteristics of aggressive, hyperactive and aggressive hyperactive boys. *Journal of the American Academy of Child Psychiatry,* **23**, 280–4.

McGee, R., Williams, S. & Silva, P.A. (1985). Factor structure and correlates of ratings of inattention, hyperactivity and antisocial behaviour in a large sample of 9-year-old children from the general population. *Journal of Consulting and Clinical Psychology,* **53**, 480–90.

McGee, R.M., Williams, S., Share, D.L., Anderson, J. & Silva, P.A. (1986). The relationship between specific reading retardation, general reading backwardness, and behavioural problems in a large sample of Dunedin boys: a longitudinal study from five to eleven years. *Journal of Child Psychology and Psychiatry,* **27**, 597–610.

McGee, R.M., Feehan, M., Williams, S., Partridge, F., Silva, P.A. & Kelly, J. (1990). DSM-III disorders in a large sample of adolescents. *Journal of the American Academy of Child and Adolescent Psychiatry,* **29**, 611–19.

McGee, R.M. Partridge, F., Williams, S. & Silva, P.A. (1991). A twelve-year follow-up of preschool hyperactive children. *Journal of the American Academy of Child and Adolescent Psychiatry,* **30**, 224–32.

Nichols, P.L. & Chen, T.C. (1981). *Minimal Brain Dysfunction: A Prospective Study.* Hillsdale: NY, Erlbaum.

Pelham, W.E.J., Gnagy, E.M., Greenslade, K.E. & Milich, R. (1992). Teacher ratings of DSM-III-R symptoms for the disruptive behavior disorders. *Journal of the American Academy of Child Adolescent Psychiatry,* **31**, 210–18.

Rahim, S.I.A. & Cederblad, M. (1984). Effects of rapid urbanisation on child behaviour and health in a part of Khartoum, Sudan. *Journal of Child Psychology and Psychiatry,* **25**, 629–41.

Richman, N., Stevenson, J.E. & Graham, P.J. (1975). Prevalence of behaviour problems in 3-year-old children: an epidemiological study in a London borough. *Journal of Child Psychology and Psychiatry,* **16**, 277–87.

Richman, N., Stevenson, J.E. & Graham, P.J. (1982). *Preschool to School: A Behavioural Study*. London: Academic Press.

Rowe, K.J. & Rowe, K.S. (1992a). The relationship between inattentiveness in the classroom and reading achievement (Part A): methodological issues. *Journal of the American Academy of Child and Adolescent Psychiatry,* **31**, 349–56.

Rowe, K.J. & Rowe, K.S. (1992b). The relationship between inattentiveness in the classroom and reading achievement (Part B): an explanatory study. *Journal of the American Academy of Child and Adolescent Psychiatry,* **31**, 357–68.

Rutter, M. (1976). Isle of Wight studies, 1964–74. *Psychological Medicine,* **6**, 313–32.

Rutter, M. (1988). Epidemiological approaches to developmental psychopathology. *Archives of General Psychiatry,* **45**, 486–95.

Rutter, M. (1989*a*). Isle of Wight revisited: twenty-five years of child psychiatric epidemiology. *Journal of the American Academy of Child and Adolescent Psychiatry,* **28**, 633–53.

Rutter, M. (1989*b*). Attention deficit disorder/hyperkinetic syndrome: conceptual and research issues regarding diagnosis and classification. In *Attention Deficit Disorder. Clinical and Basic Research,* eds. T. Sagvolden & T. Archer, pp. 1–24. Hillsdale New Jersey: Lawrence Erlbaum.

Rutter, M., Tizard, J. & Whitmore, K. (1970). *Education, Health and Behaviour*. London: Longmans.

Sandberg, S.T., Wieselberg, M. & Shaffer, D. (1980). Hyperkinetic and conduct problem children in a primary school population: some epidemiological considerations. *Journal of Child Psychology Psychiatry*, **21**, 293–311.

Satin, M.S., Winsberg, B.G., Monetti, C.H., Sverd, J. & Foss, D.A. (1985). A general population screen for attention deficit disorder with hyperactivity. *Journal of the American Academy of Child Psychiatry*, **24**, 756–64.

Schachar, R., Rutter, M. & Smith, A. (1981). The characteristics of situationally and pervasively hyperactive children: implications for syndrome definition. *Journal of Child Psychology and Psychiatry,* **22**, 373–92.

Schleifer, M., Weiss, G., Cohen, N., Elman, M., Cvejic, H. & Kruger, E. (1975). Hyperactivity in preschoolers and the effect of methylphenidate. *American Journal of Orthopsychiatry,* **45**, 38–50.

Schmidt, M.H., Esser, G. Allehoff, W., Geisel, B., Laught, M. & Woerner, W. (1987). Evaluating the significance of minimal brain dysfunction – results of an epidemiological study. *Journal of Child Psychology and Psychiatry,* **25**, 803–21.

Semrud-Clikeman, M., Biederman, J., Sprich-Buckminster, S., Lehman, B.K., Faraone, S.V. & Norman, D. (1992). Co-morbidity between ADDH and learning disability: a review and report in a clinically referred sample. *Journal of the American Academy of Child and Adolescent Psychiatry,* **31**, 439–48.

Shapiro, S.K. & Garfinkel, B.D. (1986). The occurrence of behaviour disorder in children: the interdependence of attention deficit disorder and conduct disorder. *Journal of the American Academy of Child and Adolescent Psychiatry*, **25**, 809–19.

Shekim, W.P., Kashani, J., Beck, N., Cantwell, D., Martin, J., Rosenberg, J. & Costello, A. (1985). The prevalence of attention deficit disorders in a rural midwestern community sample of nine-year-old children. *Journal of the American Academy of Child Psychiatry,* **24**, 765–770.

Shen, Y-C., Wang, Y-F. & Yang, X-L. (1985). An epidemiological investigation of minimal brain dysfunction in six elementary schools in Beijing. *Journal of Child Psychology and Psychiatry,* **26**, 777–87.

Szatmari, P., Offord, D.R. & Boyle, M.H. (1989*a*). Ontario Child Health Study: prevalence of attention deficit disorder with hyperactivity. *Journal of Child Psychology and Psychiatry,* **30**, 219–30.

Szatmari, P., Offord, D.R. & Boyle, M.H. (1989*b*). Correlates, associated impairments and patterns of service utilization of children with attention deficit disorder: findings from the Ontario Child Health Study. *Journal of Child Psychology and Psychiatry,* **30**, 205–17.

Szatmari, P., Boyle, M.H. & Offord, D.R. (1989*c*). ADDH and conduct disorder: degree of diagnostic overlap and differences among correlates. *Journal of the American Academy of Child and Adolescent Psychiatry,* **28**, 865–72.

Szatmari, P., Offord, D.R., Siegel, L.S., Finlayson, M.A.J. & Tuff, L. (1990). The clinical significance of neurocognitive impairments among children with psychiatric disorders: diagnosis and situational specificity. *Journal of Child Psychology and Psychiatry,* **31**, 287–99.

Taylor, E. (1986). Overactivity, hyperactivity and hyperkinesis: problems and prevalence. In *The Overactive Child,* ed. E. Taylor, pp. 1–18, Oxford: Blackwell Scientific Publications.

Taylor, E. & Sandberg, S. (1984). Hyperactive behaviour in English school children: a questionnaire survey. *Journal of Abnormal Child Psychology,* **12**, 143–56.

Taylor, E., Schachar, R., Thorley, G., Wieselberg, M. (1986*a*). Conduct disorder and hyperactivity I: separation and hyperactivity of antisocial conduct in British child psychiatric patients. *British Journal of Psychiatry,* **149**, 760–7.

Taylor, E., Everitt, B., Thorley, G., Schachar, R., Rutter, M. & Wieselberg, M. (1986b). Conduct disorder and hyperactivity: II. A cluster analytic approach to the identification of a behavioural syndrome. *British Journal of Psychiatry,* **149**, 768–77.

Taylor, E., Schachar, R., Thorley, G., Wieselberg, M., Everitt, B. & Rutter, M. (1987). Which boys respond to stimulant medication? A controlled trial of Methylphenidate in boys with disruptive behaviour. *Psychology Medicine,* **17**, 121–43.

Taylor, E., Sandberg, S., Thorley, G. & Giles, S. (1991). *The Epidemiology of Childhood Hyperactivity. Institute of Psychiatric Maudsley Monograph.* London: Oxford University Press.

Trites, R.L. & Laprade, K. (1983). Evidence for an independent syndrome of hyperactivity. *Journal of Child Psychology and Psychiatry,* **24**, 573–86.

Velez, N., Johnson, J. & Cohen, P. (1989). A longitudinal analysis of selected risk factors for childhood psychopathology. *Journal of American Academy of Child and Adolescent Psychiatry,* **28**, 861–4.

Verhulst, F., Berden, G.F.M.G. & Sanders-Woudstra, J.A.R. (1985). Mental health in Dutch children: II. The prevalence of psychiatric disorder and relationship between measures. *Acta Psychiatrica Scandinavica,* **72** *(suppl. 342).*

Verhulst, F.C. & Koot, H.M. (1992). *Child Psychiatric Epidemiology. Concepts, Methods and Findings*. Newbury Park: Casage Publications.

Vikan, A. (1985). Psychiatric epidemiology in a sample of 1510 ten-year-old children: I. Prevalence. *Journal of Child Psychology and Psychiatry*, **26**, 55–75.

Wang Yu-feng, Shen Yu-cum, Gu Bo-mei, Jia Mei-Xiang & Zhang Ai Lin (1989). An epidemiological study of behaviour problems in school children in urban areas of Beejing. *Journal of Child Psychology and Psychiatry* **30**, 907–12.

Whitaker, A., Johnson, J., Shaffer, D., Rapoport, J.L., Kalikow, K., Walsh, B.T., Davies, M., Braiman, S. & Dolinks, A. (1990). Uncommon trouble in young children: prevalence estimates of selected psychiatric disorders in a nonreferred adolescent population. *Archives of General Psychiatry* **47**, 487–96.

World Health Organization (WHO). (1978). *International Classification of Diseases*, 9th edn. Geneva: WHO.

World Health Organization (WHO). (1988). *International Classification of Diseases*, 10th edn. Draft of Chapter V. Categories F00–F99. Mental, behavioural and developmental disorders. Geneva: WHO.

3

Clinical aspects

Seija Sandberg, Ruth Day and Gotz Eric Trott

INTRODUCTION

Children hardly ever refer themselves for psychiatric help. Instead, this usually happens because someone else is troubled by their behaviour, or concerned about their unhappiness. Behaviour that persistently transgresses accepted limits is the commonest single reason for a referral to child mental health service: the children may be aggressive to others, or destructive of property, or break the rules of society. This should not be taken to suggest that every disruptive child is suffering from an illness; the vast majority of defiant and unruly children never find their way to medical services, nor would the services have the capacity to treat them. For some children, however, rule breaking is part of personal maladjustment. They show definite problems in personal development: they may be persistently miserable, or have no close friends, or are unable to learn.

Disorders characterised by hyperactive behaviour are important because they are common and often disabling. Their validity is supported by the consistent appearance of hyperactivity as a component in factor analytical studies of behaviour rating scales, common patterns in their natural history, and similarities of outcome. Hyperactive disorders are of particular interest because of the long-held belief that they form a biologically determined group. This idea has persisted ever since Still's (1902) descriptions of 'defects of moral control'. It has never been confirmed or disproved. Reviews have generally concluded that no biological cause has been found, except in a very few instances of structural damage to the brain. This conclusion has always been qualified by the inadequacy of the evidence and the unsatisfactory nature of the diagnostic definitions. There also continues to exist some doubt regarding the discriminative validity between hyperactivity and other disorders of disruptive conduct (see also Chapter 6 in this volume).

The nature of the supposed deficit in hyperactivity is still unknown. Correspondingly, there are wide differences between individual clinicians regarding the definition of hyperactivity disorder and the frequency with which the diagnosis is applied. The detailed comparison of diagnostic approaches to the same case histories by UK and US clinicians by Prendergast *et al.* (1988), succinctly demonstrated some important systematic differences: the US diagnosticians applied the label much more widely than their colleagues from the UK. However, even without resorting to international or cross-Atlantic comparisons, similar phenomena are easy to find: In any given centre of child psychiatry, or behavioural neurology, it is easy to observe that the diagnosis is used much more frequently by clinicians who believe that biologically rooted deficits often contribute to children's disruptive behaviour, and by those who generally more often use pharmacological treatments. Such differences in theoretical orientation to patient care are responsible for much unnecessary confusion in the communications between clinicians.

Many UK clinicians see little reason to use the concept of hyperactivity. As they prefer not to use the stimulant drugs anyway, they see no pressing therapeutic reason for making the diagnosis. If questioned, they would point to the lack of demonstrated aetiological or prognostic homogeneity in children with hyperactivity disorder. They do, of course, see children who behave in restless and impulsive ways, but classify them as showing 'conduct disorder'. By contrast, some US clinicians interpret the definitions of the American Psychiatric Association's Diagnostic and Statistical Manual (1980, 1987), in such a way that 'conduct disorder' refers primarily to delinquency, and 'hyperactivity' refers to the impulsively antisocial acts that make up most of the disruptive behaviour of children. The result is that hyperactivity is the commonest psychiatric diagnosis of childhood, and stimulants are the commonest treatment. Some European clinicians reject hyperactivity, but prefer to diagnose 'minimal brain dysfunction' (MBD), for which hyperactive behaviour is one piece of evidence, among many others.

These differences in clinical practice between different countries have led to common and heterogeneous groups of children; differently named, but overlapping greatly. Nevertheless, the boundaries are differently defined. When we add to this the likely differences between individual centres in their referral patterns, and the possible differences between cultures in what adults see as problems in children, it is not surprising that each clinical tradition tends to go its own way. Neither is it too surprising if scientific observers, when confronted with a welter of over-inclusive and incommensurable definitions, conclude that the whole area is best ignored. This cynicism is understandable, but just as unhelpful as the approaches based on untested theories.

Based on the evidence largely from a series of their own studies Taylor (1986*a*, *b*), and Sandberg (1986) concluded that much of hyperactive behaviour, at least as rated by adults, is situationally specific but aetiologically non-specific. Furthermore, the results have clearly pointed towards lack of usefulness of a traditional medical model of common hyperactivity, while at the same time supporting the validity of a much more restricted and limited concept of hyperkinetic disorder.

The concept of hyperkinetic disorder has been primarily based upon clinical research. Its characteristics and associations in several studies include: pervasiveness and severity of hyperactivity; a lowered IQ, and, after allowing for that, a poor performance on psychological tests of attention; motor clumsiness; a high frequency of language impairment and other forms of developmental delay; an early onset, nearly always in the years before entry to school; accident proneness and poor relationships with peers; a substantial response to stimulant medication; and an adverse outcome in terms of psychosocial adjustment during adolescence. Associations with social class and adversities of family life have been less clear.

In the attempt to arrive at unified criteria of how to define a clinically valid concept of hyperkinetic disorder, rules of what aspects to include and what to exclude have been developed. These have then been applied in epidemiological studies where samples of subjects are at least free of the distortions created by unknown referral biases. The common approach to defining clinically relevant groups has been through using a two-stage approach, with a large number of unselected children being assessed by behaviour questionnaires, usually completed by parents and teachers. Children scoring above the cut-off on the pre-determined scales of hyperactivity, behaviour problems, anxiety, etc., have then been examined in depth by using standardised methods resembling clinical assessments.

In spite of careful assessment procedures, prevalence rates for a clinically relevant diagnostic entity of hyperkinetic disorder have varied from 0.1% on the Isle of Wight (Rutter, Tizard & Whitmore, 1970), to 0.4% in rural Norway (Vikan, 1985), and to 5.7% in Beijing (Shen, Wang & Yang, 1985). Two issues are notable regarding the results obtained by ostensibly similar research designs. First, there is a surprising level of agreement between the studies, based on widely differing societies, regarding proportions of children scoring high on the hyperactivity dimensions of the parent and teacher questionnaires. Therefore, the primary reason for the different prevalence figures does not lie in the adults in one society attributing more of the children's behaviour to hyperactivity than in another. Secondly, it is to be noted that the clinical diagnostic criteria were based on different diagnostic schemes: hyperkinetic syndrome as defined by the ICD-9 in the UK and Norwegian studies, and ADDH as defined by the DSM-III in the Chinese study. In this context it is worth noting a Swedish study by Gillberg, Carlström & Rasmussen (1983), even though it was directed at minimal brain dysfunction (MBD) rather than hyperactivity. A questionnaire screen for motor and perceptual impairments was followed by a detailed assessment of selected groups using multiple measures and explicit cut-offs. The tentative point-prevalence rate for hyperkinetic syndrome (30 per 1000) was the same as that suggested for ADDH in the DSM-III Diagnostic Manual (American Psychiatric Association, 1980). (For a fuller discussion of epidemiological evidence, see Chapter 2.)

DIAGNOSTIC CONCEPT OF HYPERKINETIC DISORDER

Defining a case

As clearly illustrated in the epidemiological study by Taylor *et al.* (1991), there are many levels of a definition of hyperactivity disorder, with the figures of prevalence varying accordingly: the dimension of behaviour such as pervasive hyperactivity (as rated present by both parent and teacher on a questionnaire) applied to about 9% of boys in the population; DSM-III diagnosis of ADDH (based largely on teacher assessments of behaviour) was applicable to about 17%; however, only about 1.7% qualified for the ICD-9 diagnosis of hyperkinetic syndrome. The problem of case definition is not just confined to epidemiological research; the same issues and dilemmas are met in everyday clinical work dealing with diagnosis and treatment.

There are many reasons underlying the difficulties in defining the concept of hyperkinetic disorder: First, the behaviours that are supposed to characterise the disorder: inattention, overactivity and impulsiveness, can have different meanings to different people. Thus, 'over-activity' as a rating may refer to an excess of motor movements, or to a qualitative change in the pattern of activity, for example. Likewise, inattentiveness may mean 'difficulty concentrating', 'not listening' or 'day-dreaming'. 'Impulsiveness' poses a particular problem because it may mean over-rapid tempo (which is obviously similar to over-activity), or an over-dependence on immediate gratification (which is a theory about cause), or an acting-out of antisocial impulses (which is part of conduct disorder).

Secondly, overactivity and inattentiveness can each have many causes: Overactivity is a feature of anxious, fidgety children; of children who are depressed and agitated; of mania; of autism; and is seen in some children whose development is otherwise normal. Children can also be referred to clinics with the complaint of over-activity, but turn out to suffer from conditions widely other than hyperkinetic disorder. Such alternative, albeit rare, diagnoses include obsessional neurosis, Tourette's syndrome, Sydenham's chorea, schizophrenia, ataxic cerebral palsy, and disintegrative psychosis. 'Inattentive behaviour' is a non-specific complaint about most children with psychiatric disorder of any type.

A third difficulty for case definition is that there are no clear dividing lines between normal and abnormal levels of activity and attention. The range of 'normal variation' is very wide; though even this remark begs the question of the sources of that variation and its acceptable limits. The problem is substantial, though, of course, it is not confined to hyperactivity. Many important biological variables, such as blood pressure, are distributed continuously in the population and arbitrary levels of case definition have been required in the early stages of their study. Ultimately, the answer will depend upon determining the level at which there is significant impairment.

Fourthly, a difficulty, linked to that above, concerns problems in determining the number of dimensions to be used. Quay (1979), for example, has taken a leading part in arguing that a dimension of 'inattentiveness–immaturity' should be given primary importance rather than the one of overactivity. An added complexity is that of hyperactive behaviour frequently being specific to a single situation, such as school (Sandberg, 1986). Up to now it has not been clear to what extent this is due to an error in ratings, or how far children are actually behaving differently in different situations. It is possible that hyperactivity as seen at home is a different dimension from that seen in school (Goodman & Stevenson, 1989*a*, *b*).

In order to overcome the problems presented by the issue of 'situation specificity' of hyperactivity, many researchers and clinicians have found it useful to consider pervasiveness of hyperactivity across situations, and its persistence over time, as the necessary explicit criteria for a 'case'. The reasons for this practice are that pervasiveness and persistence are both indicators that a significant quality of the child's behaviour is being measured.

Fifthly, there is the issue of age and gender effects upon motor activity and attention. Boys are far more often identified as hyperactive than girls; so are younger children as compared with children approaching teenage years. Should we therefore apply different case definition criteria for boys and girls, and for pre-school age children and young teenagers, for example?

And finally, the ambiguity created by mixed symptom pictures and the overlapping of conditions needs to be faced. A traditional approach to clinical case definition, based on a categorical ordering of symptoms, faces many dilemmas when dealing with hyperactivity. However, given that symptoms of hyperactivity are commonly measured as scores or dimensions of behaviour, it is not necessary for categorical ordering to involve all-or-none dichotomisation into the 'presence' or 'absence' of a disorder. It may be more realistic to conceive of the degree to which a case fits into a category. A diagnosis can also be conceived of as a prototype, so that it is possible to quantify the number of features in common between a case and a prototype of the condition (e.g. Horowitz *et al.*, 1981).

There is now reasonably good evidence from four British studies (two clinical and two epidemiological), to suggest that a combination of pervasive hyperactivity (present in more than one situation, and noted by more than one observer), with onset before the age of 6 years, accompanied by lower IQ, more neurodevelopmental abnormalities, high frequency of early language impairment or other forms of developmental delay, accident prone behaviour and markedly poor peer relationships does form a distinct disorder (Sandberg, Rutter & Taylor, 1978; Schachar, Rutter & Smith, 1981; Taylor *et al.*, 1986*b*; Taylor *et al.*, 1991). Furthermore, these are also the characteristics that predict a beneficial response to stimulant medication, with pervasiveness and early onset of hyperactivity being the most significant ones.

The above constellation of symptoms helps us to decide on whether or not a child is likely to suffer from a clinically significant disorder, and also point a way towards choosing an appropriate treatment with some knowledge of the likely short-term prognosis. As responsible clinicians we should also be concerning ourselves with the issue of minimising any long-term handicaps that the disorders we treat are prone to give rise to. In the case of childhood hyperactivity, the most likely negative long-term consequences involve poor scholastic performance and behavioural disturbance involving aggression and delinquency. Furthermore, this prediction is much strengthened by the combination of hyperactivity and aggressive conduct disorder in the first place (Loeber, 1990; Magnusson, 1987; McGee, Williams & Silva, 1984*a*, *b*; Offord *et al.*, 1979). The importance of early onset hyperactivity as a predictor of psychiatric disorder during school years was also highlighted by the findings of a longitudinal study from age 3 to 8 years undertaken by Richman, Stevenson & Graham (1982). Thus, it is reasonable to conclude that the combination of hyperactivity and inattention, with an early onset, is predictive of continuing psychiatric problems; and also, that it is the combination of these features with aggressiveness that is most strongly predictive.

Behavioural components

The essential task of a clinical assessment is to establish whether or not there is adequate evidence of a 'behavioural syndrome' of hyperactivity. This can be defined by the presence of overactivity and attentional problems, without reference to any particular aetiological hypothesis. This procedure, however, though at the outset appearing fairly straightforward, has to be carried out in the context of a number of ambiguities of definitions and measurement. The main ones of these involve the heterogeneity of behaviours that are supposed to characterise the syndrome: criteria for what constitutes abnormal overactive/inattentive behaviours, and the very definition of poor attention.

Overactivity

Regarding heterogeneity and differences of the key behaviours, the question how to define and measure overactivity is a pertinent one. Apart from being a part of hyperactivity disorder, excessive motor overactivity may be observed as restlessness in anxiety, as psychomotor agitation in depression, as excessive energy and talkativeness of mania, and in the hyperkinesis of autism. The overactive behaviour also varies with age; restlessness, common in hyperactive school-age children, tends to decrease by early adolescence. Likewise, it is normal for toddlers to be a lot more active than children of school age. This means that a child's age needs to be taken into account when judging what is an abnormally high level of motor activity. A further problem is that there is no clear dividing line between normal and abnormal activity levels. Individual children vary greatly with regard to their usual level of activity, and it is because of this that activity level is generally accepted as one of the main features of normal temperamental variation in childhood (Buss & Plomin, 1975). Another aspect of motor activity in children is its tendency to fluctuate from one situation to the next. Thus, it is normal for children to run around on the school playground but sit quietly in church, or when watching their favourite television programme, for example. Rather than the absolute amount of motor activity, it is the inappropriateness of it in relation to the context and the demands of the social situation that matters.

In spite of these ambiguities of definition and measurement, all major diagnostic categorisations used at present agree that excessive locomotor activity is part of hyperkinetic disorder. Direct observations and mechanical recordings of activity have demonstrated that children who are rated as hyperactive by parent and teacher questionnaires, for example, do make more movements than others (Taylor *et al.*, 1991). Such excess of locomotor activity applies across situations from set tasks in the classroom to those allowing children a choice of activity; from meal times at home to quiet play and watching television as well as to playing with other children (as established by detailed interviews of teachers and parents). Children rated as hyperactive have also been found to make more movements during their sleep as shown by prolonged recordings of activity (Porrino *et al.*, 1983). The demonstration that high level of activity in a hyperactive child is not confided to only inattentive off-task activity has helped the shift from 'Attention Deficit Disorder' in DSM-III to 'Attention Deficit Hyperactivity Disorder' in DSM-III-R.

Inattention

Similar and different aspects of inattention, compared to those regarding overactivity, pose problems in its use as a diagnostic feature: as with overactivity, inattention is a very common expression of psychiatric disturbance in childhood. For example, poor concentration is reported by parents and teachers as being present in the majority of children with a psychiatric disorder of any kind (e.g. Richman *et al.*, 1982; Rutter *et al.*, 1970; Shaffer, 1980). Thus, poor attention in itself is not a useful characteristic pointing to a specific diagnosis.

There is also a major difficulty of how to infer attention from what can be observed of the child's behaviour. Indeed, children may display 'inattentiveness' for numerous different reasons. These include boredom, daydreaming, preoccupation with worries, or finding their tasks too difficult. Just observing the child's behaviour would also make it difficult to decide whether, for example, a child who is looking out of the classroom window is watching what is going on outside, or in fact working out in his head how to write the next line of his essay. Likewise, it is quite impossible to know if a child who is staring at the book in front of him is processing what he is reading, or not reading at all, but thinking of what he is going to do when he gets out of school.

Direct observations, however detailed, all share the same limitation of how to infer inattention from the outward behaviour if the result of the attentional behaviour is not known. This problem can be largely overcome by the use of psychological tests of attention. However, they in turn are open to other limitations: For example, a poor performance on any given test may mean that the child was unable to perform well, or it may simply mean that he was not trying. (This problem is not unique for attention tests, it can just as well occur with other psychometric or reading tests. However, with the assessments of attention there is the additional issue of the tests mostly involving tedious and seemingly meaningless tasks.)

Another difficulty in interpreting the results of psychometric attention tests is to distinguish between behaviours involved in paying attention to the task and the processing of the incoming information by the brain. The central processing in turn involves a variety of separate activities (Douglas, 1983; Taylor, 1986*a*, *b*). Thus, when assessing the various functions, it is necessary to employ different tasks. For example, 'selective attention' is measured by assessing the child's ability to focus on some stimuli while excluding others. 'Sustained attention' is measured in terms of the ability to maintain attention in spite of boredom, frustration or distraction. There are also tasks for which it may be necessary to divide one's attention in order to integrate different sources of information, while other tasks require efficient exploration of the environment and systematic sampling of stimuli.

The evidence that children rated as hyperactive show inattentive behaviour in many situations is not in dispute. Their inattentiveness is present in the activities they choose at home as well as in tasks set by teacher at school. It can also be objectively recorded by an outside observer (Schachar, Sandberg & Rutter, 1986; Taylor *et al*., 1991). By 'inattentiveness of behaviour' here is meant lack of persistence in activities ('short attention span'), a great deal of off-task behaviour, frequent changes in activity, and orienting to task-irrelevant aspects of the environment ('distractibility').

The above description of inattentive behaviour does, however, need to be qualified with some reservations. Mere 'inattentiveness' is not a sufficient term; there are many ways of being inattentive in behaviour. The Taylor *et al.* (1991) study identified at least three separate types of behavioural inattentiveness: the hyperactive pattern of pervasive restlessness and distractibility; the rather inert and apathetic picture seen in the 'pure inattentiveness' as identified by teachers; and the distractibility of some anxious and unhappy children. The findings clearly indicate that the types are too different to be all grouped together and considered under the single umbrella term of attention deficit. It is also possible that the different types of inattentiveness may turn out to require separate kinds of remedial action.

A further issue regarding inattentiveness is that, apart from the term used as a behavioural description, it has other meanings: the word can also be used to refer to a score on a psychological test such as Continuous Performance Test, for example; or to an inferred psychological process. The various concepts of inattention, as well as the means of quantifying them, and the significance of scores obtained by different tests, are discussed in depth in Chapter 4 of this volume.

In the first place, the points requiring to be dealt with in the present context are those that are of immediate relevance for the clinical assessment of hyperactivity. These involve being familiar with the individual tests of attention and the corresponding terminology referring to different aspects of attention concept. In brief, these are: the test of 'central vs. incidental learning' aimed to assess the child's ability for selective attention (Hagen & Hale, 1973), and the test of 'sustained attention' (Erlenmeyer-Kimling & Cornblatt, 1978). There is indeed considerable evidence to suggest that central learning is impaired in hyperkinetic disorder (Taylor *et al.*, 1991). The conventional suggestion has been that in hyperactive children central learning, i.e. the ability to learn the relevant material is hampered, but learning of the irrelevant material, i.e. 'incidental learning' is correspondingly better, on the supposition that the children show an ineffective deployment of their cognitive resources. This conclusion, however, has not been supported by systematic studies (Douglas, 1988). Of the few different tests designed to assess the child's ability to sustain attention, the 'continuous performance test' (CPT) (Erlenmeyer-Kimling & Cornblatt, 1978), is perhaps the best known one. On this test, number of scores, all referring to different aspects of attention, can be computed on the basis of the child's performance. These concern the ratio of correct responses vs. total number of responses, latency time before responding, duration of maximum attention, etc. The results obtained in different studies regarding the importance of sustained attention as a key deficit in hyperactivity disorder have been contradictory: hyperactive children make more errors than other children with even comparable levels of overall psychiatric disturbance (Taylor *et al.*, 1991; Werry, Reeves & Elkind, 1987), but none of the deficits shown has proved to be a function of the test length. This means that the ability to maintain test performance over time is not the crucial process limiting the achievement of hyperactive children.

Impulsiveness

Impulsiveness is one of three key characteristics of the DSM-IV diagnostic definition of ADHD (with increased motor activity and inattention being the other two). For a number of reasons, however, it has not been included as part of the ICD-10 definition of 'hyperkinetic disorder'. One of these, is that the term 'impulsiveness' means different things to different people; this makes using it in behaviour questionnaires particularly problematic. And, even more important are the reasons relating to the fact that at present there is little agreement among clinicians or researchers on what are the relevant and most significant aspects of impulsiveness, and how to recognise and measure them.

One of the most commonly used tests is that of 'matching familial figures'

(MFF) (Kagan *et al.*, 1964), and its revised version 'MFF-20' (Cairns & Cammock, 1978). Scores are obtained for the number of errors made and for the time taken before responding. Swift inaccurate responses can be interpreted as one form of 'impulsiveness'. Studies using the MFF or MFF-20 have, however, provided inconsistent findings. The inconsistency has particularly concerned the extent to which the speed and inaccuracy of responding actually go together. Studies by both Firestone & Martin (1979), and Sandberg *et al.* (1978) found that pervasively hyperactive children made more errors on the MFF than did controls with other types of disordered behaviour, but that in neither study did they take any less time with their answers than the controls did. Boys qualifying for the clinical diagnosis of 'hyperkinetic syndrome', in the Taylor *et al.* (1991) East London survey, were both faster and more inaccurate than the boys with the diagnosis of conduct disorder, or the normal controls.

Further evidence of the complexities inherent in examining impulsiveness comes from studies that have measured the reaction time during traditional psychological tests: children suffering from ADDH have been shown to be slower in responding when pacing of the test is controlled by the experimenter (Sykes, Douglas & Morgenstern, 1973), and during automated tests (Klorman *et al.*, 1988). Therefore it is by no means obvious that hyperactive children are simply speeded up; to the contrary, they may even take longer to process information.

Sergeant (1981, 1988*b*) examined the idea of impulsivity considered as 'inefficient information processing with fast, inaccurate control'. He found that children with ADDH can and do make fast, accurate responses on occasion. Indeed, when they respond slowly, they are more likely to be wrong than when they respond quickly. These results indicate that hyperactive children are not impulsive in their cognitive processing. Furthermore, the long latency times on the MFF are largely determined by the children's choice about how long to spend, not by their capacity to go quickly. A long latency is not always an index of the amount of effort spent: the time may be spent on fidgeting or amusing oneself as well as figuring out the right answer. This means that simply teaching children to slow down would not be a sufficient remedial action. But, if one wants to get the answer right first time, then the decision to take a long time over it is adaptive. In this sense, the children are regulating themselves inefficiently when they respond quickly and make mistakes.

The term 'inefficiently' is only valid if we use it to refer to getting the answer right first time. However, this may not be the primary aim of children. Indeed, provided they are allowed to go on guessing after an error they may well prefer that strategy; by quick, multiple guessing they might in fact hit the right answer as rapidly as by laborious thought. Perhaps 'hyperactive' approach in such situations is maintained because of its effectiveness in increasing the rate of gain of reward. Even if this is not the case 'impulsive' behaviour still cuts down the time spent in delay before action, and delay could be unpleasant for children who are hyperactive and prefer immediate gratification.

A clear distinction, however, needs to be drawn between behavioural manifestations of impulsivity and the cognitive processes that could be linked to them. Impulsive behaviour – badly timed, intrusive on others, and accident-prone certainly exists in children with behaviour problems, but it is just as common in non-hyperactive conduct disorder as it is in pervasive hyperactivity. On the other hand, hyperactive behaviour is specifically linked to an unregulated and often maladaptive style of approach during problem-solving tasks; a style that reflects children's decision-making rather than a deficiency in processing information. This is the important feature behind the statement that hyperactive children are impulsive.

DIAGNOSTIC CRITERIA FOR HYPERKINETIC DISORDER

Inattentive restlessness gives the definition of hyperactivity; but the recognition of a valid disorder needs more than simply the presence of some degree of hyperactivity. A recent epidemiological study carried out in East London (Taylor *et al.*, 1991), for example, demonstrated that the then contemporaneous DSM-III definition of ADDH was only a helpful starting point, but unusable as such in clinical practice. The main reasons for this were that, when its criteria were applied in general populations of children of primary school age, about one boy in six would qualify for the diagnosis. Furthermore, besides being very common, the diagnosis would not imply current social impairment or significant educational problems in a large majority of children so classified. At best, it would only serve as a serious risk factor for later development.

Hyperkinesis also needs to be distinguished from inattentiveness without hyperactivity (ADD). The two types of behavioural disturbance are so different that it would be very dubious to consider them as variants of one condition (Taylor *et al.*, 1991). The ADD group has a different pattern of symptoms and different neurodevelopmental and psychosocial correlates. When occurring on its own, ADD is associated with a lower IQ and delayed language development, but unlike hyperkinetic disorder, it is not associated with test scores indicating inattentiveness once IQ has been allowed for. Its association with low family socio-economic status is similar to that of children with mild intellectual retardation, and unlike that of hyperkinesis. In the Taylor *et al.* (1991) survey, a rating of 'poor housecraft', as noted on the children's early developmental records, could refer to impoverished early environment. All in all, the pattern of associations suggests that ADD and hyperkinetic disorder arise and develop independently from one another.

Other patterns of hyperactive behaviour still remain ambiguous in terms of their place in diagnostic classification procedures. A common one is that involving lesser degrees of hyperactivity, more than the non-hyperactive conduct disorder but less than hyperkinetic disorder. On present evidence, this fits better with the non-hyperactive conduct disorder. Another presentation is that of serious situation-specific hyperactivity (i.e. hyperactivity that occurs only at home, or only at school, for example). The suggestion from a recent twin study by Goodman & Stevenson (1989*a*, *b*), is that hyperactivity confined to the home may warrant a status of a disorder on its own.

The definition of 'hyperkinetic disorder' that emerged from the epidemiological survey by Taylor *et al.* (1991) is close to the ICD-10 definition (WHO, 1988, 1992), Barkley's (1982) criteria, and the criteria put forward by Sergeant (1988*a*,*b*). The diagnosis of hyperkinetic disorder requires the definite presence of abnormal levels of inattention and restlessness that are pervasive across situations and persistent over time, that can be demonstrated by direct observation, and that are not due to other disorders such as autism or affective disorders.

Impairment of attention is manifested by prematurely breaking off from tasks and leaving activities unfinished. The children change frequently from one activity to another, seemingly losing interest in one task because they become diverted to another (although laboratory studies do not generally show an unusual degree of sensory or perceptual distractibility). These deficits in persistence and attention should be diagnosed only if they are excessive for the child's age and IQ.

Overactivity implies excessive restlessness, especially in situations requiring relative calm. It may, depending upon the situation, involve the child running and jumping around, getting up from a seat when he or she was supposed to remain seated, excessive talkativeness and noisiness, or fidgeting and wriggling. The standard for judgement should be that the activity is excessive in the context of what is expected in the situation and by comparison with other children of the same age and IQ. This behavioural feature is most evident in structured, organised situations that require a high degree of behavioural self-control.

The associated features are not sufficient for the diagnosis or even necessary, but help to sustain it. Disinhibition in social relationships, recklessness in situations involving some danger, and impulsive flouting of social rules (as shown by intruding on or interrupting others' activities, prematurely answering questions before they have been completed, or difficulty in waiting turns) are all characterisitic of children with the disorder. Learning problems and motor clumsiness occur with undue frequency, and should be noted separately when present: they should not, however, be part of the actual diagnosis of hyperkinetic disorder.

Symptoms of conduct disorder are not exclusion criteria for the main diagnosis, but their presence or absence constitutes the basis for the main subdivision for the disorder.

All the following must be present for the ICD-10 diagnosis of hyperkinetic disorder (Taylor *et al.*, 1991; World Health Organisation, 1992):

1. **Demonstrable abnormality of attention and activity at home,** for the age and developmental level of the child, as evidenced by at least three of the following **attention problems:**

(a) short duration of spontaneous activities
(b) often leaving play activities unfinished
(c) over-frequent changes between activities
(d) undue lack of persistence at tasks set by adults
(e) unduly high distractibility during study, e.g. homework or reading assignment

and by at least two of the following **activity problems:**

(a) continuous motor restlessness (running, jumping, etc.)
(b) markedly excessive fidgeting and wriggling during spontaneous activities
(c) markedly excessive activity in situations expecting relative stillness (e.g. meal times, travel, visiting, church)
(d) difficulty in remaining seated when required

2. **Demonstrable abnormality of attention and activity at school or nursery** (if applicable), for the age and developmental level of the child, as evidenced by at least two of the following **attention problems:**

(a) undue lack of persistence at tasks
(b) unduly high distractibility, i.e. often orienting towards extrinsic stimuli
(c) over-frequent changes between activities when choice is allowed
(d) excessively short duration of play activities

and by at least two of the following **activity problems:**

(a) continuous and excessive motor restlessness (running, jumping, etc.) in situations allowing free activity
(b) markedly excessive fidgeting and wriggling in structured situations
(c) excessive levels of off-task activity during tasks
(d) unduly often out of seat when required to be sitting

3. **Directly observed abnormality of attention or activity.** This must be excessive for the child's age and developmental level. The evidence may be any of the following:

(a) direct observation of the criteria in 1 or 2 above, i.e. not solely the report of parent and/or teacher
(b) observation of abnormal levels of motor activity, or off-task behaviour, or lack of persistence in activities, in setting outside home or school (e.g. clinic or laboratory)

(c) significant impairment of performance on psychometric tests of attention

4. Does not meet criteria for pervasive developmental disorder, mania or depressive or anxiety disorder

5. Onset before the age of 6 years

6. Duration of at least 6 months

7. IQ above 50

Eventually, assessment instruments should develop to the point where it is possible to take a quantitative cut-off score on reliable, valid and standardised measures of hyperactive behaviour in the home and classroom, corresponding to the 95th percentile on both measures. Such criteria would then replace 1 and 2 above.

DIAGNOSTIC CRITERIA FOR HYPERACTIVITY ATTENTION DEFICIT DISORDER

The problems that were identified in the DSM-III scheme were partly resolved by the revision into DSM-III-R, and further so by the DSM-IV (American Psychiatric Association, 1987, 1994). Certainly DSM-IV makes it clear that hyperactivity (rather than attention deficit alone) is the core of the disorder. The key problems of the scheme in terms of identifying excessive numbers of children as disordered, because of the inclusion of some unremarkable types of behaviour as symptoms, and due to the lack of discriminative validity largely stemming from the emphasis on impulsivity, have continued to outlive the revisions. Furthermore, the rule of DSM-III to give preference to teachers' observations of behaviour has in DSM-IV been replaced by the need to demonstrate some impairment on the child's functioning at least in two settings, usually the home and school. This requirement goes some way, but only some way, towards the criterion of 'pervasiveness across situations', one of the key features of the ICD diagnosis.

Diagnostic features

The essential feature of attention-deficit/hyperactivity disorder is a persistent pattern of inattention and/or hyperactivity–impulsivity that is more frequent and severe than is typically observed in individuals at a comparable level of development (Criterion A). Some hyperactive–impulsive or inattentive symptoms that cause impairment must have been present before age 7 years, although many individuals are diagnosed after the symptoms have been present for a number of years (Criterion B). Some impairment from the symptoms must be present in at least two settings (e.g. at home and at school or work) (Criterion C). There must be clear evidence of interference with developmentally appropriate social, academic, or occupational functioning (Criterion D). The disturbance does not occur exclusively during the course of a pervasive developmental disorder, schizophrenia, or other psychotic disorder and is not better accounted for by another mental disorder (e.g. a mood disorder, anxiety disorder, dissociative disorder, or personality disorder) (Criterion E).

Diagnostic criteria

A. Either (1) or (2)

(1) six (or more) of the following symptoms of **inattention** have persisted for at least 6 months to a degree that is maladaptive and inconsistent with developmental level:

Inattention

(a) often fails to give close attention to details or makes careless mistakes in schoolwork, work or other activities
(b) often has difficulty sustaining attention in tasks or play activities
(c) often does not seem to listen when spoken to directly
(d) often does not follow through on instructions and fails to finish schoolwork, chores, or duties in the workplace (not due to oppositional behaviour or failure to understand instructions)
(e) often has difficulty organising tasks and activities
(f) often avoids, dislikes, or is reluctant to engage in tasks that require sustained mental effort (such as schoolwork or homework)
(g) often loses things necessary for tasks or activities (e.g. toys, school assignments, pencils, books, or tools)
(h) is often easily distracted by extraneous stimuli.
(i) is often forgetful in daily activities

(2) six (or more) of the following symptoms of **hyperactivity–impulsivity** have persisted for at least 6 months to a degree that is maladaptive and inconsistent with development level:

Hyperactivity

(a) often fidgets with hands or feet or squirms in seat
(b) often leaves seat in classroom or in other situations in which remaining seated is expected
(c) often runs about or climbs excessively in situations in which it is inappropriate (in adolescents or adults, may be limited to subjective feelings of restlessness)

(d) often has difficulty playing or engaging in leisure activites quietly
(e) is often 'on the go' or often acts as if 'driven by a motor'
(f) often talks excessively
Impulsivity
(g) often blurts out answers before questions have been completed
(h) often has difficulty awaiting turn
(i) often interrupts or intrudes on others (e.g. butts into conversations or games)

B. Some hyperactive–impulsive or inattentive symptoms that caused impairment were present before age 7 years.
C. Some impairment from the symptoms is present in two or more settings (e.g. at school (or work) and at home).
D. There must be clear evidence of clinically significant impairment in social, academic, or occupational functioning.
E. The symptoms do not occur exclusively during the course of a pervasive development disorder, schizophrenia, or other psychotic disorder and are not better accounted for by another mental disorder (e.g. mood disorder, anxiety disorder, dissociative disorder, or a personality disorder).

CORRELATES

Perinatal risk factors

Evidence from recent epidemiological studies suggests that factors in prenatal development, rather than injury during or after birth, are of most importance in the initiation of severe degrees of hyperactive behaviour. Thus, a large study by Nichols & Chen (1981) focusing on the later outcome of children with birth complications found that 'hyperkinetic impulsive' behaviour at the age of 7 years was only weakly predicted by complications of pregnancy and delivery. Instead, maternal smoking during pregnancy, low foetal heart rate during labour, and a small head circumference at birth were the strongest early risk factors. The results of the East London survey of 6- and 7- year-old school boys by Taylor *et al*. (1991) likewise showed that of the factors recorded in the children's obstetric histories, features considered by the present state of knowledge to be fairly minor, correlated significantly with presence of pervasively hyperactive behaviour early in the child's school career. These involved admission into a special care unit because of the baby's 'jitteriness', or delay in establishing respiration; or evidence of neonatal hypoxia in a baby of normal birth-weight and unremarkable delivery. It might therefore almost be argued that such features are more of an indication of a pre-existing constitutional abnormality than the cause of some brain damage to follow.

The role of organic brain dysfunction

It is well established that a relatively high rate of neurodevelopmental problems is associated with pervasive hyperactivity of an early onset (Sandberg *et al.*, 1978; Taylor *et al.*, 1986*a*, 1991). Whether this is due to some identifiable form of brain pathology remains an open question as assessing this still presents difficulty due to the lack of unambiguous indicators of organic brain dysfunction. We also know that the presence of pre- and perinatal complications in the child's history is not a satisfactory defining feature. This is because, in most cases, perinatal complications do not give rise to brain damage (Nichols & Chen, 1981; Stewart *et al.*, 1987).

The role of neurodevelopmental immaturities, the so-called 'neurological soft signs', as specific markers of organic brain pathology, remain uncertain (Shaffer *et al.*, 1983, 1985). As such, they cannot be taken as definite signs/indicators of organic brain damage, however slight, though sometimes this will be the case. The reverse is also true: substantial brain damage or disease can occur without this being evident in detectable abnormalities, major or minor, hard or soft signs, on the clinical neurological examination (Rutter, Chadwick & Schachar, 1983).

Added to this is the evidence that exists for important associations between child psychiatric disorder of any kind and neurodevelopmental abnormalities indicated by 'soft signs' (Shaffer *et al.*, 1983), or by developmental delays in functions such as language (Howlin & Rutter, 1987). It thus becomes clear that such neurodevelopmental associations are by no means confined to the specific diagnosis of hyperactivity disorder. Indeed, Shaffer *et al.* (1985) found that neurological soft signs were most strongly associated with anxiety disorders as evident in adolescent years. In conclusion, therefore, the for many, old-times favourite concept of minimal brain dysfunction syndrome or 'MBD' as a synonym for hyperactivity disorder is best forgotten and buried for good. The role of biologically determined processes in hyperactivity disorder is fully discussed in Chapter 7 of this volume.

Cognitive impairment

The link between hyperactivity disorder and cognitive impairment is strong. It is also specific in the sense that the same does not appear to hold for conduct disorder without hyperactivity. It is, however, not specific in the sense of referring to a deficit in a single test or a particular inferred process. On the contrary, the cognitive deficit in hyperactivity disorder implies a fairly generalised impairment of the very high level control processes of self-regulation and inhibition, rather than a failure in the elementary stage of perception, attention and motor response (Douglas, 1988). In keeping with this, the hyperkinetic children in the Taylor *et al.* (1991) study did poorly on several different tests, some measuring attention and some assessing different aspects of IQ.

A note of caution regarding specific learning problems is relevant here. Any excess of specific, rather than generalised, learning problems in groups of children suffering from hyperactivity disorder, is very likely to be a reflection of selective referral procedures: specialised research/clinical centres may well attract referrals of children with the combination of hyperactivity and specific learning problems, while the less tightly defined helping agencies would receive the disturbed children of lower overall cognitive ability and more widespread learning disabilities. Studies based on population rather than clinic-based samples have also found general rather than specific learning disabilities associated with hyperactivity (McGee *et al.*, 1986; Sergeant, 1988*b*; Szatmari, Offord & Boyle, 1989).

Family and other psychosocial associations

There are many psychosocial associations of hyperkinetic disorder as has been suggested by the work of Gillberg *et al.* (1983), and Schachar *et al.* (1981). The study by Taylor *et al.* (1991) was also able to identify some fairly specific patterns of maladaptive parent–child relationship as being associated both with presence of hyperkinetic disorder, and especially its persistence over time. The role of psychosocial factors, both in terms of maintaining existing hyperactive behaviour, as well as possibly contributing to the initial cause of it, has been more fully explored in Chapter 8 of this volume. Therefore, only a brief synopsis is given here as a way of summary of the likely mechanisms.

The interactions between child constitution and family environment may operate in a different way at different developmental stages. Taylor (1986*a*, *b*) has argued that a deprived and unstimulating atmosphere makes it harder for a young child to develop good attending skills, and is therefore a risk factor for inattentiveness. It does not necessarily lead to hyperactivity. For this to happen, the presence of relevant constitutional factors appears to be required as the main initiators. That this is the case, is suggested by the early onset of hyperactive behaviour, its links with neurodevelopmental delays, its heritability and susceptibility to pharmacological effects. However, the natural course of development would favour the decrease of hyperactive behaviour. When this does not happen, it is likely that the main perpetuating factors at work are the unhelpful reactions of other people, usually the child's family members. Hyperactivity tends to evoke hostile reactions in adults, contributing to ineffective coping style in parents, and to make the child unpopular among siblings and peers. The extent to which this happens is modulated by the presence of additional stresses, such as parental psychiatric disorder or marital discord, taxing the resources of the family. The resulting negative relationships contribute a main part of the risk predicting the likelihood of persisting problems in the child's personal and social adjustment and educational progress.

DEVELOPMENTAL ASPECTS OF SYMPTOM PRESENTATION

Infancy

Some mothers report that their child's hyperactivity was noticeable already during pregnancy; the baby's movements were particularly strong and intensive. Likewise, over a half of the children later diagnosed as hyperactive have been reported to show extreme restlessness during infancy (Rapoport *et al.*, 1979). Other problems at this age commonly include being easily aroused by external stimuli, being prone to colic and sleep problems, and reacting strongly to changes in feeding routine (Greenhill, 1985; Weiss & Hechtman, 1979). Hyperactive children have also been described as non-cuddly babies (Campbell, 1979). Fairly typical are also delays in speech acquisition and in toilet training (Schain & Royhard, 1975).

Pre-school age

The majority of hyperactive children exhibit considerable problems by the time they reach pre-school years, but only few are referred for expert help (Campell *et al.*, 1986). This is partly due to relatives and professionals (such as family doctors and health visitors) commonly attributing the hyperactive child's difficulties to shortcomings in the parents' skills of child-rearing. Hyperactivity at this age may be equated with a 'lively temperament' and 'normal boisterousness'. Due to their increased locomotor activity the children are exposed to a number of risks, especially as they do not seem to recognise danger, or learn from past experiences (Stewart & Olds, 1973). This makes them accident prone and liable to suffering from frequent minor injuries and accidental poisoning. Parents also frequently describe their young hyperactive child as requiring little sleep, and being prone to frequent temper tantrums whenever their wishes are thwarted (Prior, Leonard & Wood, 1983).

The hyperactive child's lack of consideration for the feelings of others is noticeable already during preschool years. This, in turn, leads to the child being avoided by his peers which conveys the early experience of social rejection. The hyperactive child is less often invited to play in other children's homes and may even be asked to leave his kindergarten or nursery school. Both the motor restlessness and interpersonal difficulties are more noticeable in structured situations as opposed to free play (Cohen & Minde, 1983; Conners, 1990; Schleifer *et al.*, 1975). The hyperactive pre-schooler's striking characteristics are his increased restlessness which has an obvious quality of aimlessness, and his inability/lack of will to follow instructions, as well as apparent lack of concern for the feelings of others. Furthermore, the symptoms of hyperactivity and conduct problems appear to be particularly intermingled in very young children; the parents of 3-year-olds complain most about discipline and peer problems (Jenkins, Bax & Hart, 1980).

School age

The peculiarities of the hyperactive child become especially evident in the school situation (Richman *et al.* 1982; Fischer *et al.*, 1984). While during the pre-school years hyperactivity may be viewed as a 'natural urge' for freedom and movement that others should make allowances for, in the school context it usually becomes disturbing enough as to call for professional help. The child's lack of concentration and inability to work in an organised fashion lead to impediments in memory and learning. It is particularly the learning of abstract constructs and the recognition of socially desirable behaviour patterns that are affected. Also, the ability to write is impeded by behavioural impulsiveness; all this adding to the sense of frustration and failure on the child. Hyperactive children require considerable practice in achieving reasonable handwriting skills, and it is particularly with joined-up writing where their difficulties in managing consistency of form become apparent (Trott, 1993).

Classroom situations, where the child is part of a larger group, but where independent work is usually required, often require the greatest effort from a hyperactive child (Whalen, Henker & Swanson, 1987). It is especially when not managing to keep up with the work that the child finds a temptation to channel his hyperactivity into the role of a class clown. At break times, however, one may observe that the hyperactive child is mostly alone, or at best on the fringe of a group. This is because the impetuous behaviour is often experienced as annoying by the other children who begin to avoid the child's company. It is therefore not surprising that the teachers do not necessarily see such children as needing medical or psychological help, but see them as naughty and lazy instead. To the hyperactive child, school becomes a place for constant failure, reprimand by teacher and rejection by fellow pupils.

It is not only the school situation that is problematic for a hyperactive child, many difficulties also need to be overcome in the context of the family. The child's restless and disruptive behaviour may make the parents more reluctant to engage in usual social contacts, such as extended family and friends, as they try to fend off criticism about their parenting abilities. This, in turn, contributes to the family's social isolation and can magnify the existing interpersonal tensions. In the child, the intensified parental supervision can lead to feeling infantilised and being further impaired in acquiring social skills needed to cope with peer pressures. There may also be harbouring rivalries with the sibling group who resent the extra attention the hyperactive child receives. The child's poor scholastic performance is likely to contribute further to feelings of disappointment in his parents which may in turn be conveyed to the child as excessive criticism. (For a full discussion on the problems of hyperactive children at school, see Chapter 11 in this volume.)

Adolescence

While the motoric overactivity and restlessness decrease with advancing age (Loney, Kramer & Milich, 1981), impulsiveness and inattentiveness remain (Weiss & Hechtman, 1986). Increasing academic demands during the adolescent years highlight the difficulties of the hyperactive child even further. Unsuccessfully resolved battles over homework contribute to further deterioration of the parent–child relationship (Greenhill, 1990), and the adolescent 'accumulates increasing evidence' of his poor self-worth. The outwardly restless and disruptive behaviour is sometimes largely an attempt to cover up the underlying feelings of worry and sadness, which may be completely misinterpreted by parents (Trott & Boehm, 1992). Antisocial behaviour is particularly common among teenagers whose earlier problems have included both hyperactivity and learning difficulties (Ackerman, Dykman & Peters, 1977; Lambert, Hartsough & Sassone, 1987). When antisocial behaviour also involves aggressiveness, the likelihood of the hyperactive youngster coming into conflict with the law is greatly accentuated (Gittelman *et al.*, 1985). In the few cases where the young person also ends up with psychiatric contact, the label of personality disorder may well be attached to him with several negative connotations for future outcome.

CLINICAL ASSESSMENT

After the rather theoretical considerations of hyperkinetic disorder, we shall now move to dealing with the more practical issues of clinical assessment and finish off with a summary of clinical management. We do this by first addressing how the doctor can determine whether a child has a significant hyperactivity, and in the latter part of the section focus on the assessment of a child who has pervasive innate hyperactivity (hyperkinetic disorder).

As hyperactivity is an expression of a complex interaction of social, psychological and biological factors, its management in order to be effective, must take into account the contribution of each one of these. The initial assessment therefore must tease out the relative importance of these factors in any one child. This is established through history, examination, observation and relevant reports. It is important to realise that parents and teachers may call a variety of children's behaviours hyperactivity. However, they can also misjudge the severity of any hyperactivity due to lack of knowledge of what is normal at a particular age.

Determining whether a child has clinically significant hyperactivity

History of the problem

An account of the child's behaviour from a parent or primary caretaker should elicit:

(i) What is it that the child does that is causing concern, and is this inappropriate for the age?
(ii) When and where does this behaviour occur?
(iii) From what age has it been noticeable?
(iv) How does the child play with other children?
(v) Is the child on any medication which might be causing hyperactivity?
(vi) Is there evidence of family disturbance or behavioural mismanagement to account for the child's behaviour?

What is the behaviour being described?

Typically parents will report a child who is always on the go, never sits still, is restless and fidgety, with poor concentration, an inability to follow through instructions, and who is easily distractible. More recent hypotheses suggest that the underlying deficit is one of poor inhibitory control. This is exemplified by impulsivity and dishibition, acting before thinking of the consequences. These features of the disorder often get the child into trouble. However, misdeeds or conduct disorder should be seen as distinct from hyperactivity. If they are the presenting complaint, the features of hyperactivity, distractibility and difficulty sustaining attention need to be elicited before a diagnosis of hyperkinetic disorder can be made, as opposed to, or in addition to, one of conduct or behaviour disorder.

Parents will list symptoms as above and it is often difficult to gauge the significance of these. It can be helpful to ask them to describe particular episodes of behaviour including the antecedents, the parental response, and the way the situation was resolved. Asking what the child concentrates best at, and for how long he does so, can also be illuminating. Poor concentration in the absence of restlessness and hyperactivity is insufficient for the diagnosis and may, for example, indicate anxiety or learning difficulties. A report of hyperactivity in a toddler is particularly difficult to interpret; on more detailed questioning it may be apparent that the parents are reporting the normal exploratory and testing behaviour of the 1–2 year old, and that their expectations of a child's ability to sit and play are unrealistic. In addition, mishandling may have led to tempers which are cited as further evidence of hyperactivity. Observation in the consulting room may reveal a child who plays perfectly normally, but as soon as he moves from his seat the parents respond with shouted reprimands leading to a temper tantrum. For a more comprehensive assessment, a systematic standardised interview such as PACS (the parental account of children's symptoms) (Taylor *et al.*, 1986*a*), is a valuable clinical tool as it provides detailed and reliable information about the child's behaviour at home.

When and where does the described behaviour happen?

Is the child active, distractible, impulsive in all situations, or only at home or alternatively at school? Does he behave 'fine' when he stays with Granny? Are there tasks or activities on which he concentrates well? The child who is hyperactive in all situations and does not attend well to any task is described as having a pervasive hyperactivity which is more likely to be an innate, biologically determined disorder or behavioural trait. The child who is hyperactive at school, but not at home (apart perhaps when schoolwork is brought out), is more likely to have learning difficulties, global or specific. These make it very difficult for him to engage in class work, hence the poor concentration. It is, however, important to ask the parents quite carefully about behaviour at home, as occasionally it becomes clear that the child has shown hyperactivity and distractibility at home but that these have been accepted as unremarkable. The demands that the classroom makes, bring his innate difficulties to light.

Hyperactivity described in the home, and not a problem in school, must make one seriously consider family disturbance and/or behavioural mismanagement, or alternatively the parent's inability to tolerate a normal activity level. A school report can be very helpful because sometimes the child is showing some features of the disorder in school. These may be tolerated by the teacher or controlled by the child, a feat which can only be sustained in the structured setting of school and not in the less structured home setting.

A child with a disposition to be active, distractible and impulsive, may behave much better in an environment which is positive and rewarding of good behaviours. This should be seen as the 'baseline state' – that which can be achieved with good management, and the state one would bear in mind when considering whether the addition of medication was justified.

From what age has the behaviour been noticeable?

What was the child's temperament like as a baby and toddler? Excessive activity level, low persistence of pursuing objects with which to play, strong intensity of response and demandingness are often reported as being present in the younger children. However, it is also clear that negative temperamental characteristics, are by themselves, weak predictors of later problems. Power of prediction is increased by combining knowledge of such child characteristics with the parental characteristics; for example, the existence of negative, critical and commanding styles of child management. This emphasises again the inter-play of innate and behavioural factors in creating significant problems. Some hyperactive school children will only have had mild difficulties reported pre-school. The increase in the severity of symptoms reflects the increased demands on concentration and sitting still that school imposes. If there really is a clearly described onset at age of 4 years or above, then it is important to enquire about any changes in home or school circumstances. An abrupt late onset is more likely to be environmentally induced than innate. Children with language or learning difficulties may show a deterioration in their behaviour and ability to concentrate as the schoolwork they are exposed to gets more demanding. This should be responded to by pitching educational demands at a level the child can cope with, rather than treating the hyperactivity.

How does the child play with other children?

Children with significant hyperactivity invariably find it difficult to play constructively with their peers. They are commonly described as not popular, being left out of games, going out to play for a short while and either returning home soon afterwards, or going off on their own. The child himself, especially when older, is usually painfully aware of and saddened by the fact that he has no friends. Reports that a child plays well with his peers makes the diagnosis of hyperkinetic disorder unlikely.

Medication

It is always important to check that the child is not on any medication which might be causing or worsening the hyperactivity. Phenobarbitone is notorious for this but is fortunately little used nowadays. Some other anti-convulsants can have a similar effect in particular children.

Family structure and functioning

If it seems that the child doesn't have an innate pervasive hyperactivity, but that what is being described is situation-specific hyperactivity or a behavioural disturbance, it is important to try to elicit evidence of family dysfunction, behavioural mismanagement or specific learning difficulties to account for this.

Observation of behaviour

Characteristically the hyperactive child moves around the consulting room, trying one activity after another, often at a speed. The younger child can be destructive in his activity but the older child may play constructively, albeit in a fleeting manner, replacing objects after use. The child may constantly interrupt the conversation between doctor and parent, sometimes asking questions or making comments which might be considered impertinent or socially inappropriate. When encouraged to sit and draw, the child may rush off a drawing and then be out of his seat, or if forced to stay, be fidgety and squirmy, fiddling with all available objects. It is hard to sustain the diagnosis of hyperkinetic disorder in a child who comes in and sits and draws for a long period of time without interrupting the doctor/parent conversation. It can be informative deliberately not to address the child after the first introductions in order to see just how long he can sustain his concentration. The parents often express amazement at how well the child has behaved. Sometimes, in such situations, the parents intervene in a negative or disparaging manner, rapidly leading to a clear deterioration in the child's willingness to co-operate, which often can be retrieved by the doctor adopting a more positive, encouraging tone, hence demonstrating that the problem is primarily one of parent/child interaction. Such dysfunctional pattern of interaction is in some cases the result of earlier active/impulsive child behaviour which has since resolved.

Another scenario witnessed in the consulting room is a child's behaviour suddenly deteriorating when faced with a particular task, for example, drawing, writing or reading. Concentration goes and the child becomes restless, negative, and even destructive. This should make one consider whether the child is unable to perform the particular task, and that the changed behaviour may be due to awareness of the difficulty. It is easy to say, 'didn't co-operate' and 'not testable'; however, it is much more likely that the difficulty of the task is leading to the deterioration of behaviour. This can be checked by attempting to regain the child's co-operation by giving a task the child definitely can do. This situation is commonly seen when testing hyperactive children with specific difficulties in writing, spelling or drawing. Again, 'the best state' that can be achieved by 'good behavioural management' should be considered as the 'baseline' when considering whether the use of medication is indicated.

Persistent hyperactivity in the consulting room has been shown to be related to a poorer performance in measures of general intelligence, attention, cognitive style, motor clumsiness and to predict favourable response to stimulant drugs (Luk, Thorley & Taylor, 1987).

Behaviour reports from other sources

A report of behaviour in other situations, particularly school, can be helpful. It can be very difficult for parents to convey just exactly what it is that teachers are concerned about, and a report direct from the teacher can be invaluable. Questionnaires, in particular the Conners Teacher questionnaire, have been shown to correlate highly with clinically relevant hyperactivity. However, they tend to result in over-reporting; perhaps in order to get help for a child whom teachers are worried about, or perhaps as the result of a misconception that defiant or aggressive children are by definition hyperactive. The value of questionnaires can be enhanced by asking for a description of particular episodes and a record of how often these episodes occur in a stated period of time. (These issues are systematically covered in a structured Teacher Interview (Sandberg, 1986), described in Taylor *et al.*, 1991.)

The procedure of clinical assessment

In carrying out the clinical assessment of a child in order to establish the possible diagnosis of hyperkinetic disorder, the main tasks to undertake are: physical examination, weighing up aetiological evidence, establishing developmental history, carrying out necessary investigations, establishing cognitive profile, checking for learning difficulties, looking for maintaining factors, and establishing the level of overall impairment.

Examination of the child: physical and neurological

The child's height and head circumference should be measured, and the child examined for any evidence of dysmorphic features suggestive of intra-uterine insult or specific syndromes, for example, foetal alcohol or Williams Syndrome. An excess of minor physical abnormalities has been reported in hyperactive children, but this is a non-specific sign and occurs in other developmental and psychiatric disorders. A formal neurological examination should be undertaken looking for hard neurological signs, which are rarely found, and for soft neurological signs, which reflect neurological immaturity and are commonly present. The significance of such soft signs is, however, non-specific and their main importance is to indicate the need for a detailed look at the child's motor skills. Hard neurological signs, such as ataxia, disordered eye movement, absent reflexes, significant asymmetry in tone and reflexes should lead to more sophisticated neurological examination and investigations.

Aetiological evidence

Current theories about the aetiology of pervasive hyperactivity suggest a biological pre-disposition which possibly has a genetic basis. The likelihood of this pre-disposition exhibiting itself is affected by the parents' capacity to constructively manage the child's emergent difficult temperament. In addition, it is thought that the pre-disposition may be enhanced by adverse factors during pregnancy and birth, such as smoking or alcohol consumption, intra-uterine growth retardation, perinatal asphyxia or pre-term delivery. Most children with pervasive hyperactivity do not have a history of significant adverse perinatal events. More formal studies have suggested that any slight increase in incidence of these events can be accounted for by the younger age and the socio-economic status of the mothers, both of which are independently pre-disposing factors to perinatal adversity and hyperactivity. A genetic pre-disposition to hyperactivity in the mothers may also contribute to the low socio-economic status and the age of child bearing.

Overall, it is considered that less than 5% of children with hyperactivity have evidence of brain damage. In clinical practice the commonest of these would be foetal alcohol syndrome and encephalitis. Very rarely neuro-degenerative disorders may present with a deterioration in the ability to concentrate and a fall off in rate of learning in the absence of hard neurological signs. San Filioppo-type of mucopolysaccharidosis can present in this way and can be diagnosed by urine analysis for mucopolysaccharides (Cleary & Wraith, 1993). If a child has associated learning difficulties, the aetiology of this will need to be sought, for example, Fragile X (Bregman, Leckman & Ort, 1988).

Developmental history

An account should be taken of the details of the pregnancy, labour, delivery and neonatal period, but this is largely to discount the significance of any reported event as the primary aetiology of the child's hyperactivity. The one exception would be heavy drinking, especially if the child showed physical features of the fetal alcohol syndrome. In the postnatal period, significant neurological illnesses such as meningitis or encephalitis or onset of troublesome seizure disorder can be of importance, especially if the symptoms date from this time. Head injuries are often found to post-date the onset of hyperactivity.

Enquiring as to whether other family members have, or had, a similar behaviour style may lead to a statement such as 'granny says that his father (uncle) was just like him when young'. This is, of course, very hard to interpret. Occasionally it is apparent that one or other parent still has an active, impulsive style of behaving. For example, one parent rang up the hospital asking for a further supply of methylphenidate on the day it ran out, and with insufficient money to complete the phone call!

Investigations

There are no laboratory or electrophysiological tests that help in diagnosis of hyperkinetic disorder. CT scans are invariably normal (Shaywitz *et al.*, 1983), and while EEG analysis has in some cases shown greater slow wave activity (Werry, 1979), this is not useful in making the diagnosis of an individual child. Investigations such as chromosome studies may be done if the child has learning difficulties, and neurological investigations may be neccssary if the child has hard signs. In the absence of those, pressure to do investigations should be resisted as equivocal results may be yielded which will result in confusion. For example, occasional spikes in the EEG is a finding in many normal children (Engel, Leuders & Chutorian, 1977), but can be difficult to explain away, or ignore, in a child with hyperactivity. Other aspects of history may make further investigations desirable in selected cases: there may have been exposure to a source of lead pollution which justifies carrying out lead estimates on samples of blood, and also an environmental samples such as dust. (For a fuller discussion on investigations for biological processes, please see Chapter 7 in this volume.)

Cognitive profile

Children with hyperactivity reflect the entire spectrum of intellectual ability. Many children present with evidence of academic failure and it is extremely important to get some measure of the child's intellectual ability with which attainments can be compared. Hyperactivity can certainly be worsened by placing a child in an academic setting with which he/she cannot cope. Knowledge of the child's basic ability will help teachers and parents to pitch academic work and expectations at an attainable and therefore rewarding level. Whenever appropriate, formal intellectual assessment should be undertaken by a psychologist attached to the clinic, or to the child's school. The Wechsler Intelligence Scale for Children (Wechsler, 1949) has the merit of distinguishing between the various aspects of cognition, and of supplying a profile which may reveal particular strengths and weaknesses in the child's capabilities. During the test situation, a note can be taken of the child's ability to concentrate, his approach to solving problems, and of his response to praise and encouragement.

Learning difficulties: reading/spelling, language, clumsiness

Children with an innate pervasive hyperactivity have an increased incidence of other developmental difficulties. Barkley (1982) reports an incidence of between 19 and 26% using strict criteria for definition. The physician can get some idea of the child's reading and spelling difficulties by using one of the standardised tests (e.g. the Schonell Graded Word Reading and Spelling Test (Schonell & Schonell, 1950)). If there is a marked discrepancy between attainments and ability, it is probable that the child has a specific difficulty. It is very tempting to assume that the failure to learn is due to the hyperactivity and poor concentration. However, often this is not the whole explanation, and it is important to acknowledge the child's underlying difficulties with reading and spelling and to devise an appropriate remedial programme with some probability for the child to experience success.

Language delay in young children is associated with an increase in temper tantrums and behaviour disorders; however, the majority of these resolve with the development of language (Woodard & Lansdown, 1988). This is possibly because the development of language helps a child to structure his play, as well as enabling him to express himself verbally, rather than solely through actions. The majority of older children with language disorders are not hyperactive (Taylor *et al.*, 1991), but in a few children the conditions co-exist. It is important to be aware of this because using long explanations of why and why not are less likely to be helpful. The child may appear fluent when he is generating the conversation, but may struggle when asked to generate language in response to specific demands. The child may become much less fluent, for example, when being asked to describe pictures or answer questions.

Many children who are hyperactive appear clumsy, and it is often difficult to decide how much of this is due to their rushed approach to tasks and how much is a true incoordination. However, some clearly have great difficulty with gross motor tasks such as kicking, catching a ball and riding a bike. This can be an additional reason for not joining in street or playground activities. Some children will be clumsy in fine motor tasks, finding dressing and eating awkward. Yet others will have a specific difficulty with drawing and/or writing (constructional dyspraxia). A clue to this is that the child will be able to match shapes very much better than he can draw them. The importance of recognising all these difficulties is that acknowledgement and help can reduce the child's frustration and improve his capacity to concentrate and attend.

Maintaining factors

Low socio-economic status, family dysfunction and marital discord, negative, critical and controlling parental attitudes can all make the child's predisposition to hyperactivity worse (Taylor *et al.*, 1991), and need to be evaluated, particularly with a view to trying to modify them as part of the management.

Parents may well state that various foods or food additives cause, or contribute to, their child's hyperactivity. There is no evidence that food substances or additives cause significant hyperactivity (Harley *et al.*, 1978). There is some evidence that, in a minority of hyperactive children, some additives may increase irritability and hence lead to a deterioration in behaviour (Egger *et al.*, 1985). Therefore, when parents give clear accounts of some colouring adversely affecting their child's behaviour, this should be noted.

Impairment

Establishing the level of overall impairment caused by hyperactivity on the child's functioning is particularly important when deciding what management strategies are justified. One of the most useful ways of doing this is to get some assessment of the impact of hyperactivity on the child's functioning within the family, with peers and at school.

In school, the teacher may report that, with the correct balance of controls and rewards, the child is able to settle in the classroom and make the expected academic progress. Alternatively, school may indicate that the child is not settling and not learning in the classroom. It is then important to try and appraise how much this might reflect anxiety and uncertainty in the teacher. A report card full of negatives suggests that the attitude/approach of the teacher may not be conducive to success. At home, the amount of disruption to the family's lifestyle is a useful guide. The child may be accommodated by being allowed to let off steam in the garden. This may not be possible if the child is living in a flat with no opportunity to play out, consequently the child's behaviour may be more disruptive. Families may alter their lifestyle by restricting visitors and by removing breakables from the house. The child's ability to play with peers is an important marker of the severity of difficulties. A child who is accepted by peers and joins in with their activities in a constructive way is unlikely to have a severe pervasive hyperactivity. If the child is being left out of group activities and has no friends, this is an indication for intervention.

CLINICAL MANAGEMENT

Whether or not hyperactivity occurring on its own suffices as the reason for referral to a specialist service, especially child psychiatry, depends on a number of reasons, besides the availability of services. These are to do with the extent that hyperactivity is seen as a medically relevant condition by parents, teachers and family practitioners, and the likelihood that some therapeutic consequences would actually follow.

In general, children are more commonly sent to a specialist service if their problems are severe and include other disabilities. In the case of hyperactivity, these accompanying conditions are usually either conduct disorder or learning difficulties. These are both conditions which are recognised by the authorities as meriting therapeutic input or special facilities. This phenomenon is also likely to be behind the figures, indicating particularly high overlaps between hyperactivity and conduct disorder, or learning problems. Only diagnosing conduct disorder when hyperactivity and conduct disorders co-exist is not wrong as such, but the practice does overlook the contribution of hyperactivity to the poorer long-term prognosis of conduct disorder (Schachar & Wachsmuth, 1991).

Other reasons for the under-recognition of hyperactivity stem from the beliefs of parents and teachers. Parents may well be critical of the behaviours that their hyperactive children show, but do not regard them as a problem requiring medical attention; or even if they do, they see it mainly as naughtiness and defiance. This may be partly a result of advice received; some general practitioners are likely to dismiss hyperactive behaviour being in any way a valid reason for medical intervention and tell the parents that it is their child rearing methods that need revising.

Several issues are involved in deciding the most appropriate therapeutic strategies, short and long-term. These have been well reviewed in the past by Prior & Griffin, 1985; Schachar & Tannock, 1993; Taylor, 1986*a*, *b*), and are fully discussed in Chapter 12 of this volume. In short, the consistent conclusion has been that although stimulant medication is often the most effective short-term treatment, long-term management requires a combination of treatment strategies of which medication is only one, and not by any means the most important one. Little is known about the long-term benefits of medication and we do know that family adversities and maladaptive patterns of parent–child interaction play an important part in the course of the disorder irrespective of their role in the initial aetiology (Weiss & Hechtman, 1986). It appears that drugs may bring about a short-term improvement in the family functioning

(Gittelman-Klein, 1987; Schachar *et al.*, 1987). These results therefore suggest that combinations of behavioural and pharmacological approaches are likely to be most beneficial.

The old notion, that the response of hyperactive children to stimulant medication was to do with some 'paradoxical' calming effect needs no longer to confuse us. The work undertaken by Rapoport and her colleagues (Rapoport *et al.*, 1978) clearly demonstrated that this was simply a mistaken assumption: stimulants, such as methylphenidate and dextroamphetamine, tend to improve attention and reduce activity level in all people, children and adults, irrespective of whether or not they are hyperactive. However, the one clear difference between children and adults concerns the side-effects of the drug: dysphoria is more common in childhood and euphoria in adult life.

A carefully conducted and methodologically sound study by Taylor *et al.* (1986*a*,*b*; 1987) used a double-blind cross-over trial of mehylphenidate and placebo in a group of boys referred to a psychiatric clinic for antisocial, disruptive and overactive behaviour. A good response (as defined by a difference of behaviour between methylphenidate and placebo conditions) was predicted by higher levels of inattentive and restless behaviour, impaired performance on tests of attention, clumsiness, younger age, and by the absence of overt anxiety.

Practical guidelines for management

The final section provides a brief summary of important points, especially from the point of view of a paediatrician. Firstly, we want to emphasise that it is always helpful to acknowledge the very real nature of the child's problems both to the parent and the child. It is also vital to describe to the parent, in language they understand, the nature of the difficulty, discussing the contribution of biological factors, learning difficulties, and the relevant social or psychological factors at home and at school. Even if the child's hyperactivity appears largely biologically determined the contributory role of environmental factors should be recognised, both from the point of view of maintaining the behaviour and as assets in the management. Rewarding good behaviours and enhancing self-esteem is of extreme importance. Parents may need to have appropriate responses to specific situations modelled for them. It is also crucial to make sure the child is in an educational setting where he/she can achieve, and where any general or specific learning difficulties are acknowledged. It is important for teachers to appreciate that they have a significant influence on the child's behaviour and that correct management can make a difference. It can be helpful to devise a routine at home and at school in which the child has the opportunity to let off steam safely and has targets for periods of attention which are then rewarded. If the impact of the hyperactivity on the child or on his family is more severe then consideration should be given to the use of psychological or behavioural strategies with or without the use of pharmacological treatment. However, if medication is used, it should always be combined with good behavioural management. It is important that the use of medication does not lead to the idea that the behaviour is totally biologically based and therefore unresponsive to environmental contingencies. If medication reduces the hyperactivity even a little, this can nevertheless be sufficient to make other strategies more effective.

The commonest medication used is methylphenidate (MP); in doses around 0.5–1.0 mg/kg, usually divided for morning and mid-day. Factors which predict the likelihood of a child responding to MP are the pervasiveness and severity of the hyperactivity and impaired concentration. MP can induce tics and their presence would be a contra-indication to its use. There is still debate as to whether MP can worsen seizures or cause them in susceptible individuals. This effect is rarely seen clinically but MP should be introduced cautiously in children with seizures. MP can affect appetite and in larger doses may slow down growth, it is therefore important to monitor height and weight at regular intervals. Most importantly, the effect of an adequate dose of MP is seen within days and, if there is no effect after 3 weeks, the drug should be discontinued.

SUMMARY

This chapter has set out to define a group of children whose hyperactivity constitutes a primary disorder distinct from the overactivity or restlessness that may be seen as a secondary phenomenon in conduct disorder or anxiety. This hyperkinetic disorder is defined by pervasive hyperactivity, onset before the age of seven years, greater frequency of low IQ and specific developmental disorders, accident proneness and poor peer relationships. The definition and measurement of overactivity, inattentiveness and impulsiveness is discussed. There is no clear association of hyperkinetic disorder with perinatal risk factors or abnormal neurological signs. There are no diagnostic tests for this disorder and diagnosis is a matter of eliciting through history and observation the combination of behaviours described of sufficient severity to warrant this diagnosis. The contribution of family/social factors and appropriateness of management must be taken into account when trying to decide just how much of the child's disorder is innate/biological, and how much might be amenable to social and behavioural intervention. Beneficial response can be predicted on the pervasiveness, severity and early onset of hyperkinetic disorder. It is important to define a group of children who are disabled by their hyperactivity as the long-term outlook untreated is not good. Although it is not yet clear that management affects the outcome, (as discussed in detail in Chapter 13), it is this group that therapeutic endeavours should be focused on.

Stimulant drugs are valuable for the most severe cases that do not respond to simpler measures and therefore require a referral to a specialist provision (Taylor *et al.*, 1987). Even though a valid argument could be made for increasing the use of stimulant drugs (such as methylphenydate) in the treatment of hyperactivity disorder in the UK and some other European countries, it is not to say that the usage should be increased to the levels seen in many US practices.

Especially within the realms of primary health care, behavioural therapies and advice to parents is the preferred means of intervention (Yule, 1986). However, on the present evidence it could be argued that stimulants should probably be used more widely in specialist child–psychiatric and behavioural–paediatric centres, though there is yet no case for expanding their use in primary care. This is because the necessary monitoring of the treatment requires specialist expertise. Also, it is to be noted that successful treatment of hyperactive children needs more than the reduction of hyperactivity: difficulties in the child's interpersonal relationships are crucial targets of therapy. Comprehensive review of current therapeutic approaches and guidance for their use are the focus of Chapter 12 by Schachar, Tannock and Cunningham in this volume.

Dietary treatments may be indicated for those hyperactive children who also suffer from frequent accompanying physical symptoms such as headaches (Egger *et al.*, 1985). Our present knowledge regarding the indications and the benefits of diet therapies is, however, still fairly rudimentary for providing clinical advice on a general level.

Although there is little doubt about the beneficial effects of current treatments of hyperactivity in the short term, their long-term effects in terms of promoting healthy psychological development remains uncertain, and largely untested. Considering the fairly extensive scale of demand for therapeutic resources, at present often largely placed on teachers in mainstream schools, it is vital that some more systematic redevelopment of existing services is carried out if hyperactive children and their families are truly to benefit.

This would still leave the issue of preventative services entirely unattended, and for this need to be met, extra resources and further research to guide them are likely to be called for. At present, the problems often seem to be noted, for example, by health visitors and nursery teachers, but there is little guidance towards any helpful remedial action. It is conceivable that, with some outside support, simple behavioural therapies and advice on common parenting problems could be easily implemented by professionals who already monitor children's health and development.

REFERENCES

Ackerman, P., Dykman, R. & Peters, J. (1977). Teenage status of hyperactive and nonhyperactive learning disabled boys. *American Journal of Orthopsychiatry,* **47**, 577–96.

American Psychiatric Association (1980). *Diagnostic and Statistical Manual of Mental Disorders.* Second Edition. Washington, DC: APA.

American Psychiatric Association (1987). *Diagnostic and Statistical Manual of Mental Disorders.* Third Edition – Revised. Washington, DC: APA.

American Psychiatric Association (1994). *Diagnostic and Statistical Manual of Mental Disorder.* Fourth Edition. Washington, DC: APA.

Barkley, R.A. (1982). Guidelines for defining hyperactivity in children. In *Advances in Clinical Child Psychology, Vol. 5,* eds. B.B. Lahey, & A.E. Kazdin, pp. 153-80. New York: Plenum.

Bregman, J.D., Leckman, J.F. & Ort, S.I. (1988). Fragile X syndrome: genetic predisposition to psychology. *Journal of Autism and Developmental Disorders,* **18**, 343–54.

Buss, A.H. & Plomin, R. (1975). *A Temperament Theory of Personality Development.* New York: John Wiley.

Cairns, E. & Cammock, T. (1978). Development of a more reliable version of the Matching Familiar Figures Test. *Developmental Psychology,* **14**, 555–60.

Campbell, S.B. (1979). Mother–infant interaction as a function of maternal ratings of temperament. *Child Psychiatry and Human Development,* **10**, 67–76.

Campbell, S.B., Breaux, A.M., Ewing, L.J. & Szumowski, E.K. (1986). Correlates and predictors of hyperactivity and aggression: a longitudinal study of parent-referred problem pre-schoolers. *Journal of Abnormal Child Psychology,* **14**, 217–34.

Cleary, M.A. & Wraith, J.E. (1993). Management of mucopolysacharidosis type III. *Archives of the Diseases of Children,* **69**, 403–6.

Cohen, N. & Minde K. (1983). The 'hyperactive syndrome' in kindergarten children: comparison of children with pervasive and situational symptoms. *Journal of Child Psychology and Psychiatry,* **24**, 443–55.

Conners, C.K. (1969). A teacher rating scale for use in drug studies with children. *American Journal of Psychiatry,* **126**, 884–8.

Conners, C.K. (1970). Symptom patterns in hyperkinetic, neurotic, and normal children. *Child Development,* **41**, 667–82.

Conners, K. (1990). Diagnosis of attention deficit hyperactivity disorder. In *Attention Deficit Hyperactivity Disorder,* eds. K. Conners & M. Kinsbourne, München: MMV Medizin Verlag.

Douglas, V. (1983). Attentional and cognitive problems. In *Developmental Neuropsychiatry,* ed. M. Rutter, pp. 280-329. New York: Guilford Press.

Douglas, V.I. (1988). Cognitive deficits in children with attention deficit disorder with hyperactivity. In *Attention Deficit Disorder: Criteria, Cognition, Intervention.* A book supplement to the *Journal of Child Psychology and Psychiatry*, No. 5, eds. L.M. Bloomingdale & J. Sergeant, pp. 65-82. Oxford: Pergamon Press.

Egger, J., Carter, C.M., Graham, P.J., Gumley, D. & Soothill, J.F. (1985). Controlled trial of oligoantigentic treatment in the hyperkinetic syndrome. *Lancet,* **i**, 540–5.

Engel, M., Leuders, H. & Chutorian, A.M. (1977). The significance of focal EEG spikes in epileptic and non-epileptic children. *Annals of Neurology,* **2**, 257–8.

Erlenmeyer-Kimling, L. & Cornblatt, B. (1978). Attentional measures in a study of children at high-risk for schizophrenia. *Journal of Psychiatric Research,* **14**, 93–8.

Firestone, P. & Martin, J.E. (1979). An analysis of the hyperactive syndrome: a comparison of hyperactive, behavior problem, in asthmatic and normal children. *Journal of Abnormal Child Psychology,* **7**, 261–73.

Fischer, M., Rolf, J.E., Hasazi, J.E. & Cummings, L. (1984). Follow-up of a pre-school epidemiological sample: cross-age xxxx and prediction of later adjustment with internalizing and externalising dimensions of behaviour. *Child Development,* **55**, 137–50.

Gillberg, C., Carlström, G. & Rasmussen, P. (1983). Hyperkinetic disorders in seven-year-old children with perceptual, motor and attentional deficits. *Journal of Child Psychology and Psychiatry,* **24**, 233–46.

Gittelman, R., Manuzza, S., Shenker R. & Bonagura, N. (1985). Hyperactive children almost grown up. *Archives of General Psychiatry,* **42**, 937–47.

Gittelman-Klein, R. (1987). Pharmacotherapy of childhood hyperactivity: An update. In *Psychopharmacology: The Third Generation of Progress,* ed. H.Y. Meltzer, pp. 1215-24. New York: Raven Press.

Goodman, R. & Stevenson, J. (1989*a*). A twin-study of hyperactivity – I. An examination of hyperactivity scores and categories derived from Rutter Teacher and Parent Questionnaires. *Journal of Child Psychology and Psychiatry,* **30**, 671–89.

Goodman, R. & Stevenson, J. (1989*b*). A twin study of hyperactivity – II. The aetiological roles of genes, family relationships and perinatal adversity. *Journal of Child Psychology and Psychiatry,* **30**, 691–709.

Greenhill, L.L. (1985). The Hyperkinetic Syndrome. In *The Clinical Guide to Child Psychiatry*, eds. D. Shaffer, A.A Ehrhardt, & L.L. Greenhill, pp. 251–75. New York: The Free Press.

Greenhill, L.L. (1990). Attention deficit hyperactivity disorder in children. In *Psychiatric Disorders in Children and Adolescents*, eds. B.D. Garfinkel, G.A. Carlson & E.B. Weller, Philadelphia: Saunders.

Hagen, J.W. & Hale, E.A. (1973). The development of attention in children. *In Minnesota Symposia on Child Psychology, Vol. 7,* ed. A.D. Pick, Minneapolis: University of Minnesota.

Harley, J.P., Ray, R.S., Tomasi, L., Eichman, P.L., Matthews, C.G., Chun, R., Cleeland, C.S. & Traisman, E. (1978). Hyperkinesis and food additives: Testing the Feingold hypothesis. *Pediatrics,* **61**, 818–28.

Horowitz, L.M., Wright, J.C., Lowenstein, E. & Parad, H.W. (1981). The prototype as a construct in abnormal psychology: I. A method for deriving prototypes. *Journal of Abnormal Psychology,* **90**, 568–74.

Howlin, P. & Rutter, M. (1987). The consequences of language delay for other aspects of development. In *Language Development and Disorders,* eds. W. Yule & M. Rutter, *Clinics in Development Medicine*, No. 101/102. London: MacKeith Press.

Jenkins, S., Bax, M. & Hart, H. (1980). Behaviour problems in preschool children. *Journal of Child Psychology and Psychiatry*, **21**, 5–18.

Kagan, J., Rosman, B.L., Day, D., Albert, J. & Phillips, W. (1964). Information processing in the child and the significance of analytic and reflective attitudes. *Psychological Monographs,* 78, No. 1.

Klorman, R., Brumaghim, J.T., Salzman, L.F., Strauss, J., Borgstedt, A.D., McBride, M.C. & Loeb, S. (1988). Effects of methylphenidate on attention deficit hyperactivity disorder with and without aggressive/non compliant features. *Journal of Abnormal Psychology,* **97**, 413–22.

Lambert, N., Hartsaugh, C. & Sassone, D. (1987). Persistence of hyperactivity symptoms from childhood to adolescence. *American Journal of Orthopsychiatry,* **57**, 22–31.

Lewine, J.D., Borgstedt, A.D. & Goldstein, M.G. (1988). The contributions of event-related potentials to understanding effects of stimulants on information processing in attention deficit disorder. In *Attention Deficit Disorder: Criteria, Cognition, Intervention*, eds., L.M. Bloomingdale & J. Sergeant. A Book Supplement to the *Journal of Child Psychology and Psychiatry*, No. 5. Oxford: Pergamon Press.

Loeber, R. (1990). Development and risk factors of juvenile antisocial behaviour and delinquency. *Clinical Psychology Review,* **10**, 1–41.

Loney, J., Kramer, J. & Milich, R. (1981). The hyperactive child grows up: Predictors of symptoms, delinquency, and achievement at follow-up. In *Psychosocial Aspects of Drug Treatment for Hyperactivity*, eds., K.D. Gadow & J. Loney, pp. 381–415. Westview: Boulder, CO.

Luk, S.L., Thorley, G. & Taylor, E. (1987). Gross overactivity – a study by direct observation. *Journal of Psychopathology and Behavioural Assessment*, **9**, 173–82.

McGee, R., Williams, S. & Silva, P.A. (1984*a*). Behavioral and developmental characteristics of aggressive, hyperactive and aggressive–hyperactive boys. *Journal of the American Academy of Child and Adolescent Psychiatry*, **23**, 270–79.

McGee, R., Williams, S. & Silva, P.A. (1984*b*). Background characteristics of aggressive, hyperactive and aggressive–hyperactive boys. *Journal of the American Academy of Child and Adolescent Psychiatry*, **23**, 280–84.

McGee, R.M., Williams, S., Share, D.L., Anderson, J. & Silva, P.A. (1986). The relationship between specific reading retardation, general reading backwardness, and behavioural problems in a large sample of Dunedin boys: a longitudinal study from five to eleven years. *Journal of Child Psychology and Psychiatry,* **27**, 597–610.

Magnusson, D. (1987). *Individual Development in an Interactional Perspective* (Vol. 1. Series: Paths Through Life, ed. D. Magnusson). Hillsdale, NJ: Lawrence Erlbaum.

Nichols, P.L. & Chen, T.C. (1981). *Minimal Brain Dysfunction: A Prospective Study.* Hillsdale, NY: Erlbaum.

Offord, R.R., Sullivan, K., Allen, N. & Abrams, N. (1979). Delinquency and hyperactivity. *Journal of Nervous and Mental Diseases,* **167**, 734–41.

Porrino, L.J., Rapoport, J.L., Behar, D., Sceery, W., Ismond, D.R. & Bunney, W.E. (1983). A naturalistic assessment of the motor activity of hyperactive boys. I. Comparison with normal controls. *Archives of General Psychiatry,* **40**, 681–87.

Prendergast, M., Taylor, E., Rapoport, J.L., Bartko, J., Donnelly, M., Zametkin, A., Ahearn, M.B., Dunn, G. & Wieselberg, H.M. (1988). The diagnosis of childhood hyperactivity. *Journal of Child Psychology and Psychiatry,* **29**, 289–300.

Prior, M. & Griffin, M. (1985). *Hyperactivity: Diagnosis and Management.* London: Heinemann.

Prior, M., Leonard, A. & Wood, G. (1983). A comparison study of preschool children diagnosed as hyperactive. *Journal of Pediatric Psychology*, **8**, 191–207.

Quay, H.C. (1979). Classification. In *Psychopathological Disorders of Childhood*, 2nd edn, eds. H.C. Quay & J.S. Werry, pp. 1–34. New York: Wiley.

Rapoport, J., Buchsbaum, M.S., Zahn, T.P., Weingartner, H., Ludlow, C. & Mikkelsen, E.J. (1978). Dextroamphetamine: cognitive and behavioral effects in normal prepubertal boys. *Science,* **199**, 560–3.

Rapoport, J.L., Quinn, P.O., Burg, C. & Bartley, L. (1979). Can hyperactives be identified in infancy? In *Hyperactivity in Children*, ed. R.L. Trites, Baltimore: University Park Press.

Richman, N., Stevenson, J.E. & Graham, P.J. (1982). *Preschool to School: A Behavioural Study.* London: Academic Press.

Rutter, M., Chadwick, O. & Schachar, R. (1983). Hyperactivity and minimal brain dysfunction: epidemiological perspectives on questions of cause and classification. In *The Child at Psychiatric Risk*, ed. R.E. Tarter, pp. 80-107. New York: Oxford University Press.

Rutter, M., Tizard, J. & Whitmore, K. (eds.) (1970). *Education, Health and Behaviour.* London: Longman.

Sandberg, S.T. (1986). Overactivity: behaviour or syndrome? In *The Overactive Child*, ed. E. Taylor, pp. 41–72. London: The MacKeith Press/Blackwell.

Sandberg, S.T., Rutter, M. & Taylor, E. (1978). Hyperkinetic disorder in clinic attenders. *Developmental Medicine and Child Neurology*, **20**, 279–99.

Schachar, R. & Tannock, R. (1993). Effectiveness of long-term treatment of childhood hyperactivity with psychostimulants. A methodological critique and review (unpublished manuscript).

Schachar, R.J. & Wachsmuth, R. (1991). Family dysfunction and psychosocial adversity: comparison of attention deficit disorder, conduct disorders, normal and clinical controls. *Canadian Journal of Behavioral Science*, **23**, 332–48.

Schachar, R., Rutter, M. & Smith, A. (1981). Characteristics of situationally and pervasively hyperactive children: implications for syndrome definition. *Journal of Child Psychology and Psychiatry*, **22**, 375–92.

Schachar, R., Sandberg, S. & Rutter, M. (1986). Agreement between teachers' ratings and observations of hyperactivity, inattentiveness and defiance. *Journal of Abnormal Child Psychology*, **14**, 331–45.

Schachar, R., Taylor, E., Wiselberg, M., Thorley, G. & Rutter, M. (1987). Changes in family function and relationships in children who responded to methylphenidate. *Journal of the American Academy of Child and Adolescent Psychiatry*, **26**, 728–32.

Schain, R.J. & Royhard, C.L. (1975). Observations on effects of a central stimulant drug (methylphenidate) in children with hyperactive behavior. *Pediatrics* **55***:* 709–16.

Schleifer, M., Weiss, G., Cohen, N., Elman, M., Cveije, H. & Kruger, E. (1975). Hyperactivity in preschoolers and the effect of methylphenidate. *American Journal of Orthopsychiatry*, **45**, 38–50.

Schonell, T.J. & Schonell, F.E. (1950). *Diagnostic and Attainment Testing, including a Manual of Tests, Their Nature, Use, Recording and Interpretation.* Edinburgh: Oliver and Boyd.

Sergeant, J. (1981). *Attentional Studies in Hyperactivity.* Rijksuniversiteit te Groningen: Groningen.

Sergeant, J. (1988*a*). From DSM-III attentional deficit disorder to functional defects. In *Attention Deficit Disorder: Criteria, Cognition, Intervention,* eds. L.M. Bloomingdale & J. Sergeant. A Book Supplement to the *Journal of Child Psychology and Psychiatry*, No. 5. pp. 183-98. Oxford: Pergamon Press.

Sergeant, J. (1988*b*). RDC for hyperactivity/attention disorder. *In Attention Deficit Disorder: Criteria, Cognition, Intervention,* eds. L.M. Bloomingdale & J. Sergeant. A Book Supplement to the *Journal of Child Psychology and Psychiatry*, No. 5. pp.1–18. Oxford: Pergamon Press.

Shaffer, D. (1980). An approach to the validation of clinical syndromes in childhood. In *The Ecosystem of the 'Sick' Child,* eds. S. Salzinger, J. Antrobus & J. Glick. London: Academic Press.

Shaffer, D., O'Connor, P.A., Shafer, S.Q. & Prupis, S. (1983). Neurological 'soft signs', their origins and significance for behaviour. In *Development Neuropsychiatry,* ed. M. Rutter, pp. 144-163. New York: Guilford Press.

Shaffer, D., Schonfeld, I., O'Connor, P.A., Stockham, C., Trautman, P., Shafer, S. & Ng, S. (1985). Neurological soft signs: their relationship to psychiatric disorders and intelligence in childhood and adolescence. *Archives of General Psychiatry,* **42**, 342–51.

Shaywitz, B.A., Shaywitz, S.E., Byrne, T., Cohen, D.J. & Rothman, S. (1983). Attention deficit disorder: quantitative analysis of CT. *Neurology,* **33**, 1500–3.

Shen, Y-C., Wang, Y-F. & Yang, X-L. (1985). An epidemiological investigation of minimal brain dysfunction in six elementary schools in Beijing. *Journal of Child Psychology and Psychiatry,* **26**, 777–87.

Stewart, A.L., Reynold, E.O.R., Hope, P.L., Hamilton, P.A., Baudin, J., Costelloe, A.M. de

L., Bradford, B.C. & Wyatt, J.S. (1987). Probability of neurodevelopmental disorders estimated from ultrasound appearance of brains of very preterm infants. *Developmental Medicine and Child Neurology,* **29**, 3–11.

Stewart, M.A. & Olds, S.W. (1973). *Raising a Hyperactive Child.* New York: Harper & Row.

Still, G.F. (1902). The Coulstonian Lectures on some abnormal psychical conditions in children. *Lancet,* **i**, 1008–12; 1077–82; 1163–8.

Sykes, D.H., Douglas, V.I. & Morgenstern, G. (1973). Sustained attention in hyperactive children. *Journal of Child Psychology and Psychiatry,* **14**, 213–20.

Szatmari, P., Offord, D.R. & Boyle, M.H. (1989). Ontario Child Health Study: prevalence of attention deficit disorder with hyperactivity. *Journal of Child Psychology and Psychiatry,* **30**, 219–30.

Taylor, E.A. (1980). Development of attention. In *Scientific Foundations of Developmental Psychiatry,* ed. M. Rutter, pp. 185–97. London: Heinemann Medical.

Taylor, E.A. (1986*a*). Overactivity, hyperactivity and hyperkinesis: problems and prevalence. In *The Overactive Child*, ed. E.A. Taylor, pp. 1–18. Oxford: Blackwell Scientific Publications.

Taylor, E.A. (1986*b*). Attention deficit. In *The Overactive Child*, ed. E.A. Taylor, Clinics in Developmental Medicine No. 97, pp. 73–106, Oxford: Blackwell Scientific Publications.

Taylor E.A., Sandberg, S., Thorley, G. & Giles, S. (1991). *The Epidemiology of Childhood Hyperactivity.* Institute of Psychiatric Maudsley Monograph. London: Oxford University Press.

Taylor, E.A., Schachar, R., Thorley, G. & Wieselberg, M. (1986*a*). Conduct disorder and hyperactivity: I. Separation of hyperactivity and antisocial conduct in British child psychiatric patients. *British Journal of Psychiatry,* **149**, 760–7.

Taylor, E.A., Everitt, B., Thorley, G., Schachar, R., Rutter, M. & Wieselberg, M. (1986*b*). Conduct disorder and hyperactivity: II. A cluster analytic approach to the identification of a behavioural syndrome. *British Journal of Psychiatry,* **149**, 768–77.

Taylor, E.A, Schachar, R., Thorley, G., Wieselberg, H.M., Everitt, B. & Rutter, M. (1987). Which boys respond to stimulant medication? A controlled trial of methylphenidate in boys with disruptive behaviour. *Psychological Medicine,* **17**, 121–43.

Trott, G.E. (1993). *Das hyperkinetische Syndrom des Kindes- und Jugendalters. Therapeutische Moglichkeiten und deren Evaluation.* Leipzig: Heidelberg. Ambrosius Barth.

Trott, G.E. & Boehm, K. (1992). *Hyperkinetische Kinder als Jugendliche,* in press.

Vikan, A. (1985). Psychiatric epidemiology in a sample of 1510 ten-year-old children: I. Prevalence. *Journal of Child Psychology and Psychiatry,* **26**, 55–75.

Wechsler, D. (1949). *Wechsler Intelligence Scale of Children (Manual).* New York: Psychological Corporation.

Weiss, G. & Hechman, L.T. (1979). The hyperactive child syndrome. *Science*, **205**, 1348–54.

Weiss, G. & Hechtman, L.T. (1986). *Hyperactive Children Grown Up.* New York: Guilford Press.

Werry, J.S. (1979). Organic factors. In *Psychopathological Disorders of Childhood*, 2nd edn, eds. H.C. Quay & J.S. Werry, pp. 90–133. New York: Wiley.

Werry, J.S., Reeves, J.C. & Elkind, G.S. (1987). Attention deficit, conduct, oppositional and anxiety disorders in children: I. A review of research on differentiating characteristics; II. Clinical characteristics. *Journal of the American Academy of Child and Adolescent Psychiatry,* **26**, 133–55.

Whalen, C.K., Henker, B. & Swanson, J.M. (1987). Natural social behavior in hyperactive children: Dose effects of methylphenidate. *Journal of Consulting and Clinical Psychology,* **55**, 187–93.

Woodard, M. & Lansdown, R. (1988). Language and communication. *In Problems of Preschool Children,* eds. N. Richman & R. Lansdown, pp. 55–74. Chichester: John Wiley & Sons.

World Health Organization (1988). *ICD-10: 1988 Draft of Chapter V. Categories F00–F99. Mental, Behavioural and Developmental Disorders.* Geneva: World Health Organisation Division of Mental Health

World Health Organization (1992). *International Classification of Diseases – ICD-10.* Geneva: WHO.

Yule, W. (1986). Behavioural treatments. In *The Overactive Child,* ed. E.A. Taylor, Clinics in Developmental Medicine No. 97. pp. 219–35. London: The MacKeith Press/Blackwell.

4

The role of attention

Jaap J. Van der Meere

INTRODUCTION

The goal of this chapter is to present a review of research into attentional aspects of hyperactivity disorder. Before starting with the review, some issues, which are not mutually exclusive, will be discussed. The issues concern the appropriateness of the paradigms commonly used to study attention and the accuracy of the methods of identifying hyperactivity in children.

Many attempts have been made to validate the clinical concept of hyperactivity disorder in the laboratory. However, since the manifestation of the primary symptoms of hyperactivity (inattention, impulsivity and overactivity) largely depend on the types of environments in which the children are observed, the laboratory approach may be criticised because of the limited range of situations in which the children's behaviour is studied. In addition, experimental task demands may be highly sophisticated, so that extensive training is needed before the actual experiment can start. Moreover, in order to keep the children 'on the track', they are commonly not left to perform the task alone. When all these factors are taken into account, it could be argued that the symptoms of hyperactivity may have been 'filtered out' by the time the laboratory experiment starts. Consequently, one may question the extent to which an attention deficit in hyperactivity disorder, as indicated by teachers and parents and defined by clinical diagnostic procedures, can be accounted for by laboratory data.

Barkley (1991) recently examined the degree of ecological validity of laboratory experiments of hyperactivity. In his attempt to formulate a set of ecological criteria he was forced to rely primarily on parent and teacher ratings of symptoms because so few studies were available for comparing the laboratory findings with direct observations in natural settings. Since, in general, low correlations are reported between laboratory measures of attention, impulsivity and activity on the one hand and teacher and parent ratings on the other, one may conclude that laboratory experiments have little ecological validity. However, this argument is not without problems.

First, it is doubtful whether parent and teacher ratings are the golden standard for ecological validity, since parents and teachers may use undifferentiated concepts in their subjective ratings. This has been demonstrated by Vaessen & Van der Meere (1990). They showed that many children rated by their teachers as hyperactive were in fact clumsy, as measured by the Test of Motor Impairment (Stott, Moyes & Henderson, 1984); or learning disabled, as measured by a Dutch revised version of the Primary Mental Ability Test (Thurstone, 1938). Furthermore, the learning disabled and clumsy children were not rated as hyperactive by their parents and/or observers during standardised laboratory observations. Hence, low correlations between laboratory measures and hyperactivity ratings by parents and teachers may reflect the heterogeneity of hyperactive samples under study, instead of reflecting the degree of the ecological validity of laboratory measures *per se*. This brings us to the problem of the appropriateness of selection procedures. As already mentioned, key behaviours of hyperactive children vary across situations. A number of studies suggest that a child may be hyperactive at home but not at school, or vice versa, or hyperactive at home and school but not in a third situation (Lambert, Sandoval & Sassone, 1978; Kazdin, Esveldt-Dawson & Loar, 1983; Vaessen & Van der Meere, 1990; Sandberg, Rutter & Taylor, 1978; Schachar, Rutter & Smith, 1981). If both the teacher and the parents consider the child to be hyperactive, the child may be termed as showing pervasive hyperactivity. If only one of the informants considers the child hyperactive, the child is considered to show situational hyperactivity. Methodologically speaking, the degree of agreement is not obvious unless it is clear which part of the variance between teachers and parents is explained by the child's behaviour pattern, and which part of the variance is accounted for by the variability and individual response bias of the teachers and parents themselves. If this requirement is met, then the disagreement between sources of information is not necessarily a problem. In fact, agreement/disagreement between informants may provide important information about severity of the symptoms, and is therefore an essential factor needing to be clarified in sample selection procedures. With the exception of the study by Rapoport *et al.* (1986), differences between situational and pervasive hyperactivity have been reported for the age of onset of neurodevelopmental immaturities, task accuracy (Sandberg *et al.*, 1978), prognosis (Campbell, Endman & Bernfeld, 1977; Schachar *et al.*, 1981; Schleifer *et al.*, 1975), motor impulsivity (Cohen & Minde, 1983), activity level, attention, minor neurological deficits (Luk, Leung & Yen, 1991), and for stimulant drug response (Pliszka, 1989; Taylor *et al.*, 1986). Given these findings, the low correlations between laboratory measures and questionnaire ratings of hyperactivity as meant by Barkley (1991), may be largely due to lack of differentiation between children with situational and pervasive hyperactivity. In order to get a better grip on the issue of situational and pervasive hyperactivity, however, we must go further than the school–home comparison which remains an oversimplification of discrimination of childhood behaviour. Following Barkley's advice (1982), it would seem more useful to refer to the occurence of hyperactive behaviour within multiple defined settings. It is therefore suggested that clustering of hyperactive cases around different situational dimensions (such as highly structured versus free play, and social interaction versus alone), may be a way of identifying subgroups of hyperactive children.

Secondly, there is the problem of co-morbidity and its influence on group selection. A number of studies have demonstrated that hyperactivity disorder shows considerable overlap with conduct disorder, depression and anxiety disorders (including post traumatic stress disorder), learning disorders, Gilles de la Tourette syndrome and others. Maurer & Stewart (1980), for instance, reported that 80% of a clinical sample of children with hyperactivity disorder had at least one other psychiatric disorder. (For a review of co-morbidity see Barkley, 1990.) Although the extent of co-morbidity is dependent on the range and reliability of the instruments used (Vaessen & Van der Meere, 1990), there is no doubt about its existence. It is therefore reasonable to assume that the low correlations between laboratory measures and ratings of hyperactivity are at least partly due to this co-morbidity. Hence the optimal design in cognitive research is the comparison of hyperactive children varying in degree of pervasiveness of the symptoms, with the type(s) of co-morbidity studied being clearly specified. The research diagnostic Criteria (RDC), as proposed by Sergeant (1988*a*), are a good starting point. These criteria are designed for research in which precisely defined groups are required for a meaningful interpretation of data. However, one may argue that, in clinical practice, it is inappropriate to select subjects on the basis of strict criteria because care should be given to all children who need it. Nevertheless, it can be argued that diagnosis for clinical as well as for research purposes will benefit from the choice of a model in which the dimensions of deviant behaviour are most clearly highlighted (Vaessen & Van der Meere, 1990).

The argument up to now has focused on the fact that correlations between laboratory measures of cognition, and parent and teacher ratings of hyperactivity have generally been low because of the heterogeneity and the comorbidity of the samples used in the studies. The next question concerns the type of hyperactive behaviour that is relevant for studies carried out in the laboratory condition; and the appropriateness of the tasks most frequently used to study these behaviours.

As stated before, parents and teachers consider hyperactive children as inattentive, overactive and impulsive. Barkley (1990) has suggests that in order to help conceptualise the disorder, greater weight should be given to impulsivity and overactivity, rather than to inattention when ranking the importance of the primary symptoms. However, content overlap between items is clearly the case (Dienske & Sanders-Woutstra, 1988), and it is doubtful whether entirely distinct constructs of attention, activity and impulsivity can unequivocally be operationalised in terms of observable behaviour in the laboratory (Gittelman, 1988; Kalverboer, 1988). Furthermore, since parent and teacher evaluations are liable to be subjective, it may be the case that neither evaluation reflects the child's actual behaviour in the specific (school or home) situation, rather than being based on global impressions (Lambert *et al.*, 1978); with the result that attention and activity are often indistinguishable and treated as one factor (McGee, Silva & Williams, 1984). Hence, it appears safe to conclude that, at the moment, the exact relationship between activity, impulsivity and inattention is unknown. Part of this problem stems from the so-called 'lack of positive transfer' between research approaches. Overactivity has been studied using the ethological approach in a wide range of situations: at school, at home and in the laboratory (for a review see, Barkley, 1990), without any reference to cognitive abilities. Instead, the cognitive characteristics have primarily been studied in the laboratory, using traditional tests such as the matching familiar figures test (MFT), Porteus mazes, figures embedded test, Stroop, etc.; but again without reference to the overt behaviour of the child during experimentation. Thus, it seems that there is a gap to be bridged not only between subjective teacher and parent reports on the one hand and laboratory measures on the other but also between research traditions themselves.

Moreover, as has been argued elswere (Sergeant & Van der Meere, 1989; 1990*a*,*b*), these traditional tests (MFFT, Porteus mazes, figures embedded test, stroop, etc.) can be seen as only the 'first generation' of cognitive tests. Such tests measure a complex web of cognitive abilities. As a consequence, poor task performance may be caused by numerous and unknown factors which make test results difficult to interpret. The author has reason to believe that the 'information processing approach' may be more helpful in identifying the assumed cognitive deficits of hyperactive children. The main advantage of this approach is that cognition is unravelled in its elementary parts, thus making it possible to locate the assumed cognitive (attention) deficit in a particular clinical condition more presisely. Regarding the question of ecological validity, the author believes that a combination of attention assessments, based on the information processing approach, and 'on-line' systematic behavioural observations, is required in order to make teacher and parent reports more objective, compared with correlating heterogeneous measures of cognitive abilities (i.e. traditional tests) with parent and teacher hyperactivity questionnaire ratings (Alberts & Van der Meere, 1992; Kalverboer, 1988, 1990). (For a more detailed discussion about information processing theory and its ecological relevance the reader is referred to Sergeant & Van der Meere (1994).)

The author now wishes to proceed with a review of research into cognitive aspects of hyperactivity disorder. The review is centred around the state/process distinction as it is presented in recent models of information processing theory (Sanders, 1983; Mulder, 1986). The state/process distinction can best be conceptualised as a continuum (Hockey, Coles & Gaillard, 1986). Processes are defined as discrete and short-term events (elementary operations) that mediate between stimulus and response. State fluctuations are not directly involved in information processes but modulate the elementary operations. Important state factors are time-on-task, incentives, feedback and presence/absence of the experimenter. Although there are no generally agreed methods of distinguishing between direct effects on elementary cognitive operations and indirect effects via energetic (state) mechanisms, it is assumed that basic attention abilities, such as orienting and selective attention, are best studied if factors that influence the subject's state are kept as constant as possible during experimentation. Hence, tasks purporting to measure such abilities have to be short, and training as well as the presence of the experimenter is needed (Gaillard, 1988). The results of this type of investigation are evaluated in the first section of the review. The concept of impulsivity in hyperactivity disorder will be discussed in the second section. The influence of state factors on task performance is the theme of the third section, and the fourth section reviews psychophysiological attention research in hyperactivity disorders.

In a salutory paper by Taylor (1983), the relationship between drug response and diagnostic validity of hyperkinetic disorder was examined critically. Taylor pointed out that methylphenidate has not provided the favourable outcome that one would wish to see from an effective therapy. However, this drug has shown short-term effects on task performance. If the employment of information processing paradigms points in a certain direction with respect to the processing deficiency of the hyperactive child, and if drug action specifically affects this processing deficiency, then these findings together may be considered as converging evidence at least. Therefore, in each section of this chapter where an attention construct is discussed, the results regarding hyperactivity disorder will be linked with these methylphenidate (MPH) studies, whenever possible. (For a more in-depth discussion about MPH and laboratory findings, the reader is referred to Sergeant & Van der Meere (1991)).

BASIC ATTENTION ABILITIES

One main characteristic of the hyperactive child is task inefficiency. Whether this task inefficiency is caused by attentional dysfunctions, such as difficulties in orientation, reorientation, encoding, focused and divided attention abilities, is the central theme of this first section. For the purposes of this section, error scores and reaction times (RT) are defined as the dependent variables of the tasks.

Orientation

There is ample evidence that spatial cues are very important for organising and guiding attention (Posner, 1988). In this type of study cues can be informative (valid), non-informative (invalid), or neutral. The typical finding is that RT for detection is faster on valid trials than on neutral trials, and slower on invalid trials than on neutral trials. These two effects are often referred to as the benefits and costs of allocating attention.

Studies using cuing techniques have revealed that hyperactive and control children are not different in the time taken to direct attention towards cues (Pearson & Lane, 1990). Moreover, hyperative children show the same level of benefits in the valid cue position, and RT costs in the invalid cue position, as controls (Burke, 1990; Swanson *et al.*, 1990). Besides varying the type of cues (valid, invalid and neutral), Burke (1990), and Swanson *et al.* (1990), have also varied the temporal relation between cue and target (the stimulus onset asynchrony, SOA). Both studies reported that hyperactive children made more errors only with long SOA intervals. Hence, SOA and not cuing, is the crucial factor in hyperactivity disorder. The question of SOA, i.e. presentation rate of events and hyperactivity disorder, will be further discussed in the third section of this chapter.

Re-orientation

In the study referred to above, Pearson & Lane (1990), compared hyperactive and non-hyperactive children for the time required to 'get back on track after switching gears' in a dichotic listening task. Subjects were instructed to detect targets in the message received by one ear, and to ignore the message received by the other ear. After about ten seconds, a signal instructed them either to remain on the same ear, or else to re-orient to the other ear. The onset of the target series varied from 0.5 to 3.5 seconds. Once the hyperactive children were thrown off course by the switch, they never re-oriented. This was especially so at longer delay intervals. Hence, the results of this study also indicate that the rate of presentation of events is a crucial factor in studying the attention deficits of hyperactivity disorder.

The effect of switching attention between modalities in hyperactive and non-hyperactive children was studied by Zahn, Kruesi & Rapoport (1991). In their task, the subjects were instructed to respond to a tone with the right hand and to a light with the left hand. Reaction times were sorted by preceding stimulus: Ipsimodal sequences (tone–tone; light–light) were compared to cross-modal (tone–light; light–tone) sequences. No group differences were found with respect to either type of sequence.

Information uptake

Information uptake, or encoding, can be subdivided into three types: that of codes at the physical, name and semantic level. Theoretically, each dimension forces the individual to process the stimulus at a different cognitive level, or depth, in order to accurately perform the task (Craik & Lockhart, 1972; Posner & Boies, 1971). Three types of encoding tasks have been used to study hyperactivity disorder. The first is Sternberg's (1969) stimulus degradation task. In this task, children are required to identify targets in a target-degraded and a target-non-degraded condition. Encoding time is defined as the difference in response latency between the degraded and non-degraded condition. The second is the 'depth-of-processing task' (Craik & Lockhart, 1972). Here, an incidental recall task for the stimulus words is given immediately following the encoding phase. Craik and his colleagues have argued that information which is more extensively (deeply) processed will leave a relatively stronger memory trace and is more likely to be recalled in a free recall task. It is assumed that the less errors the more deeply the information has been processed. The third is Posner's letter-matching task (Posner & Mitchell, 1967). Under physical identity (PI) matching, subjects are instructed to indicate when two letters look exactly the same (a–a). Under name-identity (NI) matching, subjects are instructed to indicate when the two letters have the same name (A–a). Encoding time is defined here as the difference in response latency between the PI and the NI conditions.

The three types of encoding tasks have failed to show differences between hyperactive and control children at the various levels of encoding (Ballinger, Varley & Nolen, 1984; Balthazor, Wagner & Pelham, 1991; Benezra & Douglas, 1988; Borcherding *et al.*, 1988; Malone, Kershner & Siegel, 1988; Peeke *et al.*, 1984; Reid & Borkowsky, 1984; Sergeant & Scholten, 1985*a*). The results can also be taken to indicate that methylphenidate and D-amphetamine (the treatments of choice in hyperactivity disorder), have no effects on encoding, with only one exception (Weingartner *et al.*, 1980). Thus, the available evidence seems to rule out encoding as the attentional deficit in hyperactivity disorder. In fact, it has been demonstrated many times that the basic abilities of encoding and retrieval of verbal and nonverbal information are intact in hyperactivity disorder (e.g. Douglas, 1988). However, there is some evidence that hyperactive children have some problems in encoding stimuli in parallel (Wilding, 1994), and a study by Douglas & Benezra (1990) suggests that deficits do become apparent on word lists requiring organised and deliberate rehearsal strategies. This has been explained in terms of impaired self-regulatory processing. The matter of self-regulatory processing will be further discussed in the third section of the chapter.

Focused attention

Focused attention in the visual modality in hyperactivity disorder has been studied by Van der Meere & Sergeant (1988*a*). In this study the subjects were instructed to pay attention to the top-left to bottom-right (relevant) diagonal of a display but to ignore the other (irrelevant) diagonal. In half of the trials a target appeared in the relevant diagonal and a 'yes' response was required. A 'no' response was required if the target was not presented in the relevant diagonal. Foils were presented in less than 10% of the trials in the relevant diagonal. A focused attention deficit could be assumed if responses to foils were more pronounced in the hyperactive group than in peer controls. This was not the case: that is to say, hyperactive children responded to foils to the same extent as the control group did. Hence, this study demonstrated that hyperactive children are not abnormally distractable. In addition, a methylphenidate study by De Sonneville, Njiokiktjien & Hilhorst (1991), using the same focused attention paradigm demonstrated that the error rate for foil signals did not improve during treatment with methylphenidate.

Focused attention in the auditory modality has been studied using the dichotic listening task. Here, subjects are instructed to focus attention to one ear and to ignore the stimulus presented at the other ear. No differences in task performance between hyperactive and control children have been found in this type of task (Davidson & Prior, 1978; Douglas & Peters, 1979; Pelham, 1979). Only with a high event rate has the dichotic listening task differentiated hyperactive children from controls (Loiselle *et al.*, 1980). Hence, not focused attention but again, event rate seems to play a crucial role in the attentional performance of children with hyperactivity disorder.

In fact, there are a surprising number of failures in the attempts to show that hyperactive children are abnormally distractible (for an extensive review see Douglas, 1983). On the contrary, many studies using external distractors (radio music, noise, etc.), have shown that hyperactive children are not hindered, but may in fact benefit from this type of distraction during test performance (Browning, 1967; Zentall, Zentall & Barack, 1978). This was recently confirmed by Abikoff, Szeibel & Courtney (1990). They reported that hyperactive children working on an arithmetic task produced significantly more correct responses under a music condition than in a speech or silence condition. The finding that hyperactive children benefit from distraction has led to the formulation of the self-stimulation hypothesis in hyperactivity disorder (Zentall & Zentall; 1983; Zentall & Meyer, 1987). This issue will be further discussed in section three of this chapter.

Capacity

Capacity refers to the idea that the cognitive system is limited by the availability of central processing capacity. Two paradigms have been used to measure information processing capacity in hyperactive children. The first is the double task paradigm. Here, subjects are instructed to divide their attention between two simultaneous tasks. According to this paradigm, limitations arise when two mental tasks have to be performed at the same time. The first assumption of the paradigm is that task efficiency is positively related to the amount of available resources. The second assumption is that tasks, when performed simultaneously, will compete for processing resources. Only when groups do not differ in performance on the primary task, and when performance on the primary task does not vary as result of load manipulations on the secondary task, can performance on the secondary task be interpreted as reflecting the resources remaining after those needed for the primary task have been expended. If these requirements are met, then it is justified to interpret greater impairment of secondary task performance of the hyperactive group in terms of a smaller attentional capacity.

The dual task paradigm has been employed in hyperactivity research by Schachar & Logan (1990*a*). In their study the primary task was a simple forced-choice reaction time task. The letters O and X were presented on a screen. Subjects were instructed to respond by pressing corresponding response buttons, mapped with O and X, with the fingers of the left hand. The secondary task, which involved a 55 dB tone of 100 ms duration, required the subjects to respond by pressing a third key with a finger of the right hand. The tone was generated on half of the trials. The temporal overlap between the onset of the primary and secondary task was varied. Schachar and Logan argued that the greater the temporal overlap, the less the capacity left for the secondary task and the greater the secondary-task response delay. This study indicated that the extent of interference between the primary and secondary tasks, over the range of temporal overlap, was the same in hyperactive children and controls. Consequently, it was concluded that hyperactive children do not have a deficient information processing capacity.

The dual task paradigm has also been used in so-called ecologically relevant task conditions. In the Vaessen (1990*a*) study, the primary task was walking over a balance beam. The secondary task involved pressing a button attached to either the left or right thumb, in response to a high or a low pitched tone respectively. No difference in the secondary task performance between hyperactive and control children was observed. In another study by the same author (Vaessen, 1990*b*), the primary task was a traffic task. The experimental location was set up on a pavement near a road with medium to high traffic intensity (400–700 vehicles per hour). The child started at an imaginary curb and had to cross over a distance of 9 metres to the other curb, representing the opposite side of the imaginary road. The latter curb was at a safe distance of 4 metres from the real road. The child had an adequate view of the traffic on the real road. Hence, real traffic was used as stimulus material, and the child had to cross the imaginary street in the same way and with the same time interval as when crossing the real street. The secondary task was a digit recall task. The digits had to be memorised during the period in which the child had to observe the traffic and detect a suitable gap. The digits were to be repeated by the child on reaching the other side of the imaginary road. It was emphasised that the child should cross as soon as the last car he had been waiting for had passed. It appeared that, particularly in a difficult recall condition, hyperactive children consistently accepted shorter gaps in the traffic to cross the street. The results could be interpreted as indicating that the primary task interacted with the secondary task, and therefore, the requirements of the dual task paradigm were not fully met in this study. Consequently, no direct conclusions in terms of capacity limitations may be drawn from this particular experiment.

Another capacity measure employed in hyperactivity research is the Sternberg (1969) memory recognition task. Here subjects are instructed to divide attention between simultaneously presented input. Increasing the cognitive load (consonant letters) will lead to slower processing. This is reflected in a linear increase in reaction time. This increase, in turn, is an index of the information processing capacity (Schneider & Shiffrin, 1977; Shiffrin & Schneider, 1977; Sanders, 1983). Following this paradigm, a limitation in capacity could be assumed in hyperactivity disorder, if, because of cognitive overload, the increase in reaction time and errors was more pronounced in the hyperactive group than in peer controls. With one exception (Leung & Connolly, 1994) a number of studies have indicated that this is not the case with children either currently suffering from hyperactivity or with those with a past diagnosis of hyperactivity disorder (Coons, Klorman & Borgstedt, 1987; Sergeant & Scholten, 1985*a*; Van der Meere & Sergeant, 1987; Van der Meere, Van Baal & Sergeant, 1989).

Consequently, the dual task and the Sternberg task findings demonstrate that hyperactive children have no capacity problem. Methylphenidate studies have likewise indicated that capacity measures, as defined in terms of both the dual task paradigms and the Sternberg paradigm, are not affected by the stimulant drug (De Sonneville *et al.*, 1991; Carlson *et al.*, 1991).

In summary, the majority of studies have failed to demonstrate that children suffering from hyperactivity disorder have an inability in orienting, reorienting, encoding, focused attention, or divided attention. The argument that it is the paradigm itself that may account for the negative findings does not hold, given that cuing techniques (Akhtar & Enns, 1989), distraction tasks (Enns & Girgus, 1985), and capacity measures (Kail, 1990) are sensitive to age. The work in this area has also brought to light information processing deficits in various clinical groups other than those suffering from hyperactivity (for a review, see Sergeant & Van der Meere (1990*a*,*b*)).

Motor-related processes

There is some evidence that task inefficiency of hyperactive children is caused by dysfunctional processes located at the output (motor) side of information processing. Sergeant & Van der Meere (1988) reported that, during a visual search task, hyperactive children corrected their errors as frequently as the control children did but failed to adjust their response speed after a mistake. In a subsequent visual search study by Van der Meere, Van Baal & Sergeant (1989), hyperactive children were instructed to react either in the direction of the target location (i.e. a compatible response), or in the opposite direction from the target location (i.e. an incompatible response). The finding of delayed incompatible responses of hyperactive children was interpreted in terms of a motor decision problem. Also, the finding that presentation rate of stimuli play a crucial role in the attentional performance of children with hyperactivity disorder, points in the direction of a motor-related dysfunction given that motor timing/preparation is more difficult with either a fast or a slow event rate of stimuli. Event rate has been shown to play a crucial role during orientation, reorientation and dichotic listening tasks (discussed above), and in paired associate learning tasks (Conte *et al.*, 1986; Dalby *et al.*, 1977), and visual search tasks (Chee *et al.*, 1989; Van der Meere, Vreeling & Sergeant, 1992; Van der Meere, Stemerdink & Gunning, 1995*a*). Also, the study by Zahn *et al.* (1991), revealed that hyperactive children have difficulties with motor timing/preparation. In this study, reaction times were examined while varying the length and regularity of the preparatory intervals. The results showed that, in the regular series, reaction times were delayed more at long intervals for the hyperactive group. In the irregular series, an additional effect was reported. The findings indicate a greater lack of preparation of the hyperactive group on trials on which a shorter interval is followed by a long interval. Problems of motor timing/preparation of hyperactive children have also been reported by Cappella, Gentile & Juliano (1977).

Since experimental findings point in the direction of an information processing deficiency in hyperactivity disorder being located at the output side of the information processing, it is important to note that a positive influence by methylphenidate on response processes has been demonstrated by Frowein (1981) in adults, and by De Sonneville *et al.* (1991) in children. The 'motor hypothesis' highlights the admonishment by Douglas (1988) that researchers should not neglect the long history of clinical and research interest in motor control deficiencies in hyperactive children. Motor control and impulsivity is the theme of the next section.

MOTOR CONTROL AND IMPULSIVITY

Impulsivity is a loosely defined concept in the literature concerning hyperactivity disorder (Milich & Kramer, 1985; Taylor, 1989). The concept includes, among others, social responsibility, risk-taking and task inappropriate responding (for reviews, see Douglas, 1983, 1988; Barkley, 1990). The present review focuses on the concept of task inappropriate responding.

Many procedures for operationalising impulsivity in terms of task inappropriate responding have been developed in the laboratory. A current operationalisation of impulsivity consists of fast but inaccurate responding on tests such as the matching familiar fgures test, the children's embedded figure test, the Wisconsin card sorting test, the porteuz mazes, the Stroop and errors of commission on the continuous performance test. As stated earlier, these tests are not appropriate measures in describing the mechanisms underlying task inefficiency (defined here as fast but inaccurate responding). That is to say, poor performance on these tests may reflect any combination of poor quality of information processing such as hasty scanning of the stimulus material, rapid decision making or lack of planning, and/or difficulties in response inhibition *per se*. In addition, the test findings are rather inconsistent (for a review, see Barkley, Grodzinsky & Du Paul, 1992). Many information processing studies show that hyperactive children are slow-inaccurate performers rather than fast-inaccurate performers (Van der Meere & Sergeant, 1987, 1988*a*,*b*,*c*; Van der Meere, Van Baal & Sergeant, 1989; Van der Meere, Wekking & Sergeant, 1991; Van der Meere, Vreeling & Sergeant, 1992). Moreover, hyperactive children tend to slow down even when they are asked to perform as quickly as possible (Kalverboer & Brouwer, 1983; Milich & Kramer, 1985; Sergeant & Scholten, 1985*b*; Stevens, Stover & Backus, 1970; Pelham, 1979). Hence, impulsivity defined as fast-inaccurate responding has little validity in hyperactivity disorder.

The ability to withhold responses to distractors

With some exceptions (Ceci & Tisman, 1984; McIntyre, Blackwell & Denton, 1978; Radosh & Gittelman, 1981; Rosenthal & Allen, 1980; Zentall & Shaw, 1980), the plethora of studies using external distractors (radio music, noise, colour discrepancy, peripheral pictures, foils, etc.) have failed to show that hyperactive children are unable to withhold responses to distractors (for reviews, see Douglas, 1983; Van der Meere & Sergeant, 1988*a*). On the contrary, task performance of hyperactive children may even improve in the presence of a distractor (see subsection focused attention). Consequently, the concept of impulsivity, defined in terms of distractibility, has little validity in hyperactivity disorder. In addition, the findings suggest that hyperactive children are able to generate an internal stop signal and subsequently withhold responding, if required.

Ability to inhibit a response after a stop signal

In children suffering from hyperactivity disorder, this ability has been measured using the stop-task of Logan, Cowan & Davis (1984). It involves engaging the subjects in a forced choice letter discrimination task with the need to respond to an occasional stop signal. The signal instructs the subjects to inhibit their response. The main independent variable of the stop task is the interval between the stop signal and response signal. If the stop signal occurs early enough, all subjects are able to inhibit. Plotting the probability of inhibition against the stop signal delay generates an 'inhibition function'. Schachar & Logan (1990*b*) demonstrated that the slope of the inhibition function is much flatter in hyperactive children than in the controls. Inpaired inhibition in hyperactive children is also found on the Go/No-Go task (Trommer *et al.* (1988). Methylphenidate has been shown to improve response inhibition in the stop task (Tannock *et al.*, 1989), and in the Go/No-Go task (Trommer, Hoeppner & Zecker, 1991).

It is questionable whether the stop-task findings reflect an inability to withhold responding in hyperactive children. The stop-signal paradigm assumes a race between the response signal process and the stop signal process. Stopping or responding depends upon which process will win the race. The proportion of responses which escape inhibition increases with the stop signal delay. Consequently, the stop signal findings in studies of hyperactive children may be explained in terms of a slow motor inhibition instead of a failure to inhibit responding *per se*. There are three reasons for assuming that this possibility is more likely. First, there is increasing evidence that children with hyperactivity disorder are slow motor processors (see section one). Secondly, there is increasing evidence that hyperactive children are able to withhold responses to distractors (see above). And, thirdly, experimental findings indicate that hyperactive children, like their peer controls, are able to inhibit automatized responses if they are instructed to do so (Van der Meere & Sergeant, 1988*a*). Further evidence that it is more appropriate to interpret the stop-signal findings in terms of slow motor processing, than inhibition, comes from a recent study of Van der Meere, Stemerdink & Gunning (submitted for publication).

In this study, the author and his colleagues investigated whether children are able to stop and change a response set if required. This executive control function was examined using a variant of Sternberg's memory search paradigm which includes a response bias. The task consisted of two response probability conditions, a baseline condition and a response bias condition. In the baseline condition the target probability was 50%. In the response bias condition the target probability was 30%. Subjects were required to press a 'yes' response button if a target appeared on a screen. Otherwise a 'no' response was required. Specifically, the response bias condition required executive control involving both the ability to adjust a response set towards the most frequent response type, and at the same time being able to stop and change response set if the infrequent response type was required. If hyperactive children lack executive control then fast inaccurate responding would be expected in the response bias condition. This was not the case. The findings indicate that, although slower, children with hyperactivity were comparable with their controls in their ability to stop and change their response set in the response bias condition. Hence, this study gave no indication of hasty scanning or difficulty in 'stop and change' response set in the hyperactive group. This finding is comparable with the findings of the reorienting and dual task experiments, as discussed earlier, which have indicated no problems in switching from one course of action to another.

In a recent study we found that the ability to inhibit a response in ADHD children decreases in conditions with fast and slow presentation rates of stimuli. No problems with responses inhibition were found in a condition with a medium presentation rate (Van der Meere, Stemendink & Gunning, 1995*a*). Hence, again, presentation rate of stimuli is a crucial factor in ADHD.

Ability to withhold responding in order to receive reinforcement

The differential reinforcement of low rate responding (DRL) procedure was devised to measure this construct (Gordon, 1979). In this test the subjects are instructed to respond after a set time interval in order to receive reinforcement. Gordon (1979), and McClure & Gordon (1984), showed that hyperactive children are unable to withhold responding as evidenced by the large number of anticipatory responses. However, Daugherty & Quay (1991), and Loge, Staton & Beatty (1990), reported no differences in DRL performance between hyperactive and normal children. Apart from such inconsistencies in findings, one may question how far the anticipatory responding of hyperactive children totally reflects an inability to delay gratification. If it does, then hyperactive children may be expected to make more anticipatory responses during reinforcement than during response cost conditions. Solanto (1990) showed, however, that the number of anticipatory responses during DRL in hyperactive and in control children is equally affected by reinforcement and response costs. Furthermore, it has been suggested that hyperactive children delay averse responses rather than that they are impulsive or reward maximisers

(Sonuga-Barke *et al.*, 1992). The findings of Roth *et al.* (1991) are also of importance with respect to this issue. In order to measure the efficacy of inhibitory motor processes, they used the delayed motor reaction time task (Leubuscher & Roth, 1983). Like the DRL, this task requires the suppression of an immediate response to an imperative signal. After presentation of a visual signal (white bar) on the video screen, a delayed (800 ms) motor response is required. Correctness of the delay is fed back by auditory signals. The more accurate the delay of the motor response, the smaller the time window becomes (range from 600 to 150 ms). The results indicated that children with signs of allergy (about half of the sample showing symptoms of hyperactivity disorder) performed with less temporal stability than the controls. It is, however, to be noted that since less temporal stability of performance was observed in the absence of reinforcement, the results are at odds with the delayed gratification hypothesis but are compatible with the motor deficiency hypothesis as put forward by the author and his colleagues.

The sensation-seeking component of impulsivity seems to offer a more promising explanation. Daugherty & Quay (1991) administered a response perseverance task and the DRL task to groups of children with hyperactivity and related disorders. The performance of the subjects differed on the perseveration task but not on the DRL. The perseverance task consisted of a series of doors presented sequentially in a pre-programmed order of winning and losing doors. The probability of a winning door appearing decreased by 10% with each succeeding set of ten doors. The dependent measure was the total number of doors opened before giving up. The results supported the hypothesis that subjects suffering from conduct disorder or conduct disorder with hyperactivity would persevere while responding to a game in which the probability of winning decreases as the game is played. For a review of the inability to withhold responding in so-called risk-taking conditions in hyperactivity disorder, see Douglas (1983).

In summary, the studies reviewed seem to indicate that it is rather questionable whether hyperactive children strictly speaking suffer from an inability to withhold responses. Given the findings that hyperactive children are delayed in their response-related processes, it may be concluded that the motor hypothesis is not covered by the impulsivity concept of fast-inaccurate responding. The author and his colleague Sergeant, (Sergeant & Van der Meere, 1989; Sergeant & Van der Meere, 1990*a,b*), have argued that a state regulation problem may account for loss of motor control. The findings of Daugherty & Quay (1991) may also be interpreted in terms of a state-regulation dysfunction. The concept of state-regulation dysfunction in children suffering from hyperactivity disorder is the theme of the next section.

THE CONCEPT OF STATE

A non-optimal arousal state has a long tradition as a physiological mechanism underlying hyperactivity (for reviews, see Douglas, 1983, 1988). According to this theory, in order to normalise their arousal level, hyperactive children require stimulants, benefit from extraneous distraction and are sensation seekers (Zentall & Zentall, 1983). It, however, requires to be pointed out here that the 'unitary state' concept in cognitive psychology has in the past been criticised for the following two main reasons. First, the uni-dimensionality and non-specificity of arousal cannot explain the lack of correlation between different measures of energy mobilisation. Secondly, the unitary state concept of arousal gives no clarification of the different patterns of autonomic activity observed in subjects during different tasks (Lacey, 1967). This dissatisfaction has led to the postulation of a variety of cognitive multi-state models. Although there remain a fundamental set of questions concerning the basis of energetical constructs in psychophysiology, anatomy and biochemistry of the brain and the nervous system (Hockey *et al.*, 1986), there are strong arguments for distinguishing arousal and activation as different physiological states. Tucker & Williamson (1984) have suggested that arousal and activation are concerned, respectively, with the alerting effect of sensory activity and the control of motor readiness. Arousal is located in the fronto-limbic forebrain and activation in the basal ganglia (Pribram & McGuinness, 1975). Important neurotransmitters in the arousal system are noradrenaline and serotonin. The primary neurotransmitters in the activation system are dopamine and acetylcholine (Tucker & Williamson, 1984). In addition, arousal and activation are affected by different drugs, e.g. barbiturates affect arousal whereas amphetamine affects activation (Frowein, 1981).

Pribram & McGuinness (1975), Mulder (1986) and Sanders (1983), have postulated a third energetic system, i.e. the effort system. This system, in turn, is under the control of an evaluation system (Sanders, 1983). The latter mechanism scans the subject's arousal and activation state. A suboptimal state as identified by the evaluation mechanism may be compensated for by effort. The hippocampus is believed to be involved in such compensatory control (Gray, 1982; Pribram & McGuinness, 1975). The effort mechanism is influenced by motivational factors such as knowledge of results, absence–presence of the experimenter and pay-off. Figure 4.1 presents the Sanders model.

The model has received support from the results of neural network simulation studies (Molenaar & Van der Molen, 1986), developmental studies (Van der Molen, 1990), and psychophysiological studies (Mulder, 1986) (see also

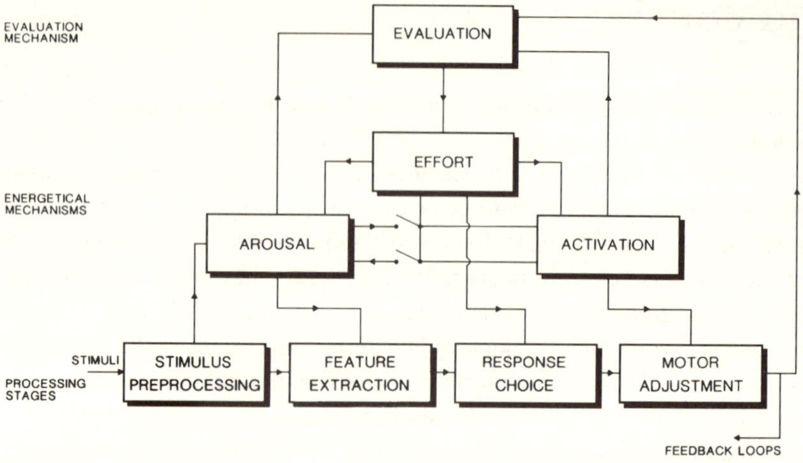

Fig. 4.1

p. 135). Therefore, the multi-state approach may be of great value in future studies since it may help to specify the assumed cognitive deficits in hyperactivity disorder (Sergeant & Van der Meere, 1989, 1990*a*;*b*).

Using the model of Sanders (see Fig. 4.1), task inefficiency in children with hyperactivity disorder may be considered to be caused by limitations located at the elementary level of information processing, or at the state level, or in a combination of both levels. In the first section of this chapter, a variety of tasks considered to measure the efficiency of information processing at the first level of the model were discussed. These tasks are characterised by short duration, lack of use of incentives, and by children working in the presence of an experimenter. Hence, it may be assumed that, in these experiments, the influence of state factors has been kept as constant as possible. The evidence available so far suggests that hyperactive children have a deficit on the motor side of the information processing chain. The motor processing deficit manifests itself as slow-inaccurate responding, instead of fast-inaccurate responding. These are unexpected findings in so-called impulsive children (see p. 123). Consequently, another explanation is needed to account for the hypothesised motor processing dysfunction in hyperactive children. The author believes that the postulation of deficit in the regulation of activation/effort is a good working hypothesis. As can be seen from Fig. 4.1, the Sanders model connects motor processes with the effort/activation state of the subject. Hence, in terms of the model, it is possible that the motor dysfunction in hyperactive children actually involves an activation/effort dysfunction. This would mean that hyperactive children respond slowly and inaccurately because of a 'state' condition which is inadequate. Four types of state manipulations will be discussed: time-on-task, presentation rate of stimuli, pay-off and absence–presence of the experimenter.

Sustained attention

A deficit in sustained attention is considered to be the prime characteristic of hyperactivity disorder (Douglas 1983; 1988). The consistent finding of poor performance on a continuous performance test (CPT), characterised by the detection of fewer targets and more omissions, is generally considered as proof of the assumed sustained attention deficit. However, as the author has pointed out elswhere (Van der Meere & Sergeant, 1988*b*), the main argument against this interpretation is that an 'overall' CPT performance difference between hyperactive and control children is not sufficient for validation, since a sustained attention deficit implies a deficit originating during the course of the task. Consequently, a sustained attention deficit is demonstrated only when hyperactive children show a greater decline in performance over a period of time than do the controls.

According to the literature on vigilance, (for a review, see Van der Meere & Sergeant, 1988*b*), there are two different types of sustained attention deficits, depending on whether time-on-task exerts its influence on arousal or activation. The factor considered responsible for the performance decline depends in turn on the task parameters of the vigil. If the subject is required to discriminate a target from a non-target represented in working memory at a high event rate, then arousal is affected. If few working memory processes are involved, and the event rate is low, the performance decrement is thought to result from changes in the activation level.

CPTs with a fast event rate of stimuli

So far, the majority of CPT studies in hyperactivity disorder have employed a high event rate. Hence, in terms of the vigilance paradigm these studies have tested the arousal hypothesis. With four exceptions (Dykman, Ackerman & Oglesby, 1979; Hooks, Milich & Pugzles Lorch, 1994; Sykes, Douglas & Morgenstern, 1973; Seidel & Joschko, 1990), the plethora of studies show that in a wide variety of prolonged tasks, initial differences in task accuracy between hyperactive children and controls are present right from the beginning. However, even more important is the finding that hyperactive children do not differ from the controls in terms of decline in task performance in the course of the task (McLaren, 1990; Leung & Connolly, 1994; Michael *et al.*, 1981; Nuechterlein, 1983; O'Dougherty *et al.*, 1988; O'Dougherty, Neuchterlein & Drew, 1984; Kupietz, 1990, Prior *et al.*, 1985; Schachar *et al.*, 1988; Sergeant, 1988*b*; Solanto, Wender & Lynch, 1990; Van der Meere & Sergeant, 1988*b*). The findings of Rapoport *et al.* (1980) are also noteworthy with respect to this issue. They reported a comparable time decrement effect and improvement in performance by D-amphetamine in hyperactive, control children and college students over time. Hence, according to the model of Sanders, hyperactive children do not suffer from a sustained attention deficit in terms of an inadequate arousal state.

So far, sustained attention abilities have been discussed in terms of the extent of decline in task efficiency over time under conditions with a fast presentation rate of stimuli. However, also the finding that in conditions with a fast presentation rate of stimuli, hyperactive children and controls do not differ in either the rate of acquisition of a divided attention skill in a testing period of six hours (Van der Meere & Sergeant, 1988*c*), nor in the rate of changing that skill measured in focused attention conditions (Van der Meere & Sergeant, 1988*a*), is at odds with the assumed sustained attention deficit in hyperactivity disorder. Furthermore, also school-like paper and pencil tasks which are self-paced have failed to differentiate between hyperactive and normal children in terms of performance decline in the course of the task (Gunning, 1992; Van der Meere, Wekking & Sergeant, 1991).

CPTs with a slow presentation rate of stimuli

The author and his colleagues have tested the underactivation hypothesis in hyperactivity disorder using a slow event rate vigilance task. In our first experiment, the task was performed during experimenter present and experimenter absent conditions. Two hypotheses were proposed. First, if hyperactive children have a sustained attention deficit, they will exhibit a greater decrement in performance over time than the control group. Secondly, if motivational factors are responsible for the deficit, the decrement in task performance will be minimal during the experimenter present condition and maximal during the experimenter absent condition. Both hypotheses were confirmed in this experiment. That is to say, the sustained attention deficit was prominent in hyperactive children especially while working in the absence of the experimenter. This finding supports the under-activation/effort hypothesis in hyperactivity disorder and underlines the need for external control in such children (see Barkley, 1991).

The same study demonstrated that the deficit disappears when hyperactive children are placed on methylphenydate (MPH) medication (Van der Meere *et al.*, 1995*a*, *b*, *c*). Studies by Draeger, Prior & Sanson (1986), and Power (1992) have likewise reported that task efficiency (and activity) level of hyperactive children is sensitive for experimenter presence/absence. However, the drawback of the former study was that it did not examine the effects of experimenter presence and absence over a non-interrupted period of time. The latter study did not include a control group, and hence, it cannot be known if the reported findings are specific for hyperactivity disorder. Recently, Gomez and Sanson (1994) compared attentional performance of hyperactive children with and without CD on a cancellation task under three conditions: when performing the task alone, with mother present and with the experimenter present. Results indicated that attentional scores of hyperactive children with CD were normalized when the experimenter was present; this was not so marked for hyperactive children without CD. Unfortunately, no reference was made concerning time-on-task, but also this study underlines the importance of external control in hyperactivity.

In a second experiment of the author and his colleagues, hyperactive children with and without conduct disorder (CD) were compared on the slow event rate vigilance task, performed under reward and non-reward conditions. Both groups of children were receiving medication: MPH was the predominant medication in the pure hyperactive group, whereas tricyclics, lithium and carbamazepine were more frequently used in the mixed group. The results indicated that, in spite of the active treatment, the children suffering from the mixed disorder showed a deficit of sustained attention in the non-reward condition. In the reward condition the deficit disappeared for a short period of time. This finding suggests that children with a mixed hyperactivity-conduct disorder suffer from an activation/effort disturbance. No difference in task performance was found between children with a pure hyperactivity disorder and the controls. It can therefore be argued that MPH improved the CPT performance of the hyperactive children to the level found in normal children (Van der Meere *et al.*, 1995*a*, *b*, *c*).

In summary, the answer to the question of whether the CPT is a valuable research tool for use with children with ADHD (see Corkum & Siegel, 1993), depends on a few factors. The evidence available so far indicates that hyperactive children do not suffer from a sustained attention deficit in prolonged task conditions when stimuli are presented at a high rate of sequence, or when the children are allowed to adapt their own speed of performing. According to the model of Sanders, these negative findings do not support the presence of an arousal deficiency in hyperactivity disorder. However, a sustained attention deficit does emerge in hyperactive children in CPT conditions when a slow presentation rate is used. In children with hyperactivity minus CD, this is especially the case in conditions of experimenter absence. In children with a mixed hyperactivity and conduct disorder this is especially the case in the absence of reward. According to the model of Sanders, the positive findings are in favour of a non-optimal activation state as a physiological basis of hyperactivity disorder. They also support the idea that the motor hypothesis in hyperactive children, as discussed in section one, is in fact reflecting a non-optimal activation state. So far, the focus has been on changes of task accuracy over time. The theme of the next section is changes of activity level over time.

Unfortunately, observational studies of hyperactive children's behaviour during CPT are scarce. Sykes *et al.* (1971) reported an increased restlessness between first and second test sessions in hyperactive children when compared to controls. Their results seem to suggest that hyperactive children are more restless when required to perform the same task twice. It is, however, not possible to know whether the increased activity in the second session was due to difficulties in sustained attention or due to differences in recovery of activity level between the sessions. Draeger *et al.* (1986) reported that, in the absence of the experimenter, task accuracy was lower and activity level higher in the hyperactive group. Unfortunately, the activity level was not measured within a non-interrupted condition, but as in the Sykes *et al.* study, between successive conditions. Hence, studies have failed to show that hyperactive children become more restless in the course of a non-interrupted period. Alberts & Van der Meere (1992) presented behavioural observation data of hyperactive and control children during a 36-minute CPT task. Five categories of body activity were measured: auto-manipulations, arm, leg and trunk movements, and position shifts. Visual behaviour was measured in terms of frequency and duration of looking away from the screen. The data indicated that bodily activity tended to be more pronounced in hyperactive children than in controls. More important, however, was the finding that both groups showed the same increase in body movements and the same decrease in task efficiency in the course of the experiment. However, in the course of the experiment, hyperactive children did start to look away more frequently from the monitor than the controls did. An analysis of the temporal relations between (the onset and offset of) periods of looking away and the occurrence of omission errors indicated that looking away did not negatively interfere with the task performance. The authors speculated that looking away from the screen may have reflected self-stimulation in order to compensate for the assumed non-optimal activation state of hyperactive children.

To summarise the evidence dealt with so far, it is to be noted that task performance of hyperactive children is sensitive to event rate manipulations during tasks involving orienting, reorienting dichotic listening, paired associate learning and visual search as pointed out in the first section of this chapter. Also the CPT findings, discussed above, indicate that event rate is a crucial factor in the performance of hyperactive children. These findings together with behavioural observations lead to the suggestion that hyperactive children have a non-optimal activation /effort state: their task performance decreases when the stimulus rate or event rate decreases or when the experimenter is absent, and conversely, their task performance increases when the presentation rate of stimuli increases or when the experimenter is sitting beside the child, or when the child is placed on methylphenidate. Using a metaphor, the engine is intact (i.e. the basic information processing capacity is intact), but there is a problem with the supply of petrol (i.e. the utilisation of the cognitive capacity depends on state factors such as incentives, event rate and presence/absence of the experimenter, etc.). Consequently, this review strongly supports the sensation-seeking concept as a relevant factor in hyperactivity disorder as formulated by Zentall & Zentall (1983), and the suggestion made by Douglas & Peters (1979), that hyperactive children have an inability to modulate their physiological state according to task and situation demands. However, the concept of a 'non-optimal state' in hyperactivity disorder, as put forward by the author and his co-workers, differs in an important way from its previous definitions in that it is more precisely based on the theoretical model by Sanders. That is, slow and inaccurate responses of hyperactive children are caused by an non-optimal activation/effort state which manifests itself in slow motor preparation and execution processes.

So far, the review has largely concentrated on interpreting the research on inattention in terms of reaction time measures (the second generation of cognitive tests). How far the non-optimal activation state in hyperactivity disorder is supported by psychophysiological measures (the third generation of cognitive tests), is the topic of the next section.

PSYCHOPHYSIOLOGICAL MEASURES

Evoked potentials

It has been claimed that various (endogenous) components of the evoked reaction on potentials (ERP) reflect more precisely the timing and duration of cognitive processing than does reaction on time (RT) (Mulder, 1986). Four components which are important in hyperactivity disorder will be discussed here: the N2, P3b, CNV and the Nd. The N2 is a negative peak starting around 200 msec after stimulus onset. Two negative components can be distinguished in this range: the MMN and the N2b (Naatanen & Gaillard, 1983). The MMN is modality specific and reflects an automatic mismatch process between input and template. The N2b is not modality specific and occurs only when the stimulus is attended to. It has been suggested that this component reflects an early process related to sensory encoding (Van Dellen *et al.*, 1984).

The P3b latency indexes the stimulus evaluation time and is relatively independent of response selection and production (Brookhuis *et al.*, 1981; Mulder *et al.*, 1984). The CNV is a slow negative shift, developing over the foreperiod of a stimulus presentation and consists of two negative components: the early CNV or O(rientation)-wave, and the terminal CNV or E(expectancy)-wave (Gaillard, 1977; 1978). The terminal CNV seems to reflect the level of motor preparation and is similar to the readiness (bereitschafts) potential preceding voluntary movements (Deecke, Grozinger & Kornhuber, 1976). The Nd is obtained by subtracting ERPs to unattended stimuli from ERPs to attended stimuli. The Nd also contains two separate components: an early phase (Nde) with a sensory specific maximum and a later phase (Ndl) with a more anterior (frontal) distribution (Naatanen & Michie, 1979). This Ndl may reflect the further ongoing stimulus evaluation.

In an extension of Sanders' model, Mulder (1986) considers amplitude variations as measures of arousal, effort, and activation. Peak latencies are measures of the duration of basic (input, central and output) processing. For a critical discussion of Mulders' model, presented in Fig. 4.2, the reader is refered to Kok (1990).

The RT research has directed us to an output-activation/effort-related problem in the hyperactive child. This section deals with different measures thought to reflect arousal, activation and effort in an attempt to assess whether conclusions based on RT measures hold for electrophysiological measures in terms of Mulder's model.

The (input) arousal hypothesis

Grunewald-Zuberbier, Grunewald & Rasche (1975) and Grunewald -Zuberbier *et al.* (1978) reported a great alpha attenuation (i.e. measure of phasic arousal) after warning signals in hyperactive children. In addition, smaller N2 amplitudes have also been reported (Camman, 1985; Satterfied & Braley, 1977; Satterfield & Schell, 1984; Satterfield *et al.*, 1988). Moeover, Satterfield *et al.*, (1988) reported an abnormal processing negativity (Nd) in hyperactivity

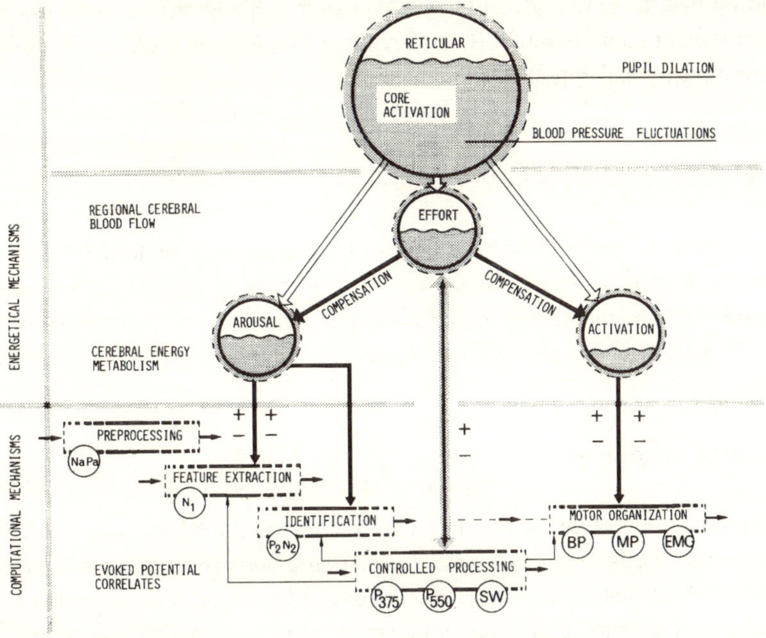

Fig. 4.2

disorder. Larger negative slow waves over frontal sites in children with attentional problems were reported by Friedman *et al.* (1986). Given these findings, an (arousal) selective attention deficit may not be excluded from further consideration.

The (output) activation hypothesis

A series of ERP studies point in the direction of an output related dysfunction in hyperactivity disorder. With some exceptions (Brumaghim *et al.*, 1987; Holcomb, Ackerman & Dykman, 1985; Loiselle *et al.*, 1980), the majority of studies indicate that hyperactive and control children differ with respect to post-P3b (motor-related) processes. In addition, these studies show that methylphenidate affects post-P3b processes (Brumaghim *et al.*, 1987; Callaway, 1983; 1984; Coons, Klorman & Borgsted, 1987; Coons *et al.*, 1981; Hink *et al.*, 1978; Fitzpatrick *et al.*, 1988; Klorman *et al.*, 1979; Peloquin & Klorman, 1986).

With respect to CNV findings, it appeared that hyperactive children have a smaller CNV after a warning signal (Grunewald-Zuberbier *et al.*, 1978). The finding that the amplitude of the CNV (motor preparation) has been increased by stimulant administration (Coons *et al.*, 1981; Kopell *et al.*, 1974) confirms the output-related hypothesis.

The effort hypothesis

The consistent finding that hyperactive children have a smaller P3b amplitude (Holcomb *et al.*, 1986; Loiselle *et al.*, 1980), is consistent with the effort hypothesis. The fact that methylphenidate increases the P3b amplitude (Coons *et al.*, 1981; Strauss *et al.*, 1984; Michael *et al.*, 1981) confirms this hypothesis.

Cardiac response

In the period between the warning and the imperative signal, a triphasic heart rate response has been observed. This response consists of an initial deceleration followed first by an acceleration and then by a second deceleration which reaches a minimum at the time of presentation of the reaction time signal. It is suggested that this final cardiac deceleration is related to both stimulus anticipation and motor preparation. The anticipatory deceleration has been extensively studied to investigate preparatory processes in information processing tasks (for reviews, see Pribram & McGuinness, 1975; Van der Molen *et al.*, 1987). A smaller anticipatory deceleration in combination with a normalisation of the cardiac response after the administration of methylphenidate has been reported in hyperactivity and related disorders (Dykman *et al.*, 1983; O'Dougherty *et al.*, 1988; Porges *et al.*, 1980; Porges *et al.*, 1975; Sroufe *et al.*, 1973; Zahn *et al.*, 1978).

Neurochemical level

Neurochemical studies lend further support to the motor output deficiency hypothesis in hyperactivity. The basal ganglia, particularly the corpus striatum, are involved in the organisation of motor behaviour (activation) (Mulder, 1986; Sanders, 1983). Most of the brain's dopamine is found within the nigrostriatal system and both dopamine and norepinephrine are associated with fronto-striatal circuits (Tucker & Williamson, 1984). There is evidence that hyperactivity is associated with a dysfunction of the fronto-striatal system. Neurochemical studies have led to explanations of hyperactivity that are based on dysfunction of monoaminergic systems, especially dopamine (Shaywitz, Cohen & Bowers, 1977) and perhaps to a lesser extent norepinephrine (Zametkin & Rapaport, 1987). (See also Sagvolden & Archer, 1989.) Schneider & Roeltgen (1991) observed poor attention and hyperactivity in animals who received chronic low doses (CLD) of 1-methyl-4-phenyl-1,2,3,6,-tetrahydropyridine (MPTP). MPTP is a neurotoxin that selectively damages dopaminergic innervation of the dorsal striatum and disrupts the functioning of the fronto-striatal axis. A reduced glucose metabolism of the striatum has been reported in children with hyperactivity disorder (Lou, Henrikson & Bruhn, 1990; Lou *et al.*, 1989). (See also Zametkin, Nordahl & Gross, 1990 for further discussion on this issue.)

However, altered metabolism of serotonin which is an important neurotransmitter in the arousal system (Tucker & Williamson, 1984) has also been suggested as a potential aetiology of hyperactivity (Zametkin & Rapoport, 1987). Thus, an altered metabolism of a single neurotransmitter does not seem an adequate explanation of hyperactivty.

In summary, the interpretation of evoked potentials and heart rate studies in terms of Mulder's model leads to the conclusion of an activation-effort dysfunction in hyperactivity. However, the arousal hypothesis is not to be dismissed. Also neurochemical studies point in the direction of an output-related dysfunction (i.e. a dysfunction of monoaminergic systems), but again, the arousal hypothesis (i.e. an altered metabolism of serotonin) is not to be dismissed.

EPILOGUE

There is growing evidence that hyperactive children are delayed in cognitive processes just preceding the overt motor action, i.e. response decision and response organisation processes. It is probably of interest to the present argument that the later a cognitive stage is in the suggested sequence of cognitive stages, the more its active processes refer to 'presetting the stage' prior to the presentation of the stimulus (Sanders, 1983). Hence, the output-related processing disturbance may hinder the hyperactive child also in the execution of so-called input-related processes such as orientation and re-orientation.

An attempt has been made here to explain the output hypothesis in terms of a state regulation (activation and effort) problem. This regulation problem is demonstrated especially during slow event rate tasks, and may be reduced by manipulating both external control and motivation (incentives). However, the term state regulation is still loosely defined and deserves more investigation using a chain of approaches: the behavioral observation approach, the reaction time approach, together with the electrophysiological and neurochemical approach. In addition, the term may be unspecific. By this it is meant that cognitive dysfunctions found in clinical groups other than those involving hyperactivity, may also be explained in terms of a dysfunction in the energetical regulation of motor control (Sergeant & Van der Meere, 1990*a*). Further research, especially that based on longitudinal data, is needed to help clarify these issues. The present theoretical review of the role of attention in hyperactivity disorder can hopefully be used to make specific predictions about the patterns of deficits encountered.

The final question to answer is how to relate the laboratory findings as reviewed here with the clinical concept of hyperactivity disorder. The diagnostic label is derived from behavioural descriptions by parents, teachers and clinicians which are highly subjective and imprecise. Laboratory findings show that children with a so-called attention deficit are able to orient, re-orient, divide and focus their attention. In addition, such children do not differ from controls with respect to the rate of the acquisition of attentional skills. These are unexpected findings in children with a so-called attention deficit. However, laboratory findings indicate that task efficiency of hyperactive children is highly sensitive to state manipulations, such as presentation rate and external control. So, the first conclusion to be drawn is that the diagnostic term is incorrect and should be changed to the label of (S)tate (R)egulation (D)eficit. Whether this state regulation deficit is due to a suboptimal arousal, activation or effort level is an important issue, but the issue is unimportant with respect to this conclusion.

The second conclusion to be drawn is that we may present the parents and teachers with the wrong questions. The question is not whether a hyperactive child is easily distracted or not, or whether the child is able to sustain his/her attention for a long period. The question is whether the symptoms of hyperactivity disorder emerge in conditions which are believed to tap the state of the child. The author's experience with parents of hyperactive children is that they describe that the symptoms are manifestated in boring conditions. Thus their claim is that if the child is really motivated, the symptoms will disappear. Such a description perfectly fits the majority of laboratory findings. In summary, the trait of the hyperactive child is his state regulation deficit!

REFERENCES

Abikoff, H. Szeibel, P.J. & Courtney, M.E. (1990). The effects of auditory distractors on the academic performance of ADHD and normal boys. Poster Presented at the Annual Meeting of the American Academy of Child and Adolescent Psychiatry, Chicago, Ill.

Akhtar, N. & Enns, J.T. (1989). Relations between covert orienting and filtering in the development of visual attention. *Journal of Experimental Child Psychology,* **48**, 315–34.

Alberts, E. & Van der Meere, J.J. (1992). Observations of hyperactive behaviour during vigilance. *Journal of Child Psychology and Psychiatry*, **33**, 1355–64.

Ballinger, C.T., Varley, C.K. & Nolen, P.A. (1984). Effects of methylphenidate on reading in children with attention deficit disorder. *American Journal of Psychiatry,* **141**, 1590–3.

Balthazor, M., Wagner, R.K. & Pelham, W.E. (1991). The specificity of the effects of stimulant medication on classroom learning-related measures of cognitive processing for attention deficit disorder children. *Journal of Abnormal Child Psychology,* **19**, 35–52.

Barkley, R.A. (1982). Guidelines for defining hyperactivity in children. In *Advances in Clinical Child Psychology,* Vol. 5, eds. B.B. Lahey & A.E. Kazdin, pp. 95–137. New York: Plenum Publishing Corporation.

Barkley, R.A. (1990). *Attention Deficit Hyperactivity Disorder. A Handbook for Diagnosis and Treatment.* New York: The Guilford Press.

Barkley, R.A. (1991). The ecological validity of laboratory and analogue assessment methods of ADHD symptoms. *Journal of Abnormal Child Psychology,* **19**, 149–78.

Barkley, R.A., Grodzinsky, G. & Du Paul, G.J. (1992). Frontal lobe functions in attention deficit disorder with and without hyperactivity: a review and research report. *Journal of Abnormal Psychology,* **20**, 163–88.

Benezra, E. & Douglas, V.I. (1988). Short-term serial recall in ADDH, normal, and reading disabled boys. *Journal of Abnormal Child Psychology,* **16**, 511–26.

Borcherding, B., Thompson, K., Kruesi, M., Bartko, J., Rapoport, J.L. & Weingartner, H. (1988). Automatic and effortful processing in attention deficit hyperactivity disorder. *Journal of Abnormal Child Psychology,* **16**, 333–46.

Brookhuis, K.A., Mulder, G., Mulder, L.J.M., Gloerich, A.B.M., van Dellen, H.J., van der Meere, J.J. & Ellermann, H.H. (1981). Late positive components and stimulus evaluation time. *Biological Psychology*, **13**, 107–23.

Browning, R.M. (1967). Effects of irrelevant peripheral visual stimuli in minimally brain damaged children. *Journal of Consulting Psychology,* **31**, 371–6.

Brumaghim, J.T., Klorman, R., Strauss, J., Lewine, J.D. & Goldstein, M.G. (1987). Does methylphenidate affect information processing? Findings from two studies on performance and P3b latency. *Psychophysiology,* **24**, 361–73.

Burke, R.S. (1990). A cognitive-developmental approach to studying attention deficits. In *The development of Attention: Research and Theory*, ed. J.T. Enns, pp. 365–81. North-Holland: Elsevier Science Publishers BV.

Callaway, E. (1983). The pharmacology of human information processing. *Psychophysiology,* **20**, 359–70.

Callaway, E. (1984). Human information-processing: some effects of methylphenidate, age, and scopolamine. *Biological Psychiatry,* **19**, 649–62.

Camman, F. (1985). Evoked potentials in children with impaired and normal powers of concentration. In *Psychophysiological Approaches to Human Information Processing*, eds. F. Klix., R. Neetenen & K. Zimmer, pp. 269-78. North Holland: Elsevier Science Publishers BV.

Campbell, S.B., Endman, M.W. & Bernfeld, G. (1977). A three-year follow-up of hyperactive preschoolers into elementary school. *Journal of Child Psychology and Psychiatry,* **18**, 239–50.

Cappella, B., Gentile, J.R. & Juliano, D.B. (1977). Time estimation by hyperactive and normal children. *Perceptual and Motor Skills,* **44**, 787.

Carlson, C.L., Pelham, W.E., Swanson, J.M. & Wagner, J.L. (1991). A divided attention analysis of the effects of methylphenidate on the arithmetic performance of children with attention deficit hyperactivity disorder. *Journal of Child Psychology and Psychiatry,* **32**, 463–71.

Ceci, S.J. & Tisman, J. (1984). Hyperactivity and incidental memory: evidence for attentional diffusion. *Child Development,* **55**, 2192–203.

Chee, P., Logan, G., Schachar, R., Lindsay, P. & Wachsmuth, R. (1989). Effects of event rate and display time on sustained attention in hyperactive, normal, and control children. *Journal of Abnormal Child Psychology,* **17**, 371–91.

Cohen, N.J. & Minde, K. (1983). The hyperactive syndrome in kindergarten children: comparison of children with pervasive and situational symptoms. *Journal of Child Psychology and Psychiatry,* **24**, 443–55.

Conte, R., Kinsbourne, M., Swanson, J., Zirk, H. & Samuels, M. (1986). Presentation rate effects on paired associate learning by attention deficit disordered children. *Child Development,* **57**, 681–87.

Coons, H.W., Klorman, R. & Borgstedt, A.D. (1987). Effect of methylphenidate on adolescents with a childhood history of attention deficit disorder: 2. *Journal of the American Academy of Child Psychiatry,* **26**, 368–74.

Coons, H.W., Peloquin, L.J., Klorman, R., Ryan, R.M., Bauer, L.O., Perlmutter, R.A. & Salzman, L.F. (1981). Effects of methylphenidate on young adults vigilance and event-related potentials. *Electroencephalography and Clinical Neurophysiology,* **51**, 373–87.

Corkum, P.V. & Siegel, L.S. (1993). Is the continuous performance task a valuable research tool for use with children with attention deficit hyperactivity disorder? *Journal of Child Psychology and Psychiatry*, **34**, 1217–39.

Craik, F.I.M. & Lockhart, R.S. (1972). Levels of processing: a framework for memory research. *Journal of Verbal Learning and Verbal Behavior,* **11**, 671–84.

Dalby, D.T., Kinsbourne, M., Swanson, J.M. & Sobel, M.P. (1977). Hyperactive children's use of learning time: correlation by stimulant treatment. *Child Development,* **48**, 1448–53.

Daugherty, T.K. & Quay, H.C. (1991). Response pervasiveness and delayed responding in childhood behavior disorders. *Journal of Child Psychology and Psychiatry,* **32**, 453–61.

Davidson, E.M. & Prior, M.R. (1978). Laterality and selective attention in hyperactive children. *Journal of Abnormal Child Psychology,* **6**, 475–81.

Deecke, L., Grozinger, B. & Kornhuber, H.H. (1976). Voluntary finger movement in man: cerebral potentials and theory. *Biological Cybernetics,* **23**, 99–119.

De Sonneville, L.M.J., Njiokiktjien, C. & Hilhorst, R.C. (1991). Methylphenidate-induced changes in ADDH information processors. *Journal of Child Psychology and Psychiatry,* **32**, 285–95.

Dienske, H. & Sanders-Woudstra, J.A.R. (1988). A critical and conceptual consideration of attention deficit and hyperactivity from an ethological point of view. In *Attention Deficit Disorder: Criteria, Cognition, Intervention*, eds. L.M. Bloomingdale & J.A. Sergeant, pp. 43–64. Oxford: Pergamon Press.

Douglas, V.I. (1983). Attentional and cognitive problems. In *Developmental Neuropsychiatry,* ed. M. Rutter, pp. 280–328. New York: Guilford Press.

Douglas, V.I. (1988). Cognitive deficits in children with attention disorder with hyperactivity. In *Attention Deficit Disorder: Criteria, Cognition, Intervention*, ed. L.M. Bloomingdale & J.A. Sergeant, pp. 65-83. Oxford: Pergamon Press.

Douglas, V.I. & Benezra, E. (1990). Supraspan verbal memory in attention deficit disorder with hyperactivity normal and reading disabled boys. *Journal of Abnormal Child Psychology,* **18**, 617–38.

Douglas, V.I. & Peters, K.G. (1979). Toward a clearer definition of the attentional deficit of hyperactive children. In *Attention and the Development of Cognitive Skills*, eds. G.A. Hale & M. Lewis, pp. 173–247. New York: Plenum Press.

Draeger, S., Prior, M.R. & Sanson, A.V. (1986). Visual and auditory attention performance in hyperactive children: competence or compliance. *Journal of Abnormal Child Psychology,* **14**, 411–24.

Dykman, R.A., Ackerman, P.T., Holcomb, P.J. & Boudreau, A.Y. (1983). Physiological manifestations of learning disabilities. *Journal of Learning Disabilities,* **16**, 46–53.

Dykman, R.A., Ackerman, M.A. & Oglesby, D.M. (1979). Selective and sustained attention in learning disabled and normal boys. *Journal of Nervous and Mental Disease,* **167**, 288–97.

Enns, J.T. & Girgus, J.S. (1985). Developmental changes in selective and integrative visual attention. *Journal of Experimental Child Psychology,* **40**, 319–337.

Fitzpatrick, P., Klorman, R., Brumaghim, J.T. & Keefover, R.W. (1988). Effects of methylphenidate on stimulus evaluation and response processes: Evidence from performance and event-related potentials. *Psychophysiology,* **25**, 292–304.

Friedman, D., Cornblatt, B. Vaughan, H. & Erlenmeyer-Kimling, L. (1986). Event–related potentials in children at risk for schizophrenia during two versions of the continuous performance test. *Psychiatric Research,* **18**, 161–77.

Frowein, H.W. (1981). Selective drug effects on information processing. Thesis, Enschede: Sneldruk Boulevard.

Gaillard, A.W.K. (1977). The late CNV wave: preparation versus expectancy. *Psychophysiology,* **14**, 563–68.

Gaillard, A.W.K. (1988). The evaluation of drug effects in laboratory tasks. In *Psychopharmacology and Reaction Time,* eds. I. Hindmarch, B. Aufdembrinke & H. Ott, pp. 15–24. Chichester: John Wiley and Sons.

Gittelman, R. (1988). The assessment of hyperactivity: The DSM-III approach. In *Attention Deficit Disorder: Criteria, Cognition, Intervention*, eds. L.M. Bloomingdale & J.A. Sergeant, pp. 9–29. Oxford: Pergamon Press.

Gomez, R. & Sanson, A.V. (1994). Effects of experimenter and mother presence on the attentional performance and activity of hyperactive boys. *Journal of Abnormal Child Psychology*, **22**, 517–29.

Gordon, M. (1979). The assessment of impulsivity and mediating behaviors in hyperactive and nonhyperactive children. *Journal of Abnormal Child Psychology,* **7**, 317-26.

Gray, J.A. (1982). *The Neurophysiology of Anxiety. An Enquiry into the Functions of the Septo-Hippocampal System.* New York: Oxford University Press.

Grunewald Zuberbier, E., Grunewald, G. & Rasche, A. (1975). Hyperactive behavior and EEG arousal reactions in children. *Electroencephalography and Clinical Neurophysiology,* **38**, 149–59.

Grunewald-Zuberbier, E., Grunewald, G., Rasche, A. & Netz, J. (1978). Contingent negative variation and alpha attenuation responses in children with different abilities to concentrate. *Electroencephalography and Clinical Neurophysiology,* **44**, 37–47.

Gunning, B. (1992). A controlled trial of clonidine in hyperkinetic children. Thesis. Erasmus University Rotterdam.

Hink, R.F., Fenton, W.H., Tinklenberg, J.R., Pfefferbaum, A. & Kopell, B.S. (1978). Vigilance and human attention under conditions of methylphenidate and secobarbital intoxication. *Psychophysiology,* **15**, 116–25.

Hockey, G.R.J., Coles, M.G.H. & Gaillard, A.W.K. (1986). Energetical issues in research on human information processing. In *Energetics and Human Information Processing*, eds. G.R.J. Hockey, A.W.K. Gaillard & M.G.H. Coles, pp. 3–22. Dordrecht: Martinus Nijhoff Publishers.

Holcomb, J.P., Ackerman, P.T. & Dykman, R.A. (1985). Cognitive event related brain potentials in children with attention and reading deficits. *Psychophysiology,* **6**, 656–67.

Holcomb, P.J., Ackerman, P.T. & Dykman, R.A. (1986). Auditory event related potentials in attention and reading disabled boys. *International Journal of Psychophysiology,* **3**, 263–73.

Hooks, K., Milich, R. & Pugzles Lorch, E. (1994). Sustained and selective attention in boys with attention deficit hyperactivity disorder. *Journal of Clinical Child Psychology*, **23**, 69–77.

Kail, R. (1990). More evidence for a common, central constraint on speed of processing. In *The Development of Attention Research and Theory*, ed. J.T. Enns, pp. 159–173. North Holland: Elsevier Science Publishers B.V.

Kalverboer, A.F. (1988). Hyperactivity and observational studies. In *Attention Deficit Disorder. Criteria, Cognition, Intervention*, eds. L.M. Bloomingdale & J.A. Sergeant, pp. 29–42. Oxford: Pergamon Press.

Kalverboer, A.F. (1990). Introduction: developmental biopsychology and the study of behavioral deviance in childhood. In *Developmental Biopsychology. Experimental and Observational Studies in Children at Risk*, ed. A.F. Kalverboer, pp.1–17. Ann Arbor: The University of Michigan Press.

Kalverboer, A.F. & Brouwer, W.H. (1983). Visuomotor behaviour in preschool children in relation to sex and neurological status. *Journal of Child Psychology and Psychiatry*, **24**, 65–88.

Kazdin, A.E., Esveldt-Dawson, K. & Loar, L.L. (1983). Correspondence of teacher ratings and direct observations of classroom behavior of psychiatric inpatient children. *Journal of Child Psychology and Psychiatry,* **11**, 549–64.

Klorman, R., Brumaghim, J.T., Salzman, L.F., Strauss, J., Borgstedt, A.D., McBride, M.C. & Loeb, S. (1979). Effects of methylphenidate on attention deficit hyperactivity disorder with and without agressive/noncompliant features. *Journal of Abnormal Child Psychology,* **16**, 41322.

Kok, A. (1990). Internal and external control: a two factor model of amplitude change of event-related potentials. *Acta Psychologica,* **74**, 20335.

Kopell, B.S., Wittner, W.K., Lunde, D.T., Wolcott, L.J. & Tinklenberg, J.R. (1974). The effects of methamphetamine and secobarbital on the contingent negative variation amplitude. *Psychopharmacologia,* **34**, 55–62.

Kupietz, S.S. (1990). Sustained attention in normal and in reading disabled youngsters with and without ADDH. *Journal of Abnormal Child Psychology,* **18**, 357–72.

Lacey, J.I. (1967). Somatic response patterning and stress: Some revisions of activation theory. *In Psychological Stress*, ed. M.H. Appley & R. Turnbull, pp. 14–42. New York: Appleton Century Crofts.

Lambert, N.M., Sandoval, J. & Sassone, D. (1978). Prevalence of hyperactivity in elementary school children as function of social system definers. *American Journal of Orthopsychiatry,* **48**, 446–63.

Leubuscher, H.J. & Roth, N. (1983). A computer-controlled conditioning procedure in man. *In Psychophysiology*, eds. R.Sinz & M. Rosenzweig, pp. 151–57. Jena: Fischer Verlag.

Leung, P.W.L. & Connolly, K.J. (1994). Attentional difficulties in hyperactive and conduct-disordered children: a processing deficit. *Journal of Child Psychology and Psychiatry*, **7**, 1229–45.

Logan, G.D., Cowan, W.B. & Davis, K.A. (1984). On the ability to inhibit simple and choice reaction time respones: A model and a method. *Journal of Experimental Psychology: Human Perception and Performance,* **10**, 276–91.

Loge, D.V., Staton, R.D. & Beatty, W.W. (1990). Performance of children with ADHD on tests sensitive to frontal lobe dysfunction. *Journal of the American Academy of Child and Adolescent Psychiatry,* **29**, 540–45.

Loiselle, D.L., Stamm, J.S., Maitinsky, S. & Whipple, S. (1980). Evoked potential and behavioural signs of attentive dysfunctions in hyperactive boys. *Psychophysiology,* **17**, 193–201.

Lou, H.C., Henriksen, L. & Bruhn, P. (1990). Focal cerebral dysfunction in developmental disabilities. *Lancet,* **338**, 8–11.

Lou, H.C., Henriksen, L., Bruhn, P., Brner, H. & Nielsen, J.B. (1989). Striatal dysfunction in attention deficit and hyperkinetic disorder. *Archives Neurology,* **46**, 48–52.

Low, M.D. & Stoilen, L. (1973). CNV and EEG in children: Maturational characteristics and findings in the MCD syndrome. *Electroencephalography, Clinical Neurophysiology supplement,* **33**, 139.

Luk, S.L., Leung, P.W.L. & Yuen, J. (1991), Clinic observations in the assessment of pervasiveness of childhood hyperactivity. *Journal of Child Psychology and Psychiatry,* **32**, 833–50.

McLaren, J. (1990). Selective and sustained attention in hyperactive, oppositional and normal children. Unpublished doctoral dissertation Dalhousie University, Halifax.

Malone, M.A., Kershner, J.R. & Siegel, L. (1988). The effects of methylphenidate on levels of processing and laterality in children with attention deficit disorder. *Journal of Abnormal Child Psychology,* **16**, 379–96.

Maurer, R.G. & Stewart, M.A. (1980). Attention deficit without hyperactivity in a child psychiatric clinic. *Journal of Clinical Psychiatry,* **41**, 232–33.

McClure, F.D. & Gordon, M. (1984). Performance of disturbed hyperactive and non-hyperactive children on an objective measure of hyperactivity. *Journal of Abnormal Child Psychology,* **12**, 561–72.

McGee, R., Silva, P.A. & Williams, S. (1984). Background characteristics of aggressive, hyperactive and aggressive–hyperactive boys. *Journal of the American Academy of Child Psychiatry,* **23**, 280–4.

McIntyre, C.W., Blackwell, S.L. & Denton, C.L. (1978). Effects of noise distractability on the spans of apprehension of hyperactive boys. *Journal of Abnormal Psychology,* **6**, 483–92.

Michael, B.M., Klorman, R., Salzman, L.F., Borgstedt, A.D. & Dainer, K.B. (1981). Normalizing effects of methylphenidate on hyperactive children's performance and evoked potentials. *Psychophysiology,* **18**, 665–71.

Milich, R., & Kramer, J. (1985). Reflections on impulsivity: an empirical investigation of impulsivity as a construct. In *Advances in Learning and Behavioral Disabilities*, Vol. 3, eds. K.D. Gadow & I. Bialer, pp. 57-94. Greenwich, CT: JAI Press.

Molenaar, P.C.M. & Van der Molen, M. (1986). Steps to a formal analysis of the cognitive-energetic model of stress and human performance. *Acta Psychologica,* **62**, 237–61.

Mulder, G. (1986). The concept and measurement of mental effort. In *Energetics and Human Information Processing*, eds. G.R.J. Hockey, A.W.K. Gaillard & M.G.H. Coles, pp. 175–98. Dordrecht: Martinus Nijhoff Publishers.

Mulder, G., Gloerich, A.B.M., Brookhuis, K.A., Van Dellen, H.J. & Mulder, L.J.M. (1984). Stage analysis of the reaction process using brain-evoked potentials and reaction time. *Psychological Research,* **46**, 15–32.

Näätänen, R. & Gaillard, A.W.K. (1983). The orientation reflex and the N2 deflection of the event-related potential (ERP). In *Tutorials in Event-Related Potential Research: Endogenous Components*, eds. A.W.K. Gaillard & W. Ritter, pp. 119–41. Amsterdam: North Holland.

Näätänen, R. & Michie, P.T. (1979). Early selective attention effects on the evoked potential: a critical review and reinterpretation. *Biological Psychology,* **8**, 81–136.

Nuechterlein, K.H. (1983). Signal detection in vigilance tasks and behavioural attributes among offspring of schizophrenic mothers and among hyperactive children. *Journal of Abnormal Psychology*, **92**, 4–28.

O'Dougherty, M., Neuchterlein, K. & Drew, B. (1984). Hyperactive and hypoxic children: signal detection, sustained attention and behaviour. *Journal of Abnormal Psychology,* **93**, 178–91.

O'Dougherty, M., Berntson, G.G., Boysen, S.T., Wright, F.S. & Teske, D. (1988). Psychophysiological predictors of attentional dysfunction in children with congenital heart defects. *Psychophysiology,* **25**, 305–15.

Pearson, D.A. & Lane, D.M. (1990). Reorientation in hyperactive and non-hyperactive children: evidence for developmentally immature attention? In *The Development of Attention: Research and Theory*, ed. J.T. Enns, pp. 345–63. North Holland: Elsevier Science Publishers B.V.

Peeke, S., Halliday, R., Callaway, E., Prael, R. & Reus, V. (1984). Effects of two doses of methylphenidate on verbal information processing in hyperactive children. *Journal of Clinical Psychopharmacology,* **4**, 82–8.

Pelham, W.E. (1979). Selective attention deficits in poor readers. Dichotic listening, speeded classification, and auditory and visual and incidental learning tasks. *Child Development,* **50**, 1050–61.

Peloquin, L.J. & Klorman, R. (1986). Effects of methylphenidate on normal children's mood, event-related potentials, and performance in memory scanning and vigilance. *Journal of Abnormal Psychology,* **95**, 88–98.

Pliszka, S.R. (1989). Effect of anxiety on cognition, behaviour, and stimulant response in ADHD. *Journal of the American Academy of Child and Adolescent Psychiatry,* **28**, 882–87.

Posner, M.J. (1978). *Chronometric Explorations of Mind.* Hillsdale, NJ: Lawrence Erlbaum Associates.

Posner, M.I. (1988). Structures and functions of selective attention. In *Clinical Neuropsychology and Brainfunction: Research, Assessment*, eds. T. Boll & D.K. Bryant, pp. 173–202. Washington DC: APA.

Posner, M.I. & Boies, S.J. (1971). Components of attention. *Psychological Review,* **78**, 391–408.

Posner, M.I. & Mitchell, R.F. (1967). Chronometric analysis of classification. *Psychological Review,* **74**, 392–409.

Porges, S.W. (1984). Physiological correlates of attention: a core process underlying learning disorders. *Pediatric Clinics of North America,* **31**, 371–85.

Porges, S.W. & Smith, K.M. (1980). Defining hyperactivity: psychophysiological and behavioral strategies. In *Hyperactive Children: The Social Ecology of Identification and Treatment*, eds. C.K. Whalen & B. Henker, pp. 75–04. New York: Academic Press.

Porges, S.W., Walter, G.F., Korb, R.J. & Sprague, R.L. (1975). The influence of methylphenidate on heart rate and behavioural measures of attention in hyperactive children. *Child Development,* **46**, 727–33.

Power, T.J. (1992). Contextual factors in vigilance testing of children with ADHD. *Journal of Abnormal Child Psychology,* **20**, 579–95.

Pribram, K.H. & McGuinness, D. (1975). Arousal, activation and effort in the control of attention. *Psychological Review,* **2**, 116–49.

Prior, M., Sanson, A. Freethy, C. & Geffen, G. (1985). Auditory attentional abilities in hyperactive children. *Journal of Child Psychology and Psychiatry,* **26**, 289–304.

Radosh, A. & Gittelman, R. (1981). The effect of appealing distractors on the performance of hyperactive children. *Journal of Abnormal Child Psychology,* **9**, 179–89.

Rapoport, J.L., Buchsbaum, M.S., Weingartner, H., Zahn, T.P., Ludow, C. & Mikkelsen, E.J. (1980). Dextroamphetamine – its cognitive and behavioral effects in normal and hyperactive boys and normal men. *Archives of General Psychiatry,* **37**, 933–43.

Rapoport, J.L., Donnely, M., Zametkin, A. & Carrougher, J. (1986). Situational hyperactivity in a US clinical setting. *Journal of Child Psychology and Psychiatry,* **27**, 639–46.

Reid, M.K. & Borkowski, J.G. (1984). Effects of methylphenidate (Ritalin) on information processing in hyperactive children. *Journal of Abnormal Child Psychology,* **12**, 169–86.

Rosenthal, H.R. & Allen, T.W. (1980). Intratask distractibility in hyperkinetic and nonhyperkinetic children. *Journal of Abnormal Child Psychology,* **8**, 175–87.

Roth, N., Beyreiss, J., Schlenzka, K. & Beyer, H. (1991). Coincidence of attention deficit disorder and atopic disorders in children: empirical findings and hypothetical background. *Journal of Abnormal Child Psychology,* **19**, 1–13.

Sagvolden, T. & Archer, S (1989). *Attention Deficit Disorder. Clinical and Basic Research.* Hillsdale NY: Lawrence Erlbaum Ass. Inc.

Sandberg, S.T., Rutter, M. & Taylor, E. (1978). Hyperkinetic disorder in clinic attenders. *Developmental Medicine and Child Neurology,* **20**, 279–99.

Sanders, A.F. (1983). Toward a model of stress and human performance. *Acta Psychologica,* **53**, 61–97.

Satterfield, J.H. & Braley, B.W. (1977). Evoked potentials and brain maturation in hyperactive and normal children. *Electroencephalography and Clinical Neurophysiology,* **43**, 43–51.

Satterfield, J.H. & Schell, A.M. (1984). Childhood brain function differences in delinquent and non-delinquent hyperactive boys. *Electroencephalography and Clinical Neurophysiology,* **57**, 199–207.

Satterfield, J.H., Schell, A.M., Nicholas, T. & Backs, R.W. (1988). Topographic study of auditory event-related potentials in normal boys and boys with attention deficit disorder with hyperactivity. *Psychophysiology,* **25**, 591–606.

Schachar, R. & Logan, G. (1990*a*). Are hyperactive children deficient in attentional capacity? *Journal of Abnormal Child Psychology,* **18**, 493–513.

Schachar, R. & Logan, G.D. (1990b). Impulsivity and inhibitory control in normal development and childhood psychopathology. *Developmental Psychology,* **26**, 710–20.

Schachar, R., Rutter, M. & Smith, A. (1981). Characteristics of situationally and pervasively hyperactive children: implications in syndrome definition. *Journal of Child Psychology and Psychiatry,* **22**, 375–92.

Schachar, R., Logan, G.D., Wachsmuth, R. & Chajczyk, D. (1988). Attaining and maintaining preparation: a comparison of attention in hyperactive, normal, and disturbed control children. *Journal of Abnormal Child Psychology,* **16**, 361–70.

Schleifer, M., Weiss, G., Cohen, N., Elman, M., Cvejic, H. & Kruger, E. (1975). Hyperactivity in preschoolers and the effect of methylphenidate. *American Journal of Orthopsychiatry,* **45**, 38–50.

Schneider, J.S. & Roeltgen, D.P. (1991). Chronic low dose MPTP-induced cognitive impairments in primates: a possible model for the cognitive disturbances of attention deficit disorders. *Journal of Child Neurology*, **6**, 82–9.

Schneider, W. & Shiffrin, R.M. (1977). Controlled and automatic human information processing: I. Detection, search, and attention. *Psychological Review,* **84**, 1–66.

Seidel, W.T. & Joschko, M. (1990). Evidence of difficulties in sustained attention in children with ADDH. *Journal of Abnormal Child Psychology,* **18**, 217–29.

Sergeant, J.A. (1988*a*). RDC for hyperactivity/attention disorder. In *Attention Deficit Disorder: Criteria, Cognition, Intervention*, eds. L.M. Bloomingdale & J.A. Sergeant, pp. 1–8. Oxford: Pergamon Press.

Sergeant, J.A. (1988*b*). From DSM attentional deficit disorder to functional defects. In *Attentional Deficit Disorder: Criteria, Cognition, Intervention*, eds. L.M.Bloomingdale & .A. Sergeant, pp. 183–98. Oxford: Pergamon Press.

Sergeant, J.A. & Scholten, C.A. (1985*a*). On data limitations in hyperactivity. *Journal of Child Psychology and Psychiatry,* **26**, 111–24.

Sergeant, J.A. & Scholten, C.A. (1985*b*). On resource strategy limitations in hyperactivity: cognitive impulsivity reconsidered. *Journal of Child Psychology and Psychiatry,* **26**, 97–109.

Sergeant, J.A. & Van der Meere, J.J. (1988). What happens after a hyperactive commits an error? *Psychiatric Research,* **24**, 157–64.

Sergeant, J.A. & Van der Meere, J.J. (1989). The diagnostic significance for ADD(H) classification, a future DSM. In *Attention Deficit Disorder and Hyperkinetic Syndrome*, eds. T. Sagvolden, H.M. Borggrevink & T. Archer, pp. 149–63. New York: Lawrence Erlbaum Associates.

Sergeant, J.A. & Van der Meere, J.J. (1990*a*). Convergence of approaches in localizing the hyperactivity deficit. In *Advances in Clinical Child Psychology*, eds. B.B. Lahey & A.E. Kazdin, pp. 207–46. New York: Plenum Press.

Sergeant, J.A. & Van der Meere, J.J. (1990*b*). Additive factor method applied to psychopathology with special reference to childhood hyperactivity. *Acta Psychologica,* **74**, 277–96.

Sergeant, J.A. & Van der Meere, J.J. (1991). Theoretical implications of attention problems, attention deficit hyperactivity disorder, and ritalin actions. In *RITALIN. Theory and Patient Management*, eds. L.L. Greenhill & B.B. Osmanpp, pp. 1–15. New York: Mary Ann Liebert, Inc. Publishers.

Sergeant, J.A. & Van der Meere, J.J. (1994). Towards an empirical child psychopathology. In *Disruptive Behaviour Disorders in Childhood*, ed. D.K. Routh, pp. 59–86. New York: Plenum Press.

Shaywitz, B. A., Cohen, D.J. & Bowers, M.B. (1977). CFS monoamine metabolites in children with minimal brain dysfunction – evidence for alteration of brain dopamine. *Journal of Pediatrics*, **90**, 67–71.

Shiffrin, R.M. & Schneider, W. (1977). Controlled and automatic human information processing: perceptual learning, automatic attending, and a general theory. *Psychological Review*, **84**, 127–90.

Solanto, M.V. (1990). The effects of reinforcement and response cost on a delayed response task in children with attention deficit hyperactivity disorder: a research note. *Journal of Child Psychology and Psychiatry*, **31**, 803–8.

Solanto, M.V., Wender, E.H. & Lynch, E.M. (1990). The continuous performance test as a measure of attention and impulsivity in attention deficit hyperactivity disorder. Poster presented at the annual meeting of the American Academy of Child and Adolescent Psychiatry. Chicago. Ill.

Sonuga-Barke, E.J.S., Taylor, E., Sembi, S. & Smith, J. (1992). The effect of delay of choice. *Journal of Child Psychology and Psychiatry*, **33**, 387–98.

Sroufe, L.A. Sonies, B.C., West, W.D. & Wright, F.S. (1973). Anticipatory heart rate deceleration and reaction time in children with and without referral for learning disability. *Child Development*, **44**, 267–73.

Sternberg, S. (1969). Discovery of the processing stages: extentions of the Donder`s method. In *Attention and Performance*, Vol. 2, ed. W.G. Kosters, pp. 276–315. Amsterdam: Noord Holland.

Stevens, D.A., Stover, C.F. & Backus, J.T. (1970). The hyperkinetic child: effects of incentives on the speed of rapid tapping. *Journal of Consulting and Clinical Psychology*, ***34***, 56–9.

Stott, D.H., Moyes, F.A. & Henderson, S.E. (1984). *Test of Motor Impairment*. Guelph, Ontario, Canada: Brook Educational Publishing Ltd.

Strauss, J., Lewis, J.L., Klorman, R., Peloquin, L.J., Perlmutter, R.A. & Salzman, L.F. (1984). Effects of methylphenidate on young adults' performance and event related potentials in a vigilance and a paired-associates learning test. *Psychophysiology*, **21**, 609–61.

Swanson, J.M., Shea, C., McBurnett, K., Potkin, S.G., Fiore, C. & Crinella, F. (1990). Attention and hyperactivity. In *The Development of Attention: Research and Theory*, ed. J.T. Enns, pp. 383–403. North Holland: Elsevier Science Publishers B.V.

Sykes, D.H., Douglas, V.I., Weiss, G. & Minde, K.K. (1971). Attention in hyperactive children and the effect of methylphenidate (Ritalin). *Journal of Child Psychology and Psychiatry*, **12**, 129–39.

Sykes, D.H., Douglas, V.I. & Morgenstern, G.L. (1973). Sustained attention in hyperactive children and the effect of methylphenidate (Ritalin). *Journal of Child Psychology and Psychiatry*, **12**, 129–*39*.

Tannock, R., Schachar, R.J., Carr, R.P., Chajczyk, D. & Logan, G.D. (1989). Effects of methylphenidate on inhibitory control in hyperactive children. *Journal of Abnormal Child Psychology*, **17**, 473–91.

Taylor, E. (1983). Drug response and diagnostic validation. In *Developmental Neuropsychiatry*, ed. M. Rutter, pp. 348–68. New York: Guilford Press.

Taylor, E. (1989). Some research issues in Attention Deficit. In *Attention Deficit Disorder. Current Concepts and Emerging Trends in Attentional and Behavioral Disorders of Childhood*, eds. L.M. Bloomingdale & J. Swanson, pp. 313–333. Oxford: Pergamon Press.

Taylor, E., Schachar, R., Thorley, G. & Wieselberg, M. (1986). Conduct disorder and hyperactivity. I. Separation of hyperactivity and antisocial conduct in British child psychiatric patients. *British Journal of Psychiatry,* **149**, 760–77.

Thurstone, L.L. (1938). Primary mental abilities. *Psychometric Monographs*, 1.

Trommer, B.L., Hoeppner, J.B., Lorber, R. & Armstrong, K.J. (1988). The go–no-go paradigm in attention deficit disorder. *Annals of Neurology,* **24**, 610–14.

Trommer, B.L., Hoeppner, J.B. & Zecker, S.G. (1991). The go–no-go test in attention deficit disorder is sensitive to methylphenidate. *Journal of Child Neurology, 6* (suppl.), 126–29.

Tucker, D.M. & Williamson, P.A. (1984). Asymmetric neural control systems in human self-regulation. *Psychological Review,* **91**, 185–215.

Vaessen, W. (1990*a*). Ecological validity of hyperactivity studies. Two field experiments with carefully selected hyperactive and clumsy children. Thesis, University of Groningen, The Netherlands.

Vaessen, W. (1990*b*). Performance of hyperactive children in a traffic task: a validation study. I*n Developmental Biopsychology: Experimental and Observational Studies in Children at Risk*, ed. A.F. Kalverboer, pp. 95–114. Ann Arbor: The University of Michigan Press.

Vaessen, W. & Van der Meere, J.J. (1990). Issues in the selection of hyperactive/ADD(H) children for experimental clinical studies. In *Developmental Biopsychology: Experimental and Observational Studies in Groups 'at risk'*, ed.A.F. Kalverboer, pp. 21–37. Ann Arbor: The University of Michigan Press.

Van Dellen, H.J., Brookhuis, K.A., Mulder, G., Okita, T. & Mulder, L.J.M. (1984). Evoked potential correlates of practice in a visual search task. In *Clinical and Experimental Neuropsychophysiology*, eds. D. Papakostopoulos, S.Butler & L.Martin, pp. 132–56. London: Croom Helm.

Van der Meere, J.J. & Sergeant, J.A. (1987). A divided attention experiment with pervasively hyperactive children. *Journal of Abnormal Child Psychology,* **15**, 379–91.

Van der Meere, J.J. & Sergeant, J.A. (1988*a*). A focused attention experiment in pervasively hyperactive children. *Journal of Abnormal Child Psychology,* **16**, 627–39.

Van der Meere, J.J. & Sergeant, J.A. (1988*b*). Controlled processing and vigilance in hyperactivity: time will tell. *Journal of Abnormal Child Psychology,* **16**, 641–55.

Van der Meere, J.J. & Sergeant, J.A. (1988*c*). Aquisition of attention skill in pervasively hyperactive children. *Journal of Child Psychology and Psychiatry,* **29**, 301–10.

Van der Meere, J.J., Van Baal, M. & Sergeant, J.A. (1989). The additive factor method: a differential diagnostic tool in hyperactive and learning disability. *Journal of Abnormal Child Psychology,* **17**,409–22.

Van der Meere, J.J., Wekking, E. & Sergeant, J. (1991). Sustained attention and pervasive hyperactivity. *Journal of Child Psychology and Psychiatry,* **32**, 275–84.

Van der Meere, J.J., Vreeling, H.J. & Sergeant, J.A. (1992). A motor presetting experiment in hyperactive, learning disabled and control children. *Journal of Child Psychology and Psychiatry,* **33**, 1347–54.

Van der Meere, J.J., Stemerdink, B.A. & Gunning W.B. (1995*a*). Effects of presentation rate of stimuli on response inhibition in ADHD children with and without tics. *Perceptual and Motor Skills*, **81**, 259–62.

Van der Meere, J.J., Hughes, K. A., Borger, N. & Sallee, F.R. (1995*b*). The effect of reward on sustained attention in ADHD children with and without CD. In *Eunethydis*: *European Approaches to Hyperkinetic Disorder*, ed. J.A. Sergeant, pp. 241–53. Zurich: Trümpi and Partner.

Van der Meere, J.J., Shalev, R.S. Burger, N. & Gross-Tsur, V. (1995*c*). Sustained attention, activation and MPH in ADHD. *Journal of Child Psychology and Psychiatry*, **36**, 697–703.

Van der Molen, M.W. (1990). Energetics of cognitive development. *In Developmental Psychology Behind the Dikes*, eds. W. Koops and H. Soppe, pp. 123-40. Delft: Eburon.

Van der Molen, M.W., Somsen, R.J.N., Jennings, J.R., Nieuwboer, R.T. & Orlebeke, J.F.

(1987). A psychophysiological investigation of cognitive- energetical relations in human information processing: a heart rate/additive factors approach. *Acta Psychologica,* **66**, 251–89.

Weingartner, H., Rapoport, J.L., Buchsbaum, M.S., Bunney, W.E., Ebert, M.H., Mikkelsen, E.J. & Caine, E.D. (1980). Cognitive processes in normal and hyperactive children and their response to amphetamine treatment. *Journal of Abnormal Psychology,* **89**, 25–37.

Wilding, J. (1994). Attentional problems in the classroom and parallel procesing ability. *British Journal of Developmental Psychology*, **12**, 539–53.

Zahn, T.P., Kruesi, M.J.P. & Rapoport, J.L. (1991). Reaction time indices of attention deficit in boys with disruptive behavior disorders. *Journal of Abnormal Child Psychology,* **19**, 233–52.

Zahn, T.P., Little, B. & Wender, (1978). Pupillary and heart rate reactivity in children with minimal brain dysfunction. *Journal of Abnormal Child Psychology,* **6**, 135–47.

Zametkin, A.J., Nordahl, T.E. & Gross, M. (1990). Cerebral glucose metabolism in adults with hyperactivity of childhood onset. *The New England Journal of Medicine,* **323**, 1361–6.

Zametkin, A.J. & Rapoport, J.L. (1987). The neuropharmacology of attention deficit disorder with hyperactivity: where have we come in 50 years? *Journal of the American Academy of Child and Adolescent Psychiatry*, **26**, 676–86.

Zentall, S.S. & Meyer, M.J. (1987). Self-regulation of stimulation for ADD-H children during reading and vigilance task performance. *Journal of Abnormal Child Psychology,* **15**, 519–36.

Zentall, F.S. & Shaw, J.H. (1980). Effects of classroom noise on performance and activity of second-grade hyperactives and control children. *Journal of Educational Psychology,* **71**, 830–40.

Zentall, S.S. & Zentall, T.R. (1983). Optimal stimulation: a model of disordered activity and performance in normal and deviant children. *Psychological Bulletin,* **94**, 446–71.

Zentall, S.S., Zentall, T.R. & Barack, R.B. (1978). Distraction as a function of within-task stimulation for hyperactive and normal children. *Journal of Learning Disabilities,* **11**, 13–21.

5

Developmental perspectives

Sheryl Olson

INTRODUCTION

There is a growing consensus that knowledge of normal developmental processes is essential for understanding the nature of childhood behaviour disorders (Achenbach, 1974; Cicchetti, 1984; 1990; Rutter & Garmezy, 1983; Sroufe & Rutter, 1984). In this chapter, developmental perspectives are brought to bear on questions concerning the ontogenesis and course of childhood hyperactivity. Despite the fact that hyperactivity is one of the most densely researched childhood behaviour disorders, its developmental precursors are poorly understood. We are only beginning to disentangle the complex tapestries of biological, emotional, cognitive–developmental, familial and social–ecological factors that mark individual pathways to this disorder and to its multiform outcomes in later life.

The term 'developmental perspectives' refers to a rich set of concepts derived from the study of normal and abnormal development. The most basic context for understanding childhood disorders is the age or cognitive-developmental level of the child. Normal processes of development involve complex quantitative and qualitative transformations in children's physical, cognitive, emotional and behavioural functioning, with increasing differentiation and hierarchical integration as age progresses. Thus, atypical or 'deviant' development can only be defined in relation to what is known to be normal for a given age group. For example, negativism, temper tantrums, and attention-seeking, relatively commonplace in toddlers, would have very different meaning in school-age children or adolescents. Once a behaviour disorder is defined, the age of the child affects how it is perceived and interpreted by adults, the manner in which symptomatic behaviours are expressed, and the probable course of the disorder (Campbell, 1989). Moreover, the developing cognitive emotional and behavioural characteristics of the child determine what types of clinical interventions may be optimally effective (Kendall, Lerner, & Craighead, 1984).

Beyond concern with normative, age-related trends, developmental perspectives also encompass questions of individual development that are vitally important to the psychopathologist. The concept of developmental issues or tasks is useful for examining continuities in individual adaptation over the course of time (Erickson, 1963; Sroufe, 1979; Sroufe & Rutter, 1984). At each different age period, there are adaptational challenges that are central to the development of competent social and emotional functioning. Successful adaptation provides the child with increased behavioural flexibility, providing a foundation for the growth of normal competence (Block & Block, 1980; Waters & Sroufe, 1983). Conversely, adaptational failures at any level may predispose the child to develop behaviour disorders at later stages of development, although this progression is far from inevitable and is unlikely to occur in a simple, linear manner (cf. Cicchetti & Rizley, 1981). Also, the manner in which adaptational failures mark pathways to specific childhood behaviour disorders is not well understood.

Finally, the process of individual development is characterised by complex transactions between child and environment. Current models stress that behavioural deviance is the product of a continuous, dynamic interplay between qualities that individual children bring to their social interactions and characteristics of the immediate caregiving environment and its broader social-ecological context (Sameroff & Chandler, 1975). Concepts of risk (factors which increase the chance of developing behaviour disorders), vulnerability (factors which intensify the effects of risk) and protection (factors which ameliorate risk) are important for understanding the individual paths that children take in developing behaviour disorders (Anthony, 1987; Garmezy, 1983; Rutter, 1983, 1987).

In the current chapter, these concepts are applied to our knowledge of the early developmental precursors and course of childhood hyperactivity. First, however, defining features of the hyperactive syndrome will be briefly outlined in the following section.

OVERVIEW OF CLINICAL AND ASSOCIATED FEATURES

Diagnostic criteria

The clinical features of hyperactivity, known as attention deficit hyperactivity disorder in the current diagnostic nomenclature (DSM-IV;APA, 1994), have proven difficult to define. Many different definitions of hyperactivity have been suggested throughout its history, and as Barkley (1982) has emphasised, none of them has been highly operational. Moreover, due to overlap between features of hyperactivity and related disorders, some have even questioned whether it should be considered a discrete syndrome.

The publication of DSM-III (APA, 1980) marked increasing consensus that deficits in attention/concentration were central features of hyperactivity, also with age-inappropriate levels of impulsivity and overactivity. In the latest revision of the DSM (APA, 1994), there are two broad groups of primary symptoms: inattention (e.g. fails to attend to details; has difficulty sustaining attention in task or in play; easily distracted) and hyperactivity–impulsivity (e.g. fidgety; often out of seat; highly active and talkative; often interrupts; has difficulty waiting turn). To receive a diagnosis of ADHD, children must show at least six symptoms from either the inattention or hyperactivity–impulsivity groups. The diagnosis also requires that symptoms appear before the age of seven and persist for a minimum of six months. Moreover, these symptoms must be present in at least two different settings, and there must be clear evidence of significant impairment in social or academic functioning. Hyperactivity has been consistently found to be over-represented in boys, by ratios of 4:1 to 9:1 in clinical samples (Ross & Ross, 1982).

Primary characteristics

The primary or core features of ADHD have been well-established clinically, and in numerous research studies comparing hyperactive children with normal peers (for reviews see Ross & Ross, 1976, 1982; Whalen & Henker, 1980; Whalen, 1989). One primary characteristic is that of overactivity. Hyperactive children are often described by parents and teachers as fidgety, 'always on the go', restless, and accident-prone (Whalen, 1989). Qualitative features are paramount, in that the overactivity of ADHD children appears disorganised, haphazard, and contextually inappropriate in contrast to the goal-directed behaviour of highly active but normal peers. However, measurement of overactivity in ADHD children has proven to be less than straightforward. Different measurement techniques, such as mechanical devices, direct observations and behaviour ratings, show modest levels of agreement at best (Barkley & Ullman, 1975) and symptoms of overactivity in hyperactive children show substantial levels of individual and situational variability (Goyette, Conners,& Ulrich, 1978; Schachar, Rutter & Smith, 1981; Zentall, 1984). Generally, hyperactive children are more likely to manifest problems with overactivity in highly structured task situations than in more relaxed or informal settings (Jacob, O'Leary & Rosenblad, 1978; Porrino et al., 1983; Zentall, 1980), making the school classroom environment an ideal context for observing symptomatic behaviour.

Attentional problems comprise a secondary primary characteristic of ADHD. Parents of hyperactive children complain that they never listen, and have difficulty playing alone and sticking to single activities. Teachers complain that ADHD children are frequently 'off task' in classroom situations, and that they have difficulty following directions and completing assignments. Due to the multidimensional nature of the attention construct, and to subtleties involved in the measurement of attentional processes, however, efforts to pin-point specific attentional deficits in hyperactive children have often met with frustration. One of the most widely supported hypotheses is that ADHD children are deficient in the ability to maintain their attention over time in structured task situations (Douglas & Peters, 1979; Douglas, 1983; Barkley, 1988). For example, on measures of sustained attention such as the continuous performance test, ADHD children have been shown to make more errors and to respond more slowly than normal and psychiatric controls (Douglas, 1983). However, some studies have cast doubt on the notion that the attentional performance of ADHD children actually deteriorates over time, as would be required to substantiate a deficit in sustained attention (e.g. Schachar et al., 1988). Moreover, in both natural settings and on sustained attention tasks in the laboratory, it is very difficult to separate attentional deficits from problems of motivation, co-operation, or fluctuations in mood.

Finally, deficiencies in inhibitory control comprise the third core characteristic of ADHD. Problems of impulse control manifest themselves in diverse situations; the hyperactive child may intrude upon the games of peers, have difficulty waiting his turn to play, behave in 'silly' ways that are situationally inappropriate, interrupt others, call out answers before the question is finished, or even run into traffic to retrieve a wayward toy. However, as with the concept of inattention, impulsivity is a complex, multidimensional construct that has proven difficult to operationalise: different laboratory measures of impulsivity typically show negligible to low intercorrelations with one another and with reports of hyperactive symptoms by teachers and parents (Milich & Kramer, 1984; Olson, 1989). As Whalen (1989) has lamented, '...there is a consensus that hyperactive children have problems with impulsivity and inhibitory control, but these problems are manifested and measured in diverse and different ways, and it is difficult if not impossible to predict performance in one area on the basis of measure derived from another (p.143)'. An additional complication is that impulsivity problems are common to many different types of childhood behaviour problems (Biedermah, Newcorn & Sprich, 1991), most notably disturbances of conduct.

Patterns of co-morbidity

Conduct disorders have been found to frequently co-occur with hyperactivity (Hinshaw, 1987; Szatmari, Boyle & Offord, 1989). For example, Hinshaw (1987) reviewed studies that had classified children into subtypes, and concluded that 30–90% of children who were classified ADHD were also classified as having conduct disorder. The high degree of correspondence between these two disorders, coupled with lack of evidence indicating that ADHD and conduct disorders show distinctive aetiological patterns or long-term prognoses, have led some to question whether ADHD is a distinct syndrome (e.g. Prior & Sanson, 1986; Rutter, 1982). One approach to this problem has been to subdivide ADHD youngsters according to the presence and severity of concomitant conduct problems (Loney & Milich, 1982; Stewart *et al.*, 1981). Generally, children with combined symptom patterns have more broad-ranging and severe adaptational problems than children with 'pure' ADHD. For example, children with the mixed subtype have been found to show higher rates of social maladjustment in family and peer settings, as well as poor long-term outcomes and a greater incidence of parental psychopathology, than children with hyperactive but not aggressive features (Anderson, *et al.*, 1987; Hinshaw, 1987; Werry, Reeves & Elkind, 1987; Schachar & Wachsmuth, 1990; Szatmari *et al.*, 1989). Children with 'pure' hyperactivity tend to show more cognitive and neurodevelopmental difficulties and poorer school achievement than those with features of conduct disorder (Reeves *et al.*, 1987; Taylor *et al.*, 1986). There is also some evidence that they have a more favourable response to stimulant medication than those with mixed symptom patterns (Loney, 1987: Matier *et al.*, 1991).

Academic problems

Academic failure and underachievement are also common problems of ADHD children, as evidenced by poor grades and achievement test scores, teacher evaluations, placement in special classes, and failure to be promoted to the next grade (Edelbrock, Costello & Kessler, 1984; McGee & Share, 1988). Specific learning disabilities have been found to be over-represented among hyperactive children (Cantwell & Satterfield, 1978; Lambert & Sandoval, 1980; Schachar *et al.*, 1981); however, estimates of the proportion of hyperactive children who are also learning disabled vary widely between studies, reflecting heterogeneity in sample composition and diagnostic criteria (Semrud-Clikeman *et al.*, 1992; Shaywitz & Shaywitz, 1988; Whalen, 1989). Although the presence of learning and academic problems in hyperactive children has been well established, it is unclear whether these problems are attributable to deficits in motivation, attention, impulse control, problem solving, or some combination of these factors (McGee & Share, 1988).

Problems in social relationships

Hyperactive children tend to show pervasive problems in social adjustment (Whalen & Henker, 1985). Relative to other children, they have few friends and experience high rates of peer rejection (Johnston, Pelham & Murphy, 1985; Klein & Young, 1979; Pelham & Bender 1982; Whalen *et al.*, 1983). Several studies have suggested that the behaviour of hyperactive children catalyses negative interactions with others. For example, sibling dyads that contain a hyperactive child show more negative interaction than others (Mash & Johnston, 1983); similar patterns have been found for peer interactions with and without the presence of a hyperactive child (Cunningham & Siegel, 1987; Clark *et al.*, 1988). Similarly, teachers and parents tend to be more directive and controlling with hyperactive children than with normal children (Mash & Johnston, 1982; Whalen, Henker & Dotemoto, 1980, 1981). However, adults' responses to hyperactive children become less controlling and more positive as ADHD symptoms improve with either age (Mash & Johnston, 1982; Barkley, Karlsson & Pollard, 1985) or stimulant medication (Barkley, 1985; Humphries, Kinsbourne & Swanson, 1978; Whalen *et al.*, 1981), indicating that the negative response styles of adults are 'elicited' in part by difficult or annoying child behaviour.

Several potential explanations for the social maladjustment of hyperactive children have been proposed, including specific deficits in social knowledge, attributional style, and social reasoning (Whalen, Henker & Granger, 1990). Currently, however, there are no clear answers, necessitating further research into this important question.

Hyperactivity: a disorder of self-regulation

In summary, hyperactive children show considerable heterogeneity in their symptom pictures, and their adaptational difficulties tend to span many different life contexts. The pervasiveness of these problems, coupled with their task and situational variability, has led many to question whether hyperactive children possess a generalised deficit in the integration of cognitive, affective and motor functions in response to varying situational demands. An emerging consensus is that the diverse problems of adaptation shown by hyperactive children share a common thread; they all reflect deficits in self-regulation (Barkley, 1989; Douglas & Peters, 1979; Douglas, 1983; Kendall & Braswell, 1985). Self-regulation is a complex, superordinate construct subject to many different theoretical and empirical perspectives. One approach focuses upon affect regulation, particularly modulation of fear and anger (e.g. Rothbart, 1989; Thompson, 1994). Infants show clear individual differences in emotional arousability and intensity which remain moderately stable through early development (Fox & Calkins, 1993; Kagan *et al.*, 1984). Moreover, emotional arousability and intensity have been associated with aggressive and disruptive behaviour in children (Brody, Stoneman, & Burke, 1988; Fabes & Eisenberg, 1992; Teglasi & McMahon, 1990), suggesting that modulation of strong emotional arousal is an important component of social competence (Eisenburg *et al.*, 1994). Another major approach to understanding self-regulation emphasises aspects of cognitively mediated behavioural inhibition, often assessed in isolation of social interaction using specific laboratory tasks. For example, 'Self-control' has been variously operationalised as the ability to inhibit immediate responding to achieve a goal or comply with a request (Kagan, *et al.*, 1964), wait for a desired object or goal (Mischel & Patterson, 1974), plan ahead (Porteus, 1965), inhibit overt motor movements in response to situational demands (Maccoby *et al.*, 1965), and organise and sustain attention in response to situational demands (Douglas & Peters, 1979). As Kopp (1987) has noted, common to all definitions is the requirement that children flexibly adapt to life situations that have different standards of conduct associated with them: 'Thus it is permissible to shout in a playground but not in a classroom, to run across a meadow but not a street, and to respect another's possessions whether the person is present or absent (1987, p.34)'. Similarly, Barkley (1981, 1989) has argued that ADHD children have a generalised deficit in rule-governed behaviour, defined as the ability of language or other symbol system to serve as discriminative stimuli for contextually appropriate responding. Hence, their behaviour is under the control of immediately occurring contingencies, not rules, which could explain the poor problem-solving, impulsivity, non-compliance, and socially inappropriate behaviour so commonly observed in these children. In the following sections, the construct of self-regulation will be used as a context for examining earliest developmental precursors of hyperactivity.

Early developmental precursors

It is widely believed that hyperactivity has its onset in early childhood, even though the majority of cases are not diagnosed until the school-age years. Indeed, a requirement of diagnosis is that symptoms appear before the age of seven (APA, 1980, 1987). Ironically, however, the early development of hyperactivity has been grossly underresearched. Relatively little is known about developmental pathways in infancy and early childhood which lead to full expression of the syndrome in later life. One way to approach this question is by examining the early development of self-regulatory competence, defined broadly as the ability to modulate affective responses, impulses, and attention in accordance with situational demands. As discussed above, there are cogent arguments for viewing hyperactivity as a disorder of self-regulation. Thus, knowledge of factors which influence the normal and abnormal development of self-regulatory skills can provide a foundation for exploring early developmental pathways to hyperactivity.

Normative development of self-regulation

Achieving flexible levels of self-control is a major developmental task for the preschool-age child (Block & Block, 1980; Flavell, 1977, 1985; Kopp, 1982; Sroufe, 1983). Self-regulation provides an important foundation for the growth of normal social and academic competence. Young children who have difficulty managing their impulses, appraising the demands of different life situations, and organising environmental stimuli efficiently are at risk for a host of behavioural and learning problems in the school-age period, chief among them the attention deficit disorders (Campbell & Ewing, 1990). Despite the clear importance of the construct, however, we know relatively little about the early developmental course of self-regulation.

The work of Kopp and her colleagues stands as a notable exception. In a review article integrating diverse theoretical and empirical perspectives, Kopp (1982, 1989) placed the antecedents of self-regulation in a developmental framework. The most salient feature of her model is that the development of self- regulation is closely linked to the growth of higher-order cognitive processes. Self-regulatory competence emerges gradually in a series of discontinuous developmental phases which parallel the maturation of different cognitive skills. The role of the caregiving environment is also critical, in that it mediates the extent to which the child successfully negotiates developmental challenges inherent in each different phase. Because issues relative to each phase have different implications for understanding how normal development can go awry, these challenges will be briefly reiterated here.

Neurophysiological maturation (0–3 months)

In the earliest months of life, 'control' takes the form of modulation of arousal states. Individual infants differ in the capacity to modulate arousal: for example, some infants are easily distressed, and have difficulty self-soothing or being soothed by caregivers. Caregivers can facilitate effective arousal modulation by responding sensitively to the child's communications (e.g., adjusting their behaviour to the state of the child), and by providing routines which mark transitions between different states of arousal.

Sensorimotor modulation (3–12 months)

During this phase, infants are capable of adjusting their voluntary motor behaviour in response to environmental stimuli, e.g. reaching for an interesting toy, or responding to the vocalisations and smiles of caregivers. According to Kopp, these modulations help infants organise their interactions efficiently with the social and physical world, which sets the stage for more complex levels of control with advancing age. The ability to modulate sensorimotor behaviour is thought to reflect individual differences in biological predispositions (such as activity levels) as well as patterns of caregiver stimulation and the availability of play objects.

Control (12-18 months)

Towards the end of the first year, there is an important transitional phase in the development of self-regulation. Because of their rapidly maturing cognitive and motoric abilities, infants become aware of social demands and are able to adjust their behaviour accordingly. For example, although control is limited to the immediate stimulus environment, infants of this age are capable of complying with simple caregiver requests ('give Mommy a kiss') and prohibitions ('no, baby!'). The child's increased capacity for locomotion and intense need to explore the environment leads to a natural escalation in caregiver demands. During this critical transition phase, individual differences in control may be facilitated by caregiver sensitivity to the child's preferred style of engaging the social and physical environment; for example, if the child is highly active, to what extent can the caregiver 'channel' this activity into constructive rather than conflicted interactions? Caregivers of toddlers also differ in their efficacy as teachers. For example, adults can facilitate the development of attention and comprehension skills by providing verbal instructions for compliance (Schaffer, 1984), and by using multiple cues and age-appropriate language to reinforce a point (Kopp, 1987).

Self-control (24 + months)

With the development of representational (symbolic) thought and recall memory, the child is able increasingly to delay immediate gratification of desires, engage in self-initiated monitoring of behaviour, differentiate self from others (Harris, 1989; Wellman, 1990), and use words for psychological states such as beliefs, desires and emotions (Bartsch & Wellman, 1994; Bretherton & Breeghly, 1982; Brown & Dunn, 1991). During this period, struggles with caregivers over autonomy isues and pride in self-help behaviours become normative. The child's behavioural flexibility in adapting to new situations is still quite limited, however, as is capacity for delay.

As cognitive skills mature into the preschool years, children become increasingly capable of self-monitoring their behaviour in response to diverse situational demands. More complex cognitive processes play an important role in self-regulatory behaviour at this age, such as internalised, self-guiding speech (Luria, 1961; Vygotsky, 1962), language used to request information and to negotiate and meaning (Dunn, 1988); and self-generated strategies aimed at planning a course of behaviour and reducing frustration. It is this expanded and flexible repertoire of coping responses that marks the achievement of true self-regulatory competence.

Although Kopp's framework focuses upon normative developmental transitions, it provides a good basis for raising the question of how individual differences in self-regulatory competence arise. Perhaps the most obvious theme is that the development of self-regulation is firmly entrenched in the caregiving system. At each different phase of early development, caregiver behaviours may facilitate or retard the child's progress in achieving internal controls, either through direct social interaction or the manner in which the caregiver structures the physical environment. To the extent that it has a disorganising effect upon the caregiving system, environmental stress may play an important role in the early development of self-regulation. A second, less obvious theme concerns individual differences in infant's biological predispositions. Individual infants vary considerably in the ability to modulate arousal, the earliest hallmark of self-regulation (see, for example, Thompson, 1994). At later ages, biologically based differences in behavioural tempo and emotional expression may have an important impact upon the development of self-regulatory competence, especially if the child's interactional style leads to conflicts with caregivers and peers (Eisenberg *et al.*, 1994; Lerner & Lerner, 1983; Teglasi & McMahon, 1990). Thus, the construct of temperament would seem critical to an understanding of the early development of self-regulation. In the following sections, these constructs are used to examine the development of individual differences in self-regulation among infants and toddlers.

Early caregiving relationships

Through processes of social interaction with their infants and the ways in which they structure the physical environment, caregivers are thought to play a critical role in the development of self-regulation (Kopp, 1982, 1989; Mahler, Pine & Bergman, 1975; Sander, 1975; Sroufe, 1991). However, due to a paucity of research, we are only beginning to understand the complex relationships between early caregiving systems and the development of individual differences in children's self-regulatory competence. Two different approaches to this question will be discussed in this section, one focusing upon the primacy of the caregiver–infant attachment relationship as a broad context for the development of self-regulation, and the other on caregiver control strategies and compliance in toddlers.

Caregiver–infant attachment relationships and self-regulation

The most important developmental task of infancy is the establishment of a positive, smoothly functioning relationship with primary caregivers. According to Bowlby (1969, 1982), early attachment relationships provide a critical context for the development of physical and emotional security. Attachment refers to a specific, enduring, and reciprocal bond between infant and caregiver. Bowlby conceived of attachment relationships as homeostatic systems which function to ensure the safety and security of the infant through regulation of physical proximity to the caregiver. Thus, if the infant is frightened or distressed, the caregiver provides protection and soothing. On the psychological level of the attached child, the availability and responsiveness of the caregiver leads to feelings of emotional security and attraction to the relationship (Bishof, 1975; Bowlby, 1982). Although the formation of attachment bonds is considered a species universal, individual attachment relationships show qualitative variations that are of clinical relevance.

In their classic studies on the Strange Situation, a laboratory paradigm designed to measure the infant's trust in the physical and emotional availability of the caregiver, Ainsworth and her colleagues (Ainsworth, Bell & Stayton, 1971; Ainsworth, *et al.*, 1978) distinguished three qualitatively different patterns of attachment. Following brief separations from the caregiver, 'secure' one-year-old infants were able to quickly re-establish and maintain positive contact with the caregiver. A substantial minority (approximately one-third in this study) were deemed 'insecure' or 'anxiously attached' in that they either ignored the caregiver on her return (insecure–avoidant) or mixed proximity-seeking with angry, ambivalent behaviour (insecure–resistant). Consistent with the hypothesis that these patterns reflect qualities of antecedent mother–infant interaction, caregiver sensitivity and responsiveness during the first year have been empirically linked to secure attachment at one year of life (Ainsworth *et al.*, 1978; Bates, Maslin & Frankel, 1985; Belsky, Taylor & Rovine, 1984). However, antecedent maternal behaviour accounts for extremely modest portions of the variance in later attachment status (Lamb *et al.*, 1985), and it is unclear whether these links reflect the influence of maternal responsiveness, or other aspects of maternal behaviour which tend to co-occur with responsiveness.

How, specifically, can knowledge of early attachment relationships inform our understanding of the development of self-regulation? One hypothesis is that quality of caregiver–infant interaction is linked to the development of cognitive/affective schemata which mediate the emergence of basic attentional, motivational and problem-solving skills. As Bretherton puts it: 'Confidence in the mother's physical and psychological availability appears to lay the groundwork for autonomous exploration and problem solving coupled with the expectation that help will be forthcoming when needed. Thus attention span and persistence, which have often been regarded as traitlike, perhaps constitutionally based, qualities, may at least be in part a product of particular relationship systems (1985, p.21)'. Assuming (as Kopp has argued) that compliance is an emergent characteristic of self-regulation, security of attachment has been empirically related to toddlers' willingness to comply with the mother and engage in constructive problem-solving (Londerville & Main, 1981; Matas, Arend & Sroufe, 1978). For example, Matas *et al.* demonstrated that children who were rated securely attached at 18 months tended to function more competently than others in a 24-month dyadic problem-solving task. In a laboratory setting, mother and toddler were given four puzzles of increasing difficulty; the most difficult tasks were only solvable with maternal assistance. Securely attached toddlers were found to be more compliant, enthusiastic, persistent and attentive to maternal suggestions that insecurely attached children. In a recent replication, Frankel & Bates (1990) found that toddlers who had been rated securely attached at 13 months spent more time 'on task' and showed less aggression and verbal negativism than insecurely attached toddlers. However, the groups did not differ in compliance to the mother, or in expressions of frustration and whiny affect. Frustration on the part of the child was closely linked to maternal directiveness; the most frustrated toddlers had mothers who issued frequent commands. Further analyses revealed that this type of dyadic interaction was linked to a generalised pattern of conflicted mother–child interaction: children who were frustrated in problem-solving tended to be demanding and troublesome at home, and had mothers who exerted high degrees of restrictive, punitive control. As infants, these children were observed to be more socially demanding than others and their mothers tended to show low levels of positive involvement with them during the first year of life.

In other studies, quality of mother–infant interaction behaviour and attachment have been viewed as antecedents of later externalising-type behaviour problems. In a large prospective study of socially disadvantaged families (the Minnesota High Risk Study), Erickson, Sroufe & Egeland (1985) found that children who had anxious-avoidant attachments to their mothers at 12 and 18 months were rated by preschool teachers as more impulsive and hostile than others. The latter ratings comprised a broad dimension of negative behaviour; a narrower hyperactivity scale did not differentiate the groups. The overall pattern of findings appeared to fit a 'multipathway' model of transmission, in that the prediction of behaviour problems from early attachment status was mediated by later aspects of parenting. For example, secure infants who eventually developed behaviour problems evidenced suboptimal patterns of mother–child interaction in the early preschool years. Cognitive characteristics of children were also important in accounting for group differences. Children who showed behaviour problems in preschool had lower scores than others on measures of cognitive competence at 24 months and language ability at 42 months, irrespective of attachment status. Similarly, follow-up assessments in the early school-age period (Renken *et al.*, 1989) and in preadolescence (Urban, *et al.*, 1991) have shown that at-risk children who have insecure early attachments tended to have poorer peer relationships and greater problems with depression and aggression than those with secure early attachments. In all cases, these predictive relationships were stronger for boys than for girls.

However, other longitudinal studies have been inconsistent in supporting a link between insecure attachment and later problems of impulsivity and aggression. Lewis, *et al.* (1984) found that quality of attachment at 12 months predicted mother reports of internalising problems at 6 years of age, but only for boys. There was a marginal relationship between early attachment status and later externalising problems in boys, and no relationship between early attachment status and any kind of psychopathology in girls. Further, predictions between attachment security and later adjustment were moderated by many different factors; insecurely attached boys who were unplanned, second born children and had experienced elevated rates of family stress were most highly at risk for later negative outcome.

Fagot and Kavanagh (1990) assessed security of attachment in 18 month-old children and related it to parent's reports of problem behaviours at 24, 27, 30 and 42 months. Children were also observed at 18 and 30 months in the home and in toddler play groups. No relationships were found between insecure attachment status and later indices of problem behaviour, although girls who had been classified insecure/avoidant at 18 months were viewed by teachers and observers as more difficult to manage and more incompetent with peers than others.

Similarly, Bates, Maslin & Frankel (1985) found that attachment security in 13-month infants was unrelated to maternal and secondary caregivers' reports of behaviour problems at age three, and to maternal reports of behaviour problems at age 5 and 6. Boys' externalising problems were related to mother's early reports of temperamental difficultness and resistance to control, whereas girls' externalising problems were related to the same temperament variables and to a general lack of early positive involvement with their mothers, as observed in the home.

Thus, attempts to link early attachment status to global measures of externalising problems have been inconsistent, failing to support a simple linear association between attachment status and later externalizing problems. The Lewis, Fagot and Bates studies differed from the Minnesota study in that in the former, attachment status was assessed at one point in time in low-risk samples. Single indices of risk have been proven much less reliable predictors of later child deviance than multiple and cumulative indices (Rutter, 1983; Sameroff *et al.*, 1993; Werner & Smith, 1982). Indeed, studies of multi-risk families have consistently shown concurrent links between inscure parent–infant attachment and early disruptive child behaviour (e.g. DeMulder & Radke-Yarrow, 1991; Lyons-Ruth *et al.*, 1987).

Finally, two later reports from the Bloomington and Minnesota groups indicate that choice of predictor and outcome measures is also important in examining links between early experience and children's later impulse control deficits. Reporting from the Bloomington Longitudinal Study, Olson, Bates & Bayles (1990) found that specific self-control deficits in 6 year-old children were associated with prior attachment history and with other antecedent mother–infant interaction variables. In this prospective study of 80 mother–child dyads, quality of mother–infant interaction was assessed in the home at age 6, 13, and 24 months, and security of attachment was assessed using a subsample at age 13 months. Measures of infant temperament and cognitive competence were also collected during the first two years, and related to later outcome status. At 6 years of age, children participated in a series of laboratory procedures designed to measure different aspects of self-regulatory competence. These included tests of cognitive impulsivity, motor inhibition, and delay of gratification, as well as indexes of off-task behaviour and resistance to temptation assessed during a 30-minute structured observation paradigm. Boys who were rated insecurely attached in infancy tended to show inferior cognitive impulse control and delay ability at age of 6 years. Patterns of early maternal control also predicted later self-control in boys: those who engaged in restrictive, punitive interactions with their mothers at age 2 tended to perform more poorly on a measure of cognitive inhibition than others. For both sexes, ability to stay task-focused during the observation was predicted by antecedent patterns of enriched mother–child verbal communication during the second year. Finally, measures of child cognitive competence at 24 months predicted a broad range of self-control competencies at follow-up, including delay ability, inhibitory control, and task orientation.

Jacobvitz & Sroufe (1987), reporting from the Minnesota High Risk Study, observed mother–child interaction at 6 months in feeding and play situations. Their main hypothesis was that early mental intrusiveness might interfere with infants' abilities to modulate their arousal states, thus creating a risk condition for the later difficulties in regulation of arousal to meet situational demands.

When children were 42 months old, levels of distractibility, inattention, and impulsivity were assessed using a laboratory barrier box paradigm, and mother–child interaction was again observed during a teaching task. At 6 years, teachers rated children for symptoms of attention deficit disorder, and two extreme groups (hyperactive/control) were designed. In addition, a variety of early health status and temperament variables were assessed between 0 and 30 months and related to age 42-month and 6-year outcomes. As hypothesised, hyperactives and controls differed according to qualities of early caregiving. As infants, children in the hyperactive group had mothers who scored highly on a rating measure of maternal intrusiveness/interference, which indexed the extent to which mothers disrupt infant's ongoing activities rather than adapting their responses to the infant's state, mood, and interests. Distractibility at 42 months was also moderately correlated with early intrusiveness, and with later hyperactivity ratings. Surprisingly however, measures of early health status and temperament did not differentiate the groups.

In summary, although relevant empirical studies have been sparse and inconsistent, aspects of early caregiving have been prospectively linked to children's later self-regulatory capabilities. Even so, associations between early caregiving and later impulse control problems have been quite modest, and their clinical relevance is uncertain. In addition, the reasons for these associations remain unclear. Sroufe's hypothesis (Sroufe, 1991) that intrusive caregiving interferes with early modulation of arousal deserves further attention, as it is consistent with theories of self-regulation (Kopp, 1982, 1989; Sander, 1975) and hyperactivity (Douglas, 1983). It is puzzling that aspects of temperament did not relate to hyperactivity in this study, as many of the temperament measures included by Jacobvitz and Sroufe bore direct relevance to the construct of arousal modulation. Only linear relationships between early temperament and later hyperactivity were examined, though, indicating the importance of searching for interactional or transactional effects in further work.

Additional work is also needed to specify how maternal intrusiveness might affect risk of later hyperactivity. Sroufe (1991) has argued that insensitive maternal care is a primary causal agent in developmental pathways to hyperactivity, disrupting the child's ability to learn effective techniques for modulating arousal and sustaining attention. As the child grows, he or she may perceive little control over emotionally arousing situations, which in turn may account for later difficulties in attention modulation. However, this theory focuses upon only one aspect of the hyperactive syndrome, inattention. It is unclear how problems of impulsivity and overactivity might result from early intrusive maternal care, particularly in the absence of temperamental vulnerabilities that the child brings to caregiving interactions.

Qualities of early caregiving could also be associated with children's self-regulatory abilities because they stimulate the development of cognitive and linguistic competence. For example, in the Olson *et al.* (1990) study, the patterns of verbally stimulating and nonrestrictive caregiving that predicted children's later self-control were closely related to superior child cognitive competence at earlier age levels (Olson, Bates & Bayles, 1984; Olson, Bayles & Bates, 1986). Moreover, cognitive and linguistic deficits have been found consistently to co-vary with problems of hyperactivity and aggression in young children (Bates *et al.*, 1985; Campbell *et al.*, 1982; Erickson *et al.*, 1985; Moffitt, 1990; Pianta & Caldwell, 1990; Richman, Stevenson & Graham, 1982), and some investigators have argued that cognitive and linguistic problems precede the development of disruptive behaviour disorder (Beitchman *et al.*, 1986; Schonfeld *et al.*, 1988). The extent to which early verbal competence mediates children's attentional and impulse control capabilities is an important topic for further research. Cognitive immaturity is usually conceptualised as a secondary correlate of hyperactivity, but it may play a primary role in its early development.

To conclude: much further work is needed before we can understand the role of early caregiving in the development of hyperactivity. Refinements in attachment research, such as the development of new categories of insecure attachment (Main & Hesse, 1990), and the development of methods for assessing quality of attachment during the preschool years (Cassidy & Marvin, 1989; Greenberg, Speltz & De Klyen, 1993) may facilitate these efforts. Clearly, however, there is a need to go beyond attachment constructs by incorporating socio-ecological influences in primary relationship systems, broader patterns of family relationships, and temperamental contributions to parent–child relationships.

Parent–toddler control interactions

Achieving a sense of independent mastery constitutes a major developmental task issue for toddlers. In this period of rapid cognitive, social and motor growth, it is normal for toddlers to test parental limits and resist control (McFarlane, Allen & Honzik, 1954; Richman, Stevenson & Graham, 1982). As Kopp (1982) has argued, toddlerhood marks a critical transition period in the development of self-regulation, due to these very developmental changes. The manner in which parents and toddlers resolve these normative issues may forecast continuing problems in self-regulation.

A substantial body of research indicates that highly directive, negatively toned parent–toddler interactions are associated with non-compliance and other early manifestations of self-control problems. For example, the work of Lytton and his colleagues has shown that highly directive, controlling interactional styles are associated with non-compliance and escalating cycles of conflict between parents and toddlers (Lytton & Zwirner, 1975; Lytton, 1979). Similarly, Schaffer & Crook (1979, 1980) observed control techniques used by mothers of toddlers in a laboratory play situation. Frequent use of physical control and punishment was the most important predictor of non-compliance, whereas consistent rule enforcement, encouragement of mature behaviour, and use of praise as a reward were associated with positive compliance. These findings coincide with those of other recent investigators who have reported links between highly directive maternal behaviour in task situations and toddler non-compliance and task disengagement (Crockenberg & Litman, 1990; Feldman & Sarnat, 1986; Frankel & Bates, 1990; Silverman & Ragusa, 1990). Moreover, although most previous studies have been conducted with normal samples, Campbell and her colleagues (Campbell *et al.*, 1986) have shown that this dyadic pattern also characterises clinically relevant populations of young children. Campbell *et al.* studied a group of 3 year-old children who were identified by their parents as excessively overactive, noncompliant and inattentive. Mother–child dyads were observed during free play at initial assessment, and again one year later. Relative to controls, dyadic interactions between referred children and their mothers were characterised by less positive affect, more conflict and greater directiveness. At one year follow-up, mothers were less directive in play than at intake, but those with complaints about their children continued to provide more direction than mothers of controls. Finally, mothers showed high levels of individual stability in style of interaction: those who were initially most directive tended to remain so one year later.

These combined findings have a clear analogue in studies of older hyperactive children and their parents. Generally, social interactions between hyperactive children and their mothers have been characterised by greater conflict than is seen in normal mother–child dyads (Cunningham & Barkley, 1979; Mash & Johnston, 1982). Relative to controls, hyperactive children have shown higher degrees of non-compliant, negativistic, and off-task behaviour during interactions with their mothers, particularly in high structured task situations. Mothers of hyperactive children, in turn, have been found to be more directive, intrusive, and less positively reinforcing in these situations than mothers of normal children. Parent–child conflicts occur with fathers of hyperactive children as well as mothers (Tallmadge & Barkley, 1983). However, interactions between mothers and younger hyperactive children tend to be more directive and controlling than those between dyads containing older children (Mash & Johnston, 1982; Barkley, Karlsson & Pollard, 1985). Further, hyperactive boys who receive stimulant medication are less negativistic and more compliant with their mothers in task situations, and mothers respond in kind by becoming less directive and critical (Barkley & Cunningham, 1979; Humphries *et al.*, 1978; Barkley *et al.*, 1984). Thus, directive, conflicted interactions between mothers and their hyperactive children are in part a response to high levels of difficult child behaviour: When these levels decrease developmentally or as a result of medication, interactions become less restrictive and more positively toned. On the other hand, restrictive, controlling maternal behaviour towards infants and toddlers has been identified as a stable individual difference dimension in previous research (Clarke-Stewart, 1973; Olson *et al.*, 1984; Pettit & Bates, 1984), suggesting that it would be premature to dismiss the parent's contribution as an 'epiphenomenon' of difficult child behaviour. Indeed, Silverman & Ragusa (1990) recently reported that maternal negative control *vis-à-vis* toddlers in a structured task situation predicted disruptive behaviour problems at age four even when earlier levels of negative child behaviours were statistically controlled. Clearly, a transactional model is needed.

A study by Lee & Bates (1985) illustrates the importance of examining complex transactional relationships between maternal and child behaviour in the genesis of self-regulatory problems. These authors found that 2 year-old children perceived as difficult by their mothers were more likely to have conflicted mother–child interactions than others. In the home setting, difficult children were more negative and resistant to maternal control attempts than others. Mothers of difficult children, in turn, tended to use intrusive control strategies. The more difficult the child, the more likely there would be conflict after maternal control responses, resulting in extended episodes of negative interaction. Most significantly, these troubled relationship patterns had antecedents in earlier maternal ratings of temperamental difficultness: infants who were viewed as extremely irritable and difficult to manage at 6 and 13 months were at risk for conflicted mother–child interactions at age two. It is noteworthy that most of the toddlers in the difficult group were boys, even though the number of difficult boys and girls was relatively even at earlier age points.

Similarly, in further analyses of hard-to-manage preschool children, Campbell, *et al.* (1991) found that negative maternal control was strongly predicted by levels of non-compliant and overactive child behaviour in structured task situations. Negative control was also related to a host of family contextual variables reflecting high stress (e.g. marital distress; single parenthood), and to high levels of emotional distress in mother.

In summary, there is a substantial body of literature linking maternal directiveness and problems of non-compliance in toddlers. Some theorists might view the difficulties as early precursors of later behaviour disorders. For example, according to Patterson (1982), non-compliance is a form of coercive child behaviour that is maintained by inept parental control techniques. Early conflicts around non-compliance may place children at risk for escalating cycles of coercive interactions with parents and siblings, perhaps eventuating in later patterns of peer rejection, academic failure and delinquency (Patterson, DeBaryshe & Ramsey, 1989). However, in many cases it is both normal and healthy for toddlers to show non-compliance *vis-à-vis* their parents. As Kuczynski *et al.* (1987) have emphasised, non-compliance can serve many positive developmental functions, e.g. by providing a context for the development of socially appropriate expressions of autonomy and independence. Qualitative features of non-compliance may provide a key to understanding its clinical relevance. In a longitudinal study of parent–toddler interaction, Kuczynski & Kochaska (1990) examined multiple dimensions of child non-compliance which ranged from unskilful (angry, reactive, defiant behaviour) to skilful (active negotiation with parent), in quality. Only unskilful forms of resistance were predictive of children's behaviour problems at age 5, suggesting that these distinctions are important to consider in future research. Similarly, Crockenberg & Litman (1990) found that defiance, compliance and self-assertion were separate dimensions of behaviour in 1 year-old children, in that they loaded on different factors and showed distinctive relationships with mother–child interaction in a teaching task. Child defiance was a strong and consistent correlate of maternal negative control, but this association did not hold true for other dimensions of child non-compliance.

As with the research on mother–infant attachment and children's behaviour disorders, it is unclear how conflicted mother–toddler relationships relate to emerging self-regulatory difficulties in young children, and whether these problems generalise to other situational contexts. Moreover, again paralleling the attachment studies, these dyadic patterns appear to be risk markers for generalised patterns of behavioural maladjustment in young children. Their specific relevance to hyperactivity remains to be demonstrated.

Finally, many of the studies discussed above have indicated that 'difficult' child behaviour tends to elicit upper-limit control responses from socialising agents. As suggested by the Lee & Bates (1985) study, it is quite plausible that the child's behaviour reflects early appearing temperamental traits. Therefore, the role of early temperament as an antecedent of children's self-regulatory competence is considered in the following section.

Temperament and self-regulation

The construct of temperament encompasses individual differences in responsiveness to the environment which appear early in life, show evidence of heritability, and remain relatively stable within developmental periods (Bates, 1987; Buss & Plomin, 1984). Stylistic differences in behavioural expression, the 'how' rather than the 'what' of behaviour, are central to definitions of temperament. Temperamental differences are thought to play an important role in the early development of self-regulation (Buss & Plomin, 1984; Rothbart & Derryberry, 1981; Thompson, 1986). Moreover, the aetiology of hyperactivity is believed to be at least partly rooted in diverse organic factors (c.f. Barkley, 1989) which may find expression in temperamental traits. Surprisingly, however, there is a paucity of evidence linking early temperament to individual differences in self-regulatory competence, or to the later development of impulse control disorders. Two aspects of temperamental style have received the most attention in this regard: the global concept of difficultness and the narrower concept of activity level.

Difficultness

The concept of temperamental difficultness was introduced by Thomas, Chess & Birch (1968) to explain early appearing patterns of hyperirritability and biological irregularity. The most central feature of difficultness is a generalised pattern of negative emotional arousal in the young infant (Bates, 1980, 1987). Thus, 'difficult' infants fuss and cry excessively, and are resistant to caregivers' attempts to soothe them. They may also be slow to adapt to changes in daily routine, and irregular in sleep and feeding habits. Clearly, these infants show difficulties in the modulation of arousal, which is considered a critical early antecedent of self-regulation.

There are two sources of evidence linking temperamental difficultness in infancy to later problems of self-regulation. First, retrospective reports have indicated that some hyperactive children manifest early difficulties with emotional arousal and regulation (Ross & Ross, 1982). For example, Lambert (1982) examined evidence of infant temperamental difficultness among school-age hyperactive children and controls, using retrospective interviews with parents. Dimensions of difficult infant temperament, such as negative mood, unadaptability, low persistence, and high activity level, differentiated hyperactive children from controls at the .01 level of significance. Similarly,

Campbell, *et al.* (1982) studied a group of 2–3 year-old children identified by parents as overactive, inattentive, aggressive and noncompliant. In a structured interview, mothers of 'problem' children reported more difficulties during the early infant period than other mothers. As infants, the clinical group was described as highly active, hyperirritable, unsoothable and resistant to changes in feeding routines. The reports are intriguing, but methodological problems preclude any firm conclusions. Obviously, retrospective reports are highly vulnerable to selective distortion and bias, i.e. mothers of problem children may tend to selectively recall or exaggerate negative infant characteristics. Moreover, not all hyperactive children have been described as 'difficult' in infancy. Finally, difficultness is a nonspecific risk condition that may predispose children to a wide variety of later behavioural and emotional problems, not just hyperactivity.

Secondly, infant difficultness has been linked to late externalising-type behaviour problems in several prospective longitudinal studies of non-referred children. Wolkind & DeSalis (1982) found that difficult temperament, assessed using maternal interview at 4 months, predicted child behaviour problems at 42 months. Maternal depression tended to co-occur with child behaviour problems, but only if the child had been rated as difficult in infancy. In a re-analysis of the Thomas *et al.* (1968) data, Cameron (1978) found that difficult temperament at age 1 combined with problems in parental child rearing at age 3, predicted later behaviour problems in girls, but not in boys. The most consistent evidence for a link between infant difficultness and later behaviour problems has come from the Bloomington Longitudinal Study of Bates and his colleagues (Bates *et al.*, 1982). In a large, prospective study of normal infants and their families, temperamental difficultness was assessed using a maternal report questionnaire at age 6 months (Bates, Freeland & Lounsbury, 1979), with age-adjusted forms at 13 and 24 months of age. Observational measures of difficult temperament were also collected by visiting homes to assess levels of infant and toddler irritability, as were measures of parent–child interaction at each different assessment point. Two different aspects of early difficultness were salient as predictors: global scores, which indexed frequent and intense expressions of negative affect, and a narrow 'temperament-like' dimension involving toddler activity management problems and resistance to maternal control. Early irritability and resistance to control, as reported by mothers, were the best predictors of maternal ratings of aggression and hyperactivity in the preschool years (Bates *et al.*, 1985). More recently, these predictive patterns were found to generalise to mother reported behaviour problems at age 8 (Bates *et al.*, 1990). Observational indexes of irritability were relatively weak predictors of these outcomes, as were measures of parent–infant and parent–toddler interaction. Mothers' perceptions of early activity management problems predicted later externalising but not internalising problems. However, global ratings of negative emotionality predicted internalising problems as well, necessitating further differentiation of this broad construct.

Although limited to maternal assessments of temperament and behaviour problem outcomes, these reports suggest that early indexes of negative emotionality and difficult behaviour may forecast later behaviour problems, at least in the context of the mother–child relationship. The predictive associations are quite modest, however, and their clinical relevance is unclear. Moreover, two other longitudinal reports have failed to substantiate a link between early temperament and children's later impulse control problems. Olson *et al.* (1990), drawing upon the Bloomington data base, correlated mothers' ratings of difficult temperament at 24 months with a diverse set of laboratory and observational measures of impulsivity assessed at age 6 years. No relationship was found between early temperamental difficultness and later measures of self-control, nor did temperament interact with qualities of the caregiving environment to predict impulsive responding. Similarly, in their prospective study of high- risk families, Jacobvitz and Sroufe (1987) assessed individual differences in temperamental difficultness during the newborn period using nurses' ratings, and at 3, 6, and 30 months using maternal ratings. No relationships were found between the various temperament measures and teacher assessments of hyperactivity at age 6.

Thus, relevant research is both sparse and inconsistent on the role of temperamental difficulties in the development of children's self-regulatory difficultness. Although hyperactive children have often been described as difficult infants in retrospective reports, prospective longitudinal studies have provided no support for a linear association between early difficultness and later problems of impulse control. However, difficultness may be an early marker of more general patterns of behavioural maladjustment, especially oppositional behaviour in the context of the mother–child relationship.

Due to limitations in the measurement and conceptualisation of temperament, the relationship between early difficultness and self-regulatory problems remains an open and highly researchable question. Several points are worth noting. First, temperament is not an 'immutable' characteristic of individuals: temperamental traits show only modest to moderate stability within developmental periods, indicating the importance of examining sources of discontinuity as well as continuity (Bates, 1987). The extent to which temperamental traits remain stable and predict important developmental outcomes depends upon how they transact with qualities of the caregiving environment (Crockenberg, 1986). The prevailing model of temperament–environment interaction as a 'goodness of fit' model (Lerner & Lerner, 1983; Thomas *et al.*, 1968), stressing that lack of mutual accommodation between child and caregiver, not isolated characteristics of individuals, predicts negative developmental outcomes. The amount of stress vs. support resources in the broader social environment also plays an important role in this process. It is easy to imagine how an extremely irritable infant might overwhelm the caregiving skills of a chronically stressed parent who possesses few social or economic resources, yet be quite manageable for a parent with adequate support. Indeed, Crockenberg (1981) has shown the newborn irritability predicts insecure attachment only if coupled with low maternal social support.

It is also necessary to question how interactions between difficult children and their parents might foster problems of distractibility, aggression and impulsivity. Although few researchers have addressed this question, the Lee & Bates (1985) study (discussed above), showed that difficult infants, especially boys, were at risk for highly conflicted mother–toddler interactions that may prestage the development of conduct problems. In a similar vein, Maccoby, Snow & Jacklin (1984) observed 12 month-old children interacting with their mothers in teaching tasks, with concurrent assessments of infant difficultness. Comparable measures were obtained when the children were 18 months old. Maccoby *et al.* found that mothers of boys who were temperamentally difficult at 12 months were less active in guiding them at 18 months. They speculated that this may be part of a transactional cycle, in which the child 'creates' an interpersonal environment that exacerbates negative temperamental traits. Olweus (1980) reported a similar pattern of mother–child interaction in his longitudinal study of young boys who later developed conduct problems. Although patterns of temperamental difficultness are found in both sexes, these studies clearly suggest that difficult boys are more vulnerable to parent–child relationship problems than difficult girls.

Lambert & Hartsough (1984) have argued that an additive model of risk best explains the apparent relationship between early temperamental difficultness and later hyperactivity. They studied 97 children, aged 5 to 11 years, who were identified as pervasively hyperactive, and compared their developmental progress to that of 93 matched controls. Based on retrospective interviews with parents and concurrent assessments of family functioning, the hyperactive children were found to have higher incidences of pre- and perinatal risk factors, greater evidence of early health and temperamental problems, and less optimal parental relationships (e.g. more punitive, less educationally stimulating), than the controls. All three sets of risk factors made independent contributions to diagnoses of hyperactivity, but an aggregated set of predictors explained more variance in diagnostic status than either predictor set alone.

Thus, temperamental difficultness was one of many risk factors which accumulate to predict later hyperactivity, necessitating a multifactorial and longitudinal approach to this problem. However, the additive model still leaves us questioning how constitutional vulnerabilities transact with other risk conditions to potentiate hyperactivity.

Finally, there is a need to identify specific indices of temperament that place children at risk for hyperactivity. Difficultness is probably too broad a construct to use as risk marker for specific behaviour disorders. For example, as Bates (1987) has noted, there are many reasons why infants may fuss and cry excessively. Some may be seeking stimulation, whereas others may be seeking reductions in stimulation due to autonomic overactivity. The former pattern is most convergent with concepts of conduct and impulsivity problems.

Activity level

Activity level is commonly regarded as a dimension of temperament (e.g. Buss & Plomin, 1984), even though there has been inconsistent evidence for its stability in the first year of life (Bates, 1987). Evidence linking early activity levels to clinical manifestations of hyperactivity is lacking, but several studies have shown that highly active toddlers and preschoolers have elevated rates of conflicted/coercive interactions with parents and peers. Analysing data from the Fels Longitudinal Study, Battle & Lacey (1972) identified a group of 3–6 year-old 'hyperactive' children using observation based ratings of impulsive and highly active behaviour. Active boys and girls were less compliant towards adults, and more domineering and physically aggressive towards peers than others. Billman & McDevitt (1980) found that highly active preschoolers, as rated by parents and teachers, were involved in more coercive interactions with peers than others. Similarly, Halvorson & Waldrop (1973) found that highly active toddlers, identified using actometer ratings, tended to play more vigorously and become involved in more negative peer interactions than the normally active toddlers. Finally, Buss, Block & Block (1980) found that highly active 3 year-olds, identified by actometer ratings, were less compliant, more resistant to adult control, more domineering with peers, and more impulsive, than others. In a follow-up study, Buss (1981) found that activity level assessed at age 3 predicted quality of parental control at age 5. Highly active children tended to have more conflicted interactions with parents than others, as evidenced by greater use of physical control and expressions of hostility and impatience on the part of parents.

However, the association of early activity level with later hyperactivity is questionable: stability coefficients are only in the moderate range, and it is unclear whether highly active–aggressive children are manifesting early onset of hyperactivity or more generalised patterns of negativistic behaviour (Bates, 1987). As with the construct of difficultness, longitudinal research is needed to identify specific markers of the hyperactivity syndrome (perhaps using more qualitative indices of overactivity), then examine how they change over time as a consequence of being filtered through different social systems.

DEVELOPMENTAL COURSE

Preschool predictors of hyperactivity

As children progress through the preschool years, the number of referrals for hyperactivity rises sharply; Barkley (1989) has estimated that 50% of hyperactive children manifest significant behaviour problems by the time they are 3 years old. Although studies of hyperactivity symptoms in preschoolers have been relatively rare, there is an emerging consensus that the primary features of hyperactivity can be identified at these early ages. However, diagnosis and prognosis are complicated by a host of developmental and definitional factors.

In one of the earliest studies, Schleifer *et al.* (1975) examined 28 children who were referred for symptoms of 'hyperactivity'; according to their parents, these children were unresponsive to discipline, inattentive, overactive and unable to play by themselves. The clinical group was compared with 26 matched controls on measures of impulsive responding assessed in the laboratory, and measures of social and task-relevant behaviour assessed in home and preschool settings. In the preschool setting, only 11/28 children manifested problems of hyperactivity, and thus the clinical group was subdivided into 'true' and 'situational' subgroups. Relative to controls, hyperactive children were more impulsive on a test of reflection–impulsivity, and manifested more overactive, inattentive behaviour in the preschool, but only during structured task situations. Elevated rates of physical and verbal aggression were also found in the hyperactive group. Parents of children with 'true' hyperactivity reported more parenting stress than parents of children with 'situational' hyperactivity and controls; and were observed to use more physical punishment than others. At 2-year follow-up, children in the hyperactive group continued to evidence conflicts with parents (Campbell *et al.*, 1977). Finally, in a 3-year follow-up, Campbell, Endman & Bernfeld (1977) examined the self-esteem and classroom behaviours of these children using teacher reports and direct observation. Children who were designated hyperactive (both subtypes) in preschool continued to show problems in elementary school: they were more disruptive, and to a slight degree, had lower self-esteem than controls. Children who had been designated 'true' hyperactives in preschool manifested more out of seat and off-task behaviour than the 'situationals'. Thus, although the groups were very small, these findings indicated that hyperactive symptoms could be identified early in life, and persisted across the transition to elementary school.

Similar conclusions have been reached by Campbell and her colleagues on the basis of their later, programmatic efforts to identify preschoolers at risk for hyperactivity. In their initial study, Campbell *et al.* (1982) identified a group of 46 children aged 2 to 3 years, whose parents complained of high motor activity, distractibility, tantrums, defiance and difficulty playing alone. These children were compared with controls on a broad range of measures, including parent questionnaire rating of behaviours and laboratory measures of impulsivity and inattention. Not surprisingly, parents' complaints centred upon problems in social relationships: referred children were described as highly attention-seeking, resistant to discipline, and aggressive with peers and siblings. On the Behar problem behavior questionnaire, referred children were rated highly on both the hyperactivity and aggression scales. Maternal reports of hyperactive symptoms were validated by the results of laboratory tests: during structured observations, the clinical group switched activities more often and spent less time on single activities; during structured tasks, they were more often out of seat and off-task, and showed poorer ability to delay gratification than controls. Finally, these problems generalised to other situational contexts: Campbell & Cluss (1982) observed a subsample of subjects who attended preschool and found that they were more aggressive with peers during free play and less compliant in response to teacher directives than controls.

In short, parental complaints about these children were analogous to symptoms of hyperactivity in older, clinically defined groups. As Campbell has repeatedly emphasised, however, identification of 'hyperactivity' in the preschool period is complicated by significant developmental and definitional issues. The chief difficulty concerns the normative nature of some early 'problem' behaviours. Many of the problems that parents in her study complained of, such as restlessness, defiance, and tantrums, are common during this developmental period. Thus, it was unclear how many of these problems reflected true precursors of the disorder, rather than more transient manifestations of age-specific issues. Additionally, referred children showed considerable heterogeneity in their symptom pictures, and so it was uncertain whether these problems were precursors of hyperactivity *per se*, or more generalised patterns of conduct disturbance.

A series of follow-up reports by the Campbell group has illuminated some of these questions. Although there were general improvements in symptom levels over time, at 1-year follow-up, parent–referred children continued to exhibit more active, inattentive and impulsive behaviour than controls (Campbell, *et al.*, 1984). At age 6, problems of aggression and hyperactivity were found to be strongly related to earlier assessments of negative behaviour; and symptom severity was predicted by a constellation of factors, particularly low SES and highly conflicted, directive mother–child interaction (Campbell *et al.*, 1986). Since half of the referred group continued to show chronic problems, Campbell (1987) searched for antecedent variables that discriminated those who improved from those who persisted in their maladjustment. Children with persistent problems were rated by mothers as more inattentive, disobedient and maladjusted in their peer relations (e.g. disliked, aggressive) than others. Across the age range, children with persistent problems were rated higher on measures of antisocial behaviour than those who improved, whereas children who improved tended to show steady decrements in levels of externalising symptoms over time. At age 9, children in the persistent problems group were more likely than others to receive DSM-III diagnoses of attention deficit disorder, oppositional disorder, and/or conduct disorder (Campbell & Ewing, 1990). Moreover, teachers evaluated them as having significant problems with core symptoms of hyperactivity, and with peer adjustment. Once again, continuing problems of aggression and hyperactivity, as reported by mothers, had multiple antecedents, including reports of difficult temperament in infancy, high levels of preschool externalising problems, conflicted mother–child interaction at age 3 and 4, and elevated levels of family stress. Finally, early levels of family stress and laboratory measures of inattention and overactivity were predictive of later teacher ratings of externalising problems.

These combined findings suggest several tentative conclusions. First, symptoms of hyperactivity can be identified early in life, and they persist at moderate levels across the transition to middle childhood. Although the Montreal and Pittsburgh studies were limited by very small sample sizes, their findings are consistent with other reports showing moderately high persistence of externalising symptoms from preschool to the school-age years (Achenbach, Edelbrock & Howell, 1987; Fischer *et al.*, 1984; Kohn, 1977; Richman *et al.*, 1982; Rose, Rose & Feldman, 1989). For example, in their epidemiological survey of 3 year-old children living in a London Borough, Richman *et al.* (1982) identified a subgroup who showed serious behaviour problems. When children were 8 years of age, 62% of the initial problem group remained disturbed, compared with 22% of a matched control group. Among those who persisted in their maladjustment, temper tantrums, negativism, antisocial behaviour, restlessness, overactivity, and poor social relationships were salient concerns. Boys were far more likely than girls to show problem persistence, especially in the area of antisocial behaviour. Consistent with Campbell *et al.*'s (1986) findings, boys with persistent problems were more difficult to manage, restless, and overactive as preschoolers. As preschoolers, they also had more symptoms in general, and lower levels of language competence than others.

Moderate levels of stability in symptomatic behaviour exist despite developmental changes in primary problem areas such as overactivity, inattention, and disruptiveness. Numerous studies have shown that hyperactive and normal children show clear decrements in activity level between the age of 3 and 9 (Abikoff, Gittelman-Klein & Klein 1977; Milich, 1984; Routh, Schroeder & O'Tuama, 1974). Sustained attention and motor inhibition also increase over the same time period (Levy, 1980; Milich, 1984). Apparently, children who begin with the highest number and most severe initial symptoms fail to 'catch up' with their peers (Campbell, 1987; Mash & Johnston, 1982; Richman *et al.*, 1982), evidencing patterns of cognitive and social functioning characteristic of much younger children.

However, a substantial number of 'difficult' children do not manifest behaviour problems in later childhood. The presence of chronic family adversity, such as maternal distress, mother–child conflict, and marital discord, is a powerful predictor of problem persistence in preschoolers (Campbell *et al.*, 1986; Campbell & Ewing, 1990; Egeland *et al.*, 1990; McGee, Silva & Williams, 1984; Pianta & Caldwell, 1990; Richman *et al.*, 1982). These reports are consistent with current systems models, which stress that persistent maladjustment is most likely to occur in the context of continuously and pervasively negative child-environment interactions.

Problem persistence can also be viewed from the perspective of adaptational failures. The transition to preschool requires that young children adapt to structured routines, conform to the authority of adults other than parents, and share resources and adult attention with many other peers. Hence, establishing flexible levels of self-control and positive peer relationships are central developmental tasks for the preschool-age child (Sroufe, 1979; Sroufe & Rutter, 1984).

Preschoolers at risk for continued maladjustment show pervasive deficits in self-regulatory competence and perhaps as a consequence, experience disharmonious relationships with peers (Campbell & Cluss, 1982; Campbell *et al.*, 1982; Richman *et al.*, 1982). Similarly, studies of non-referred preschool children have shown that impulsive and disruptive behaviour tends to co-occur with peer rejection (Milich *et al.*, 1982; Olson & Brodfeld, 1991; Olson, 1989; Rubin & Clark, 1983), and predicts social maladjustment in the school-age years (Ladd, Price & Hart, 1986; Olson, 1989). These early patterns may represent one developmental pathway to the pervasive patterns of social maladjustment that often characterise school-age hyperactive children.

Finally, the issue of symptom heterogeneity within the broad externalising spectrum remains unresolved. Preschoolers at risk for persistent maladjustment show a mix of negativistic and aggressive features in addition to the 'classic' characteristics of hyperactivity (Campbell *et al.*, 1982; Richman *et al.*, 1982). These symptom patterns forecast later diagnoses of attention deficit hyperactivity disorder, conduct disorder, oppositional disorder, and combinations of these problems (Campbell & Ewing, 1990). Small sample sizes have precluded efforts to examine the long-term developmental sequelae of narrow-band syndromes, but a growing consensus is that a combination of hyperactive and aggressive features places children at greatest risk for serious and persistent maladjustment. This is clearly an issue for further systematic study.

Long-term outcome and predictors

Although hyperactivity was once thought to reflect a maturational disorder that children 'outgrew' in adolescence (Laufer & Denhoff, 1957), accumulating evidence from follow-up studies of school-age hyperactives has put this notion to rest. It is abundantly clear that hyperactive children are at elevated risk for a host of adaptational difficulties in later life, ranging from problems in self-esteem and social relationships to serious criminality.

The most concentrated efforts to examine the long-term course of hyperactivity have come from Weiss and her colleagues at Montreal Children's Hospital, who followed a group of 104 hyperactive children into adolescence and early adulthood (Weiss & Hechtman, 1986). At primary school-age, hyperactive subjects were quite similar in the nature of their 'core' problems (attentional problems, overactivity, impulsivity), but varied considerably in family backgrounds and the extent to which they manifested concomitant conduct and learning problems. At 5-year follow-up, 91 (mean age 13) former hyperactive children were interviewed and compared with normal controls who were selected at the time and matched for age, SES, IQ, and sex (Weiss *et al.*, 1971). Ratings of initial symptoms decreased over time, but probands continued to demonstrate higher levels of primary symptoms than controls. Adolescents in the hyperactive group were described as immature, low in self-esteem, and as having difficulty maintaining goals. Academic problems were especially salient: the hyperactive group had higher rates of academic failure and were more impulsive than controls. Twenty-five per cent had engaged in antisocial behaviour.

At 10-year follow-up (mean age 19), 50% of the probands still had significant problems of the original syndrome, particularly restlessness and impulsivity (Weiss *et al.*, 1979). Relative to controls, former hyperactive subjects showed a variety of problems in social and academic spheres: for example, they had completed less education, achieved lower grades in school, experienced more car accidents, and manifested poorer social adjustment (e.g. personality trait disorders, fewer friends) and poorer self esteem. Similarly, at 15-year follow-up (Weiss *et al.*, 1985), more than half of the hyperactive adults had retained at least one major symptom of the disorder. Restlessness seemed especially prominent, and was observable during the interview situation. The group as a whole had more suicide attempts and poorer social adjustment than controls. As at previous age levels, risk of later psychiatric disturbance mainly involved the antisocial spectrum: 23% of the probands received a DMS-III diagnosis of antisocial personality disorder. However, the authors noted that one-third of these cases involved mild symptoms that may not have been considered antisocial by other diagnosticians.

Finally, differences in work record were also found: adults who had been hyperactive were rated more negatively by their supervisors, although they tended to be economically self-sufficient and did not differ from controls in annual income. Hyperactive adults also quit their jobs or were laid off more frequently than controls, and reported greater difficulties in carrying out assigned tasks. Interestingly, however, they did not attribute these difficulties to residual symptoms of the disorder such as distractibility or restlessness. The findings regarding work record converged with those of Borland & Heckman (1976), whose follow-up analyses revealed that adults with a history of hyperactivity achieved lower work status and suffered more frequent job changes than their sibling who had not been hyperactive as children.

Lambert and her colleagues (Lambert, 1988) have reported findings similar to those of the Weiss group in their follow-up studies of hyperactive children as adolescents and young adults. Their subjects were 166 adolescents aged 17 to 18 years, who had received a medical diagnosis of hyperactivity in childhood, and whose parents and teachers also considered them to be hyperactive. Hyperactive individuals had significantly poorer educational and conduct outcome than controls, as evidenced by attendance in special schools, failure to complete high school, placement in foster care or residential settings, rates of adjudicated delinquency, and use of hard drugs. A combination of hyperactivity and aggression in childhood was a better predictor of adolescent conduct disorder than either symptom alone. This was not the case for poor educational outcomes, which were predicted by either or both symptoms of hyperactivity and aggression.

Because the greatest long-term mental health risk for hyperactive children appears to be in the area of antisocial spectrum disorders, the relationship between initial hyperactivity and later antisocial outcomes has been the focus of several follow-up reports. Gittelman and her colleagues (Gittleman *et al.*, 1985) followed up 101 male adolescents aged 16 years, who had received a childhood diagnosis of hyperactivity. Follow-up assessments were conducted by the interviewers who were blind to subjects' early diagnostic status. Although there was a gradual attrition in the severity of symptoms over time, 31% of the probands were given a DSM-III diagnosis of ADD, in comparison with 3% of the controls. Both conduct disorder and substance use disorders were over-represented in the clinical group, and tended to aggregate with continued symptoms of hyperactivity. The most interesting aspect of this report concerned a developmental progression in patterns of co-morbidity: boys whose symptoms of hyperactivity had not remitted were four times more likely to develop conduct disorder in adolescence than others. Moreover, two thirds of those who eventually developed conduct disorders progressed to drug and/or alcohol abuse.

Satterfield (Satterfield, Hoppe & Schell, 1982) also reported high rates of antisocial behaviour in adolescents with a childhood history of hyperactivity. Following a group of 110 young adults (mean age 17) who had received a childhood diagnosis of hyperactivity and 88 normal controls, Satterfield *et al.* found striking differences between probands and controls in rates of adjudicated antisocial behaviour. Only serious offences, defined as 'robbery', 'burglary', 'grand theft auto', and 'assault with a deadly weapon', were examined. Since the control group had higher SES levels than the probands, comparisons were made with SES groups. The percentage of hyperactive individuals arrested at least once for a serious offence ranged from 38%–58% across SES groups, in comparison with 2–11% for the controls. Moreover, probands had multiple arrest rates of 25–45% across SES groups, in comparison with 0–6% for controls. Finally, 25% of the probands had been admitted in institutions for delinquent behaviour, compared with only one subject in the control group.

Loney, Kramer & Milich (1981) found that initial levels of aggression (defined broadly as angry affect, aggressive interpersonal behaviour and community rule violations) were better predictors of hyperactive and antisocial symptoms in adolescence than symptoms of hyperactivity alone. A combination of aggressive and hyperactive features in childhood predicted the worst adolescent outcomes. As adolescents, children with 'pure symptoms of hyperactivity tended to manifest problems of academic under-achievement (Paternite & Loney, 1980). A small group of subjects were also followed up to the age of 21 years, and compared with their brothers (Loney *et al.*, 1983). The authors found that 45% of the former hyperactive subjects met the criteria for antisocial personality disorder, compared with 18% of the brothers. Former hyperactive subjects differed most from their brothers in the area of crimes against persons: significantly more of the hyperactive group had concealed a weapon, threatened to assault another person, or been in a fight where weapons were used.

Reporting from a large longitudinal study of New Zealand boys, Moffitt (1990) also found important differences between hyperactive children with and without histories of antisocial behaviour. At the age of 13, four groups were identified on the basis of self-reported delinquent behaviour and a clinical diagnosis of hyperactivity: hyperactive + delinquent, hyperactive only, delinquent only, and non-disordered. Correlates of delinquency, such as antisocial behaviour problems, verbal IQ deficits, reading problems and family adversity, were traced across childhood. The mixed hyperactivity/delinquent group showed the highest rates of aggressiveness, family adversity and neurophysiological deficits, along with the greatest potential for sustained antisocial behaviour. Children with symptoms of hyperactivity alone showed only mild antisocial behaviour at follow-up, and had normal IQs, reading scores and family backgrounds. In comparing patterns of adaptation across time, Moffitt found that the mixed symptom group had a distinctive developmental trajectory. Antisocial behaviour and symptoms of hyperactivity were present in the preschool years, escalated at school entry, and remained stable into adolescence. Patterns of antisocial behaviour consistently co-varied with verbal IQ deficits, reading failure at school, and a cumulative index of family adversity. In contrast, the delinquent only group had no verbal IQ deficits, and did not evidence antisocial behaviour or family adversity before the age of ll. These interesting findings should be viewed with caution, given that the mixed hyperactive/delinquent group was very small. However, they are consistent with other reports suggesting that boys with symptom co-morbidity are at very high risk for persistent and serious antisocial behaviour (e.g. Hinshaw, 1987; Magnusson & Bergman, 1990), and they suggest new information concerning the long-term developmental trajectories of at-risk children.

In summary, the 'core' symptoms of hyperactivity persist into adolescence and early adulthood but diminish in severity over time (Thorley, 1984; Whalen & Henker, 1986). Behavioural manifestations of core symptoms also differ between childhood and adolescence; for example, the unfocused overactivity so commonly reported in hyperactive children tends to be expressed as sedentary restlessness in later life (Gittleman & Mannuzza, 1985; Weiss & Hechtman, 1986). However, the most salient concerns of hyperactive adolescents and young adults do not centre upon core symptoms, but upon global patterns of educational, occupational and interpersonal maladjustment. Although risk of later psychiatric disorder clearly loads into the antisocial spectrum, rates of actual antisocial behaviour in hyperactive individuals vary considerably between studies, reflecting heterogeneity in both initial sample selection and diagnostic criteria at follow-up (Cantwell, 1986; Weiss & Hechtman, 1986).

Given the substantial variability in later life outcomes among hyperactive children, what factors differentiate those who improve from those who continue to evidence maladjustment? Because childhood hyperactivity is associated with pervasive problems of interpersonal and educational adjustment, it is unclear whether adolescent and adult outcomes are attributable to antecedent symptoms of hyperactivity, associated features such as family dysfunction, conduct disorder, or learning disabilities, or some combination of these factors (Cantwell, 1986). Indeed, predictive studies of long-term outcome status (e.g. Hechtman *et al.*, 1984; Loney *et al.*, 1981; Paternite & Loney, 1980) have consistently identified very global antecedent correlates of poor outcomes such as low IQ, low SES, childhood aggression, and family instability. Disappointingly, long-term adjustment has generally been found to be unrelated to either the type or duration of treatment (Aman, 1984; Paternite & Loney, 1980).

Based on analyses of their 10-year follow-up data, Weiss & Hechtman (1986) concluded that particular adult outcomes are not well predicted by specific antecedent variables, but by additive combinations of personal and social-familial characteristics. Moreover, different combinations of predictors appear to be salient for different outcome measures. For example, academic status was best predicted by a combination of childhood IQ, SES, initial measures of hyperactive symptoms and childrearing practices, whereas emotional adjustment was predicted by mental health status of family members in combination with low frustration tolerance and emotional instability in childhood. Similarly, in her extensive analyses of long-term predictors of outcome status in hyperactive children, Lambert (1988) concluded that there are general characteristics of hyperactive children (such as severity of initial symptoms and concomitant aggression) that predispose children to maladjustment in later life, but also specific pathways to educational, mental health, conduct, and substance use outcomes. Lambert and her colleagues have adopted an expanded developmental approach to the prediction of later life outcomes by considering infancy and preschool predictors as well as those characterising the school age period. Different pathways to outcome within the same disorder were marked by differentially weighted combinations of individual, environmental and developmental factors. For example, factors operating during infancy and preschool, such as the presence of difficult temperament and poor health status, were more important predictors of adolescent mental health status than those operating during the school- age years. Conversely, home environment and family interaction during the elementary school years were superior predictors of later academic achievement.

Finally, the search for predictors of long-term adaptation in hyperactive individuals has focused on negative outcomes. Given that as many as 25–50% of hyperactive children are judged to be functioning normally in later life, it would be worthwhile to search for factors that ameliorate risk and lead to positive psychosocial outcomes (Whalen, 1989). In the context of assessing treatment effects, Weiss & Hechtman (1986) asked their adult subjects to identify what was most helpful to them in their childhood years. Caring, positive relationships with significant others emerged as consistent themes. Most often these relationships were with parents, but teachers, tutors, counsellors, and friends were also mentioned. Similar conclusions were reached by Werner & Smith (1982) who followed a subgroup of children with learning problems and hyperactive features from age 10–18. Parenting variables, especially consistency of discipline and respect for the child, differentiated those who improved from those whose maladjustment persisted. Social support and caring family relationships have been repeatedly identified as general protective factors in children at risk for a broad range of adverse psychiatric outcomes (Werner & Smith, 1982; Werner, 1993; Garmezy, 1983; Rutter, 1987). Further research is needed to specify how interpersonal support affects long-term outcomes in hyperactive children.

In conclusion, risk factors associated with negative outcome in hyperactive individuals appear to be additive within developmental periods and cumulative across time (Lambert, 1988). However, more complex analyses of risk should also be conducted, such as examining whether certain factors (e.g., the presence of antisocial behaviour and family adversity) combine multiplicatively rather than addictively in the prediction of later outcome status (Rutter, 1987). The picture that is emerging is that there are multiple developmental pathways to hyperactivity, and to later life outcomes once a diagnosis has been made. Explaining inter- and intra-individual variability in the life paths of hyperactive children is the most important direction for further research.

REFERENCES

Abikoff, H., Gittelman-Klein, R. & Klein, D. (1977). Validation of a classroom observation code for hyperactive children. *Journal of Consulting and Clinical Psychology,* **45**, 772–83.

Achenbach, T. (1974). *Developmental Psychopathology.* New York: The Ronald Press.

Achenbach, T.M., Edelbrock, C. & Howell, C. (1987). Empirically-based assessment of the behavior problems of 2–3 year old children. *Journal of Abnormal Child Psychology,* **15**, 629–50.

Ainsworth, M.D.S., Bell, S.M. & Stayton, D.J. (1971). Individual differences in strange situation behavior of one year olds. In *The Origins of Human Social Relations,* ed. H.R. Schaffer, pp. 17–57. London: Academic Press.

Ainsworth, M.D.S., Blehar, M.C., Waters, E., & Wall, S. (1978). *Patterns of Attachment: A Psychological Study of the Strange Situation*. Hillsdale, NJ: Erlbaum.

Aman, M.G. (1984). Hyperactivity: nature of the syndrome and its natural history. *Journal of Autism and Developmental Disorders,* **14**, 39–56.

American Psychiatric Association (1980). DSM-III: *Diagnostic and Statistical Manual of Mental Disorders,* Third edition. Washington, DC: American Psychiatric Association.

American Psychiatric Association (1987). *Diagnostic and statistical manual of mental disorders* (3rd Edition). Washington, DC.

American Psychiatric Association (1994). DSM-IV: *Diagnostic and Statistical Manual of Mental Disorders,* Fourth edition. Washington, DC: American Psychiatric Association.

Anderson, J.C., Williams, S., McGee, R. & Silva, P.A. (1987). DMS-111 disorders preadolescent children: prevalence in a large sample from the general population. *Archives of General Psychiatry,* **44**, 69–76.

Anthony, E.J. (1987). Risk, vulnerability, and resilience: an overview. In *The Invulnerable Child,* eds. E. J. Anthony & B.J. Cohler, pp. 3–48. New York: Guilford.

Barkley, R.A. (1982). Specific guidlines for defining hyperactivity in children. In *Advances in Clinical Child Psychology*, eds. B.B. Lahey and A.E. Kazdin. Vol 5, pp. 137–80. New York: Plenum.

Barkley, R.A. (1985). The social behaviour of hyperactive children: Developmental changes, drug effects, and situational variation. In *Childhood Disorders*, eds. R. McMahon and R. Peters, New York: Brunner/Mazel.

Barkley, R.A. (1989). The problem of stimulus control and rule-governed behaviour in children with attention deficit disorder with hyperacitivity. In *Emerging Trends in Research on Attention Deficit Disorders*, eds. J. Swanson and L. Bloomingdale. New York: Plenum.

Barkley, R.A. (1988). Attention deficit disorder with hyperactivity. In *Behaviour Assessment of Childhood Disorders*, eds. E.J. Mash & L.G Terdal, pp. 69–104. New York: Guilford.

Barkley, R.A. & Cunningham, C.E. (1979). The effects of methylphenidate on the mother–child interactions of hyperactive children. *Archives of General Psychiatry*, **36**, 201–8.

Barkley, R.A. & Ullman, D.G. (1975). A comparison of objective measure of activity and distractibility in hyperactive and nonhyperactive children. *Journal of Abnormal Child Psychology,* **3**, 231–44.

Barkley, R.A., Karlsson, J. & Pollard, S. (1985). Effects of age on the mother–child interactions of ADD-H and normal boys. *Journal of Abnormal Child Psychology,* **13**, 631–8.

Barkley, R.A., Karlsson, J., Strezelecki, E. & Murphy, J. (1984). Effects of age and Ritalin dosage on the mother–child interactions of hyperactive children. *Journal of Consulting and Clinical Psychology,* **52**, 750–58.

Barkley, R.A., Karlsson, J., Pollard, S. & Murphy, J. (1985). Developmental changes in the mother–child interactions of hyperactive boys: effects of two dose level of Ritalin. *Journal of Child Psychology and Psychiatry,* **26**, 705–15.

Bartsch, K. & Wellman, H.M. (1989). Young children's attribution of action to beliefs and desires. *Child Development,* **60**, 946–64.

Bartsch, K. & Wellman, H. (1994). *Children Talk about the Mind.* Oxford: Oxford University Press.

Bates, J.E. (1980). The concept of difficult temperament. *Merrill-Palmer Quarterly,* **26**, 299–319.

Bates, J.E. (1987). Temperament in infancy. In *Handbook of Infant Development,* ed. J.D.

Osofsky *2nd edn.*, pp. 1101–49. New York: Bates, J.E. Wiley & Bayles, K. (1988). The role of attachment in the development of behaviour problems. In *Clinical Applications of Attachment*, eds. J. Belsky & T. Nezworski, pp. 253–99. Hillsdale, NJ: Lawrence Erlbaum Associates.

Bates, J.E., Bayles, K., Bennett, D., Ridge, B. & Brown, M. (1990). Origins of externalising behaviour problems at eight years of age. In *Development and Treatment of Childhood Aggression*, eds. D. Pepler & K. Rubin, pp. 93–120. Hillsdale, NJ: Erlbaum.

Bates, J.E., Freeland, C.A.B. & Lounsbury, M.L. (1979). Measurement of infant difficultness. *Child Development,* **50**, 794–803.

Bates, J.E., Maslin, C.A. & Frankel, K. (1985). Attachment security, other–child interaction, and temperament as predictors of behaviour problem ratings at age three years. In: *Growing Points of Attachment Theory and Research*, eds. I. Bretherton & E. Waters, pp. 167–93. Monographs of the Society for Research in Child Development, **50**, 209.

Bates, J.E., Olson, S. L., Pettit, G. & Bayles, K. (1982). Dimensions of individuality in the mother–infant relationship at 6 months of age. *Child Development,* **53**, 445–61.

Battle, E.S., & Lacey, B. (1972). A context for hyperactivity in children over time. *Child Development,* **43**, 757–73.

Beitchman, J.H., Nair, R., Clegg, M., Ferguson, B. & Patel, P.G. (1986). Prevalence of psychiatric disorders in children with speech and language disorders. *Journal of the American Academy of Child and Adolescent Psychiatry,* **28**, 528–35.

Belsky, J., Taylor, D.G. & Rovine, M. (1984). The Pennsylvania Infant and Family Development Project, III: The origins of individual differences in mother–infant attachment: maternal and infant contributions. *Child Development,* **55**, 718–28.

Billman, J. & McDevitt, S.C. (1980). Convergence of parent and observer ratings of temperament with observations of peer interaction in nursery school. *Child Development,* **51**, 395–400.

Bishof, N. (1975). A system approach toward the functional connections of attachment and fear. *Child Development,* **46**, 801–17.

Block, J.H. & Block, J. (1980). The role of ego control and ego resiliency in the organisation of development. In *Minnesota Symposia on Child Psychology*, ed. W.A. Collins, Vol. 13, pp. 39–101. Hillsdale, N.J.: Erlbaum.

Borland, B.L. & Heckman, H.K. (1976). Hyperactive boys and their brothers: a 25-year follow-up study. *Archives of General Psychiatry,* **33**, 669–75.

Bowlby, J. (1969). *Attachment and loss: Vol. 1 Attachment*, New York: Basic.

Bowlby, J. (1982). *Attachment and Loss: Vol. 1 Attachment* (2nd edn.). New York: Basic.

Bretherton, I. Attachment theory: Retrospect and prospect (1985). In *Growing Points of Attachment Theory and Research*, eds. I. Bretherton & E. Waters pp. 3–35. Monographs of the Society for Research in Child Development, **50**, 209.

Bretherton, I. & Breeghly, M. (1982). Talking about internal states: the acquisition of an explicit theory of mind. *Developmental Psychology,* **18**, 906–21.

Brody, G.H., Stoneman, Z. & Burke, M. (1988). Child temperament and parental perceptions of individual child adjustment: an intrafamilial analysis. *American Journal of Orthopsychiatry,* **58**, 532–42.

Brown, J.R. & Dunn, J. (1991). You can cry, mum: the social and developmental implications of talk about internal states. *British Journal of Developmental Psychology,* **9**, 237–56.

Buss, A.H. & Plomin, R. (1984). *Temperament: Early Developing Personality Traits.* Hillsdale, NJ: Erlbaum.

Buss, D.M. (1981). Predicting parent–child interactions from children's activity level. *Developmental Psychology,* **17**, 59–65.

Buss, D.M., Block, J.H. & Block, J. (1980). Preschool activity level: personality correlates and developmental implications. *Child Development,* **51**, 401–8.

Cameron, J.R. (1978). Parental treatment, children's temperament, and the risk of childhood behavior problems: 2. Initial temperament, parental attitudes, and the incidence and form of behavior problems. *American Journal of Orthopsychiatry*, **48**, 140–7.

Campbell, S.B. (1987). Parent–referred problem three-year-olds: Developmental changes in symptoms. *Journal of Child Psychology and Psychiatry,* **28**, 835–45.

Campbell, S.B. (1989). Developmental perspectives. In *Handbook of Childhood Psychopathology*, eds. T.M. Ollendick & M. Hersen, pp. 5–28. New York: Plenum Press.

Campbell, S.B. & Cluss, P. (1982). Peer relations in young children with behaviour problems. In *Peer Relationships and Social Skills in Childhood,* eds. K.H. Rubin & H. S. Ross, pp. 323–53. New York: Springer-Verlag.

Campbell, S.B. & Ewing, L.J. (1990). Follow-up of hard-to-manage preschoolers: Adjustment at age 9 and predictors of continuing symptoms. *Journal of Child Psychology and Psychiatry,* **31**, 871–89.

Campbell, S.B., Endman, M. & Bernfeld, G. (1977). A three year follow-up of hyperactive preschoolers into elementary school. *Journal of Child Psychology and Psychiatry,* **18**, 239–50.

Campbell, S.B, Schleifer, M., Weiss, G. & Perlman, T. (1977). A two-year follow-up of hyperactive preschoolers. *American Journal of Orthopsychiatry,* **47**, 149–62.

Campbell, S.B., Szumowski, E.K., Ewing, L.J., Gluck, D. & Breaux, A.M. (1982). A multidimensional assessment of parent-identified behavior problem toddlers. *Journal of Abnormal Child Psychology,* **10**, 569–629.

Campbell, S.B., Breaux, A.M., Ewing, L.A. & Szumowski, E.K. (1984). A one-year follow-up study of parent-referred 'hyperactive' preschoolers. *Journal of the American Academy of Child Psychiatry,* **23**, 243–9.

Campbell, S.B., Breaux, A.M., Ewing, L.A. & Szumowski, E.K. (1986). Correlates and predictors of hyperactivity and aggression: a longitudinal study of parent-referred problem preschoolers. *Journal of Abnormal Child Psychology*, **14**, 217–34.

Campbell, S.B., Ewing, L.J., Breaux, A.M. & Szumowski, E.K. (1986). Parent-referred problem three-year-olds: follow-up at school entry. *Journal of Child Psychology and Psychiatry,* **27**, 473–88.

Campbell, S.B., Pierce, E.W., March, C. & Ewing, L. (1991). Noncompliant behavior, overactivity, and family stress as predictors of negative maternal control with preschool children. *Development and Psychopathology,* **3**, 175–90.

Cantwell, D.P. (1986). Attention deficit disorder in adolescents. *Clinical Psychology Review,* **6**, 237–47.

Cantwell, D.P. & Satterfield, J.H. (1978). The prevalence of academic underachievement in hyperactive children. *Journal of Pediatric Psychology,* **3**, 168–71.

Cassidy, J. & Marvin, R.S. with The MacArthur Working Group on Attachment. (1989). Attrachment organisation in three and four year olds: coding guidelines. Unpublished scoring manual.

Cicchetti, D. (1984). The emergence of developmental psychology. *Child Development,* **55**, 1–7.

Cicchetti, D. (1990). Perspectives on the interface between normal and atypical development. *Development and Psychopathology*, **2**, 329–33.

Cicchetti, D. & Rizley, R. (1981). Developmental perspectives on the etiology, intergeneration transmission, and sequelae of child maltreatment. *New Directions for Child Development,* **11**, 31–56.

Clark, M.L., Cheyne, J.A., Cunningham, C.E. & Siegel, L.S. (1988). Dyadic peer interaction and task orientation in attention-deficit-disordered children. *Journal of Abnormal Child Psychology*, **16**, 1–15.

Clarke-Stewart, K.A. (1973). Interactions between mothers and their young children: Characteristics and consequences. *Monographs of the Society for Research in Child Development*, 38 (no. 153).

Crockenberg, S.B. (1981). Infant irritability, mother responsiveness, and social support influences on the security of mother–infant attachment. *Child Development,* **52**, 857–65.

Crockenberg, S.B. (1986). Are temperamental differences in babies associated with predictable differences in caregiving? In *Temperament and Social Interaction during Infancy and Childhood. New Directions for Child Development*, eds. J.V. Lerner & R. Lerner, pp. 53–71. No. 31, San Francisco: Jossey-Bass.

Crockenberg, S.B. & Litman, C. (1990). Autonomy as competence in 2-year-olds: Maternal correlates of child defiance, compliance, and self-assertion. *Developmental Psychology,* **26**, 961–71.

Cunningham, C.E. & Barkley, R.A. (1979). The interactions of normal and hyperactive children with their mothers in free play and structured task. *Child Development,* **50**, 217–24.

Cunningham, C.E. & Siegel, L.S. (1987). Peer interactions of normal and attention-deficit disordered boys during free play. Cooperative task, and simulated classroom situations. *Journal of Abnormal Child Psychology,* **15**, 247–68.

DeMulder, E.K. & Radke-Yarrow, M. (1991). Attachment with affectively ill and well mothers: concurrent behavioural correlates. *Development and Psychopathology,* **3**, 227–42.

Douglas, V.I. (1983). Attention and cognitive problems. In: *Developmental Neuropsychiatry*, ed. M. Rutter, pp. 280–329. New York: Guilford Press.

Douglas, V.I. & Peters, K.G. (1979). Toward a clearer definition of the attention deficit of hyperactive children. In *Attention and the Development of Cognitive Skills*, eds. G.H. Hale & M. Lewis, pp. 173–248. New York: Plenum.

Dunn, J. (1988). *The Underpinnings of Social Understanding*. Cambridge, MA: Harvard University Press.

Edelbrock, C., Costello, A. & Kessler, M.D. (1984). Empirical corroboration of attention deficit disorder. *Journal of the American Academy of Child and Adolescent Psychiatry,* **23**, 285–90.

Egeland, B., Kalkoske, M., Gottesman, N. & Erickson, M.F. (1990). Preschool behavior problems: stability and factors accounting for change. *Journal of Child Psychology and Psychiatry,* **31**, 891–909.

Eisenberg, N., Fabes, R.A., Nyman, M., Bernzweig, J. & Pinuelas, A. (1994). The relations of emotionality and regulation to children's anger-related reactions. *Child Development,* **65**, 109–28.

Erickson, E.H. (1963). *Childhood and Society* (2nd edn.). New York: Norton.

Erickson, M.F., Sroufe, L.A. & Egeland, B. (1985). The relationship between quality of attachment and behaviour problems in preschool in a high-risk sample. In *Growing Points of Attachment Theory and Research*. Monographs of the Society for Research in Child Development, 50 No. 209, eds. I. Bretherton & E. Waters, pp. 147–65.

Fabes, R.A. & Eisenberg, N. (1992). Young children's coping with interpersonal anger. Child Development, **63**, 116–28.

Fagot, B. & Kavanagh, (1990). The prediction of antisocial behavior from avoidant attachment classifications. *Child Development,* **61**, 864–73.

Feldman, S.S. & Sarnat, L. (1986). Israeli town and kibbutz bottlers' compliance and adults' control attempts. *Merrill-Palmer Quarterly*, **32**, 365–82.

Fischer, M., Rolf, J., Hasazi, J.E. & Cummings, L. (1984). Follow-up of a preschool epidemiological sample: cross-age continuities and predictions of later adjustment with internalising and externalising dimensions of behaviour. *Child Development,* **55**, 137–50.

Flavell, J.H. (1977). *Cognitive Development.* Engelwood Cliffs, NJ: Prentice-Hall.

Flavell, J.H. (1985). *Cognitive Development* (2nd edn.). Englewood Cliffs, NJ: Prentice-Hall.

Fox, N. & Calkins, S.D. (1993). Pathways to aggression and social withdrawal: Interactions among temperament, attachment, and regulation. In *Social Withdrawal, Inhibition, and Shyness in Childhood*, eds. K.H. Rubin and J.B. Asendorpf, pp. 81–100. Hillsdale, NJ: Lawrence Erlbaum.

Frankel, K. & Bates, J.E. (1990). Mother–toddler problem solving: antecedents in attachment, home behaviour, and temperament. *Child Development,* **61**, 820–31.

Garmezy, N. (1983). Stressors of childhood. In *Stress, Coping and Development in Children*, eds. N. Garmezy & M. Rutter, pp. 43–84. New York: McGraw-Hill.

Gittleman, R. & Mannuzza, S. (1985). Diagnosing ADD-H in adolescents. *Psychopharmocology Bulletin,* **21**, 237–42.

Gittleman, R., Mannuzza, S., Shenker, R. & Bonagura, N. (1985). Hyperactive boys almost grown up: psychiatric status. *Archives of General Psychiatry,* **42**, 937–47.

Goyette, C.H., Conners, C.K. & Ulrich, R.F. (1978). Normative data for the revised Conners parent and teacher rating scales. *Journal of Abnormal Psychology,* **6**, 221–36.

Greenberg, M.T., Speltz, M.L. & DeKlyen, M. (1993). The role of attachment in the early development of disruptive behaviour problems. *Development and Psychology*, **5**, 191–214.

Halverson, C.F. & Waldrop, M. (1973). The relations of mechanically recorded activity level to varieties of preschool play behaviour. *Child Development,* **44**, 678–81.

Harris, P.L. (1989). *Children and Emotion.* Oxford: Basil Blackwell.

Hechtman, L., Weiss, G., Perlman, T. & Amsel, R. (1984). Hyperactives as young adults: initial predictors of adult outcome. *Journal of the American Academy of Child Psychiatry,* **23**, 250–61.

Hinshaw, S.P. (1987). On the distinction between attentional deficits/hyperactivity and conduct problems/aggression in child psychopathology. *Psychological Bulletin,* **101**, 443–63.

Humphries, T., Kinsbourne, M. & Swanson, J. (1978). Stimulant effects on cooperation and social interaction between hyperactive children and their mothers. *Journal of Child Psychology and Psychiatry,* **19**, 12–22.

Jacob, R.G., O'Leary, K.D. & Rosenblad, C. (1978). Formal and informal classroom settings: Effects on hyperactivity. *Journal of Abnormal Child Psychology,* **6**, 47–59.

Jacobvitz, D. & Sroufe, L.A. (1987). The early caregiver–child relationships and attention deficit disorder with hyperactivity in kindergarten: a prospective study. *Child Development,* **58**, 1496–504.

Johnston, C., Pelham, W.E. & Murphy, H.A. (1985). Peer relationships in ADDH and normal children. A developmental analysis of peer and teacher ratings. *Journal of Abnormal Child Psychology,* **13**, 80–100.

Kagan, J., Rosman, B.L., Day, D., Albert, J. & Phillips, W. (1964). Information processing in the child: significance of analytic and reflective attitudes. *Psychological Monographs,* 78 (No. 578).

Kagan, J., Reznick, J.S., Clarke, C., Snidmanm N. & Garcia-Coll, C. (1984). Behavioural inhibition to the unfamiliar. *Child Development,* **55**, 2212–25.

Kendall, P.C. & Braswell, L. (1985). *Cognitive-Behavioral Therapy for Impulsive Children.* New York: Guilford.

Kendall, P.C. Lerner, R. & Craighead, W.E. (1984). Human development and intervention in childhood psychopathology. *Child Development,* **55**, 71–82.

Klein, A. & Young, R.D. (1979). Hyperactive boys in their classroom: assessment of teacher and peer perceptions, interactions, and classroom behaviours. *Journal of Abnormal Child Psychology,* **7**, 425–42.

Kohn, (1977). *Social Competence, Symptoms, and Underachievement in Childhood: A Longitudinal Perspective*. Washington, D.C.: Winston.

Kopp, C.B. (1982). Antecedents of self-regulation: a developmental perspective. *Developmental Psychology,* **18**, 199–214.

Kopp, C.B. (1987). The growth of self-regulation: Caregivers and children. In *Contemporary Topics in Developmental Psychology*, ed. N. Eisenberg, pp. 34–56. New York: Wiley.

Kopp, C.B. (1989). Regulation of distress and negative emotions: a developmental view. *Developmental Psychology,* **25**, 343–54.

Kuczynski, L. & Kochanska, G. (1990). Development of children's non-compliance strategies from toddlerhood to age 5. *Developmental Psychology,* **26**, 398–408.

Kucznski, L., Kochanska, G., Radke-Yarrow, M. & Girnius-Brown, O. (1987). A developmental interpretation of young children's non-compliance. *Developmental Psychology,* **23**, 799–806.

Ladd, G., Price, J. & Hart, (1986). Predicting preschoolers' peer status from their playground behaviours. *Child Development,* **59**, 986–92.

Lamb, M., Thompson, R.A., Gardner, W. & Charnov, E.L. (1985). *Infant–mother attachment.* Hillsdale, NJ: Lawrence Erlbaum Associates.

Lambert, N.M. (1982). Temperament profiles of hyperactive children. *American Journal of Orthopsychiatry,* **52**, 458–67.

Lambert, N.M. (1988). Adolescent outcomes for hyperactive children: perspectives on general and specific patterns of childhood risk for adolescent educational, social, and mental health problems. *American Psychologist,* **43**, 786–99.

Lambert, N.M. & Hartsough, C.S. (1984). Contribution of predispositional factors to the diagnosis of hyperactivity. *American Journal of Orthopsychiatry,* **54**, 97–109.

Lambert, N.M. & Sandoval, J. (1980). The prevalence of learning disabilities in a sample of children considered hyperactive. *Journal of Abnormal Child Psychology,* **8**, 33–50.

Lauffer, M.W. & Denhoff, E. (1957). Hyperactive behavior syndrome in children. *Journal of Pediatrics*, **50**, 463–74.

Lee, C.L. & Bates, J.E. (1985). Mother–child interaction at age two years and perceived difficult temperament. *Child Development,* **56**, 1314–25.

Lerner, J.V. & Lerner, R.M. (1983). Temperament and adaptation across the life span. In *Life Span Development and Behavior*, eds. P. Baltes & O.G. Brim, Vol. 5. New York: Academic Press.

Lerner, J.V., Nitz, K., Talwar, R. & Lerner, R.M. (1989). On the functional sigificance of temper and mental individuality: a developmental conceptual view of the concept of good ness of fit. In *Temperament in Childhood*, eds. G.A. Kohnstamm, J.E. Bates & M. Rothbort, pp. 509–22, New York: Wiley.

Levy, F. (1980). The development of sustained attention (vigilance) and inhibition in children: Some normative data. *Journal of Child Psychology and Psychiatry,* **21**, 77–84.

Lewis, M., Feiring, C., McGuffog, C. & Joskir, J. (1984). Predicting psychopathology in six-year-olds from early social interactions. *Child Development,* **55**, 123–36.

Londerville, S. & Main, M. (1981) Security of attachment, compliance, and maternal training methods in the second year of life. *Developmental Psychology,* **17**, 289–99.

Loney, J. (1987). Hyperactive and aggression in the diagnosis of attention deficit disorder. In *Advances in Clinical Child Psychology*, eds. B.B. Lahey and A.E. Kazdin, Vol. 10, pp. 99–135. New York: Plenum Press.

Loney, J. & Milich, R. (1982). Hyperactivity, inattention, and aggression in clinical practice. In *Advances in Behavioural Pediatrics*, eds. M. Wolraich & D.Routh Vol. 2, pp. 113–47. Greenwich, CT: JAI Press.

Loney, J., Kramer, J. & Milich, R. (1981). The hyperkinetic child grows up: predictors of symptoms, delinquency, and achievement at follow-up. In eds. K.D. Gadow & J. Loney, pp. 381–415. *Psychosocial Aspects of Drug Treatment for Hyperactivity*: Boulder, CO: Westview Press.

Loney, J., Whaley-Klahn, M.A., Kosier, T., & Conboy, J. (1983). Hyperactive boys and their brothers at 21: predictors of aggressive and antisocial outcomes. In *Prospective Studies of Crime and Delinquency*, eds. K. VanDusen & S.A. Mednick, pp. 181–207. Boston: Kluwer-Nijhoff Publishing.

Luria, A.R. (1961). *The Role of Speech in the Regulation of Normal and Abnormal Behavior.* New York: Liveright.

Lyons-Ruth, K., Zoll, D., Connell, D., & Grunebaum, H.V. (1987). Family deviance and family disruption in childhood: associations with maternal behavior and infant maltreatment during the first years of life. *Development and Psychopathology,* **1**, 219–36.

Lytton, H. (1979). Disciplinary encounters between young boys and their mothers and fathers: Is there a contingency system? *Developmental Psychology,* **15**, 256–68.

Lytton, H. & Zwirner, H. (1975). Compliance and its controlling stimuli observed in a natural setting. *Developmental Psychology,* **11**, 769–79.

McCall, R.B. (1986). Issues of stability and continuity in temperament research. In *The study of temperament: Changes, Continuities, and Challenges*, eds. R. Plomin & J. Dunn, pp. 13–23. Hillsdale, NJ: Erlbaum.

McFarlane, J.W., Allen, L. & Honzik, M.P. (1954). *A Developmental Study of the Behaviour Problems of Normal Children Between Twenty-one Months and Fourteen Years.* Berkeley: University of California Press.

McGee, R. & Share, D.L. (1988). Attention deficit disorder–hyperactivity and academic failure: what comes first and what should be treated? *Journal of the American Academy of Child and Adolescent Psychiatry,* **27**, 318–25.

McGee, R., Silva, P.A. & Williams, S. (1984). Perinatal, neurological, environmental and developmental characteristics of seven-year-old children with stable behaviour problems. *Journal of Child Psychology and Psychiatry,* **25**, 573–86.

Maccoby, E., Dowley, E., Hagen, J. & Degerman, R. (1965). Activity level and intellectual functionong in normal preschool children. *Child Development*, **36**, 761–70.

Maccoby, E.E., Snow, M.E. & Jacklin, C. (1984). Children's disposition and mother–child interaction at 12 and 18 months: a short-term longitudinal study. *Developmental Psychology,* **20**, 459–72.

Magnusson, D. & Bergman, L.R. (1990). A pattern approach to the study of pathways from childhood to adulthood. In *Straight and Devious Pathways from Childhood to Adulthood*, eds. L. Robins and M. Rutter. Cambridge, England: Cambridge University Press.

Mahler, M., Pine, F. & Bergmen, A. (1975). *The Psychological Birth of the Human Infant.* New York: Basic Books.

Main, M. & Hesse, E. (1990). Adult lack of resolution of attachment-related trauma related to infant disorganised/disoriented behavior in the Ainsworth Strange Situation. In *Attachment in the Preschool Years: Theory, Research and Intervention*, eds. M.T. Greenberg, D. Cicchetti, & M. Cummings, pp. 339–425. Chicago: University of Chicago Press.

Mash, E. & Johnston, C. (1982). A comparison of the mother–child interactions of younger and older hyperactive and normal children. *Child Development,* **53**, 1371–81.

Mash, E. & Johnston, C. (1983). Sibling interactions of hyperactive and normal children and their relationship to reports of maternal stress and self-esteem. *Journal of Clinical Child Psychology,* **12**, 91–9.

Matas, L., Arend, R.A. & Sroufe, L.A. (1978). Continuity of adaptation in the second year: The relationship between quality of attachment and later competence. *Child Development,* **49**, 547–56.

Matier, B.S., Halperin, J.M., Sharma, V., Newcorn, J.H. & Sathaye, N. (1991). Methylphenidate response in aggressive and nonagressive ADHD children: distinctions on laboratory measures of symptoms. *Journal of the Academy of Child and Adolescent Psychiatry*, **31**, 219–29.

Milich, R. (1984). Cross-sectional and longitudinal observations of activity level and sustained attention in a normal sample. *Journal of Abnormal Child Psychology,* **12**, 261–76.

Milich, R. & Kramer, J. (1984). Reflections on impulsivity: an empirical investigation of impulsivity as a construct. In *Advances in Learning and Behavioral Disabilities*, eds. K. Gadow & I. Bialer, Vol. 2, pp 57–94. Greenwich, CT: JAI Press.

Milich, R., Landau, S., Kilby, G. & Whitten, P. (1982). Preschool peer perceptions of the behavior of hyperactive and aggressive children. *Journal of Abnormal Child Psychology,* **10**, 497–510.

Mischel, W. (1983). Delay of gratification as process and person variable in development. In *Humor Development: An Intractional Prespective*, eds. D. Magnusson and V.C. Allen, pp. 149–65. New York: Academic Press.

Mischel, W. & Patterson, C.J. (1974). Effective plans for self-control in children. In *Minnesota Symposium on Child Psychology*, ed. A. Collins. Hillsdale, NJ: Erlbaum.

Moffitt, T. (1990). Juvenile delinquency and attention deficit disorder: Boys' developmental trajectories from age 3 to age 15. *Child Development,* **61**, 893–910.

Olson, S.L. (1989). Assessment of impulsivity in preschoolers: cross- measure convergences, longitudinal stability, and relevance to social competence. *Journal of Clinical Child Psychology,* **18**, 176–83.

Olson, S.L. (1992). Development of conduct problems and peer rejection in preschool children: a social systems analysis. *Journal of Abnormal Child Psychology,* **20**, 27–350.

Olson, S.L. & Brodfeld, P. (1991). Assessment of peer rejection and externalising behavior problems in preschool boys: a short-term longitudinal study. *Journal of Abnormal Child Psychology*, **19**, 493–503.

Olson, S.L., Bates, J.E. & Bayles, K. (1984). Mother–infant interaction and the development of individual differences in children's cognitive competence. *Developmental Psychology,* **20**, 166–79.

Olson, S.L., Bayles, K. & Bates, J.E. (1986). Mother–child interaction and children's speech progress: a longitudinal study of the first two years. *Merrill-Palmer Quarterly,* **32**, 1–20.

Olson, S.L. Bates, J.E. & Bayles, K. (1990). Early antecedents of childhood impulsivity: the role of parent–child interaction, cognitive competence, and temperament. *Journal of Abnormal Child Psychology,* **18**, 317–34.

Olson, S.L. & Hoza, B. (1993). Preschool developmental antecedents of conduct problems in children beginning school. *Journal of Clinical Child Psychology,* **22**, 60–67.

Olweus, D. (1980). Familial and temperamental determinants of aggressive behavior in adolescent boys: a causal analysis. *Developmental Psychology*, **16**, 644–60.

Paternite, C.E. & Loney, J. (1980). Childhood hyperkinesis: Relationships between symptomotology and home environment. In *Hyperactive Children: The Social Ecology of Identification and Treatment*, eds. C.K. Whalen & B. Henker, pp. 105–41. New York: Academic Press.

Patterson, G.R. (1982). *Coercive Family Processes*. Eugene, OR: Castalia.

Patterson, G.R., DeBaryshe, B.D. & Ramsey, E. (1989). A developmental perspective on antisocial behavior. *American Psychologist,* **44**, 329–35.

Pelham, W.E. & Bender, M.E. (1982). Peer relationships in hyperactive children: Description and treatment. In *Advances in Learning and Behavioral Disabilities*, eds. K. Gadow & E. Bialer, Vol. 1, pp. 365–436. Greenwich, CT: JAI Press.

Pettit, G.A. & Bates, J.E. (1984). Continuity of individual differences in the mother–infant relationship from six to thirteen months. *Child Development,* **55**, 729–39.

Pianta, R.C. & Caldwell, C.B. (1990). Stability of externalising symptoms from kindergarten to first grade and factors related to instability. *Development and Psychopathology,* **2**, 247–58.

Porrino, L.J., Rapaport, J.L., Behar, D., Sceery, W., Ismond, D.R. & Bunney, W.E. (1983). A naturalistic assessment of the motor activity of hyperactive boys. *Archives of General Psychiatry,* **40**, 681–7.

Porteus, S. (1965). *Porteus Maze Tests: Fifty Years Application*. Palo Alto, CA: Pacific.

Prior, M. & Sanson, A. (1986). Attention deficit disorder with hyperactivity: a critique. *Journal of Child Psychology and Psychiatry,* **27**, 307–19.

Reeves, J.C., Werry, J.S., Elkind, G.S. & Zametkin, A. (1987). Attention deficit, conduct, oppositional, and anxiety disorders in children. II. Clinical characteristics. *Journal of the American Academy of Child and Adolescent Psychiatry*, **26**, 144–55.

Renken, B., Egeland, B., Marvinney, D., Mangelsdorf, S. & Sroufe, L.A. (1989). Early childhood antecedents of aggression and passive-withdrawal in early elementary school. *Journal of Personality,* **57**, 257–81.

Richman, N., Stevenson, J.S. & Graham, P.J. (1982). *Preschool to School – A Behavioural Study.* London: Academic.

Rose, S.L., Rose, S.A. & Feldman, J.F. (1989). Stability of behavior problems in very young children. *Development and Psychopathology,* **1**, 5–20.

Ross, D.M. & Ross, S.A. (1976). *Hyperactivity: Research, Theory, and Action.* New York: Wiley.

Ross, D.M. & Ross, S.A. (1982). *Hyperactivity: Current Issues, Research, and Theory*, 2nd edn. New York: Wiley.

Rothbart, M. (1989). Temperament and development. In *Temperament in childhood*, eds. G.A. Kohnstamm, J.E. Bates, & M.K. Rothbart, pp. 59–76. New York: Wiley.

Rothbart, M.K. & Derryberry, D. (1981). Development of individual differences in temperament. In *Advances in Developmental Psychology*, eds. M.E. Lamb & A.L. Brown, Vol. 1, pp. 37–86. Hillsdale, NJ: Erlbaum.

Routh, D.K., Schroeder, C.S. & O'Tuama, L. (1974). Development of activity level in children. *Developmental Psychology,* 10, 163–8.

Rubin, K.A. & Clark, M.L. (1983) Preschool teachers' ratings of behvioral problems: observational, sociometric, and social-cognitive correlates. *Journal of Abnormal Child Psychology*, **11**, 273–86.

Rutter, M. (1982). Syndromes attributed to 'minimal brain dysfunction' in childhood. *American Journal of Psychiatry,* **139**, 21–33.

Rutter, M. (1983). Stress, coping, and development. In *Stress, Coping and Development in Children*, eds. N. Garmezy & M. Rutter, pp. 1–42. New York: McGraw-Hill.

Rutter, M. (1987). Psychosocial resilience and protective mechanisms. *American Journal of Orthopsychiatry,* **57**, 316–31.

Rutter, M. & Garmezy, N. (1983). Developmental psychopathology. In *Carmichael's Manual of Child Psychology*, ed. E.M. Hetherington. Vol 4, pp. 775–911 *Social and Personality Development*. New York: Wiley.

Sameroff, A.J. & Chandler, M.J. (1975). Reproductive risk and the continuum of caretaking casualty. In *Review of Child Development Research*, ed. F.D. Horowitz, Vol. 4. Chicago: University of Chicago Press.

Sameroff, A.J., Seifer, R., Baldwin, A.L. & Baldwin, C.A. (1993). Stability of intelligence from preschool to adolescence: the influence of social and family risk factors. *Child Development,* **64**, 80–97.

Sander, L. (1975). Infant and caretaking environment. In, *Explorations in child psychology*, ed. E.J. Anthony, pp. 129–66. New York: Basic Books.

Satterfield, J., Hoppe, C.M. & Schell, A.M. (1982). A prospective study of delinquency in 110 adolescent boys with attention deficit disorder and 88 normal adolescent boys. *American Journal of Psychiatry,* **139**, 797–8.

Schachar, R., Logan, G., Wachsmuth, R. & Chojczyt, D. (1988). Attaining and maintaining preparation: a comparison of attention in hyperactive, normal and disturbed control children. *Journal of Abnormal Child Psychology,* **16**, 361–78.

Schachar, R., Rutter, M. & Smith, A. (1981). The characteristic of situationally and pervasively hyperactive children: implications for syndrome definition. *Journal of Child Psychology and Psychiatry,* **22**, 375–92.

Schachar, R. & Wachsmuth, R. (1990). Hyperactivity and parental psychopathology. *Journal of Child Psychology and Psychiatry,* **31**, 381–92.

Schaffer, H.R. (1984). *The Child's Entry into a Social World.* London: Academic Press.

Schaffer, H.R. & Crook, C. (1979). Maternal control techniques in a directed play situation. *Child Development,* **50**, 989–96.

Schaffer, H.R. & Crook, C. (1980). Child compliance and maternal control techniques. *Developmental Psychology,* **16**, 54–61.

Schleifer, M., Weiss, G., Cohen, N.J., Elman, M., Cvejic, H. & Kruger, E. (1975).

Hyperactivity in preschoolers and the effect of methylphenidate. *Americal Journal of Orthopsychiatry,* **45**, 38–50.

Schonfeld, I.S., Shaffer, D., O'Connor, P. & Portnoy, S. (1988). Conduct disorder and cognitive functioning: testing three causal hypotheses. *Child Development,* **59**, 993–1007.

Semrud-Clikeman, M., Biederman, J., Sprich-Buckminster, S., Lehman, B., Faraone, S. & Norman, D. (1992). Co-morbidity between ADDH and learning disability: a review and report in a clinically referred sample. *Journal of the American Academy of child and Adolescent Psychiatry*, **31**, 439–48.

Shaywitz, S.E. & Shaywitz, B.A. (1988). Attention deficit disorder: current perspectives. In *Learning Disabilities: Proceedings of the National Conference*, eds. J.L. Kavanagh & T.J. Truss. Parkton, MD: York Press.

Silverman, I.W. & Ragusa, D.M. (1990). Child and maternal correlates of impulse control in 24-month children. *Genetic, Social and General Psychology Monographs,* **116** (4), 435–73.

Sroufe, L.A. (1979). The coherence of individual development. *American Psychologist,* **34**, 834–41.

Sroufe, L.A. (1983). Infant–caregiver attachment and patterns of adaptation in preschool: The roots of maladaptation and competence. In *Minnesota Symposia on Child Psychology*, ed. M. Perlmutter, Vol. 16, pp. 41–81. Hillsdale, NJ: Erlbaum.

Sroufe, L.A. (1991). Considering normal and abnormal together: the essence of developmental psychopathology. *Development and Psychopathology*, **2**, 335–47.

Sroufe, L.A. & Rutter, M. (1984) The domain of developmental psychopathology. *Child Development,* **55**, 17–29.

Stewart, M.A., Cummings, C., Singer, S. & DeBlois, C.S. (1981). The overlap between hyperactive and unsocialized aggressive children. *Journal of Child Psychiatry and Psychology*, **22**, 35–45.

Szatmari, P., Boyle, M. & Offord, D.R. (1989). ADDH and conduct disorder: Degree of diagnostic overlap and differences among correlates. *Journal of the American Academy of Child and Adolescent Psychiatry,* **28**, 865–72.

Tallmadge, J. & Barkley, R.A. (1983). The interactions of hyperactive and normal boys with their mothers and fathers. *Journal of Abnormal Child Psychology,* **11**, 565–80.

Taylor, E., Schachar, R., Thornley, G. & Weiselberg, M. (1986). Conduct disorder and hyperactivity: I. Separation of hyperactivity and antisocial conduct in British child psychiatric patients. *British Journal of Psychiatry*, **149**, 760–7.

Teglasi, H. & McMahon, B.H. (1990). Temperament and common behaviour problems of children. *Journal of Applied Developmental Psychology,* **11**, 331–49.

Thomas, A., Chess, S. & Birch, H. (1968). *Temperament and Behaviour Disorders in Children.* New York: New York University Press.

Thompson, R. (1986). Temperament, emotionality, and social cognition. In *Temperament and Social Interaction in Infants and Children*, eds. J.V. Lerner & R.M. Lerner, pp. 35– 52. *New Directions for Child Development, 31.*

Thompson, R.A. (1988). Emotion and self-regulation. *Nebraska Symposium on Motivation.* Lincoln: University of Nebraska Press.

Thompson, R.A. (1994). Emotion regulation: a theme in search of a definition. In *The Development of Emotion Regulation. Monographs of the Society for Research in Child Development,* ed. N.A. Fox, **59**, #240.

Thorley, G. (1984). Review of follow-up and follow-back studies of childhood hyperactivity. *Psychological Bulletin,* **96**, 116–32.

Urban, J., Carlson, E., Egeland, B. & Sroufe, L.A. (1991). Patterns of individual adaption across childhood. *Development and Psychopathology,* **3**, 445–60.

van der Meere, J. & Sargeant, J. (1988). Controlled processing and vigilance in hyperactivity: time will tell. *Journal of Abnormal Child Psychology,* **16**, 641–55.

Vygotsky, L.S. (1962). *Thought and Language.* Cambridge, MA: MIT Press.

Waters, E. & Sroufe, L.A. (1983). Social competence as a developmental construct. *Developmental Review*, **3**, 79–97.

Weiss, G. & Hechtman, L.T. (1986). *Hyperactive Children Grown Up.* New York: Guilford Press.

Weiss, G. & Hechtman, L.T. (1986). *Hyperactive Children Grown Up.* New York: Guilford Press.

Weiss, G., Hechtman, L., Milroy, T. & Perlman, T. (1985). Psychiatric status of hyperactives as young adults: A controlled fifteen year follow-up of 63 hyperactive children. *Journal of the American Academy of Child and Adolescent Psychiatry, 24, 221–7.*

Weiss, G., Hechtman, L.T., Perlman, T., Hopkins, J. & Werner, A. (1979). Hyperactives as young adults: a controlled prospective ten-year follow-up of 75 children. *Archives of General Psychiatry,* **36**, 675–81.

Weiss, G., Minde, K., Werry, J.S., Douglas, V.I. & Nemeth, E. (1971). Studies on the hyperactive child: five-year follow-up. *Archives of General Psychiatry,* **24**, 409–14.

Wellman, H.M. (1990). *The Child's Theory of Mind.* Cambridge, MA: MIT Press.

Werner, E.E. (1993). Risk, resilience, and recovery: perspectives from the Kauai Longitudinal Study. *Development and Psychopathology*, **5**, 503–16.

Werner, E.E. & Smith, R.S. (1982). *Vulnerable but Invincible.* New York: McGraw-Hill.

Werner, E.E. & Smith, R.S. (1992). *Overcoming the Odds: High Risk Children from Birth to Adulthood.* Ithaca, NY: Cornell University Press.

Werry, J.S., Reeves, J.C. & Elkind, G.S. (1987). Attention deficit, conduct, oppositional, and anxiety disorders in children. A review of research on differentiating characteristics. *Journal of the American Academy of Child and Adolescent Psychiatry,* **26**, 133–43.

Whalen, C.K. (1989). Attention deficit and hyperactivity disorders. In *Handbook of Child Psychopathology,* eds. T.H. Ollendick & M. Hersen, pp. 131–69. New York: Plenum.

Whalen, C.K. & Henker, B. (1980). *Hyperactive Children: The Social Ecology of Identification and Treatment.* New York: Academic Press.

Whalen, C.K., Henker, B. & Dotemoto, S. (1981). Teacher response to the methylphenidate VS. placebo status of hyperactive boys in the classroom. *Child Development*, **52**, 1005–14.

Whalen, C.K. & Henker, B. (1985). The social worlds of hyperactive (ADHD) children. *Clinical Psychology Review,* **5**, 447–78.

Whalen, C. & Henker, B. (1986) Group designs in applied psychopharmacology. In *Advances in Learning and Behavioural Disabilities: Methodological Issues in Human Psychopharmacology*. eds. K.D. Gadow & A. Poling, Greenwich, CT: JAI Press.

Whalen, C.K., Henker, B. & Dotemoto, S. (1980). Methylphenidate and hyperactivity: effects on teacher behaviors. *Science,* **208**, 1280–2.

Whalen, C.K., Henker, B., Dotemoto, S. & Hinshaw, S.P. (1983). Teacher response to the methylphenidate versus placebo status of hyperactive boys in the classroom. *Child Development,* **52**, 1005–14.

Whalen, C.K., Henker, B. & Granger, D.A. (1990). Social judgement process in hyperactive boys: Effects of methylphenidate and comparisons with normal peers. *Journal of Abnormal Child Psychology,* **18**, 297–316.

Wolkind, S.N. & DeSalis, W. (1982). Infant temperament, maternal mental states and child behavior problems. In *Temperamental differences in infants and young children*, eds. R. Porter and G.M. Collins, pp. 221–39. London: Pitman.

Zentall, S.S. (1980). Behavioral comparisons of hyperactive and normally active children in natural settings. *Journal of Abnormal Child Psychology*, **8**, 93–109.

Zentall, S. (1984). Context effects in the behavioral ratings of hyperactivity. *Journal of Abnormal Child Psychology,* **12**, 345–52.

6

Other disorders of conduct

Robert Soussignan and Richard Tremblay

INTRODUCTION

In North America different labels, such as hyperactivity, attention deficit disorder with hyperactivity (ADDH), and attention deficit hyperactivity disorder (ADHD) (American Psychiatric Association, 1980, 1987) (APA) are used to refer to a cluster of developmentally inappropriate level of behaviour patterns, the most prominent symptoms of which are inattentiveness, motor restlessness and impulsiveness. This condition, more common in boys (i.e. male–female ratio ranges from 2:1 to 10:1) (Szatmari, Offord & Boyle, 1989*a*; APA), is diagnosed in up to 40% of the children referred to a psychiatric clinic (Safer & Allen, 1976) and can be applied to 1–14% of all school-age children in the general population (Szatmari *et al.*, 1989*a*). In contrast, in Europe the diagnosis is in rare use, and unlike in the USA, the condition can be assigned to children with intellectual retardation (Taylor, 1988*b*). For example, the diagnosis of hyperkinetic syndrome was applied to only 1 per 1000 children in the Isle of Wight population survey (Rutter, Tizard & Whitmore, 1970), and to only 1.5% of non-retarded British clinic-referred children in the World Health Organisation study (Rutter, Shaffer & Shepherd, 1975). This disparity in cultural prevalence of hyperactivity in clinic and community samples might reflect mainly differences in clinical practices and in the choice of screening criteria (e.g. weighting of the symptoms, pervasiveness versus situationality) (Sandberg, 1981; Prendergast *et al.*, 1988). The picture is also obscured by the fact that the children with the diagnosis of ADHD/hyperactivity in the US might include many who in the UK would be diagnosed as conduct disordered (CD) only (Sandberg, Wieselberg & Shaffer, 1980). Indeed, although the clinical operational definition of ADDH/ADHD in the American diagnostic classification (DSM-III, DSM-III-R, DSM-IV) restricts this putative syndrome to developmentally inappropriate levels of overactivity, inattention and impulsivity, it has been frequently found that a great number of ADDH children also display associated disruptive behaviours, such as aggression/conduct disorder (CD) (Stewart, DeBlois & Cummings, 1980; Loney & Milich, 1982).

These divergent views have stimulated a number of empirical investigations which, in turn, have led to the validity of a broad notion of hyperactivity to be questioned (Sandberg, Rutter & Taylor, 1978; Shaffer & Greenhill, 1979 ; Milich, Loney & Landau, 1982). Thus, for example, Shaffer & Greenhill (1979) examining the postdictive, concurrent, and particularly the predictive validity of this putative syndrome, drew attention to the heterogeneity of the groups that have been studied, and to the non-specific nature of this disorder (e.g. presence or absence of conduct problems and learning disabilities). Similarly, comparisons of 'conduct disturbed' boys scoring high on measures of hyperactivity with those scoring low have failed to distinguish the two conditions on a number of neurodevelopmental and psychosocial variables, in both clinic and general population samples (Sandberg *et al.*, 1978; Sandberg *et al.*, 1980). As has been emphasised by a number of authors (e.g. Barkley, 1982; Rutter, 1984), this important controversy has clearly been confused in previous research by the lack of rigorous definitions and selection criteria, which did not really allow to ascertain what kinds of children were studied. It is thus no wonder that hyperactive children used in a great number of studies may have included children with various degrees of conduct problems and overactivity/attention deficits/impulsivity.

In the last decade, the issue of the differential diagnosis (i.e. the issue of the syndromal independence) between ADHD/hyperactivity and CD/aggression has been the focus of great concern. The general question usually addressed is whether these different constellations of disruptive behaviours (inattention, overactivity, impulsivity and aggression) constitute specific disorders, or whether they represent subtypes of a more broadly defined category in which symptoms vary only in severity. For this issue to be settled, the validity of the specificity of the disorder requires to be tested. That is to say, if a diagnostic category has meaning, it must be shown to differ in important respects, in terms of aetiology, symptomatology, course, response to treatment, or some other meaningful variables, from other diagnostic categories (e.g. conduct disorder) (Sandberg *et al.*, 1978; Rutter & Gould, 1985). To date, it is acknowledged that new research strategies will be needed to try to resolve this issue (Campbell & Werry, 1986). It therefore appears urgent to disentangle the overlap between hyperactivity and conduct disorder (Taylor, 1988*a*). More particularly, a key issue seems to be whether it is possible to differentiate children with pure and mixed externalising problems on a number of external criteria such as neurochemical, neurodevelopmental, behavioural, cognitive and psychosocial variables. The identification of homogeneous subgroups within the disruptive behaviour disorders could offer both aetiological, treatment and long-term prognostic implications.

There now exists an increasing number of studies that have tested the working hypothesis of the distinctiveness of hyperactivity/ADDH and conduct disorder/aggression (e.g. Loney & Milich, 1982; August, Stewart & Holmes, 1983; McGee, Williams & Silva, 1984; Shapiro & Garkinkel, 1986; Werry, Elkind & Reeves, 1987; Farrington, Loeber & Van Kammen, 1990, Moffitt, 1990), so it is possible to analyse the contributions of present findings to the issue of the differential validity of these two classes of behaviour.

Up to now, three areas of research have been more extensively investigated :

- Internal validation of symptomatology by multivariate empirical statistical analyses focusing on the internal consistency of the constellation of correlated behaviours;
- Empirical validity that addresses the question of whether hyperactivity could be discriminated from aggression on variables independent of the clinical symptomatology (e.g. postdictive validity involving specific aetiological correlates such as biological or psychosocial measures);
- 'Predictive' validity, with one of the questions addressed being whether either hyperactivity or aggression has any consequences for later development, and whether the outcome of hyperactive children is different from that of conduct disordered and mixed groups of children.

SCOPE OF THE REVIEW

Attentional problems, impulsivity, overactivity and aggressive behaviours are so common among children in the general population and among children referred to clinics for a variety of psychiatric problems (Rutter *et al.*, 1970), that research diagnostic criteria and external criteria are necessary to define homogeneous behavioural disorders. The existence of a set of diagnostic criteria is central to the issue of the differential diagnosis because it increases the reliability of the diagnostic categories and generates a higher level of consensus between studies (Barkley, 1982; Gittelman, 1988; Sergeant, 1988; American Psychiatric Association, 1994). At present, it is important to recognise that cross-study comparisons of hyperactivity and conduct disorder constitute a somewhat risky task because differential diagnostic criteria for these two putative disorders are not yet well established (e.g. operational definitions of behavioural descriptors; unidimensional versus multidimensional definitions of hyperactivity; degree of severity of symptoms; situationality vs pervasiveness; age of onset and duration) (Taylor, 1988*a,b*; Sergeant, 1988; Frick & Lahey, 1991; Abikoff & Klein, 1992). Furthermore, accurate matching between results is limited by considerable methodological variations on potentially critical dimensions such as (a) clinical versus non-clinical samples, (b) variations in characteristics of sample (e.g. age, sex, size, presence of associated problems), (c) identification procedures (e.g. teacher or parent questionnaire, psychiatrist chart ratings), (d) methods of assessing the symptoms (e.g. rating scales, interviews), (e) research strategies employed (dimensional versus categorical approaches), and (f) subgroups being compared. At present, only a few studies regarding the external validation of hyperactivity and conduct problems exist and this makes it difficult to use stringent exclusive criteria for the selection of studies. For example, studies that have compared only ADDH and CD, or ADDH+CD and ADDH, though not entirely suitable to the issue of the differential validity, will not be excluded from this review.

The purpose of this chapter is to analyse and briefly review studies which have compared the two classes of disruptive behaviour/disorders (hyperactivity/ ADDH/ADHD and aggression/CD), and to examine the issues of distribution, descriptive and predictive validity among community and clinical samples. However, as some of these topics have been well covered in recent reviews (Hinshaw, 1987; Werry, Reeves & Elkind, 1987; Taylor, 1988*a;* Milich & Landau, 1989; Hinshaw, 1992), we will aim to concentrate on aspects and topics not directly addressed by these recent analyses. In previous reviews, problems of classification, internal validation of putative syndromes, psychosocial (e.g. familial factors, peer measures), neurodevelopmental factors, cognitive correlates (e.g. IQ measures, achievement) have been adequately covered and therefore will not be the subject of the present analysis. Instead, we shall begin by examining the question of the prevalence of pure and mixed forms of disruptive behaviours and thereafter proceed to the issue of the descriptive validity of the symptomatology with respect to external criteria, i.e. as defined by empirical measures of the core symptoms of hyperactivity (overactivity, attention, impulsivity) and conduct problems. The question addressed is whether the use of multiple independent measures of hyperactivity/attention deficit, and of aggression/conduct disorder makes it possible to adequately differentiate these two conditions. Special attention will also be given to studies which have focused on the developmental course of hyperactivity and aggression. The studies will be analysed within two distinct conceptual frameworks of behavioural classification : dimensional (i.e. studies using multivariate and correlational analysis), and categorical (i.e. diagnostic categories and subgroups derived from rating scales). A greater emphasis will be given to categorical studies as comprehensive reviews of dimensional studies of conduct problems and hyperactivity can already be found elsewhere (see Quay, 1986; Hinshaw, 1987).

PREVALENCE RATES OF THE BEHAVIOURAL DISORDERS

It is possible in a phenomenological sense to identify children with 'pure' and 'mixed' forms of hyperactivity and aggression. As can be seen from Table 6.1, the data reported allows the proportions of children who fall into the three groups : hyperactive/ADDH (H), aggressive/CD (A), hyperactive–aggressive/ADDH-CD (H/A), to be easily estimated regardless of the child's sex. In non-selected samples, with older children excluded (i.e. Szatmari sample of 12–16 year-old children), estimates of hyperactivity range from 2% to 3.6% of child population, whereas the prevalence rates of conduct problems/aggression vary from 1.5% to 3.6%. It therefore seems reasonable to assume that the reported differences in the prevalence rates are in large part the result of methodological variations between studies (e.g. age range, size of samples, nature and number of items in the rating scales, stringency of the screening criteria). In spite of the fact that studies vary on a number of methodological aspects, it appears that the overlap between the two conditions is substantial. Prevalence rates of both aggression and hyperactivity range from 2.1% to 4.3% in different child populations. Moreover, the data also indicate that about 60% of both the hyperactive (from 40% to 65%) and of conduct disordered children (from 45% to 66%), showed a mixture of these behavioural problems. However, as it has already been emphasised (Taylor, 1988*a*,*b*), this picture may be obscured by the use of a single source of rating (e.g. teacher), which is likely to reduce the chance of finding a real distinction between conditions, due to a halo effect.

Estimates of the frequency of hyperactivity problems in clinic-referred children must be viewed with more caution because of the bias introduced by the demand and availability of services. Consequently, data reported on clinic-referred children appear to vary a good deal. In view of the large differences in the diagnostic criteria applied by different clinicians and centres to the problems of children whose referrals vary on a number of dimensions (nature of informant, diversity of sources and instruments, nature of samples, potential presence of selection biases), it is not surprising to find a good deal of discrepancy. However, the data also show a substantial overlap, particularly with conduct disorder/aggression (from 55% to 92%), meaning that conduct disordered children in clinic samples are more likely to be hyperactive than vice versa. It can be also noted that, for three out of five clinical studies, the mixed group had the highest rate for the diagnosis of hyperactivity. Thus one can assume that the probability of referral is also dictated by severity of problems, that is children with multiple/serious problems are more likely to be referred.

The recent publication of the DSM-III-R and DSM-IV classifications have provided a redefinition of hyperactivity and have generated studies on the co-morbidity of the disorders involving different disruptive behaviours. For example, in a study of 275 high-risk non-referred children, Keller *et al.* (1992) found that 19% could be diagnosed as suffering from a disruptive-type behavioural disorder (e.g. attention deficit disorder (ADD), conduct disorder (CD), oppositional defiant disorder (ODD)). More interestingly, the results also showed that 33% of the children received two of the above diagnoses.

These findings do not allow the relative contribution of the behavioural symptoms (e.g. overactivity versus inattentiveness) to the distribution of the various groups to be disentangled. However, a recent study by Goldstein (1987) of a large community sample of 5,034 children from 6 to 11 years of age showed that most of the children who were overactive were also inattentive. For boys, 76.4% of those who were overactive were also considered to be inattentive by their teacher; likewise 70.1% of the overactive girls were low in attentiveness. Of the aggressive children, 65% of the boys were also judged to be overactive, and 54.1% as low in attentiveness; whereas of aggressive girls, 67.4 % were also overactive and the same proportion were low in attentiveness. None the less, this otherwise comprehensive study used only crude measures of attentiveness, overactivity, and aggressiveness. Furthermore, no report of the reliability and validity of the teacher questionnaire was included. Thus, these findings must be replicated in studies using other methods of classification.

In clinical practice, it seems that the mixed cases are the most difficult to identify reliably. In a recent US–UK cross-national study of DSM-III and ICD-9, Prendergast *et al.* (1988) found a poor agreement within clinician panels. The British team was more likely to choose CD, while the American team preferred hyperkinetic syndrome when ICD-9 was being used. The authors concluded that the disagreements between clinicians on the presence of hyperactivity are likely to be due to their differing views about how to weight individuals symptoms, rather than how to recognise them.

In summary, the findings reported in previous studies appear to suggest a close intertwining of hyperactive and aggressive behaviours, such that most hyperactive children are also aggressive and vice versa, as well as the presence of groups of children with exclusive behavioural problems. However, the presence of 'pure' groups of conduct disordered or ADDH children is not an argument for the existence of an independent hyperactivity or conduct disorder syndrome. Moreover, the amount of overlap raises the question of whether the two behaviour disorders are truly one. Research efforts trying to resolve this issue have related closely to the question of differential validity, with claims that the meaningfulness of a clinical/behavioural syndrome has to be established through some demonstrable specificity with respect to important external criteria.

DESCRIPTIVE VALIDITY OF THE BEHAVIOURAL SYMPTOMATOLOGY

Categorical studies

Descriptive validity rests on the convergent and discriminative properties of the classification; it addresses the degree to which categories of disorders or groups of subjects are homogeneous and distinctive with respect to relevant attributes (e.g. behavioural symptoms) (see Skinner, 1981). This fundamental step requires the construct validity of the symptoms describing the categories to be tested. In studies available so far, a number of factors constitute as limitations in this sense. First, the sample composition has often been primarily based on social judgements with some adults (e.g. teacher, mother, clinician) declaring the child's behaviour deviant in terms of items of subjective judgement about inattention/overactivity/impulsivity and/or aggression. This procedure alone, although necessary for establishing clinical history, is clearly insufficient for scientific purposes because it does not guarantee the validity of the behavioural constructs employed in the diagnostic process; instead, they stem from an adult's perception rather than the actual behaviour or performance of the children. In addition, independent and objective measures of behaviour (overactivity, inattention, impulsivity) are needed in order to clarify the concepts and operational definitions of what is being measured. However, as has already been emphasised by several authors (Taylor, 1988*a*,*b*; Sergeant, 1988; Dienske & Sanders-Woudstra, 1988), clinical concepts such as 'inattention', 'overactivity' and 'impulsiveness' are heterogeneous and have many meanings. In fact, the use of a single clinical construct involves a complexity of behavioural and/or cognitive processes. In practice, however, most diagnostic descriptors, often based on behaviour questionnaires, are vague, crude and hard to quantify (e.g. 'doesn't seem to listen, needs a lot of supervision, has difficulty organising, daydreaming'). It is often difficult to translate these into

Table 6.1 *Prevalence rates of externalising behavioural disorders*

Author	Sample (Number; age; sex ratio: number boys/girls)	Instrument[a]	H %	A %	AH[b] %	H with A %	A with H %
	Non-selected children						
Trites & Laprade (1983)	Epidemiological stratified sample (9229; 4–12; –)	2 S.D. on CTRS	2	1.9	3.7	65	66
McGee *et al.* (1984)	Follow-up of a birth cohort (949; 7; 1.07:1)	2 S.D. on Rutter teacher or parent scales	2.7	3.2	4.3	61.2	57.7
Shapiro & Garfinkel (1986)	Elementary school children (303;7–13; 1.05:1)	Scores > 7 (IO) and > 4 (A) on CTRS IOWA	2.3	3.6	2.9	56.2	45
Goldstein (1987)	Health examination survey sample (5034; 6–11; 1.08:1)	Teacher questionnaire	3.2	1.5	2.1	60.5	58
Szatmari *et al.* (1989*a*)	Health examination survey sample	Diagnostic checklists					
	(1452; 4–11; 1:1)		3.6	1.8	2.5	40.4	58
	(1235, 12–16; 0.98:1)		4.7	2.7	2.3	45.9	32.5
	Selected children						
Prinz, Connor & Wilson (1981)	Elementary school children (109; – ; 3.1:1)	Global judgment of teacher and 2 S.D. on ATRS	45.9	1.8	22	32.4	92.3

Table 6.1 (*cont.*)

Author	Sample (Number; age; sex ratio: number boys/girls)	Instrument[a]	H %	A %	AH[b] %	H with A %	A with H %
Stewart *et al.* (1981)	Clinic-referred children (156; M = 9.1–10.9; 2.3 to 9.3)	Structured interview with mother	16.9	12.8	26.3	61.2	67.2
Loney & Milich (1982)	Clinic-referred children (50; 6–12)	Scores > 11 (A) on IOWA CTRS	8	16	20	71.4	55.5
Koriath *et al.* (1985)	Clinic-referred children (117; 4–13; 3.3:1)	DSM III	45.2	10.2	18.8	29	64.7
Reeves *et al.* (1987)	Clinic-referred children (101; 5–12; 3.2:1)	DSM III	38.6	5.9	34.6	47.3	85.3
Chee *et al.* (1989)	Clinic-referred boys (51; M = 8–9)	DSM III	27.4	19.6	35.3	56.2	69.2

[a]CTRS = Conners' teacher rating scale; ATRS = abbreviated teacher rating scale; IOWA = inattention-overactivity with aggression; IO = inattention–overactivity; A = aggression; SD = standard deviation. [b]A = aggressive/conduct disorder; H = hyperactive/ADDH; HA = hyperactive+aggressive/ADDH+CD.

more objective operational measures. This lack of straightforward correspondence between the clinical behavioural descriptors and external variables, designed to be conceptually 'equivalent', could be a critical factor restricting the validity of the diagnosis as based on symptoms.

To illustrate the two points introduced above, 30 categorical studies published since 1978 have been considered. Tables 6.2–6.5 present highlights of the pertinent studies on core symptoms such as overactivity, inattention, impulsivity and conduct problems/aggression in hyperactive/ADDH and conduct disordered/aggressive children. Information about IQ, sex, SES and age are reported in studies where these factors were controlled for. Although a lack of perfect control can be noted for the majority of the studies (24/30), age has been controlled for in 29 studies and IQ in 20 studies. This shortcoming is due to the fact that in some studies these variables have been used as dependent ones.

Overactivity

Overactivity or excessive/inappropriate motor activity has been assessed by diverse procedures: technological devices (mechanical recording with an actometer or a stabilimeter), direct observational measures and adult perception, for example. The question of whether hyperactive/ADHD children are more overactive than normal children has been extensively investigated in terms of objective procedures (for reviews, see Whalen, 1983; Luk, 1985). In brief, the results have indicated that there is much more evidence supporting the view that hyperactive/ADDH children display higher levels of wrist, ankle and chest activity (as measured via an actometer), and more 'out of seat' and 'in-seat movements' (via direct observation), than normal children or children with other psychiatric diagnoses (Kaspar *et al.*, 1971; Klein & Young, 1979; Porrino *et al.,* 1983; Halperin *et al.*, 1992). However, in hyperactive as well as in normal children, situational (e.g. nature of the classroom setting or degree of structure of the task), and developmental factors are important modulators of the level and patterns of motor activity (Zentall, 1980; Luk, 1985; Eaton & Enns, 1986; Soussignan, Koch & Montagner, 1988). Furthermore, it is not sufficient just to know that hyperactive children are physically more overactive or display more inappropriate activity than normal children. For diagnostic and taxonomic classification purposes it is important to compare the level of motor activity of hyperactive children with that of children suffering from other kinds of psychiatric disorder, particularly conduct disorder. This is a necessary task because it is likely that in earlier studies the findings have been partly obscured by the lack of careful distinction between exclusively hyperactive children and hyperactive children with aggressive behaviours (e.g. Barkley & Ullman, 1975).

Table 6.2 presents the studies that have compared measures of motor activity in aggressive (A), hyperactive (H), and hyperactive/aggressive (HA) children. As shown in this Table, the results of activity level, obtained in most cases by actometers/stabilimeters are rather equivocal. Though there is evidence that H and HA children could not be distinguished on the measure of motor activity level, it appears that only HA boys were physically more overactive than A boys when the distinction is based on rating scales scores (Loney & Milich, 1982; Roberts, 1990). However, there is no evidence that children with pure hyperactivity (H) are physically more overactive than aggressive (A) children (Koriath *et al.*, 1985; Halperin *et al.*, 1993). Furthermore, it is likely that most of the hyperactive children in the Firestone & Martin's study were HA because problems with aggressiveness, tantrums or oppositional behaviours had to be present since early childhood in home and at school. The negative finding of Koriath *et al.* (1985) could be related in part to large across-study differences in the mode of classification, and to the heterogeneity of sample composition. For example, in the Koriath study, the diagnostic groupings were very unbalanced in terms of sex ratio (M/F was 10/2 for conduct disorder and 21/10 for the pervasive hyperactive group), and the diagnostic criteria differed substantially from those used in other studies (oppositional disorder was included in the emotional disorder category; a distinction between situational and pervasive hyperactivity was made). Finally, the presence of very young children (4 year-olds) could also be a factor influencing the results because of diagnostic problems associated with younger (under 5 year) age (Campbell & Werry, 1986).

Observational measures provide a robust and complementary source of information in addition to actometer measurement because they can tap the situational and social inappropriateness of the motor activity. Data reported by Roberts (1990) using the systematic observation of academic and play settings (SOAPS) procedure in a clinic sample of 5 to 13 year-old boys confirmed that HA boys displayed higher locomotor activity (number of grid crossing, and proportion out of seat) in restricted academic settings compared with aggressive boys. However, in free play situations, it was the hyperactive group who displayed the highest locomotor activity.

Finally, more recently published data indicate that observed measures of body movements (squirming), and overall activity (changes of sitting, walking) distinguish children with hyperactivity (HA and H) from children with exclusively aggressive (A) behaviours in a naturalistic setting (Buitelaar *et al.*, 1994).

Based on adults' perceptions of children's behaviour there is some evidence

Table 6.2 *Comparison of measures of overactivity*

Author	Sample	Factors controlled	Instrument and mode[a] of classification	Measure[b]	Results[c]
				Motor activity recorded by actometer	
Firestone & Martin, 1979	50 children normal and clinical samples 5–12 yrs, IQ > 80	Age, IQ	Diagnosis by paediatrician and psychologist. DC		H > A = NC
Loney & Milich, 1982	37 boys, clinical sample, IQ > 70	Age, IQ sex, SES	IOWA CTRS, CRS		HA > A = PC HA = H
Koriath *et al.*, 1985	117 children clinical sample 4–13 yrs, IQ > 60	Age, IQ SES	DSM-III, DC		HA = H = A = PC
Werry *et al.*, 1987	95 children, normal and clinical samples 5–13 yrs, IQ > 69	Age IQ, sex	DSM-III, DC		HA = H > PC HA > NC
Roberts, 1990	36 boys, clinical sample 5–13 yrs, IQ > 70	Age, IQ sex	CTRS and CPRS, CRS clinic rater		HA > A HA = H
Matier *et al.*, 1992	38 children, clinical and school samples, 6–12 yrs	Age, IQ SES	DSM-III-R, DC PS(BC)		HA = H > NC
Halperin *et al.*, 1993	43 children, normal and clinical samples 6.5–13 yrs, IQ > 90	Age, IQ	DSM-III-R, DC CBLC, CTQ		H > NC, H = A A = NC

Table 6.2 (*cont.*)

Author	Sample	Factors controlled	Instrument and mode[a] of classification	Measure[b]	Results[c]
				Observation of motor activity	
Barkley *et al.*, 1989	74 children, clinical sample 6–13 yrs, IQ > 80	Age, IQ SES	DSM-III-R, DC	Out of seat, fidgets in restricted academic task	HA = H
Roberts, 1990	36 boys, clinical sample 5–13 yrs, IQ > 70	Age, IQ sex	CTRS and CPRS CRS, clinic rater	Grid crossings, out of seat	
				Free play	H > A, A = H
				Restricted academic task	HA > A, A = H
Buitelaar *et al.*, 1994	50 children, normal and clinical samples 8.2–9.6 yrs, IQ > 95	Age, IQ	DSM-III-R, DC CBCL and CTQ	Squirming, walking and changes in sitting in restricted tasks	HA = H > A = NC
				Adult perception	
McGee *et al.*, 1984	489 boys, community sample, 7 yrs	Age, sex	Rutter Parent and Teacher scales CRS	Activity level (Ps)	A = H > NC A = NC
Werry *et al.*, 1987	95 children, clinical sample 5–13 yrs IQ > 69	Age, IQ sex	DSM-III, DC	Gross motor activity (Ps)	HA > PC, HA = H > NC
				Fidgetiness (Ps)	A > PC, HA = H > NC
				Restlessness (Ps)	HA = H = PC

Table 6.2 (*cont.*)

Author	Sample	Factors controlled	Instrument and mode[a] of classification	Measure[b]	Results[c]
Reeves *et al.*, 1987	88 children, clinical sample 6–13 yrs IQ > 69	Age, IQ sex	DSM-III, DC	Motor excess:RBPC(P)	HA = H > PC = NC
Moffitt & Silva, 1988	678 children, community sample, 11 yrs	Age	SRED, Teacher and Parent Rutter scales BPCR, DISC-C, CRS	Motor hyperactivity: (P) Motor hyperactivity: (T)	HA = H > A = NC HA = H > A = NC
Soussignan *et al.*, 1992	32 boys, school sample 10–11 yrs	Age, sex SES	Teacher Rutter scale, CRS FD	Overactivity (T) Overactivity (M)	HA > A > NC HA > NC
Soltys *et al.*, 1992	61 children, clinical sample 7–12 yrs IQ > 70	Age, SES	DICA (DSM-III criteria) DC	Motor: PIC (P) hyperactivity	HA = H = A = PC

[a]DC = Diagnostic category; CRS = Category derived from rating scale; BPCR = behaviour problem checklist-revised; CPRS = Conners' parent rating scale; CTRS = Conners' teacher rating scale; CTQ = classroom teacher questionnaires; CBCL = Child Behaviour Checklist; DICA = diagnostic interview for children and adolescents; DISC-C = diagnostic interview schedule for children–child version; FD = follow-up design; PIC = personality inventory children; SRED = self-reported early delinquency; PS(BC) = psychopharmacological study (baseline condition); [b]Ps = psychologist; P = parent; M = mother; T = teacher. [c]NC = normal controls; PC = psychiatric controls; A = aggressive/conduct disorder; H = hyperactive/ADDH/ADHD; HA = hyperactive+aggressive/ADDH+CD/ADHD+CD.

suggesting that hyperactive subgroups show more overactive behaviours than aggressive or control groups when raters are parents or teachers (Moffitt & Silva, 1988; Soussignan *et al.*, 1992).

In short, it appears safe to assert that published findings are still insufficient to provide firm conclusions on the issue of whether children with pure hyperactivity differ from those with other forms of disturbed conduct on the basis of the amount of locomotor activity. From studies published so far, there is some evidence to suggest that HA children can be distinguished from aggressive or psychiatric control groups by the degree of motor activity. However, there is less evidence to support the distinction between pure hyperactivity and hyperactivity in the presence of conduct disorder.

Inattention

Comprehensive reviews of attention deficit studies in hyperactive children have been provided by a number of authors (Rosenthal & Allen, 1978; Douglas & Peters, 1979; Prior & Sanson, 1986). In the studies reviewed, attention has usually been viewed as a diffuse and broad construct which has been conceptualised in terms of several components, such as selective attention, concentration, sustained attention and vigilance (Douglas & Peters, 1979; Rosenthal & Allen, 1978).

Consequently, it has been necessary to develop diverse measures and procedures in order to assess the attentional difficulties of hyperactive children. The first kind of measures included teacher ratings of children's attentional problems, and direct observations of 'off-task' behaviour in the classroom. Although such measures are not entirely sensitive or differentiating, and fail to pinpoint the diverse components of attentional deficits, they have a greater face validity than those used in laboratory tests and therefore are useful in providing relevant information as part of the diagnostic process. As a whole, direct behavioural observations during structured classroom activities have indicated that hyperactive children spend more time 'off-task' than do controls (Klein & Young; 1979, Luk, 1985). The second type of measures are derived from various psychometric tests and laboratory procedures, and consequently are more relevant in assessing specific functions of attention and cognitive process. A variety of measures tapping distinct components of attention have been employed to examine the performance of hyperactive and control children. While results on distractibility (i.e. attention to extraneous or irrelevant stimuli during ongoing task performances) are contradictory and fail to support a selective attention deficit hypothesis, there exists considerable evidence supporting a sustained attention deficit hypothesis (Douglas & Peters, 1979). For example, studies using tests of vigilance (e.g. continuous performance test, CPT), have consistently reported that hyperactive/ADD children make more omission errors than their normal age-mates (Douglas & Peters, 1979; Campbell & Werry, 1986). Given that inattentiveness and distractibility are also commonly reported in conduct disordered children (Quay, 1979), it is necessary to verify whether part of this picture is not the result of the undifferentiated diagnostic/screening procedures of the earlier studies.

A general outline of findings from studies that have contrasted subgroups of aggressive and hyperactive children is shown in Table 6.3. The results based on CPT measures (correct responses, reaction time, omission errors) do not indicate a consistent pattern. Eight of the 11 studies failed to find differences between the diagnostic groups (Koriath *et al.*, 1985; Werry *et al.*, 1987; Shapiro & Garfinkel, 1986, Levy, Horn & Dalglish, 1987; Klorman *et al.*, 1988; Barkley *et al.*, 1989; August & Garfinkel, 1989; Matier *et al.*, 1992), while three studies indicated that children with pure hyperactivity can be distinguished from the other diagnostic groups (Chee *et al.*, 1989; Halperin *et al.*, 1990, 1993). Although it is not possible to ascertain whether a large part of these conflicting results is a consequence of the classification procedures and characteristics of the samples, the findings seem to suggest that these variables play only a limited role. However, for the time being, caution must be taken when drawing particular conclusions from studies, which though based on 'non-contaminated' samples, are nevertheless not closely comparable.

Keeping these problems in mind, it is worth pointing out a recent study by Chee *et al.* (1989), which showed that the use of experimentally manipulated variables, such as the variation in the demand for attention, made it possible to differentiate diagnostic groups. This study is particularly convincing and interesting because, contrary to the other studies, the presence of additional diagnoses (i.e. both learning and conduct disorders), the demand for sustained attention (i.e. length of stimulus exposure or display time (DT), event rate, stimulus exposure asynchrony (SOA)), and task duration among subgroups of ADDH and CD subjects were controlled for. In the first experiment it was found that ADDH boys were uniquely affected by the variation 'in demand for attention' imposed by different SOAs (rapid event rate of 1 s). However, the results are not wholly conclusive because when task duration (experiment 2) was controlled for, there was no evidence of a poorer performance at an SOA of 1 s.

A possible effect of practice to explain these differences existed because of the greater number of trials in experiment 2 (960 versus 120). Interestingly, when distinction was made between pervasive hyperactivity (ICD-9 diagnosis of hyperkinetic syndrome) and situational hyperactivity (DSM-III diagnosis of ADDH), the results suggested a more global deficit in sustained attention among children with hyperkinetic syndrome. The authors pointed out that the deficit might be associated with a greater susceptibility of hyperactive children to refractory effects.

To sum up, although the results from the existing studies are equivocal, the failure in a number of studies to manipulate potentially critical variables (e.g. duration of task, attentional demand) could largely explain the lack of convergence. The importance of contextual factors influencing the appearance of deficits and demands for task processing has already been emphasised (Douglas, 1984, 1988; Power, 1992). It therefore appears of prime importance to control and experimentally manipulate such variables in future studies focusing on the issue of differential diagnosis.

Results of observational studies presented in Table 6.3 are also conflicting. Furthermore, these findings are not really comparable with those reported above because of the large variations regarding the methods of classifying the children's behaviour (e.g. DSM-III, DSM-III-R, ICD-9, rating scales), the dependent variables and the nature of settings in studies. The work of Roberts (1987, 1990) which employed a larger number of measures in a variety of situations seems more suitable for tapping the concept of sustained attention (e.g. time spent on task, work sheet score) compared to other studies. The results of Roberts' studies showed that, in structured play settings, the hyperactive group shifted task more frequently than the aggressive group. In a structured academic task situation, the hyperactive boys (H and HA) spent a lower proportion of time on task and completed fewer worksheet items than either the aggressive (A) group or the non-referred boys. Roberts' findings also suggested that the HA children were more likely than the children in the other groups to engage in rule violating behaviours (e.g. playing with forbidden toys). This could reflect both problems of 'attitude' and 'aptitude' in hyperactive children (Milich & Landau, 1989). The data also suggest that the SOAPS procedure is a potentially relevant method of discriminating meaningful subgroups of children with externalising disorders. So, the validity of this playroom observation technique for identification purposes should be replicated in future studies. The finding of a behavioural manifestation of inattention (looking not directed towards the task) in a naturalistic setting was also evinced in a recent ethological study that provides further support that hyperactive children (H and HA) could be discriminated from the aggressive or normal children (Buitelaar *et al.*, 1994; Table 6.3).

Rating scales have also commonly been used as criterion measures to differentiate the putative syndromes. Unfortunately, such sources of data are par-

Table 6.3 *Comparison of measures of inattention*

Author	Sample	Factors controlled	Instrument and mode[a] of classification	Measure[b]	Results[c]
			Vigilance test (CPT)		
Koriath *et al.*, 1985	117 children, clinical sample 4–13 yrs, IQ > 60	Age, IQ SES	DSM-III, DC	CR	HA = H = A = PC
Shapiro & Garfinkel, 1986	303 children, school sample 7–13 yrs	Age, sex	CTRS IOWA, CRS	OE	HA = H = A = NC
Werry *et al.*, 1987	95 children, clinical sample 5–13 yrs, IQ > 69	Age, IQ sex	DSM-III, DC OE		HA = H = PC
Levy *et al.*, 1987	158 children, clinical sample 5–10 yrs, IQ > 90	Age, IQ SES, sex	DSM-III, DC	OE RT	Hs = Hm = Hmi > PC HS = Hm = Hmi = A
Klorman *et al.*, 1988	43 children, clinical sample 6–12 yrs, IQ > 80	Age, IQ SES, sex	HAS, ACTQ IOWA scale CRS, PS(BC)	OE TR	HA = H HA = H
Chee *et al.*, 1989	87 boys, clinical and school samples, M = 8–9 yrs, IQ > 80	Age, IQ sex	DSM-III, DC	RT CR	H > HA = A = NC = PC H < NC = PC
Barkley *et al.*, 1989	74 children, clinical sample 6–13 yrs, IQ > 80	Age, IQ SES	DSM-III-R, DC PS(BC)	OE CR	HA = H HA = H

Table 6.3 (*cont.*)

Author	Sample	Factors controlled	Instrument and mode[a] of classification	Measure[b]	Results[c]
August & Garfinkel, 1989	1,038 children, school sample 5–14 yrs	Age, IQ	Yale Children's Inventory, CRS	OE	HL > H = HA = NC
Halperin *et al.*, 1990	85 children, school sample M = 9 yrs, IQ > 80	Age, IQ	CTRS IOWA CRS	OE	H > HA = A = NC
Matier *et al.*, 1992	38 children, clinical and school samples 6–12 yrs	Age, IQ SES	DSM-III-R DC, PS(BC)	OE	H = HA > NC
Halperin *et al.*, 1993	43 children, normal and clinical samples 6.5–13 yrs, IQ > 90	Age, IQ	DSM-III-R, DC CBLC, CTQ	Missed targets and X-only responses	H > A = NC
				Observation of behaviour	
Sandberg *et al.*, 1978	29 boys, clinical sample, IQ > 50	Age, sex	ICD-9, DC	Index of attention/activity	A = H
Koriath *et al.*, 1985	117 children, clinical sample 4–13 yrs, IQ > 60	Age, IQ SES	DSM-III, DC	Toy changes	HA = H = A = PC

Table 6.3 (*cont.*)

Author	Sample	Factors controlled	Instrument and mode[a] of classification	Measure[b]	Results[c]
				Observation of behaviour	
Barkley *et al.*, 1989	74 children, clinical sample 6–13 yrs, IQ > 80	Age, IQ SES	DSM-III-R, DC PS (BC)	*Restricted academic task*	
				Off-task	HA = H
				Play with toys	HA = H
Roberts, 1987, 1990	56 boys, clinical and normal samples 6–12 yrs, IQ > 70	Age, IQ sex	CTRS & CPRS CRS, clinic rater	*Restricted academic task*	
				Time on-task	NC = A > HA = H
				Worksheet score	NC = A > HA = H
				Restricted play setting	
				Number of task shifts	H > A, H = HA
Buitelaar *et al.*, 1994	50 children, clinical and normal samples, M = 8.2–9.9 yrs	Age, IQ	DSM-III-R, DC CBCL & CTQ	*Restricted tasks*	
				Look at the tasks	HA = H < A = NC
				Perception of behaviour	
Loney & Milich, 1982	37 boys, clinical sample, IQ > 70	Age, IQ SES, sex	IOWA CTRS CRS	Inattention: TOST (T)	HA = H = A > PC
McGee *et al.*, 1984	489 boys community sample 7 yrs	Age, sex	Teacher or Parent RS, CRS	Attention span (Ps)	H < NC, H = AH = A
Koriath *et al.*, 1985	117 children clinical sample 4–13 yrs, IQ > 60	Age, IQ SES	DSM-III, DC	Inattention: CTRS (T)	HA = H = A = PC

Table 6.3 (*cont.*)

Author	Sample	Factors controlled	Instrument and mode[a] of classification	Measure[b]	Results[c]
Reeves *et al.*, 1987	95 children, clinical and normal samples, 6–13 yrs, IQ > 69	Age, IQ, sex	DSM-III, DC	Inattention: CTRS Attention deficit: RBPC	HA = H > PC > NC HA = H > PC > NC
Werry *et al.*, 1987	95 clinic-referred children 5–13 yrs, IQ > 69	Age, IQ sex	DSM-III, DC	Distractibility (Ps) Attention span (Ps)	HA > PC, HA = H HA = H = PC
Moffitt & Silva, 1988	678 children, community sample, 11 yrs	Age	SRED, Teacher & Parent RS DISC-C, CRS, FD	Inattention: RS (P) Inattention: RS (T)	HA = H > A = NC HA = H > A = NC
Barkley *et al.*, 1989	74 children, clinical sample 6–13 yrs, IQ > 80	Age, IQ SES	DSM-III-R, DC BC (PS)	Inattention: CTRS (T) Inattention: CBCL-TRF	HA = H H > HA
Soussignan *et al.*, 1992	32 boys, school sample, 10–11 yrs	Age, SES sex	Teacher RS CRS, FD	Inattention (T) Inattention (M)	HA > A > NC HA > A = NC
Soltys *et al.*, 1992	61 children, clinical sample 7–12 yrs, IQ > 70	Age, SES	DICA, DC	Attention span: DOT (S) Distractibility: DOT (S)	HA < H = PC HA = H > PC HA = H = A

[a]For definitions, see Table 2; HAS = home activity scale; ACTQ = abbreviated Conners' teacher questionnaire. [b]See table 6.2 for definitions, CPT = continuous performance test; DOT = dimensions of temperament; CR = correct responses; OE = omission errors; RT = reaction time; TOST = teacher Off-Task Scale; CBCL-TRF = child behavior checklist teacher report form; CTRS = revised Conners' teacher rating scale; FD = follow-up design; RS = Rutter scales; T = teacher; P = parent; Ps = psychologist. [c]For definitions, see Table 6.2, HL = ADDH+Learning disability, Hs = ADDH severe, Hm = ADDH moderate, Hmi = ADDH mild.

tially interdependent because they may share some 'source of variance' with the clinical diagnosis; that is the information that led to the diagnosis is partly derived from parent/teacher reports (Taylor, 1988*a*,*b*). Though not wholly conclusive, the findings suggest that H and HA children are generally perceived by teacher, parent or research psychologist as more inattentive than normal or psychiatric controls. However, they offer no substantial evidence to support a distinction between conduct disordered and hyperactive groups.

Taken together, data on objective attentional measures, while giving some suggestive evidence that hyperactive subgroups tended to have more attentional problems, especially on sustained attention, than the control groups (i.e. normal or psychiatric), have produced only partial support for the separation of aggressive and hyperactive subgroups of children. Further research is needed on pure and mixed forms of externalising behaviour employing carefully controlled experimental designs in order to investigate the role of task condition and situational factors which are likely to affect the performance or the behaviour of the children.

Impulsivity

Impulsivity is usually defined as an inability to inhibit responding (Prior & Sanson, 1986). The complexity and the heterogeneity of this construct have been emphasised by a number of authors (Milich & Kramer, 1984; Gittelman, 1988). It appears that at least two major problems can be discerned: the lack of independence between the constructs of impulsivity and inattention, and the difficulty of defining and operationalising the concept (Gittelman, 1988; Campbell & Werry, 1986).

Despite the uncertainty related to the lack of a clear definition of impulsivity, the concept has continued to be used as referring to a particular style of behaviour (uncontrolled behaviour suggesting possibly a deficit in avoidance learning and inhibitory control), or a type of approach to tasks involving cognitive demands (style of problem-solving activity) (Taylor, 1985). The meaning of impulsivity as a behavioural style has, in the clinical literature, been operationalised by a variety of behavioural statements (cf. descriptors in DSM-III, DSM-III-R and DSM-IV, such as 'often acts before thinking', 'often has difficulty awaiting turn', 'shifts excessively from one activity to another', 'often interrupts or intrudes on others'). The meaning of impulsivity as a style of cognitive approaches, on the other hand, has been the subject of more extensive and systematic research (Douglas & Peters, 1979). The most widely used measures of cognitive impulsivity in hyperactive children have been derived from the matching familiar figures test (MFFT) and the continuous performance test (CPT).

The MFFT is a visual matching test in which the child has to choose from an array of similar familiar figures the one picture that is identical to a standard figure. Typically, hyperactive children tend to make more errors than matched controls (e.g. Sykes, Douglas & Morgenstern, 1973), while they do not necessarily respond faster.

The CPT is a task of vigilance that requires the child to respond by pressing a lever following a target stimulus (i.e. X) preceded by a cue stimulus (i.e. A) presented at particular random intervals. A number of studies have shown that hyperactive children make more commission errors to non-signal stimuli compared with normal children; a result suggesting a failure to inhibit or control responses to stimuli to which the child knows that he/she should not react. However, although a poor inhibiting control is considered to be a central feature of ADD/hyperactivity, it has also been found to be associated with emotional disturbance (Finch & Montgomery, 1973), learning disorders (Campbell, 1974) and conduct problems (Shaffer, McNamara & Pincus, 1974). Thus, it does not seem to be a pathognomonic feature of hyperactivity disorder. Because of the lack of adequate differential diagnostic procedures in the earlier studies, it is of great importance to examine carefully the studies that have directly compared hyperactive and conduct disordered children. Studies on adult perception of the child impulsive behaviour are scarce, but the few existing findings on community and clinic samples suggest that children identified hyperactive (H and HA) by teacher, or by a psychiatrist, are not rated by psychologists as more impulsive than the aggressive groups (McGee *et al.*, 1984; Koriath *et al.*, 1985).

As can be ascertained from Table 6.4, none of the MFF-test measures of impulsivity have been shown to differentiate groups of H and HA children in terms of their cognitive style. In two studies (Sandberg *et al.*, 1978; Koriath *et al.*, 1985), H/ADDH children did have shorter latencies than A/CD children, while in one study (Loney & Milich, 1982), the HA group made more errors than the aggressive or psychiatric control groups. It is therefore of interest to note that statistically significant differences between hyperactive and aggressive groups largely pertain to two studies, in both of which the sample included boys only (Sandberg *et al.*, 1978; Loney & Milich, 1982). It is worth, however, adding that in the Halperin *et al.* (1990) study, there was a trend ($p < 0.1$) towards hyperactive children making more MFF errors than the children in the other groups. The small number of subjects (n=4) with pure hyperactivity in this particular study might explain the lack of statistical significance.

Much the same can be said about the CPT commission errors (i.e. false posi-

Table 6.4. *Comparison of measures of impulsivity*

Author	Sample	Factors controlled	Instrument and mode[a] of classification	Measure[b]	Results[c]
				MFTT	
Sandberg *et al.*, 1978	29 boys, clinical sample, IQ > 50	Age, sex	ICD-9, DC	L E	H < A H = A
Firestone & Martin, 1979	50 children, normal and clinical samples 5–12 yrs, IQ > 80	Age, IQ	Diagnosis by pediatrician and psychologist, DC	L E	H = A = PC = NC H = A > PC = NC
Loney & Milich, 1982	37 boys, clinical sample, IQ > 70	Age, IQ sex, SES	IOWA CTRS, CRS	L E	HA = H = A = PC HA > A = PC, HA = H
Koriath *et al.*, 1985	117 children, clinical sample 4–13 yrs, IQ > 60	Age, IQ SES	DSM-III, DC	L E	Ha = H < A = PC HA = H = A = PC
Werry *et al.*, 1987	95 children, normal and clinical samples 5–13 yrs, IQ > 69	Age IQ, sex	DSM-III, DC	L E	HA = H = PC HA = H = PC
Barkley *et al.*, 1989	74 children clinical sample 6–13 yrs, IQ > 80	Age, IQ SES	DSM-III-R, DC PS (BC)	L E	HA = H HA = H
August & Garfinkel, 1989	1038 children, school sample 5–14 yrs	Age, IQ	Yale Children's Inventory, CRS	L E	HL = H = HA = NC HL = H = HA = NC

Table 6.4. (*cont.*)

Author	Sample	Factors controlled	Instrument and mode[a] of classification	Measure[b]	Results[c]
				CPT	
Koriath *et al.*, 1985	117 children, clinical sample 4–13 yrs, IQ > 60	Age, IQ SES	DSM-III, DC	CE	HA = H = A = PC
Shapiro & Garkinkel, 1986	303 children, school sample 7–13 yrs	Age, sex	CTRS IOWA, CRS	CE	HA = H = A > NC
Werry *et al.*, 1987	95 children, normal and clinical samples 5–13 yrs, IQ > 69	Age, IQ sex	DSM-III, DC	CE	HA = H = PC = NC
Levy *et al.*, 1987	158 children clinic sample 5–10 yrs, IQ > 90	Age, IQ SES, sex	DSM-III, DC	CE	Hs > A, Hm = Hmi = A
Klorman *et al.*, 1988	43 children, clinical sample 6–12 yrs, IQ > 80	Age, IQ SES, sex	HAS, ACTQ IOWA scale CRS, PS (BC)	CE	HA = H
Chee *et al.*, 1989	87 boys, clinical and school samples, M = 8–9 yrs, IQ > 80	Age, IQ sex	DSM-III, DC	CE	HA = H = A = NC = PC

Table 6.4. (*cont.*)

Author	Sample	Factors controlled	Instrument and mode[a] of classification	Measure[b]	Results[c]
				CPT	
August & Garfinkel, 1989	1038 children, school sample 5–14 yrs	Age, IQ	Yale Children's Inventory, CRS	CE	HL > HA = H = NC
Barkley *et al.*, 1989	74 children, clinical sample 6–13 yrs, IQ > 80	Age, IQ SES	DSM-III-R, DC PS (BC)	CE	HA = H
Halperin *et al.*, 1990	85 children, school sample M = 9 yrs, IQ > 80	Age, IQ	CTRS IOWA CRS	CE	HA > H = A = NC
Matier *et al.*, 1992	38 children, clinical and school samples 6–12 yrs	Age, IQ SES	DSM-III-R DC, PS (BC)	CE	HA > H = NC
Halperin *et al.*, 1993	43 children, normal and clinical samples 6.5–13 yrs, IQ > 90	Age, IQ	DSM-III-R, DC CBLC, CTQ	Missed targets and X-only responses	H > A = NC

[ac]For definitions, see Table 6.2. [b]MFFT = matching familiar figures test; CPT = continuous performance test; CE = commission errors; (L) = MFF latency; (E) = MFF errors.

tive responses), in terms of their inability to validate the distinction between hyperactivity and conduct disorder. Table 6.4 shows that, when subgroups of hyperactive children are compared, only two studies out of nine indicate that the HA subgroup made more false alarms than the H subgroup (Halperin *et al.*, 1990; Matier *et al.*, 1992). On the other hand, three studies out of six reveal that children with H or HA behaviours could be differentiated from children with pure aggression (Levy *et al.*, 1987; Halperin *et al.*, 1990, 1993). The reasons for this discrepancy cannot be fully determined from the available data, but they may well be related to diverse sources of data and other methodological variations, as well as to the degree of severity of the disorder, and the issue of pervasiveness in particular. For example, two of the studies (Shapiro & Garfinkel, 1986; Halperin *et al.*, 1990) using equivalent samples (non-referred children of comparable age), and a similar mode of classification (IOWA Conners) differed notably in the rate of stimulus presentation (dependent versus independent of the child's performance), and in defining the specific index of commission errors. Indeed, in an earlier report Halperin *et al.* (1988) had suggested that commission errors (i.e. A-not-X error, X-only error, A-only error, random error) do not comprise a homogeneous measure, but rather reflect deficits in different underlying psychological processes. In their subsequent study (Halperin *et al.*, 1990) based on a random sample of school children, whose behaviour was categorised in terms of teacher rating scale scores, they provided evidence that A-not-X error only was related to dimensions of behavioural dyscontrol (impulsivity, motor hyperactivity), and to the fastest reaction time. Thus, the conflicting results previously reported could stem from a loss of meaningful information about impulsivity due to the utilisation of a composite measure.

In summary, findings on the measures of cognitive impulsivity suggest that hyperactive children tend to be more impulsive than matched normal children, but this review has failed to reveal much evidence for the differential validity of the hyperactivity and conduct disorder in terms of impulsivity. This lack of distinction could be related to impulsivity acting as a 'confounder' as suggested by Gittelman (1988), meaning that, in almost all instances, impulsivity overlaps with both hyperactivity and conduct disorder. Furthermore, there is also the possibility that the inconsistent results are partly related to the poor sensitive or discriminative power of an overall measure of commission errors in the continuous performance test (CPT). More recently, investigators used a different paradigm (i.e. the stop signal paradigm) designated to analyse differences in inhibitory control among ADHD and CD subjects (Schachar, Tannock & Logan, 1993). Their results did not indicate an inability to delay responding in children with ADHD, as had been previously argued (Sonuga-Barke, *et al.*,

1992), but a presence of deficient inhibitory control even in a situation that involved no delay. Moreover, the finding of deficient inhibitory control was evidenced only in subjects with pure ADHD. In the same way, the lack of reliability and validity of the MFF-test, as has been stressed by some investigators (Block, Block & Harrington, 1974), could also partly explain the test's inability to discriminate between the hyperactive and conduct disordered groups.

Finally, the usefulness of the construct of impulsivity in hyperactivity disorder has also been questioned on the grounds of its theoretical foundations, such as the necessity to translate the traditional perspective into a conceptual approach that emphasises information processing stages including encoding, response decision and response organisation (Sergeant, 1988). More specifically, it has been hypothesised that the deficiency of the hyperactive child is in the degree of control which is exerted over behaviour, and that energetic processes could be the candidates by which to explain their task inefficiency, not in terms of structural process deficits but rather resource strategy limitations (Sergeant & Scholten, 1985; Van der Meere & Sergeant, 1987; Sergeant, 1988). Further research clearly remains to be undertaken in order to examine these methodological and conceptual issues in groups of children with pure and mixed externalising problems. The investigators' priority for future studies should be to select appropriate measures or paradigms in order to more carefully tap the constructs of behavioural impulsiveness and inhibitory control.

Conduct problems/aggression

Empirically derived syndromes from multivariate studies have generally revealed the emergence of a conduct problem/aggression factor (Quay, 1986; Hinshaw, 1987). Conduct problems/aggression refer to behaviours that transgress social and legal norms (e.g. no adhesion to the usual rules of social exchanges) (Doke & Flippo, 1983; Quay, 1986). These behaviours are far from forming a homogeneous pattern, and consequently a number of investigators have drawn attention to the necessity to delineate subtypes of relevant aggressive behaviours in order to improve the procedures of validation (Hinshaw, 1987; Hinshaw, Heller & McHale, 1992). Developmental studies indicated that at least two categories (i.e. 'overt' and 'covert' types) of aggressive/antisocial behaviour display divergent developmental trajectories from childhood to adolescence (Loeber, 1982). Likewise, the pattern of covert antisocial acts has also emerged as an independent dimension in a number of factor analytic studies (Werry, Spague & Cohen, 1975; Glow, 1981; Taylor & Sandberg, 1984).

Overt aggressive behaviours include confrontation acts such as fighting, threatening, tantrums, defiance, bullying, while covert antisocial behaviours refer to clandestine acts such as stealing, lying, truancy, firesetting and vandalism (Loeber & Schamling, 1985; Wolff, 1985). The equivalent clinical picture of the dimension of conduct problems is that of conduct disorder (CD) in DSM-III-R, DSM-IV and ICD-10. In this context, it is striking to note that, in contrast to the DSM-III definition of ADDH, the DSM-III definition of CD was poorly structured and failed to specify the minimum number of symptoms required for the diagnosis. This point is important because it could have constituted an additional and uncontrolled source of variation apt to obscure the comparisons between a number of studies based on the DSM-III diagnoses of ADDH and CD. This possibility is suggested by Lahey *et al.* (1990) study which showed that the utilisation of DSM-III-R's list of symptoms for the diagnosis of CD, as compared with its DSM-III counterparts, appeared to be more valid in terms of being more strongly associated with police contacts, school suspension and history of antisocial personality disorder in the biological father. More recently, efforts to improve reliability and validity of the diagnoses for ADHD and CD have led investigators to propose changes to the diagnostic criteria, as now partly implemented in the DSM-IV (American Psychiatric Association, 1994). The predictive validity of the behavioural symptoms as the DSM-IV criteria for the disruptive behaviour disorder diagnoses was tested on a sample of 440 clinic-referred children and young people aged from 4 to 17 years (Frick *et al.*, 1994). The study did indeed indicate the usefulness of restrictive definitions of behaviour, such as 'lying' and 'truancy', for example, increasing the diagnostic efficiency of conduct disorder.

As the terms 'conduct disorder' and 'aggression' refer to violations of major social rules (see ICD-10, WHO, 1992) and imply conflictual interactions of the child with the social environment, adult and peer perceptions, and direct observations by investigators, are the most commonly employed means of providing relevant information on this aspect of child behaviour. Given the overall importance of the discriminative validity of behavioural symptoms in terms of defining clinical syndromes, it is surprising that so few comparative studies have focused on observed behavioural patterns. This lack of studies may stem at least partly from the difficulties in collecting reliable information by observational methods as employed in laboratory and naturalistic settings. (One of these difficulties, for example is that aggressive behaviours occur infrequently.) Although it has not so far been directly established whether subgroups of aggressive children with and without concurrent hyperactivity differ on specific patterns of aggression, there is some indirect evidence to suggest that this is the case. Recent psychopharmacological investigations have, for example, revealed that, on placebo and baseline days, ADHD boys also scoring high on aggression, displayed higher observed frequency of verbal and non-verbal aggression (physical aggression, negative verbalisations, stealing, lying) both in the classroom and playroom settings, and were more likely to respond to provocation with aggression in a laboratory task compared with ADHD boys scoring low on aggressiveness (Hinshaw *et al.*, 1989; Hinshaw, 1991; Pelham *et al.*, 1991; Murphy, Pelham & Lang, 1992). Up to now, categorical studies on patterns of aggression have largely relied on the perceptions of raters rather than on the actual observed behaviour of the child. However, it is well established that the limitations of questionnaire-based studies in the domains of hyperactivity and conduct disorder (e.g. lack of discriminative power, operation of halo effect) considerably restrict the robustness of their findings. However, as the differential validities of a number of behavioural scales (e.g. IOWA CTRS) have been established by independent observational measures (Loney & Milich, 1982; Milich & Fitzgerald, 1985; Atkins, Pelham & Licht, 1989), the remaining measurement problems mainly concern the actual independence of the raters (e.g. teacher, parent, peers), as of that of the informants who contribute to the diagnostic process. Unfortunately, the majority of the studies available so far (see Table 6.5) have failed to yield measures of aggression which are independent of the clinical symptomatology. For example, behavioural data have been derived from a diagnostic interview with parents (Stewart, Cummings & Singer, 1981; Offord *et al.*, 1979), or stem from a variety of sources, including rating scales which have also served as part of the diagnostic/screening process (August & Stewart, 1982; Thorley, 1984; Walker *et al.*, 1987). They thus need to be viewed with some caution because they are likely to be weakened by partial interdependence of data. Obviously, this does not mean that the studies are useless as such. They may nevertheless provide relevant information about the severity and the nature of conduct problems among aggressive subgroups (A and HA) of children. However, they appear to be unsuitable for examining the question of the discriminative validity.

Given the substantial overlap between the dimensions of hyperactivity and conduct problems observed in the prevalence and correlational studies (Hinshaw, 1987), one may question whether children with pure and mixed disruptive behaviour disorders can in fact be differentiated on the basis of intensity (e.g. high score on hyperactivity or frequency of aggressive acts) and the form (overt and covert aggressive acts) of their behavioural problems. In general, it has been shown that children labelled as hyperactive and aggressive by teacher, or by multiple informants, show a greater number of conduct problems and a higher rate of offending than children whose problems involve aggression only (Loney & Milich, 1982; Shapiro & Garfinkel, 1986; Moffitt & Silva, 1988; Loeber, 1988*a*; Szatmari, Boyle & Offord, 1989*b*; Pope, Bierman &

Mumma, 1989). Instruments, such as peer ratings that do not confound the two domains of interest are probably of greater value as they have been shown to be more sensitive than teacher ratings in predicting long-term adjustment (Cowen *et al.*, 1973). Though peer–teacher agreement can be substantial, particularly when raters are asked to judge child aggression (Ledingham *et al.*, 1982), it is possible that peers are more accurate than teachers in assessing the quality of the child's interactions. Unfortunately, sociometric ratings of aggression in studies comparing hyperactive and aggressive children are scarce. The available data, however, support the view that children rated as hyperactive and aggressive by their teachers are also nominated on the pupil evaluation inventory (Pekaric *et al.*, 1976) as more aggressive/disruptive than purely hyperactive or matched normal children (Johnston & Pelham, 1986; Milich & Landau, 1989; Soussignan *et al.*, 1992), but not necessarily more disruptive than children with aggression alone.

The two major patterns which have been most investigated so far are physical aggression/fighting and covert antisocial acts. As shown in Table 6.5, there is some evidence to suggest that physical aggression is more common in the HA group than in A or H groups in studies based on children referred to psychiatric clinics, or on those designated delinquent (Offord *et al.*, 1979; August & Stewart, 1982; Walker *et al.*, 1987). However, in studies using children from the general population the subgroups of aggressive children (A and HA) appear not to be distinguishable on measures of adult perception (Soussignan *et al.*, 1992). For the time being it is not really possible adequately to resolve this issue given the methodological problems already mentioned in relation to a number of studies (e.g. lack of independent criteria, differences in instruments and source of information). However, because conduct problems reported in clinically disturbed children are likely to be more severe than those reported in conduct disturbed children in the general population (see Sandberg *et al.*, 1980), it is possible that clinic referred children with mixed externalising problems (HA) are also the ones who display the poorest inhibitory control, which in turn, might lead to confrontational acts, such as fighting.

Findings on antisocial behaviour appear to be mixed, as shown in Table 6.5. However, when the studies are separated according to the source of independent information and the nature of samples the data do appear to suggest that in community samples, children classed as HA display more antisocial acts (stealing, lying, truancy) as compared with the A or H groups (Loeber, Brinthaupt & Green, 1990; Soussignan *et al.*, 1992). Interestingly, in a number of studies, it has also been found that HA children more often exhibit the pattern of both fighting and stealing than children with the diagnosis of A only (Loeber & Schmaling, 1985; Walker *et al.*, 1987). These findings are likely

Table 6.5 *Comparison of measures of aggressive and antisocial acts*

Author	Sample	Factors controlled	Instrument and mode[a] of classification	Measure[b]	Results[c]
				Physical aggression, Fighting	
Offord *et al.*, 1979	66 delinquent boys, M = 12.5 yrs	Age, IQ SES, sex	Parental interview, DC	(P)	HA > A
August & Stewart, 1982	76 boys, clinical sample, 5–13 yrs, IQ > 55	Sex	Multiple source of information, DC	(P) + (T)	HA > H
Thorley, 1984	146 children, clinical sample, 5–11 yrs IQ < 70; IQ > 70	Age, IQ SES, sex	ICD-9, DC clinical data	(C)	A > H; A = H
Walker *et al.*, 1987	35 children, clinical sample, 6–13 yrs	Age, IQ sex	DSM-III, DC	(P) + (T) + (C) (Pe)	HA > A HA > A = NC
Loeber *et al.*, 1990	210 boys, school sample	Age, sex	Teacher rating scale, CRS	(S)	HA > H, A, NC
Soussignan *et al.*, 1992	32 boys, school sample, 10–11 yrs	Age, SES sex	Teacher Rutter scale, CRS FD	(T) (M) (S)	HA = A > NC HA = A > NC A > NC, A = HA

Table 6.5 (*cont.*)

Author	Sample	Factors controlled	Instrument and mode[a] of classification	Measure[b]	Results[c]
				Laboratory measures of aggressive behaviours	
Atkins & Stoff, 1993	80 boys, clinical and normal samples 8–12 yrs	Age, sex	DSM-III-R, DC	Instrumental aggression Hostile aggression	HA = A > NC HA > NC, A = NC
				Antisocial acts	
Offord *et al.*, 1979	66 delinquent boys, M = 12.5 yrs	Age, IQ SES, sex	Parental interview, DC	Drug use (P)	HA > A
Stewart *et al.*, 1981	175 boys clinical sample 3–16 yrs, IQ > 55	Age, IQ SES	Interview with mother, DC	Lying, stealing and fire setting Damage to propriety (M)	HA = A > H = PC (B) HA, A = H = PC (G)
August *et al.*, 1983	52 children clinical sample M = 13.7/14.2 yrs IQ > 55	Age, IQ SES, sex	Interview with parents, DC	Thefts; truancy and fire setting; vandalism; Alcohol & drug use (P)	HA = H HA > H
Thorley, 1984	146 children, clinical sample, 5–11 yrs IQ<70; IQ>70	Age, IQ SES, sex	ICD-9, DC clinic data	Stealing (C) Lying; truancy	A > H H = A

Table 6.5 (*cont.*)

Author	Sample	Factors controlled	Instrument and mode[a] of classification	Measure[b]	Results[c]
				Antisocial Acts	
Walker *et al.*, 1987	35 children, clinical sample 6–13 yrs	Age, IQ sex	DSM-III, DC	Truancy; stealing; lying;vandalism; fire setting (P) + (T) + (C)	HA = A
Loeber *et al.*, 1990	210 boys, school sample	Age, sex	Teacher rating, CRS FD	Truancy (S) + (M)	HA > H, A, NC
Moffitt, 1990	435 boys, birth cohort, 15 yrs	Age, sex	SRED, Teacher & Parent RS, BPCR, DISC-C, CRS, FD	Thefts; vandalism; drug and alcohol use (S)	A = H = A = NC
Soussignan *et al.*, 1992	32 boys, school sample, 10–11 yrs	Age, SES sex	Teacher Rutter scale, CRS FD	Lying, stealing, truancy	
				(T)	HA > A = NC
				(M)	HA > A = NC
				Stealing; vandalism; alcohol and drug use (S)	HA = A = NC

[ac]For definitions, see Table 6.2. [b](P) = parent; (M) = mother; (T) = teacher; (Pe) = peer; (S) = self; (C) = clinic data; B = boys; G = girls. FD = Follow-up design.

to have important predictive validity because it has been argued that the combination of both overt and covert antisocial behaviours occurring in early adolescence is associated with an increased risk of delinquency leading to contact with the police later on (Loeber & Schmaling, 1985).

More recently, laboratory measures of aggressive behaviours have been employed. The existing research indicates that only children with CD and ADHD display higher rates of hostile aggression (person-oriented behaviour) than normal controls during experimental conditions such as a competitive game with an unknown peer (Atkins & Stoff, 1993). Furthermore, experimental research using direct measures of child–peer interaction during a competitive task is required to assess the value of this paradigm for the issue of the differential diagnosis.

In summary, while there is some suggestive evidence to support the view that children with the mixed HA disorder can be distinguished from other groups of hyperactive children on particular patterns of conduct problems (fighting, covert antisocial acts), the methodological limitations (e.g. lack of external criteria; exclusive 'diagnostic' groups not systematically compared) of the studies available so far prevent us from concluding that the two putative disorders can be discriminated on aggressive symptomatology. Further investigations are therefore required in order for this issue to be adequately examined.

Dimensional studies

Multivariate statistical approaches such as factor analyses have been used to identify dimensions/syndromes, especially those constituting of interrelated patterns of behaviour. The application of these statistical methods has produced a substantial contribution to the task of internal validation of hyperactivity and conduct disorder (Achenbach & Edelbrock, 1978). For example, in his review on 60 empirical multivariate studies published since 1970, Hinshaw (1987) pointed out that 41 of the studies revealed separate dimensions of hyperactivity/attentional deficits and conduct problems/aggression. However, substantial correlations systematically reported between the dimensions of hyperactivity and conduct problems in multivariate studies (Quay, 1979; Hinshaw, 1987) also present a challenge to the syndromal independence of these two behavioural dimensions. Thus the application of construct validation procedures by using external criteria (for a review, see Hinshaw, 1987) has been a logical step undertaken to test more carefully the hypothesis of syndromal independence. With respect to the symptomatology, studies based on clinical samples have generally shown that hyperactivity and aggression dimensions derived from medical/symptoms charts or teacher rating scales (e.g. IOWA, CTRS) are differentially correlated with both fine (wrist and ankle actometer scores) and gross motor activity (observation of locomotion when inappropriate), observed attentional difficulties (off-task, failing to attend), disruptive behaviours (e.g. physically aggressive with peers, talking back to the teacher), and with parent rated conduct problems and impulsivity (Loney, Langhorne & Paternite, 1978; Milich *et al.*, 1982; Milich & Fitzgerald, 1985). These findings are in some contrast with those reported by Lahey, Green & Forehand (1980). The lack of discriminant validity of the hyperactivity factor in the latter study is likely to be explained, on the bases of large methodological differences as compared with most other studies, and by the confounded nature of the Conners scales (CTRS) of conduct problems and hyperactivity (teacher hyperactivity and conduct problems are largely overlapping) (Trites & Laprade, 1983). Indeed, when inattention/overactivity (I/O) and aggression (A) subscales from the CTRS were empirically generated to provide independent dimensions of hyperactivity and aggression, there was stronger evidence to support the differential validity of these two externalising dimensions (Loney & Milich, 1982; Milich & Fitzgerald, 1985). More recently, using multiple observational measures of social and academic behaviours, Atkins *et al.* (1989) substantially replicated the differential patterns of association of I/O and A subscales by the use of criterion measures in a normative sample of school-aged boys. The I/O factor turned out to be uniquely related to overactivity in the classroom and playground, disorganised desks without necessary materials,and being engaged in an incorrect academic task. The A factor, on the other hand, was uniquely associated with verbal disruptive behaviour. Yet, in contrast with previous findings, IO and A dimensions could not be distinguished on measures of observed attentional problems or overt aggressive behaviours. It is of course possible that methodological differences between the studies also contributed to these divergent findings (normative versus clinic samples, nature of classroom settings and time-sample procedures). In the same way, the study by Taylor *et al.* (1986) provided further evidence suggesting a separation of hyperactivity and defiance scales derived from a semi-structured interview with the parents in a group of children referred to a clinic because of a variety of behaviour problems. Based on laboratory, clinical and observational measures, their results showed that the hyperactivity dimension was uniquely associated with greater observed motor activity, and poorer attentional performance (i.e. index of attention derived from the CPT, the maze test and the selective listening for digits). The study already mentioned by Halperin *et al.* (1988) based on a sample of normal school children provided only partial support for the independence of externalising behaviours. The inattention dimension derived from Conners Teacher Scale and from the DSM III scales was uniquely associated with omission errors on the CPT, whereas conduct problems, impulsivity and hyperactivity dimensions were correlated with 'A-not-X' commission errors. This suggests a greater overlap between hyperactivity/impulsivity and conduct problems than between inattention and conduct problems. These data also provide empirical support against a unidimensional conceptualisation of hyperactivity/ADDH (see also Bauermeister *et al.*, 1992).

Efforts to empirically validate the revised behaviour problems checklist (RBPC) against attentional measures (e.g. CPT scores) in a sample of behaviourally maladjusted boys also lent some support for the construct validity of the RBPC subscales (e.g. attention problems, excessive motor activity, conduct disorder, socialised aggression) (Raine & Jones, 1987). Attentional problems and excessive motor activity were uniquely characterised by greater variability in reaction times, whereas conduct disorder and socialised aggression were associated with a greater number of error responses. The authors hypothesised that the fluctuations in reaction times in children scoring high on attentional problems could result from a deficit in the child's allocation of attentional resources towards the task, rather than from a deficit in information processing capacity. Finally, taking a somewhat different methodological approach, Levy & Hobbes (1989) applied a factor analytic technique on measures of vigilance, spelling and reading in a sample of clinic referred boys. Two substantial factors emerged: a vigilance factor (i.e. derived from CPT and 'draw-a-line-slow' test scores), and a reading factor. The vigilance factor was more strongly related to the diagnoses of moderate and severe ADDH than to the diagnosis of CD.

In summary, despite some equivocal results, and in contrast with categorical approach, dimensional studies have provided considerable evidence in favour of a conceptual distinction between aggression/conduct problems and attention deficit/ hyperactivity.

THE DEVELOPMENTAL PERSPECTIVE OF HYPERACTIVITY AND CONDUCT DISORDER

One means to help in clarifying the issue of overlap between hyperactivity and conduct disorder is by the use of longitudinal studies of large population samples (Hinshaw, 1987). The study of a large birth cohort by repeated measures should, for example, help to identify at what ages the symptoms first start to appear, which symptoms become evident first, when do the symptoms begin to overlap, what are their long-term consequences, and what is the validity of diagnostic constructs in terms of the outcome (Verhulst & Koot, 1991).

Longitudinal studies can also ensure that the subjects who are being studied suffer from significant disorders in terms of pervasiveness and persistence, for example. However, very large samples are needed to obtain small numbers of subjects suffering from disorders which are equivalent to those found in samples of referred children.

Barkley (1981, 1990) and Loeber (1988*a*,*b*, 1990) have suggested that hyperactivity is an antecedent to conduct disorder. If hyperactivity is a neurological condition which is largely inherited, or the result of specific perinatal conditions, one would expect the overactivity symptoms to appear early, *in utero* and during early infancy (Campbell, 1990). On the other hand, conduct problems, which are generally defined with reference to social norms (opposition, antisocial behaviour) can hardly be observed before the child has a differentiated sense of self. Thus it would not, for example, be expected for a child to be defined as oppositional before the age of 9 months (Campos *et al.*, 1983). There are some indications that oppositional behaviour closely follows difficult temperament in infancy, and that both predict externalising behaviour during childhood. Bates *et al.* (1991) followed a group of boys from 6 months to the age of 8 years. The assessments of difficult temperament at 6 and 13 months (displays of negative emotions), and resistance to control at 13 and 24 months (ignoring "no-no"), all predicted externalising behaviours at the ages of 7 and 8. Other studies have reported similar results (Carey & McDevitt, 1978; Chamberlin, 1977; see also Campbell & Ewing, 1990, for a retrospective assessment of infant temperament). However, the samples from these studies were very small and were not specifically designed to chart the development of the comorbidity between hyperactivity and conduct problems. In fact, in both cases the main focus was the prediction of antisocial behaviour. Farrington *et al.* (1990) re-analysed the data from the Cambridge Study of Delinquent Development. This study followed a sample of 411 boys from a working-class area of London. They were first contacted at age 8 or 9 years in 1961–62. Assessments of hyperactivity (motor hyperactivity–impulsivity–attention deficit) and conduct problems were combined for ages 8 to 10. Measures of offending were taken up to age 25. Four groups of subjects were created based on age 8 to 10 assessments of hyperactivity and conduct problems: (i) non-hyperactive, non-conduct problem (NH-NC); (ii) non-hyperactive, conduct problem (NH-C); (iii) hyperactive, non-conduct problem (H-NC); (iv) hyperactive, conduct problem (H-C). The H-C group turned out to comprise 14% of the sample, whilst the H-NC and the NH-C groups included 8% and 10% of the sample, respectively. The H–C group had the highest percentage of juvenile and adult convictions, the H–NC group, had higher juvenile and adult convictions than the NH-NC group, but lower than the NH–C group. Both hyperactivity and conduct problems were predictive of later offending, and they also had additive effects. It was shown, however, that early hyperactivity was predictive of juvenile convictions only when associated with criminal parents or early conduct problems. Results from this study once again demonstrated (see McGee *et al.*, 1984; August *et al.*, 1983; Schachar, Rutter & Smith, 1981; Milich & Loney, 1979) that boys who suffer from both hyperactivity and conduct disorder are at a greater risk for long-term antisocial behaviour. It also showed that hyperactivity without concomitant conduct problems is a risk factor for later antisocial behaviour only when associated with adverse family background.

Within the Dunedin Multidisciplinary Health and Development Study, Moffitt (1990) employed a different analytical strategy to address the same issue. This study is based on a total birth cohort of 1037 boys and girls born in Dunedin New Zealand in 1972–1973. The first behavioural assessments were made at age 3 and subsequently every two years up to adolescence. As a result of the age 13 assessments, four groups were created based on the available information of delinquency and attention deficit including hyperactivity. The delinquency criteria were based on the actual age 13 assessments, while the attention deficit criteria were based on age 5 to 11 assessments. All the children determined as suffering from attention deficit disorder had positive assessments at both age 11 years and prior to the age of 7, thus ensuring that only the subjects with pervasive disorder were included. Moffitt (1990) reports that 85% of the subjects given the diagnosis attention deficit disorder (ADD) had three or more symptoms of hyperactivity; but it should also be noted that the particular classification scheme (DSM-III) gives priority to attention deficit and includes subjects who are not overactive. Four groups were formed based only on the boys from the total sample of 435 children: (i) delinquents with ADD (D-ADD); (ii) delinquents without ADD (D); (iii) not delinquents with ADD (ADD); (iv) not delinquents without ADD (C). There were 19 (4%) D-ADD, 52 (12%) D, and 16 (4%) ADD. Thus, there were almost equal numbers of children with ADD among the delinquents and non delinquents. However, the proportion of ADD in this study was only just over half that obtained for hyperactivity in the Farrington *et al.* (1990) survey. These differences are probably accounted for in part by the different diagnostic criteria employed. Because the DSM-III criteria were used for the Dunedin study, these results may be closer to those generally encountered in studies of referred samples. However, there are also large socio-economic and cultural differences between the two populations which could explain part of the differences in prevalence of ADD/hyperactivity.

A number of interesting differences were observed between the four groups in the Dunedin study. At the ages of 3 and 5 years the D-ADD group scored lower on motor ability than the other three groups, who in turn did not differ from one another. However, there were no statistically significant differences between the four groups in perinatal problems or birth-weight, although the D-ADD group had the worst perinatal problem score. When the children of the four groups were compared on their overall development progress between the ages of 5 and 13 years, the results indicated that those in D-ADD group scored significantly worse than the control group at each age in terms of IQ deficits, reading failure and stability of antisocial behaviour, whilst the ADD group were never significantly different from the control group for reading, verbal ability and conduct problems. Interestingly, the onset of antisocial behaviour began at a earlier age for the boys with the co-morbidity of ADD and delinquency. Thus, ADD children with, and without, conduct problems have important behavioural differences as early as the age 3 years, and these appear to continue throughout childhood.

There were two other important differences between the ADD boys with and without conduct problems: those with additional conduct problems came from family environments with more adversity and their mothers also had lower IQs. Moffitt (1990) discusses the possibility that these boys have inherited some central nervous system characteristics which would explain the poor motor and cognitive performance. It is therefore possible that the important differences between the two types of ADD boys are explained by the interaction between inherited factors (and/or acquired perinatal complications) and adverse family environment.

The intriguing result of the Moffitt (1990) study is the finding that there were no cognitive differences between the ADD group without conduct problems and the control group. In a different paper (Moffitt & Henry, 1989), the same four groups of children were compared, but this time including both boys and girls, on age 14 assessments of cognitive 'executive function', controlling for IQ. On 5 of the 15 measures, the D-ADD groups had significantly lower scores than the control group, whilst the ADD and the D groups did not differ from the control group. These results therefore suggest that only the D-ADD have cognitive deficits compared to controls. They are also in apparent contrast with the results reported by Satterfield (1987) for a group of referred hyperactive children who were followed up to adolescence. In this study, two groups of hyperactive boys were compared with a normal control group on a series of laboratory tasks (auditory event related potential 'AERP', EEG power spectra, skin resistance level) when the boys were between the ages of 6 and 12 years. The results indicated that the hyperactive boys who had not become antisocial in the follow-up period, had the most abnormal EEG and AERP findings. In contrast, the hyperactive boys who did become antisocial, did not generally differ from the normal controls in terms of their EEG and AERP results. To explain this surprising result, Satterfield suggested that hyperactive children have an optimal arousal-inhibitory level which is different from normal subjects. Thus a normal level of arousal would be abnormal for an hyperactive child. He further suggested that hyperactivity without conduct problems, but with abnormal EEG and AERP, is a result of brain dysfunction, whilst hyperactivity with conduct problems and normal EEG and AERP is the result of social/environmental factors.

As can be seen from the complexity of findings reported above, there are no simple explanations to these behavioural phenomena. Longitudinal data appear to confirm that hyperactivity with conduct problems is clearly a different entity from both hyperactivity without conduct problems and conduct problems without hyperactivity (see also Fergusson, Horwood & Lynskey, 1993). The longitudinal data also confirm the previous observations that the long-term prognosis is worst for boys with the mixed disorder of hyperactivity conduct problems. It does also seem clear that longitudinal studies are needed to further disentangle these two behavioural disorders, but it is likely that the progress will be limited until such time that we have samples which are large enough to include relatively big numbers of referred children. There is no doubt that non-referred subjects are different from referred subjects who attain clinical levels on assessments of both hyperactivity and conduct problems. Also, in order to substantially improve our understanding of the aetiology of these disorders, we will need longitudinal studies that start during the mother's pregnancy.

CONCLUSIONS

With respect to the key symptomatic features of hyperactivity and conduct disorders, the review of categorical studies has revealed a high degree of overlap between hyperactivity and conduct problems and little evidence regarding a clear separation between these two putative disorders. This tends to confirm some of the conclusions from previous reviews (Werry *et al.*, 1987; Hinshaw, 1987; Werry, 1988) where it was shown that studies examining the potential aetiological factors (i.e. psychological background, family and neurodevelopmental variables) failed to indicate a differential pattern of biological or psychosocial measures for the two categories of behaviours. However, this conclusion needs to be applied with some caution because in previous studies a number of methodological problems could be detected which are likely to have contributed to the conflicting findings (see Hinshaw, 1987; Szatmari *et al.*,

1989*b*). Indeed, recent studies involving subgroup comparisons and based on carefully controlled designs have shown some evidence that severe and pervasive form of child hyperactivity is associated with more neurodevelopmental delays, whereas conduct disorder is specifically associated with dysfunctional parent–child relationships, low socio-economic status and parental psychopathology (e.g. Biederman, Munir, & Knee, 1987; Szatmari *et al.*, 1989*b*; Schachar & Wachsmuth, 1990; Taylor *et al.*, 1991).

Regarding the symptomatology of hyperactivity and conduct disorder, the present review indicates some distinctions between subgroups in spite of some mixed findings reported in studies based on categorical approach suggesting that it is useful to distinguish the two conditions clinically and empirically. Children with hyperactivity plus aggression tend to be more overactive and 'off-task', and tend to display more overt and covert antisocial acts and poorer rule-governed behaviour than children with pure aggression. Furthermore, although definitive data are still lacking, the studies available so far offer some evidence to suggest that hyperactive children display lower levels of sustained attention and spend more time 'off-task' than aggressive children. The necessity to distinguish these two classes of behaviour empirically is also strengthened by dimensional and longitudinal studies which have provided sufficient evidence to suggest that, with respect to external criteria, overactivity/attention/impulsivity and conduct problems/aggression can be considered as partially independent dimensions. Follow-up studies have generally revealed a worse outcome for hyperactive children who also display conduct problems (e.g. higher percentage of juvenile and adult convictions). There is also a suggestion that the aetiology of the mixed disorder could be rooted in an interaction between psychosocial disadvantage (conflictual family environment) and neurodevelopmental factors (developmental immaturity, neuropsychological deficit, perinatal problems). Given that so far such evidence stems from cross-sectional studies (see Szatmari *et al.*, 1989*b*; Schachar & Wachsmuth, 1990), this hypothesis should be more carefully tested in future developmental longitudinal studies.

The somewhat divergent picture between studies derived from categorical and dimensional model must not be considered as contradictory because these two modes of classification probably serve different purposes (Quay, 1986; Werry *et al.*, 1987; Rutter & Tuma, 1988). The fact that the dimensional model tends to be based on a better methodology (more standardised instruments compared to traditional diagnosis; greater discriminative power of statistical analyses; information on intensity and degree of severity of symptom; separation of intertwined dimensions intended to validate theoretically separate childhood problems), is likely to explain the more convergent patterns of findings derived from this approach. In contrast, the categorical model appears to offer an overall picture of child behaviour because it takes into account the covariation of behavioural symptoms.

In order for the issue of discriminative validity of hyperactivity and aggression to be clarified adequately, future studies should certainly maximise the strengths of assessment strategies and resolve a number of methodological and conceptual problems mentioned in this review and also noted by other investigators (Hinshaw, 1987; Werry, 1988; Taylor, 1988*a*, *b*). These include a selection of objective and independent measures, choice of sensitive instruments and measures that do not confound the domains of interest, necessity to use designs that compare all the behavioural dimensions of interest, more explicitly defined diagnostic criteria for hyperactivity and conduct disorder including operational definition, degree of severity, etc., as well as variation in attentional demands and the importance of testing the resource strategy allocation.

REFERENCES

Abikoff, H. & Klein, R.G. (1992). Attention-deficit hyperactivity and conduct disorder: comorbidity and implications for treatment. *Journal of Consulting and Clinical Psychology,* **60**, 881–92.

Achenbach, T.M. & Edelbrock, C.S. (1978). The classification of child psychopathology: a review and analysis of empirical efforts. *Psychological Bulletin,* **85**, 1275–301.

American Psychiatric Association. (1980). *Diagnostic and Statistical Manual of Mental Disorders*, 3rd Edition. Washington, DC.

American Psychiatric Association. (1987). *Diagnostic and Statistical Manual of Mental Disorders*, 3rd Edition Revised. Washington, DC.

American Psychiatric Association. (1994). *Diagnostic and Statistical Manual of Mental Disorder*, 4th Edition (DSM-IV). Washington, DC.

Atkins, M.S., Pelham, W.E. & Licht, M.H. (1989). The differential validity of teacher ratings of inattentive/overactivity and aggression. *Journal of Abnormal Child Psychology,* **17**, 423–35.

Atkins, M.S. & Stoff, D.M. (1993). Instrumental and hostile aggression in childhood disruptive behaviour disorders. *Journal of Abnormal Child Psychology,* **21**, 165–78.

August, G.J. & Stewart, M.A. (1982). Is there a syndrome of pure hyperactivity ? *British Journal of Psychiatry,* **140**, 305–11.

August, G.J., Stewart, M.A. & Holmes, C.S. (1983). A four year follow-up of hyperactive boys with and without conduct disorders. *British Journal of Psychiatry,* **143**, 192–98.

August, G.J. & Garfinkel, B.D. (1989). Behavioral and cognitive subtypes of ADHD. *Journal of American Academy Child and Adolescent Psychiatry,* **28**, 739–48.

Barkley, R.A. (1981). *Hyperactive Children.* New York: Guilford.

Barkley, R.A. (1982). Specific guidelines for defining hyperactivity in children (Attention Deficit Disorder). In *Advances in Clinical Psychology*, vol. 4, eds. B. Lahey & A. Kazdin. New York: Plenum.

Barkley, R.A. (1990). Attention deficit disorders: history, definition, and diagnosis. In *Handbook of Developmental Psychopathology*, eds. J. Lewis & S.M. Miller, pp. 65–75. New York: Plenum Press.

Barkley, R.A. & Ullmann, D.G. (1975). A comparison of objective measures of activity and distractibility in hyperactive and nonhyperactive children. *Journal of Abnormal Child Psychology,* **3**, 231–44.

Barkley, R.A., McMurray, M.B., Edelbrock, C.S. & K. Robins (1989). The response of aggressive and nonaggressive ADHD children to two doses of methylphenidate. *Journal of American Academy of Child and Adolescent Psychiatry,* **28**, 873–81.

Bates, J.E., Bayles, K., Bennett, D.S., Ridge, B. & Brown, M.M. (1991). Origins of externalising behaviour problems at eight years of age. In *The Development and Treatment of Childhood Aggression*, eds. D.J. Pepler & K.H. Rubin, pp. 93–120. Hillsdale, NJ: Lawrence Erlbaum.

Bauermeister, J. Alegria, M., Bird, H., Rubio-Stipec, M. & Canino, G. (1992). Are attentional-hyperactivity deficits unidimensional or multidimensional syndromes? Empirical findings from a community survey. *Journal of American Academy of Child and Adolescent Psychiatry,* **31**, 423–31.

Biederman, J., Munir, K. & Knee, D. (1987). Conduct and oppositional disorder in clinically referred children with ADD: a controlled family study. *Journal of American Academy of Child and Adolescent Psychiatry,* **26**, 724–7.

Block, J., Block, Y.H. & Harrington, D.M. (1974). Some misgivings about the MFFT as a measure of reflection–impulsivity. *Developmental Psychology,* **10**, 611–32.

Buitelaar, J.K., Swinkels, S.H.N., de Vries, H., Van der Gaag, R.J. & van Hooff, J.A.R.M. (1994). An ethological study on behavioural differences between hyperactive, aggressive, combined hyperactive/aggressive and control children. *Journal of Child Psychology and Psychiatry,* **35**, 1437–46.

Campbell, S. (1974). Cognitive style and behavior problems of clinic boys : a comparison of epileptic, hyperactive, learning-disabled and normal groups. *Journal of Abnormal Child Psychology,* **3**, 307–12.

Campbell, S.B. (1990). The socialisation and social development of hyperactive children. *In Handbook of Developmental Psychopathology*, eds. M. Lewis & S.M. Miller, pp. 71–91. New York: Plenum Press.

Campbell, S.B. & Werry, J.S. (1986). Attention deficit disorder (hyperactivity). *In Psychopathological Disorders of Childhood*, eds. H.C. Quay et J.S. Werry, pp. 111–55. New York: Wiley & Sons.

Campbell, S.B. & Ewing, L.J. (1990). Follow-up of a-hard-to-manage preschoolers: adjustment at age 9 and predictors of continuing symptoms. *Journal of Child Psychology and Psychiatry,* **31**, 871–89.

Campos, J.J., Barrett, K.C., Lamb, M.E., Goldmith, H.H. & Stenberg, C. (1983). Socioemotional development. In *Handbook of Child Psychology: Infancy and Developmental Psychobiology*, Vol. 2., eds. M.M. Haith & J.J. Campos, pp. 783–916. New York: Wiley.

Carey, W.B. & McDevitt, S.C. (1978). Stability and change in individual temperament diagnosis from infancy to early childhood. *Journal of the American Academy of Child Psychiatry,* **17**, 331–7.

Chamberlin, R.W. (1977). Can we identify a group of children at age two who are at risk for the development or behavioural or emotional problems in kindergarten or first grade. *Pediatrics (Supplement),* **59**, 971–81.

Chee, P., Logan, G., Schachar, R., Lindsay, P. & Wachsmuth, R. (1989). Effects of event rate and display time on sustained attention in hyperactive, normal, and control children. *Journal of Abnormal Child Psychology,* **17**, 371–91.

Cowen, E.L., Pederson, A., Babigian, H. Izzo, L.D. & Trost, M.A. (1973). Long term follow-up of early detectable vulnerable children. *Journal of Consulting and Clinical Psychology,* **41**, 438–46.

Dienske, H. & Sanders-Woudstra, A.R. (1988). A critical and conceptual consideration of attention deficit and hyperactivity from an ethological point of view. In *Attention Deficit Disorder : Criteria, Cognition, Intervention*, eds. L.M. Bloomingdale & J.A. Sergeant, pp. 43–63. Oxford: Pergamon Press.

Doke, L.A., & Flippo, J.R. (1983). Aggressive and oppositional behavior. In *Handbook of Child Psychopathology*, eds. T.H. Ollendick & M. Hersen, pp. 323–356. New York: Plenum Press.

Douglas, V.I. (1984). Attentional and cognitive performance. In *Developmental Neuropsychiatry*, eds. M. Rutter, pp.280–329. Edinburgh: Churchill Livingstone.

Douglas, V.I. (1988). Cognitive deficits in children with attention deficit disorder with hyperactivity. In *Attention Deficit Disorder: Criteria, Cognition, Intervention*, vol. 5, eds. L.M. Bloomingdale & J.A. Sergeant, pp. 65–81. Oxford: Pergamon Press.

Douglas, V.I. & Peters, K.G. (1979). Toward a clearer definition of the attentional deficit of hyperactive children. In *Attention and the Development of Cognitive Skills*, eds. G. A. Hale & M. Lewis, pp. 173–247. New York: Plenum Press.

Eaton, W.O. & Enns, L.R. (1986). Sex differences in human motor activity level. *Psychological Bulletin*, **100**, 19–28.

Farrington, D., Loeber, R. & Van Kammen, W.E. (1990). Long-term criminal outcomes of hyperactivity–impulsivity–attention deficit and conduct problems in childhood. In *Straight and Devious Pathways from Childhood to Adulthood*, eds. L.N. Robins & M. Rutter, pp. 62–81. Cambridge: Cambridge University Press.

Fergusson, D.M., Horwood, L.J. & Lynskey, M.T. (1993). The effects of conduct disorder and attention deficit in middle childhood on offending and scholastic ability at age 13. *Journal of Child Psychology and Psychiatry,* **34**, 899–916.

Finch, A. & Montgomery, L. (1973). Reflection–impulsivity and information seeking in emotionally disturbed children. *Journal of Abnormal Child Psychology,* **1**, 358–62.

Firestone, P. & Martin, J.E. (1979). An analysis of the hyperactive syndrome: a comparison of hyperactive, behavior problem, asthmatic and normal children. *Journal of Abnormal Child Psychology,* **7**, 261–74.

Frick, P.J. & Lahey, B.B. (1991). The nature and characteristics of attention-deficit hyperactivity disorder. *School Psychology Review,* **20**, 163–73.

Frick, P.J., Lahey, B.B., Applegate, B., Kerdyck, L., Ollendick, T., Hynd, G., Garfinkel, B., Greenhill, L., Biederman, J., Barkley, R., McBurnett, K., Newcorn, J. & Waldman, I. (1994). DSM-IV field trials for the disruptive behaviour disorders: symptom utility estimates. *Journal of American Academy of Child and Adolescent Psychiatry,* **33**, 529–39.

Gittelman, R. (1988). The assessment of hyperactivity: the DSM-III approach. In *Attention Deficit Disorder: Criteria, Cognition, Intervention*, vol. 5, eds. L.M. Bloomingdale & J.A. Sergeant, pp. 9–28. Oxford: Pergamon Press.

Glow, R.A. (1981). Cross-validity and normative data on the Conners'Parent and Teacher Rating Scales. In *The Pychosocial Aspects of Drug Treatment for Hyperactivity*, eds. K.D. Gadow & J. Loney, pp. 107–150. Boulder, CO: Westview Press.

Goldstein, H.S. (1987). Cognitive development in low attentive, hyperactive, and aggressive 6– through 11– year-old children. *Journal of American Academy of Child and Adolescent Psychiatry,* **26**, 214–18.

Halperin, J.M., Wolf, L.E, O'Brien, D., Pascualvaca, D.M., Newcorn, J.H., Healey, J.M., O'Brien, J.D., Morgenstein, A. & Young, J.G. (1988). Differential assessment of attention and impulsivity in children. *Journal of American Academy of Child and Adolescent Psychiatry,* **27**, 326–9.

Halperin, J.M., O'Brien, J. D., Newcorn, J.H., Healey, J.M., Pascualvaca, D.M., Wolf, L.E. & Young, J.G. (1990). Validation of hyperactive, aggressive, and mixed hyperactive/aggressive childhood disorders: a research note. *Journal of Child Psychology and Psychiatry,* **31**, 455–60.

Halperin, J.M., Matier, K., Bedi, G., Sharma, V. & Newcorn, J.H. (1992). Specificity of inattention, impulsivity, and hyperactivity to the diagnosis of attention-deficit hyperactivity disorder. *Journal of American Academy of Child and Adolescent Psychiatry,* **31**, 190–6.

Halperin, J.M., Newcorn, J.H., Matier, K., Sharma, V., McKay, K. & Schwartz, S. (1993). Discriminant validity of attention-deficit hyperactivity disorder. *Journal of American Academy of Child Adolescent Psychiatry,* **32**, 1038–43.

Hinshaw, S.P. (1987). On the distinction between attentional deficits/hyperactivity and conduct problems/aggression in child psychopathology. *Psychological Bulletin,* **101**, 443–63.

Hinshaw, S.P. (1991). Stimulant medication and the treatment of aggression in children with attentional deficits. *Journal of Clinical Child Psychology,* **20**, 301–12.

Hinshaw, S.P. (1992). Externalising behavior problems and academic underachievement in childhood and adolescence: causal relationships and underlying mechanisms. *Psychological Bulletin,* **111**, 127–55.

Hinshaw, S.P., Henker, B., Whalen, C.K., Erhardt, D. & Dunnington, R.E. (1989). Aggressive, prosocial, and nonsocial behavior in hyperactive boys: dose effects of methylphenidate in naturalistic settings. *Journal of Consulting and Clinical Psychology,* **57**, 636–43.

Hinshaw, S.P., Heller, T. & McHale, J.P. (1992). Covert antisocial behavior in boys with attention-deficit hyperactivity disorder: external validation and effects of methylphenidate. *Journal of Consulting and Clinical Psychology,* **60**, 274–81.

Johnston, C. & Pelham, W.E. (1986). Teacher ratings predict peer ratings of aggression at 3-year-follow-up in boys with attention deficit disorder with hyperactivity. *Journal of Consulting and Clinical Psychology,* **54**, 571–2.

Kaspar, J., Millichap, J., Backus, R., Child, D. & Schulman, J. (1971). A study of the relationship between neurological evidence of brain damage in children and activity and distractibility. *Journal of Consulting and Clinical Psychology,* **36**, 329.

Keller, M.B., Lavori, P.W., Beardslee, W.R., Wunder, J., Schwartz, C.E., Roth, J. & Biederman, J. (1992). The disruptive behavioral disorder in children and adolescents: comorbidity and clinical course. *Journal of the American Academy of Child Psychiatry,* **31**, 204–9.

Klein, A.R. & Young, R.D. (1979). Hyperactive boys in their classroom. *Journal of Abnormal Child Psychology,* **7**, 425–42.

Klorman, R., Brumaghim, J.T., Salzman, L.F., Strauss, J., Borgstedt, A.D., McBride, M.C. & Loeb, S. (1988). Effects of methylphenidate on attention-deficit hyperactivity disorder with and without aggressive/noncompliant features. *Journal of Abnormal Psychology,* **97**, 413–22.

Koriath, H. Gualtieri, C.T., Van Bourgondien, M.E., Quade, D. & Werry, J.S. (1985). Construct validity of clinical diagnosis in pediatric psychiatry: relationship among measures. *Journal of the American Academy of Child Psychiatry,* **24**, 429–36.

Lahey, B.B., Green, K.D., & Forehand, R. (1980). On the independance of ratings of hyperactivity, conduct problems, and attention deficits in children: A multiple regression analysis. *Journal of Consulting and Clinical Psychology* **48**, 566–74.

Lahey, B.B., Loeber, R., Stouthmater-Loeber, M., Christ, M.A., Green, S., Russo, M.F., Frick, P.J. & Dulcan, M. (1990). Comparison of DSM-III and DSM-III-R diagnosis for prepubertal children: changes in prevalence and validity. *Journal of American Academy Child and Adolescent Psychiatry,* **29**, 620–6.

Ledingham, J.E., Younger, A., Schwartzman, A. & Bergeron, G. (1982). Agreement among teacher, peer, and self-ratings of children's aggression, withdrawal, and likability. *Journal of Abnormal Child Psychology,* **10**, 363–72.

Levy, F., Horn, K.P. & Dalglish, R. (1987). Relation of attention deficit and conduct disorder to vigilance and reading lag. *Australian and New Zealand Journal of Psychiatry,* **21**, 242–5.

Levy, F. & Hobbes, G. (1989). Reading, spelling, and vigilance in attention deficit and conduct disorder. *Journal of Abnormal Child Psychology,* **17**, 291–8.

Loeber, R. (1982). The stability of antisocial and delinquent child behaviors. A review. *Child Developement,* **53**, 1431–46.

Loeber, R. (1988a). The natural histories of juvenile conduct problems, delinquency, and associated substance use: evidence for developmental progressions. In *Advances in Clinical Child Psychology*, vol. 10, eds. B.B. Lahey & A.E. Kadzin, pp. 73–124. New York: Plenum Press.

Loeber, R. (1988b). Behavioral precursors and accelerators of delinquency. In *Explaining Criminal Behaviour*, eds. W. Buikhuisen & S.A. Mednick, pp. 51–67. Leiden: Brill.

Loeber, R. (1990). Development and risk factors of juvenile antisocial behaviour and delinquency. *Clinical Psychology Review,* **10**, 1–41.

Loeber, R., & Schamling, K.B. (1985). The utility of differentiating between mixed and pure forms of antisocial child behaviors. *Journal of Abnormal Child Psychology,* **13**, 315–36.

Loeber, R., Brinthaupt & Green, M. (1990). Attention deficits, impulsivity, and hyperactivity with or without conduct problems: relationships to delinquency and unique factors. In *Behavior Disorders of Adolescence : Research, and Policy in Clinical and School Settings*, eds. R.J. McMahon & R. de V. Peters, pp. 39–61. New York: Plenum Press.

Loney, J. & Milich, M. (1982). Hyperactivity, inattention, and aggression in clinical practice. In *Advances in Developmental and Behavioral Pediatrics*, eds. M. Wolraich & D.K. Routh, pp. 113–147. Greenwich, Conn.: JAI Press Inc.

Loney, J., Langhorne, J.E. & Paternite, C.E. (1978). An empirical basis of subgrouping the hyperkinetic/minimal brain dysfunction syndrome. *Journal of Abnormal Psychology,* **87**, 431–41.

Luk, S.L. (1985). Direct observation studies of hyperactive behavior. *Journal of American Academy Child and Adolescent Psychiatry,* **24**, 338–44.

Matier, K., Halperin, J.M., Sharma, V., Newcorn, J.H. & Sathaye, N. (1992). Methylphenidate response in aggressive and nonaggressive ADHD children: distinctions on laboratory measures of symptoms. *Journal of American Academy Child and Adolescent Psychiatry,* **31**, 219–25.

McGee, R., Williams, S. & Silva, P.A. (1984). Behavioral and developmental characteristics of aggressive, hyperactive, and agressive-hyperactive boys. *Journal of the American Academy of Child Psychiatry,* **23**, 270–9.

Milich, R. & Loney, J. (1979). The role of hyperactive and aggressive symptomatology in predicting adolescent outcome among hyperactive children. *Journal of Pediatric Psychology,* **4**, 93–112.

Milich, R. & Kramer, J. (1984). Reflections on impulsivity: an empirical investigation on impulsivity as a construct. In *Advances in Learning and Behavioral Disabilities*, vol. 3, eds. K. Gadow & I. Bialer, pp. 57–94. Greenwich, CT: JAI Press.

Milich, R. & Fitzgerald, G. (1985). Validation of inattention/overactivity and aggression ratings with classroom observations. *Journal of Consulting and Clinical Psychology,* **53**, 139–40.

Milich, R. & Landau, S. (1989). The role of social status variables in differentiating subgroups of hyperactive children. In *Attention Deficit Disorders : Current Concepts and Emerging Trends in Attentional and Behavioral Disorders of Childhood*, vol. 4, eds. J.M. Swanson & L. Bloomingdale, pp. 1–16. Monograph supplement to the *Journal of Child Psychology and Psychiatry*. Oxford: Pergamon Press.

Milich, R., Loney, J. & Landau, S. (1982). Independent dimensions of hyperactivity and aggression: a validation with playroom observation data. *Journal of Abnormal Psychology,* **91**, 183–98.

Moffitt, T.E. (1990). Juvenile delinquency and attention deficit disorder: boys'developmental trajectories from age 3 to age 15. *Child Development,* **61**, 893–910.

Moffitt, T.E. & Silva, P.A. (1988). Self-reported delinquency, neuropsychological deficit, and history of attention deficit disorder. *Journal of Abnormal Child Psychology,* **16**, 553–69.

Moffitt, T.E. & Henry, B. (1989). Neuropsychological assessment of executive functions in self-reported delinquents. *Development and Psychopathology,* **1**, 105–18.

Murphy, D.A., Pelham, W.E. & Lang, A.R. (1992). Aggression in boys with attention deficit-hyperactivity disorder: methylphenidate effects on naturalistically observed aggression, response to provocation, and social information processing. *Journal of Abnormal Child Psychology,* **20**, 451–66.

Offord, D.R., Sullivan, K., Allen, N. & Abrams, N. (1979). Delinquency and hyperactivity. *Journal of Nervous and Mental Disease,* **167**, 734–41.

Organisation Mondiale de la Santé (1993). *Classification Internationale des Maladies.* Dixième révision (CIM 10/ICD10). Descriptions Cliniques et Directives pour le Diagnostic. Paris: Masson.

Pekaric, E.G., Prinz, R.J., Liebert, D.E., Weintraub, S. & Neale, J.M. (1976). The pupil evaluation inventory: a sociometric technique for assessing children's social behavior. *Journal of Abnormal Child Psychology,* **4**, 83–97.

Pelham, W.E., Milich, R., Cummings, E.M., Murphy, D. A., Schaughency, E.A. & Greiner, A.R. (1991). Effects of background anger, provocation, and methylphenidate on emotional arousal and aggressive responding in attention-deficit hyperactivity disordered boys with and without concurrent aggressiveness. *Journal of Abnormal Child Psychology,* **19**, 407–26.

Pope, A.W., Bierman, K.L. & Mumma, G.H. (1989). Relations between hyperactive and aggressive behavior and peer relations at three elementary grade levels. *Journal of Abnormal Child Psychology,* **17**, 253–67.

Porrino, L.J., Rapoport, J.L., Behar, D., Sceery, W., Ismond, D.R. & Bunney W.E. (1983). A naturalistic assessment of the motor activity of hyperactive boys. *Archives of General Psychiatry,* **40**, 681–87.

Power, T.J. (1992). Contextual factors in vigilance testing of children with ADHD. *Journal of Abnormal Child Psychology,* **20**, 579–93.

Prendergast, M., Taylor, E., Rapoport, J. L., Bartko, J., Donnelly, M., Zametkin, A., Ahearn, M.B., Dunn, G. & Wieselberg, H.M. (1988). The diagnosis of childhood hyperactivity: a US–UK cross national study of DSM-III and ICD-9. *Journal of Child Psychology and Psychiatry,* **29**, 289–300.

Prinz, R.J., Connor, P.A. & Wilson, C.C. (1981). Hyperactive and aggressive behaviors in childhood: interwined dimensions. *Journal of Abnormal Child Psychology,* **9**, 191–202.

Prior, M. & Sanson, A. (1986). Attention deficit disorder with hyperactivity : a critique. *Journal of Child Psychology and Psychiatry,* **27**, 307–19.

Quay, H.C. (1979). Classification. In *Psychopathological Disorders of Childhood*, 2nd edn., eds. H.C. Quay & J.S. Werry, pp. 1–42. New York: Wiley.

Quay, H.C. (1986). Classification. In *Psychopathological Disorders of Childhood*, 3rd edn, eds. H.C. Quay & J.S. Werry, pp. 1–34. New York: Wiley.

Raine, A. & Jones, F. (1987). Attention, autonomic arousal, and personality in behaviorally disordered children. *Journal of Abnormal Child Psychology,* **15**, 583–99.

Reeves, J.C., Werry, J.S., Elkind, G.S. & Zametkin, A. (1987). Attention deficit, conduct, oppositional, and anxiety disorders in children: II. Clinical characteristics. *Journal of the American Academy of Child and Adolescent Psychiatry,* **26**, 144–55.

Roberts, M.A. (1987). How is playroom behavior observation used in the diagnosis of attention deficit disorder? In *The Young Hyperactive Child: Answers to Questions about Diagnosis, Prognosis, and Treatment*, ed. J. Loney, pp. 65–74. New York: Haworth Press.

Roberts, M.A. (1990). A behavioral observation method for differentiating hyperactive and aggressive boys. *Journal of Abnormal Child Psychology,* **18**, 131–42.

Rosenthal, R.H. & Allen, T.W. (1978). An examination of attention, arousal and learning dysfunctions of hyperkinetic children. *Psychological Bulletin,* **85**, 869–715.

Rutter, M. (1984). Behavioral studies: questions and findings on the concept of a distinctive syndrome. In *Developmental Neuropsychiatry*, ed. M. Rutter, pp. 259–79. Edinburgh: Churchill Livingstone.

Rutter, M. & Gould, M. (1985). Classification. *In Child and Adolescent Psychiatry: Modern Approaches*, 2nd edn., eds. M. Rutter & L. Hersov. Oxford: Blackwell.

Rutter, M. & Tuma, A.H. . (1988). Diagnosis and classification. In *Assessment and Diagnosis in Child Psychopathology*, eds. M. Rutter, A.H. Tuma & I.S. Lann, pp. 437–452. New York: Guilford Press.

Rutter, M., Tizard, J. & Withmore, K. (1970). *Education, Health, and Behavior*. New York : Wiley.

Rutter, M., Shaffer, D. & Shepherd, M. (1975). *A Multi-axial Classification of Child Psychiatric Disorders*. Geneva: World Health Organisation.

Safer, D.J. & Allen, R.P. (1976). *Hyperactive Children. Diagnosis and Management*. Baltimore: University Park Press.

Sandberg, S.T. (1981). The overinclusiveness of the diagnosis of hyperkinetic syndrome. In *Strategic Interventions for Hyperactive Children*, ed. R. Gittelman. New York: M.E. Sharpe.

Sandberg, S.T., Rutter, M. & Taylor, E. (1978). Hyperkinetic disorder in psychiatric clinic attenders. *Developmental Medicine and Child Neurology,* **20**, 279–99.

Sandberg, S.T., Wieselberg, M. & Shaffer, D. (1980). Hyperkinetic and conduct problem children in a primary school population: some epidemiological considerations. *Journal of Child Psychology and Psychiatry,* **21**, 293–311.

Satterfield, J.H. (1987). Childhood diagnosis and neurophysiological predictors of teenage arrest rates: an eight year prospective study. In *The Causes of Crime: New Biological Approaches*, eds. S.A. Mednick, T.E. Moffitt & S.A. Stack, pp. 146–67. New York: Cambridge University Press.

Schachar, R. & Wachsmuth, R. (1990). Hyperactivity and parental psychopathology. *Journal of Child Psychology and Psychiatry,* **31**, 381–92.

Schachar, R., Rutter, M. & Smith, A. (1981). The characteristics of situationally and pervasively hyperactive children: implications for syndrome definition. *Journal of Child Psychology and Psychiatry,* **22**, 375–92.

Schachar, R., Tannock, J. & Logan, G. (1993). Inhibitory control, impulsiveness, and attention deficit hyperactivity disorder. *Clinical Psychology Review,* **13**, 721–39.

Sergeant, J.A. & Scholten, C.A. (1985). On resource strategy limitations in hyperactivity: cognitive impulsivity reconsidered. *Journal of Child Psychology and Psychiatry,* **26**, 97–109.

Sergeant, J. (1988). From DSM-III attentional deficit disorder to functional defects. In *Attention Deficit Disorder : Criteria, Cognition, Intervention*, vol. 5, eds. L.M. Bloomingdale & J.A. Sergeant, pp. 183–198. Oxford: Pergamon Press.

Shaffer, D. & Greenhill, L. (1979). A critical note on the predictive validity of the "hyperkinetic syndrome". *Journal of Child Psychology and Psychiatry,* **20**, 61–72.

Shaffer, D., McNamara, N. & Pincus, J.H. (1974). Controlled observations on patterns of activity, attention, and impulsivity in brain-damaged and psychiatrically disturbed boys. *Psychological Medicine,* **4**, 4–18.

Shapiro, S.K. & Garfinkel, B.D. (1986). The occurrence of behavior disorders in children: the interdependence of attention deficit disorder and conduct disorder. *Journal of the American Academy of Child Psychiatry,* **25**, 809–19.

Skinner, H.A. (1981). Toward the integration of classification: theory and methods. *Journal of Abnormal Psychology,* **90**, 68–87.

Soltys, S.M., Kashani, J.H., Dandoy, A.C., Vaidya, A.F. & Reid, J.C. (1992). Comorbidity for disruptive behavior disorders in psychiatrically hospitalised children. *Child Psychiatry and Human Development,* **23**, 87–98.

Sonuga-Barke, E.J.S., Taylor, E., Sembi, S. & Smith, J. (1992). Hyperactivity and delay aversion-I: the effects of delay on choice. *Journal of Child Psychology and Psychiatry,* **33**, 387–98.

Soussignan, R., Koch, P. & Montagner, H. (1988). Behavioural and cardiovascular changes in children moving from kindergarten to primary school. *Journal of Child Psychology and Psychiatry,* **29**, 321–33.

Soussignan, R., Tremblay, R.E., Schaal, B., Laurent, L., Gagnon, C., Larivée, S., Leblanc, M. & Charlebois, P. (1992). Behavioural and cognitive characteristics of conduct disturbed-hyperactive boys from 6 to 11: a multiple informant perspective. *Journal of Child Psychology and Psychiatry,* **8**, 1333–46.

Stevans, T.M., Kupst, M.J., Suran, B.G., & Schulman, J.L. (1978). Activity level: a comparison between actometer scores and observer ratings. *Journal of Abnormal Child Psychology,* **6**, 163–73.

Stewart, M.A., DeBlois, C.S. & Cummings, C. (1980). Psychiatric disorder in the parent of hyperactive boys and those with conduct disorder. *Journal of Child Psychology and Psychiatry,* **21**, 283–92.

Stewart, M.A., Cummings, C. & Singer, S. (1981). The overlap between hyperactive and unsocialised aggressive children. *Journal of Child Psychology and Psychiatry,* **22**, 35–45.

Sykes, D., Douglas, V. & Morgenstern, G. (1973). Sustained attention in hyperactive children. *Journal of Child Psychology and Psychiatry,* **14**, 213–20.

Szatmari, P., Offord, D.R. & Boyle, M.H. (1989*a*). Ontario child health study: prevalence of attention deficit disorder with hyperactivity. *Journal of Child Psychology and Psychiatry,* **30**, 219–30.

Szatmari, P., Boyle, M.H. & Offord, D.R. (1989*b*). ADDH and conduct disorder: degree of diagnosis overlap and differences among correlates. *Journal of the American Academy of Child and Adolescent Psychiatry,* **28**, 865–72.

Taylor, E. (1985). Syndromes of overactivity and attention deficit. In *Child and Adolescent Psychiatry*, eds. M. Rutter & L. Hersov. Oxford: Blackwell Scientific Publications.

Taylor, E. (1988*a*). Attention deficit and conduct disorder syndromes. In *Assessment and Diagnosis in Child Psychopathology*, eds. M. Rutter, A.H. Tuma & I.S. Lann, pp. 377–407. New York: Guilford Press.

Taylor, E. (1988*b*). Diagnosis of hyperactivity: a British perspective. In *Attention Deficit Disorder: Criteria, Cognition, Intervention*, vol. 5, eds. L.M. Bloomingdale & J.A. Sergeant, pp. 141–160. Oxford: Pergamon Press.

Taylor, E. & Sandberg, S. (1984). Hyperactive behavior in English school children: a questionnaire survey. *Journal of Abnormal Child Psychology,* **12**, 143–56.

Taylor, E., Schachar, R., Thorley, G. & Wieselberg, M. (1986). Conduct disorder and hyperactivity: I. Separation of hyperactivity and antisocial conduct in British child psychiatric patients. *British Journal of Psychiatry,* **149**, 760–77.

Taylor, E., Sandberg, S., Thorley, G. & Giles, S. (1991). *Epidemiology of Hyperactivity.* Maudsley Monograph No. 20. Oxford: Oxford University Press.

Thorley, G. (1984). Hyperkinetic syndrome of childhood: clinical characteristics. *British Journal of Psychiatry,* **144**, 16–24.

Trites, R.L., & Laprade, K. (1983). Evidence for an independent syndrome of hyperactivity. *Journal of Child Psychology and Psychiatry,* **24**, 573–86.

Van der Meere, J.J. & Sergeant, J. (1987). A divided attention experiment with hyperactive children. *Journal of Abnormal Child Psychology,* **15**, 379–91.

Verhulst, F.C. & Koot, H.M. (1991). Longitudinal research in child and adolescent psychiatry. *Journal of American Academy Child and Adolescent Psychiatry,* **30**, 361–8.

Walker, J. L. Lahey, B.B., Hynd, G.W. & Frame, C.L. (1987). Comparison of specific patterns of antisocial behavior in children with conduct disorder with or without coexisting hyperactivity. *Journal of Consulting and Clinical Psychology,* **55**, 910–13.

Werry, J.S. (1988). Differential diagnosis of attention deficit and conduct disorders. In *Attention Deficit Disorder: Criteria, Cognition, Intervention*, vol. 5, eds. L.M. Bloomingdale & J.A. Sergeant, pp. 83–96. Oxford: Pergamon Press.

Werry, J.S., Sprague, R.L. & Cohen, M.N. (1975). Conners'teacher rating scale for use in drug studies with children: an empirical study. *Journal of Abnormal Child Psychology*, **3**, 215–29.

Werry, J.S., Elkind, G.S & Reeves, J.C. (1987). Attention deficit, conduct, oppositional, and anxiety disorders in children: III. Laboratory differences. *Journal of Abnormal Child Psychology*, **15**, 409–28.

Werry, J.S., Reeves, J.C. & Elkind, G.S. (1987). Attention deficit, conduct, oppositional, and anxiety disorders in children: I. A review of research on differentiating characteristics. *Journal of American Academy Child and Adolescent Psychiatry*, **26**, 133–43.

Whalen, C.K. (1983). Hyperactivity, learning problems, and the attention defict disorders. In *Handbook of Child Psychopathology*, eds. T.H. Ollendick & M. Hersen, pp. 151–99. New York: Plenum Press.

Wolff, S. (1985). Non-delinquent disturbance of conduct. In *Child and Adolescent Psychiatry*, eds. M. Rutter & L. Hersov, pp. 400–413. Oxford: Blackwell Scientific Publications.

World Health Organisation (1992). *International Classification of Diseases*. ICD-10. Geneva: WHO.

Zentall, S.S. (1980). Behavioral comparisons of hyperactive and normally active children in natural settings. *Journal of Abnormal Child Psychology*, **8**, 93–109.

7

Biological aspects

Shinichiro Kado and Ryuro Takagi

INTRODUCTION

During the 1980s, intensive biological studies on the aetiology and pathogenesis of hyperkinetic disorders were done, but there have been no major breakthroughs for several reasons. First, as an accurate definition of, and diagnostic criteria for, hyperkinetic disorder have yet to be firmly established, the conditions of the subjects studied have varied. This situation reflects the diverse terminology used in making diagnoses. The terms minimal brain damage, minimal brain dysfunction, hyperkinetic syndrome (ICD-9), attention deficit disorder with hyperactivity (ADDH of DSM-III), and attention deficit hyperactivity disorder (ADHD of DSM-III-R) have all been used, but there are subtle differences in their meanings (Schachar, 1991). In addition, the line between hyperkinetic disorders and such related conditions as conduct disorder, learning disabilities and atypical autism, often is ambiguous, which means that the subject studied may not constitute a homogeneous group.

Secondly, biochemical data on cerebral function cannot be obtained directly. The various measures used are based on data from blood or urine samples and do not necessarily reflect cerebral functions behind the blood–brain barrier (BBB). Although animal models may be helpful in obtaining some direct measures, the experimental hyperactivity, inattentiveness and impulsivity seen in species other than humans do not necessarily show the symptomatology of hyperkinetic disorders.

Thirdly, postmortem findings on the brains of hyperkinetic children have yet to be presented. Hard postmortem findings on dopamine deficiency in the substantia nigra and striatum of Parkinsonian patients have advanced our understanding of the condition and our methods of treating it, and those on hyperkinetic disorders should provide vital information for determining the location of lesion and the nature of coexisting neurotransmitters and fourthly the interpretation of biochemical measures as well as their statistical testing present difficulties. An important, but sometimes forgotten point is that there is a distinction between a target and a sampled population. The former is the population to which an investigator wishes to generalise his results and conclusions. The latter is the population from which the study sample was drawn (Colton, 1974). Random sampling is required in order to make statistical inferences from the sample to the sampled population, and common-sense judgement is needed to make inferences from the sampled to the target population (Dawson-Sanders & Trapp, 1990). Investigators often do make statistical inferences from the sampled to the target population, mistaking their arbitrarily sampled populations to be random samples. Moreover, the statistically significant difference often is overemphasised; whereas, a substantive or clinical difference is not considered seriously (Riegelman & Hirsch, 1989). The bigger the sample, the smaller the p-value; therefore, a small p-value makes a very small difference appear large.

We shall now review the existing evidence for organic aetiology of hyperkinetic disorder in terms of the likelihood of brain damage and other neurological bases, as well as the various investigatory approaches used to establish the existence of such evidence.

BRAIN DAMAGE

Until recently, hyperkinetic disorders have been assigned the places of minimal brain damage (or dysfunction) (MBD) on the brain damage continuum. Patients with minor damage or dysfunction but without overt lesions have been considered to show the clinical features of hyperkinetic disorders. This idea that brain damage or dysfunction gives rise to a uniform behavioural picture is, however, no longer valid (Rutter, 1989) because the presence of brain damage or dysfunction is associated with an increase in the risk of a wide range of psychiatric disorders of which attention deficit disorders are by no means the most prominent (Rutter, 1981).

Taylor and his associates (1991) recently conducted an epidemiological study in which they compared five samples from a population of 2462 subjects that consisted of 6- and 7-year-old boys. These samples were made up of 41 boys with pure hyperactivity, 38 with mixed hyperactivity and conduct disorder, 42 with pure conduct disorder, 31 with attention deficit, and 42 controls. No difference was found among these five groups regarding neurological signs, brain injury in early life, or complications during delivery. This evidence argues against an aetiology of minimal brain damage. Furthermore, the idea that MBD syndromes are largely explicable in terms of perinatal complications is not valid because only very weak associations have been shown between perinatal complications and the characteristic features of MBD and because the presence of reproductive abnormalities does not delineate any type of behavioural syndrome (Nichols & Chen, 1981).

Although the association of the conventional idea of MBD with hyperkinetic disorders is no longer valid, this does not mean that these disorders might not have an organic origin (Sagvolden & Archer, 1989). The relatively high rate of neurodevelopmental problems may be differentially associated with pervasive hyperactivity of early onset, and the possibility that this is caused by an identifiable form of organic brain dysfunction is a hypothesis that is worth more systematic investigation with modern methods (Rutter, 1989). Even if no overt structural change to the brain can be shown, certain functional or neurochemical changes could be inferred as having organic bases.

SOFT SIGNS

One finding that has supported the MBD hypothesis is the existence of the so-called neurological soft signs. Bender (1947) reported that when a patient's brain is damaged overtly, he or she does not necessarily present typical neurological findings, rather neurological soft signs as well as behavioural, cognitive, and emotional disorders may appear. Since then, soft signs have been seen as signs of mild brain dysfunction, the main ones being dysdiadochokinesis, mirror (contralateral associated) movements, dysgraphesthesia, astereognosis, and mild choreo-athethosis. These soft signs frequently are found in normal children as well (Rutter, Tizard & Whitmore, 1970; Shaffer *et al.*, 1983), and in adolescent males there is a relation between the soft signs and affective symptomatology (Shaffer *et al.*, 1983). In addition, it is not clear to what extent soft signs simply reflect initial co-operativeness, attention to a task, or both (Ferguson & Rapoport, 1983). Therefore, these phenomena are of limited clinical value for screening and diagnosing hyperkinetic disorders (Shaffer *et al.*, 1983).

MORPHOLOGICAL STUDIES

Several techniques have been used with subjects who have hyperkinetic disorders to determine what morphological abnormalities cause the brain dysfunction that leads to symptoms of hyperkinetic disorders. No sooner has a new method with which to investigate brain structure and function been developed than it has been applied to psychiatric disorders of children. Much has been reported on mental retardation, autism, and hyperkinetic disorders which are considered to be of organic origin; but there are no reports that show there are morphological changes in the brain associated with the pathogenesis of hyperkinetic disorders.

Computerised axial tomography (CT)

CT of the brain is one of the best methods for locating structural brain lesions. There are, however, several disadvantages (Kuperman *et al.*, 1990): low dose radiation exposure cannot be avoided. Some subjects have an allergic reaction against the intravenous iodine contrast medium. Bones cause artefacts that obscure some brain areas, particularly in the posterior fossa. Also, there is a bias that is due to the partial volume effect or to deviation of the scanning axis (Matsui & Hirano, 1977). Of these disadvantages, the most serious is exposure to low dose radiation. When a 12-year-old is irradiated during CT of the head, the probability of future development of leukaemia or a malignant tumour is estimated to be 1/100 000 (Nishizawa *et al.*, 1981).

Another methodological problem is that, from the ethical point of view, true 'normal controls' are never available; usually, 'medical controls' are used as the 'normal controls', many of whom have had abnormal medical histories or have shown abnormalities on physical examination (Kuperman *et al.*, 1990). Moreover, when comparing measures between subjects and controls, average values usually are used, which is misleading. In the absence of good data for the range of 'normal', it is important to insist that an 'abnormal' value exceed the maximum value or be below the minimum one considered part of the normal series (Ornitz, 1978).

Caparulo and his colleagues (1981), who investigated 14 ADD children with severe learning disabilities, reported that the enlargement of lateral ventricles was present in two of them. Of these two children, one had ADDH and the other ADD. Shaywitz and his group (1983) compared the brain CT findings of 35 children who had ADD with 27 medical controls. Using a quantitative technique and 'blind analysis' they found no differences between the two groups as to the width of the anterior horns of the lateral ventricles, the biventricular width of the anterior horns of the lateral ventricle, the width of the brain at the bifrontal line, the width of the left and right hemispheres at the bifrontal line, Evans' index, and the asymmetry index. Harcherik and his associates (1985) found that, for 22 children with ADD, there were no significant differences between them and the other diagnostic groups or medical controls as to total ventricular volume, right–left ventricular volume ratio, ventricular asymmetries, ventricle–brain ratios, and brain density. Nasrallah and his colleagues (1986) compared brain CTs of 24 young males with childhood histories of hyperkinesis and MBD with those of 27 controls. The test subjects had been treated with stimulants. A significantly greater frequency of cerebral atrophy was found in the test subject group but there was no difference in cerebellar atrophy frequency or in the lateral cerebral ventricle-to-brain ratio (VBR). The investigators were not able to determine whether this cerebral atrophy was the causal factor of the condition, or whether it was an effect of alcohol or a side effect of the stimulants used. In this study, sulcal widening was present in 14 of the 24 test subjects and in one of the 27 controls, but in every case the widening was mild.

Voeller (1986) conducted a brain CT study on 15 children with behavioural disturbances and obtained findings consistent with right-hemispheric damage or dysfunction. Fourteen of the subjects had ADD of DSM-III, eight of whom were diagnosed as ADDH. He found four types of CT abnormalities: large right parietal lesions (in one ADDH subject); focal atrophy or attenuation of mild degree (in two ADDH subjects); dilated right lateral ventricle (in two ADD subjects and an ADDH one); and a striking asymmetry in the size of the hemispheres, the right being smaller than the left (in two ADD subjects and an ADDH one). Moreover, the EEG findings for these subjects showed right parietal spikes (in one ADD subject), right anterior temporal spike focus (in one ADDH subject), and decreased voltage over the right parietal area (in one ADD subject). On the basis of the CT and EEG findings, Voeller noted remarkably high percentages of children in his ADD subjects with right-hemisphere deficits. Because studies done on adults indicate that right-hemisphere lesions have profound effects on attentional mechanisms, he suggested an association between right-hemisphere deficits and ADD.

In summary, none of the brain CT studies done on ADD/ADDH children, except Voeller's, have shown significant abnormalities. In Voeller's study, the criteria used to judge the asymmetry of the brain hemisphere and the degree of ventricular dilation are not clear; therefore, the fourth disadvantage of CT must be considered. Thus, for individual children, the decision to perform a CT (as with other procedures) must be based on the total clinical picture, which includes the presence of neurological findings, recent changes in clinical status, and EGG abnormalities (Harcherik *et al.*, 1985), because the risk of the probabilistic effects of low dose irradiation outweighs the benefit of making CT a routine procedure.

Magnetic resonance imaging (MRI)

MRI is a new and excellent technique that makes visible structural changes in the brain. It has several advantages over CT; It is not necessary to use radiation. Its high resolution can delineate lesions that CT can not. Artefacts caused by bones are excluded. The use of an iodine contrast medium is unnecessary. Moreover, flexible imaging parameters and imaging planes are available. There are some disadvantages for children, the main difficulties being that much more time is needed than for CT and that the form of the apparatus may cause anxiety and fear. Although MRI is currently the most promising technique for the investigation of anatomical lesions of the central nervous system, there are not very many reports of MRI findings on hyperkinetic disorders as yet.

Hynd and his colleagues (1993) conducted a MRI study and found that, in normal children, 72.7% evidenced a left-larger-than-right (L > R) pattern of asymmetry, whereas 63.6% of the ADHD children had the reverse (L < R) pattern of asymmetry of the head of the caudate nucleus. This reversal of normal asymmetry in ADHD children was due to a significantly smaller left caudate nucleus. They suggested that the ADHD children might have asymmetries in neurotransmitter systems in the caudate region. Singer and his colleagues (1993) compared MRI findings among 18 children with ADHD as well as Tourette's syndrome (TS), 19 children with TS only, and with 18 normal controls. They found that in the ADHD and TS group, the volume of the left globus pallidus was significantly smaller than the volume of the right, and that lenticular asymmetry was due to a greater right-sided predominance in the TS and ADHD group. Although it might be likely that the basal ganglia are involved in the pathogenesis of ADHD, further research is needed to get a firm conclusion.

FUNCTIONAL STUDIES

Even if CT or MRI were not to show significant structural abnormalities, there is still the possibility of discovering certain types of functional brain abnormalities by the use of electroencephalography, computerised electroencephalography, event-related potential, positron emission tomography, and single photon emission computerised tomography.

Electroencephalography (EEG)

In the 1970s, several reports on the high incidence of routine EEG abnormalities were published (Werry *et al.*, 1972; Satterfield *et al.*, 1973; Grunewald-Zuberbeiter, Grunewald & Raske, 1975). The reported incidence ranged from 35% to 95%, a wide variation. Abnormalities in basic rhythm such as slow wave dysrhythmia, arceau rhythm, and slow posterior waves in youths were more frequent than were paroxysmal abnormalities. But, when cerebral palsy and epilepsy were excluded from the analysis, the differences in the incidence of EEG abnormalities for the hyperkinetic disorder subjects and normal controls disappeared (Werry *et al.*, 1972). Voeller (1986) conducted an EEG study on 14 children with ADD, eight of whom were diagnosed as ADDH. He found right parietal spikes (in one ADD subject), right anterior temporal spike focus (in one ADDH subject), and decreased voltage over the right parietal area (in one ADD subject). On the basis of EEG and CT results, he concluded that a right hemisphere deficit was the causal factor.

The difficulty of interpreting the results of computerised electroencephalography (CEEG) done on children with hyperkinetic disorders has been pointed out (Kuperman *et al.*, 1990). It is due to the use of different clinical populations, non-standard and limited electrode placement, and different testing conditions. Continuous abnormalities found were decreased power in the alpha and beta waves, and increased power in the slow wave (Shetty, 1971; Montagu 1975; Dykman *et al.*, 1982; Callaway, Halliday & Naylor, 1983). Mann and his colleagues (1992) conducted a computerised power spectral analytical study on 25 boys with ADHD (DSM-III-R). They found increases in theta activity in frontal and central locations and a lack of beta activation in posterior and temporal locations during cognitive tasks.

CEEG analysis holds some promise, but spatial resolution is poor and the technique mainly reflects cortical function (Lou, Henriksen & Bruhn, 1990). Further research is needed before it can be decided whether these EEG abnormalities are findings specific to hyperkinetic disorders.

Event-related potential (ERP)

ERPs are completely non-invasive, and a subject can be tested repeatedly without experiencing side effects. ERP consists of several components; waves I, II, III, IV, V, Na, Pa, N1, P2, N2, and P3b. P3b is associated with concept modification and has attention to event importance (Donchin *et al.*, 1984; Sutton & Ruchkin, 1984). It has a positive polarity and occurs 300–900 ms after an event. The P3b responses are similar whether visual, auditory, or somatosensory modalities are used. Callaway and his group (1983) compared visual ERP measures for 18 hyperactive children and 18 age-matched normal controls. The N1 amplitudes were significantly larger for both the older and hyperactive children, on this measure hyperactive children appearing more mature. They also found an increase in N2 latency with age in their normal controls but a decrease in the test subjects, which suggested that the older hyperactives showed maturational lag. Courchesne's study (1987), however, reported that N2 latency decreased with age in normal children; therefore, it is difficult to interpret the available evidence about N2 latency in hyperactive children.

Satterfield and his colleagues (Satterfield & Schell, 1984; Satterfield, Schell & Backs, 1987) conducted a long-term (8-year) follow-up study of 110 delinquent and nondelinquent hyperactives and 75 normal subjects and compared their auditory evoked response potential (AERP) measures. They found that longitudinal change in N2 amplitude in the delinquent hyperactive group took place in the same way as in the normal group but this change in the non-delinquent hyperactive group followed an entirely different developmental course. They concluded that the non-delinquent hyperactive group had abnormal maturational changes, as reflected by the AERP measures, and proposed that their ADDH subjects who developed and those who did not develop serious delinquent behaviour constitute two distinct subgroups. Nevertheless, the difference in the N2 amplitude does not appear to have been substantively signifcant, even if statistically so. In another study, Satterfield *et al.* (1988) recorded AERPs from 19 electrode sites in 20 ADDH and 20 normal subjects during a two-choice discrimination task. Although it is difficult to compare their study with other AERP studies of ADDH children (including their own previous work) because of various methodological differences, an abnormally small N2 response in ADDH boys again was found; but neither the P3b amplitude nor latency differed significantly from the values for the normal subjects although abnormally small P3b amplitudes have been found in a number of studies (Holcomb, Dykman, 1983; Holcomb, Ackerman & Dykman, 1986; Loiselle *et al.*, 1980). They suggested that children with ADDH have a problem with both automatic (not under conscious control) and controlled (under voluntary control) processing.

In short, mainly because age and diagnostic criteria vary widely in studies reported so far, there is no firm evidence regarding amplitude, reaction time, and latency of ERP in hyperkinetic disorders. Furthermore, as discussed in some detail in Chapter 8, the results of psychophysiological studies appear to be related to the degree of co-morbidity with conduct disorder and also the degree of co-existing environmental stressors – both of which, possibly, exert their unique influences via emotional/motivational mechanisms.

Positron emission tomography (PET)

PET is a unique technique for the investigation of brain metabolism *in vivo* that shows brain blood flow and brain glucose utilisation. Moreover, with radioligands it can be used for the quantification and labelling of specific neurotransmitter receptors. PET studies of noradrenergic receptor status in children with ADHD may prove useful (Rasmusson *et al.*, 1990), but radiolabelled noradrenergic receptor ligands have yet to be developed (Andreasen, 1988). It must be noted that the use of PET involves a significant amount of radiation exposure (Kuperman *et al.*, 1990) and the National Institute of Health (USA) regulations do not permit its use on children (Shaywitz & Shaywitz, 1989). Thus, Zametkin and his colleagues (1990) conducted a PET study on 25 restless and inattentive adults with a definite childhood history of ADDH(DSM-III) whose children have been diagnosed as ADDH. They reported that global cerebral glucose metabolism was reduced by 8%, and the largest reductions were found in the premotor and the superior prefrontal cortex. These cortical areas are suggested to be involved in the control of attention and motor activity. This finding is interesting because it is compatible with the data derived from the CEEG study (Mann et al., 1992).

Single photon emission computerised tomography (SPECT)

Much smaller doses of radiation are given with SPECT than with PET (Lassen, Henriksen & Paulson, 1981). In SPECT, inhaled Xe gives a quantitative measure of three-dimensional regional cerebral blood flow (rCBF) and, by inference, metabolic and functional activity (Sokoloff, 1981).

Lou and his colleagues (Lou, Henriksen & Bruhn, 1984; Lou *et al.*, 1989; Lou, Henriksen & Bruhn, 1990) conducted a series of SPECT studies on 24 children with developmental learning disabilities and on 15 controls. Regional cerebral activity was low in the striatal and posterior periventricular regions and high in the occipital regions of nine subjects who had pure ADHD of DSM-III-R. Low activity in striatal and postventricular areas also was seen in eight children who had ADHD in combination with phonologic–syntactic dysphasia. Methylphenidate administration increased the blood flow to the striatal and posterior periventricular regions. In the pure ADHD group, the mean percentage of total blood flow in the striatal region decreased by 7–11%. The differences were statistically significant, but it is questionable whether they can be called clinically so.

In animal studies, experimental lesions to the striatum were shown to cause hyperactivity, deficits in attention, and memory consolidation with poor performance in cognitive tasks, so Lou and his colleagues (1989) speculated that the caudate nucleus might modulate polysensory activity via thalamic connections that are predominantly inhibitory, and that lack of striatal inhibition of polysensory activity might be part of the pathogenesis of ADHD. They also concluded that the striatum is particularly vulnerable to early cerebral hypoxic ischaemic insults because the incidence of adverse antenatal and perinatal events was high in their patient group, and the striatum is located at the border between the anterior and middle cerebral arteries.

NEUROCHEMICAL STUDIES

Results from a variety of studies suggest that monoamine neurotransmitter systems have an important role in the pathogenesis of hyperkinetic disorders. The main evidence is the clinical fact that the stimulants: D-amphetamine, methylphenidate and pemoline are very effective in treating hyperkinetic disorders. Furthermore, animals studies (e.g. Kuczenski, 1983) have shown that these stimulants act via the central monoaminergic systems to: inhibit reuptake,increase release of amine, and to some extent to inhibit monoamine oxidase (MAO) activity. All these actions serve to increase the concentrations of the monoamines noradrenaline, dopamine and serotonin at the synaptic cleft.

The action of pemoline has not been nearly so well documented, although it is clear that the early suggestion that pemoline preferentially stimulates dopamine synthesis is not supported by results of recent studies. Results indicate that pemoline reduces catecholamine turnover and that it may inhibit catecholamine uptake (Fuller *et al.*, 1978; Molina & Orsingher, 1981). While pharmacological studies are being intensively conducted, more direct evidence is being sought by the examination of monoamines, their metabolites and related enzymes in the blood, urine and cerebrospinal fluid (CSF) of children with hyperkinetic disorders (Zametkin & Rapoport, 1987), because it has been suggested that the concentrations of these materials might serve as an index of the function of that particular catecholamine system (Shaywitz & Shaywitz, 1989).

Catecholamine hypothesis

Systems based on dopaminergic transmission

The first monoamine hypothesis was that of a dopamine deficiency derived from evidence that adults who suffered from Economo's encephalitis developed Parkinson's disease; whereas children who suffered from the same disease showed attentional and motor symptoms (Raskin *et al.*, 1984). For that reason, it has been inferred that hyperkinetic disorders may develop because of a dopamine deficiency.

Abnormalities in the central dopaminergic systems have been investigated by measuring the concentrations of homovanillic acid (HVA), the main metabolite of dopamine, in the urine and CSF of children with hyperkinetic disorders. Urine HVA concentrations in ADDH groups were compared with those in control groups by several research groups but no difference was found (Wender *et al.*, 1971; Shekim, DeKirmenjian & Chapel, 1977; Shekim *et al.*, 1983). It is not easy to determine what the function of the central nervous system is from these findings because HVA in the blood and urine is derived from both central and peripheral dopamine. The contribution of brain dopamine to HVA in the blood and urine is estimated to be between 30% and 60% (Maas *et al.*, 1980), most of what remains being derived from the adrenal glad and the gut. Therefore, it is important to differentiate peripheral from central HVA. This can be done by the use of debrisoquin, a weak MAO inhibitor, which does not cross the BBB, thereby acting only on peripheral catecholamines. Prior to the use of debrisoquin, 33% of the plasma HVA was found to be derived from the brain, but post-debrisoquin 75% was (Swann *et al.*, 1980). Use of debrisoquin therefore makes it possible to investigate the plasma HVA derived primarily from the brain dopamine. Shaywitz and Shaywitz (1989) used this strategy on 20 children with ADD who received D-amphetamine, methylphenidate, or a placebo. After debrisoquin loading, D-amphetamine produced an increase in plasma HVA and urinary dopamine. They suggested that D-amphetamine and methylphenidate differ in their effects on the brain's catecholaminergic systems despite clinical similarities, D-amphetamine influencing brain dopaminergic mechanisms, perhaps by increasing the turnover of brain dopamine.

The HVA in the CSF of ADDH subjects was compared with that of controls, again no difference was found (Shetty & Chase, 1976). Shaywitz, Cohen and Bowers (1977) measured the CSF HVA of 6 MBD boys and 16 controls after probenecid loading. Probenecid is an agent that blocks the active transport of HVA. They found that the CSF HVA-to-probenecid ratio was significantly lower in the MBD subjects, and suggested that dopamine turnover might be low in MBD.

There are, however, contradictory findings. Levoamphetamine, which has little or no dopamine agonistic activity, was reported to be effective in the treatment of hyperkinetic syndrome (Arnold *et al.*, 1972); neuroleptics do not aggravate the disorder, nor do they interfere with the beneficial effects obtained by methylphenidate administration (Gittleman-Klein *et al.*, 1976; Weizman *et al.*, 1984). As to HVA, it cannot be said there is definitive evidence for a primary involvement of the dopaminergic system in the aetiology of hyperkinetic disorders.

Catecholamines also have been measured in human plasma. Ionescu and his associates (1990) studied plasma catecholamines in 12 subjects with ADDH and in 11 controls. The plasma concentrations of dopamine and adrenaline in the subjects were significantly higher than in the controls, which suggested a close relationship between the circulatory concentrations of these neurotransmitters and the pathogenesis of the ADDH. But, their study was conducted on the assumption that the majority of catecholamines circulating in the plasma originate in the CNS and that the tendency for an increase or decrease in catecholamine concentration in the plasma parallels that in the brain. Unlike the CSF, the origin of the majority of plasma catecholamines should be thought to be the peripheral nervous system.

Animal models also provide some evidence for the involvement of the dopaminergic system in the pathogenesis of hyperkinesis. Use of the neurotoxin 6-hydroxydopamine makes it possible to produce selective depletion of brain dopamine and to develop hyperactivity in the neonatal rat (Shaywitz *et al.*, 1976*a*,*b*; Lipton, McGouth & Shaywitz, 1980; Shaywitz & Shaywitz, 1982). The behaviour of these animals is said to be remarkably similar to that of children with ADD and includes hyperactivity which abates with maturity and learning deficits which persist (Shaywitz & Shaywitz, 1989). This inference, however, needs much more consideration. If it is shown to be valid, the fact that the administration of amphetamines (Shaywitz *et al.*, 1976*b*) or methylphenidate (Shaywitz, Klopper & Gordon, 1978) reverses hyperactivity could provide strong supporting evidence for dopamine hypothesis as the pathogenesis of hyperkinetic disorders. The development of such new scientific techniques as intracranial microdialysis (Ungerstedt, 1984; Church, Justice & Neill, 1987) may make it possible to evaluate the potential explanatory value of the dopaminergic system (Rasmusson *et al.*, 1990).

In contrast, pharmacological investigations have brought out contradictory findings. Carbidopa/levodopa was ineffective (Langer *et al.*, 1982) and amantadine, a dopamine agonist, did not bring about significant improvement in nine children with ADDH; whereas relatively low doses of the dopamine antagonists haloperidol, chlorpromazine, and thioridazine were modestly effective (Winsberg & Yepes, 1978). In short, there is relatively little evidence to support the dopamine hypothesis. So far, that hypothesis can not exclusively explain the pathogenesis of hyperkinetic disorders.

Systems based on noradrenaline transmission

So far, various pieces of indirect evidence support the hypothesis that central noradrenergic mechanisms function in the pathogenesis of hyperkinetic disorders. Only 60% of urinary 3-methoxy-4-hydroxyphenylglycol (MHPG), a main metabolite of noradrenaline has been reported to be derived from the brain (Maas & Leckman, 1983); therefore, it may not provide a good index of the brain noradrenergic system. Nevertheless, compared with values for controls, urinary MHPG was reported decreased in seven hyperkinetic boys (Shekim *et al.*, 1977) in 15 children with MBD (Shekim, DeKirmenjian & Chapel, 1979), in nine children with ADDH (Shekim *et al.*, 1983), and in 73 children with MBD (Yu-cun & Yu-feng, 1984). In contrast, no difference in urinary MHPG concentrations were found in nine children with MBD (Wender *et al.*, 1971) or in 13 hyperactive boys (Rapoport *et al.*, 1978) when compared to values for the controls. Moreover, increased urinary MHPG was found in ten children with ADDH (Khan & DeKirmenjian, 1981) although, in this last study, the control values for the excretion of MHPG were considerably lower than in the other reports. It should be noted, however, that prior drug use may continue to decrease MHPG for 2 weeks, or more, after discontinuation of medication (Zametkin *et al.*, 1985*c*). As the standard 'washout' period for most of the studies was only 2 weeks, the reported differences between ADDH and normal children may reflect prior drug use (Zametkin & Rapoport, 1987). Rapoport *et al.* (1978) found increased urinary noradrenaline in 13 hyperactive boys but Ionesco *et al.* (1990), who found no difference between the plasma noradrenaline levels of 12 ADDH children and 11 healthy controls, suggested that their results do not support the noradrenaline hypothesis. Urinary noradrenaline, however, is derived almost exclusively from peripheral noradrenaline because this compound normally does not cross the BBB. From these indirect findings alone, it is still too early to conclude whether the noradrenergic system has a main role in the pathogenesis of hyperactivity disorders.

Results of animal studies suggest that noradrenaline depletion produces attention deficits (Lordon *et al.*, 1980; Maas & Leckman, 1983; Mason & Fibiger, 1987) and performance deficits but normal activity is retained (Shaywitz & Shaywitz, 1989). It is not clear whether these behavioural changes are the same as those produced by the selective depletion of brain dopamine or whether they are comparable to changes seen in the hyperkinetic disorders in humans.

The outcomes of pharmacological studies on hyperactivity disorders also support the noradrenergic hypothesis. The drugs dextroamphetamine, methylphenidate, clorgyline, tranylcypromine, and desipramine are effective for treating hyperactivity disorders. The neurotransmitter content of the monoaminergic synapses is augmented non-selectively by dextroamphetamine (Rapoport, Buchsbaum & Weingartner, 1980) and methylphenidate (Rapoport *et al*., 1974*a*; Garfinkel *et al*., 1983) as well as by the MAO-A inhibitors, clorgyline and tranylcypromine (Zametkin *et al*., 1985*c*). In contrast, the tricyclic antidepressant desipramine has been found to be a relatively specific noradrenaline reuptake blocker (Garfinkel *et al*., 1983; Gastfriend, Biederman & Jellinek, 1984; Biederman, Gastfriend & Jellinek, 1986; Donnelly *et al*., 1986*b*; Riddle *et al*., 1988).

Furthermore, these agents reproducibly suppress MHPG levels in the plasma and urine. Amphetamines have been reported to reduce urinary MHPG in ADD children (Brown *et al*., 1981; Shekim *et al*., 1977, 1979; Zametkin *et al*., 1985*a,b,c*), and a reduction also has been seen in subjects who responded positively to the drug (Shekim *et al*., 1983). Administration of the tricyclic antidepressant agent desipramine resulted in decreases in both the plasma and urinary MHPG, decreases which were correlated with behavioural improvement (Donnelly *et al*., 1986*b*).

Increases in synaptic noradrenaline induced by these effective agents have been suggested to exert inhibitory feedback effects on presynaptic neurons (Rasmusson *et al*., 1990). Indeed, MAO inhibitors rapidly decrease the firing rate of locus ceruleus neurons (Blier, DeMontigny & Chaput, 1987). Increases in synaptic noradrenaline, however, could increase noradrenergic neurotransmission via postsynaptic effects. Linnoila *et al*. (1986) suggested that, although desipramine decreases CNS noradrenaline turnover, it increases the efficacy of noradrenergic neurotransmission. At this time, published results of biochemical, animal and pharmacological studies are still too contradictory to be able to interpret and draw firm conclusions regarding the role of the noradrenergic systems in hyperactivity disorders.

Systems based on serotonergic transmission

Values for 5-hydroxyindoleacetic acid (5-HIAA), a main metabolite of serotonin (5-hydroxytryptamine; 5-HT) in the CSF of ADDH subjects, were compared with those for controls, but no difference was found (Shetty & Chase,

1976). Shaywitz *et al.* (1977), who measured the CSF 5-HIAA of 6 MBD boys and 16 controls, also found no difference. The presence of 5-HT and 5-HIAA in blood has been investigated by many researchers. Bhagauan, Coleman and Coursina (1975) found decreased 5-HT concentrations in sera from 11 hyperactive children as compared with 11 controls; Coleman (1971) found that the 5-HT in the whole blood of 25 hyperactive children was lower than normal. Moreover, plasma 5-HIAA has been reported to be low (Greenberg & Coleman, 1973, 1976). More recent studies, however, have found no difference in the 5-HT of the platelets and blood of children with ADDH (Rapoport *et al.*, 1974*b*; Irwin *et al.*, 1981; Ferguson *et al.*, 1981; Haslam & Dalby, 1983). Nevertheless, most of the 5-HT in blood is not derived from the brain; peripheral 5-HT and 5-HIAA do not reflect changes in the brain serotonergic system (Naruse *et al.*, 1989). This review of the biochemical data reported for children with hyperactivity disorder shows there is little evidence that the serotonergic system functions in the pathogenesis of hyperactivity disorders.

Nemzer and his associates (1986) found that 1-tryptophan, a precursor of 5-HT, was not effective in 15 children with ADD during school time but was modestly effective at home. Fenfluramine, an agent which reduces brain 5-HT, has no effect on ADDH children (Rapoport *et al.*, 1985; Donnelly, Rapoport & Ismond, 1986*a*). The possible involvement of serotonin in the pathogenesis of hyperactivity disorders is supported by the beneficial effects of the tricyclic antidepressant agent, clomipramine (Garfinkel *et al.*, 1983) and of clorgyline which primarily inhibits MAO-A (Zametkin *et al.*, 1985*b*). In addition, methylphenidate and D-amphetamine have serotonergic agonist activity, but urinary 5-HIAA is not affected by methylphenidate (Zametkin *et al.*, 1985*a*). To date, most pharmacological findings do not support an obvious, major role for serotonergic systems in hyperactivity disorders (Weizman, Weizman & Deutsch, 1990).

Other findings

Comparisons of platelet MAO in normal and hyperactive children are inconclusive (Zametkin & Rapoport, 1987). Shekim *et al.* (1982) reported that hyperactive children have lower platelet MAO activity than normal control subjects. This finding could not be replicated by Brown and his co-workers (1984) who demonstrated lower contents of plasma amine oxidase (which lacks specific monoamine deaminisation properties) in children with ADDH, but the decrease in MAO activity reported in the normal control children between the ages of 6 and 12 was not seen in their sample of 18 ADDH children. As platelet MAO normally decreases during childhood and adolescence

(Young *et al.*, 1980), this finding is of potential interest because a relative excess of MAO in childhood could produce a relative deficiency of monoamines (Zametkin & Rapoport, 1987).

There are three types of MAO inhibitors: selective MAO-A inhibitors such as clorgyline; mixed MAO-A and -B inhibitors such as tranylcypromine; and the MAO-B inhibitor, deprenyl. They all have had immediate therapeutic clinical effects on sustained attention and classroom behaviour (Zametkin *et al.*, 1985*b*). Because the substrates for MAO-A are noradrenaline and serotonin, those for MAO-B are ß-phenylethylamines, and dopamine is metabolised by both MAO-A and MAO-B, the importance of one transmitter system over the others can not be shown (Zametkin & Rapoport, 1987).

Other neuroregulators also may have importance. For example, γ-aminobutyric acid (GABA) is considered the major inhibitory neuroregulator in the brain, but its role in hyperactivity disorders has yet to be studied. In addition, the functions of newly discovered neuropeptide neuroregulators in the brain and their roles in the pathogenesis of hyperactivity disorders are as yet unknown.

Recently, some researchers have focused on the issue of generalised resistance to thyroid hormone (GRTH), a disease caused by mutation in the thyroid receptor-β gene and characterised by reduced responsiveness of peripheral and pituitary tissues to thyroid hormone, because symptoms suggestive of ADDH have been reported in patients with GRTH (Magner *et al.*, 1980; Refetoff, 1990). Hauser and his colleagues (1993) found 19 ADHD children (70%) in 27 subjects resistant to thyroid hormone, but 5 ADHD children (20%) in 25 unaffected subjects. Resistance to thyroid hormone must inevitably interfere with brain development. In addition, thyroid receptor–thyroid hormone complex may influence catecholamine neurotransmitter systems. However, Weiss and his co-workers (1993) conducted a prospective screening study for thyroid abnormalities in 277 children with ADHD, and found that 14 children with ADHD had thyroid function test abnormalities. Nevertheless, GRTH could not be demonstrated in a detailed study of them. Also, Elia and her colleagues (1994) compared TSH, T3 and T4 values in 53 ADHD boys with those in 41 age and gender-matched normal controls, but found none in the range suggestive of global or pituitary thyroid hormone resistance.

Contradictory evidence

A large number of neuropsychopharmacological clinical studies have provided concrete evidence for probable neurotransmitter system dysfunction in hyperactivity disorders. A variety of studies on the nature of this dysfunction have been conducted that compare monoamines and their metabolites in the urine, plasma, platelets, and CSF of hyperactivity disorder subjects and normal controls. The outcomes have been disappointing so far. Most studies have not found consistently significant differences between children with hyperactivity disorder and the normal controls (Zametkin & Rapoport, 1987) nor has it been possible successfully to reproduce study results. Results of past studies of neurotransmitter and metabolite concentrations in children with hyperkinetic disorders often have been variable or contradictory; therefore, the information available is insufficient to draw conclusions regarding the status of brain transmitter systems in hyperactivity disorders. Moreover, a number of methodological difficulties limit the interpretative power of the reported studies.

First, some of the confusion may be due to the nature of the disorders studied because many may be biologically heterogeneous or have complex and unstable phenotypes (Rasmusson *et al.*, 1990). The meanings assigned to the diagnostic labels MBD, ADDH (DSM-III), ADHD (DSM-III-R), hyperkinetic syndrome (ICD-9), and hyperkinetic disorder (ICD-10), tend to vary (Schachar, 1991).

Secondly, the sample sizes in the reported studies were small. Unless the sample size is large, it is difficult to find a statistically significant difference. Furthermore, with a small sample, the probability of a second type error, the false negative, is high. Also, the issue of the valid use of statistical tests, mentioned in the introduction to this chapter, must be considered.

Thirdly, CSF studies are flawed by the unavailability of true, normal control subjects (Zametkin & Rapoport, 1987). For ethical reasons, healthy children cannot be used as the true normal controls; therefore, clinical populations of children are used (medical controls).

Fourthly, the concentrations of transmitters, precursors, or their metabolites, in peripheral tissues alone do not directly (or reliably) reflect brain transmitter status. The usefulness of blood analysis is appreciably limited because of the existence of the BBB, making it very difficult to infer the dynamics of neurotransmitters in the brain from blood samples. Analysis of the CSF provides important information about the situation behind the BBB; even so, it is information limited to the part in contact with the CSF. Other difficulties are that the CSF does not circulate as freely as the blood, its constituents mainly being transferred from the surface of the brain and the concentrations of these constituents may differ with the site from which the CSF sample is drawn. For example, HVA concentrations at the ventricle level are higher than at the lumbar level, so that when lumbar puncture is repeated, the subsequent CSF samples will have higher concentrations of HVA (Menachem *et al.*, 1989).

Probenecid often is used to study monoamine turnover in the brain because this agent blocks active transport of the acid metabolites of monoamines from the CSF. But, at the doses that can be used clinically, transport blockade is only partial, and is affected by a large number of uncontrollable variables, making interpretation of results difficult (Faull *et al.*, 1981).

Fifthly, multiple neurotransmitters that coexist in the brain interact. Nearly 100 small molecules and peptides are known to serve as neurotransmitters. These transmitters have a wide distribution but are produced by highly localised cells that together make up only a small fraction of the neurons in the brain. However, each monoaminergic system is organised into anatomical and functional subsystems that act independently, and each interacts with, is affected by, and is interconnected to other transmitter systems (Yuwiler & Freedman, 1987). For instance, serotonergic terminals synapse on some dopamine cell bodies (Dray *et al.*, 1976), noradrenergic terminals synapse on some serotonergic cell bodies (Baraban & Aghajanian, 1981), and dopaminergic terminals synapse on some noradrenergic cell bodies (Simon, LeMoal & Calas, 1979). Moreover, opiate receptors occur on terminals of serotonergic neurons (Parenti *et al.*, 1983). It is likely that a disturbance in one transmitter system would affect the activities of the other systems; therefore, it is understandable that dextroamphetamine, methylphenidate, and, probably, pemoline would affect multiple neurotransmitter systems (Zametkin & Rapoport, 1987).

Another level of complexity is shown by the fact that the release of neurotransmitters has negative feedback because of autoreceptors stimulation in general; but, in some systems there is a positive feedback mechanism (Yuwiler & Freedman, 1987). There is also another type of interaction via a precursor and a rate-limiting enzyme. For example, because dopamine is the precursor in the synthesis of noradrenaline, it is most unlikely that the function of one transmitter can be changed without altering another transmitter as tyrosine hydroxylase activity (the rate limiting step for the synthesis of dopamine) is clearly regulated by noradrenaline levels (Cooper, Bloom & Roth, 1982). Specific antidepressants do alter both the noradrenaline and serotonin receptor numbers, functions, or both. Desipramine, the most selective noradrenaline reuptake blocker, reduces 5-HIAA; whereas, zimelidine, a serotonin reuptake blocker, reduces CSF MHPG as well as 5-HIAA (Potter *et al.*, 1985). Animal studies (Halaris, Belendiuk & Freeman, 1975; Nurse, Russell & Taljaard, 1985) have shown that desipramine alters α-adrenoreceptor-mediated release of dopamine in the nucleus accumbens as well as dopamine uptake. Moreover, dopamine itself affects the α- and ß-adrenergic neurons, although it is less potent than adrenaline, noradrenaline, and isoproterenol (Goldberg, Volkman & Kohli, 1978).

Because of this very complicated situation, a single transmitter defect hypothesis cannot be valid. A new area of investigation concerns the interactions among neuropeptides and the so-called transmitters. The most promising types of research at this time are in-depth studies of patients' responses to stimulants and physiological studies that use brain imaging techniques (Zametkin & Rapoport, 1987).

GENETIC INHERITANCE

As the genetic aspects of the hyperactivity disorder have been covered in some detail in Chapter 11 of this volume by Jim Stevenson, only a rather brief summary of the relevant studies will be presented in the context of this chapter.

Twin studies

Cunningham and Barkley (1978) reported a monozygotic (MZ) twin pair concordant for ADD. Lopez (1965) compared four MZ twin pairs with six dizygotic (DZ) pairs, all the MZ pairs being concordant for ADD as compared to one DZ pair. Only two of the DZ pairs were of the same sex, and the sample size was very small. Willerman (1973) studied 93 sets of same-sexed twins and found a higher activity level correlation for MZ than DZ twins. Heffron, Martin and Welsh (1984) reported on three pairs of MZ twins. All six individuals met the criteria for ADD of DSM-III. They concluded that these three cases of MZ twins with ADD support a genetic aetiology for ADD, but their sample size was very small. They also reported results that complicate all twin studies; twins are at higher risk for premature birth, intrauterine compromise, and abuse factors – all of which affect their psychiatric presentation.

Goodman and Stevenson (1989) investigated a large representative sample of 13 year-old twins and found that MZ pairs were more alike than same-sex DZ pairs in objective measures of attentiveness and in parent and teacher ratings of hyperactivity. A comparison of recognised and unrecognised MZ pairs indicated that parents and teachers rated twins as more similar when perceived as 'identical' rather than 'non-identical'. Allowing for this stereotyping, underlying genetic differences appear to account for 30% to 50% of the inter individual variations in trait measures of childhood hyperactivity and inattentiveness (roughly half the explainable variance). Further research is needed on much younger sets of twins with hyperactivity disorders defined by ICD-10.

Family studies

A number of family studies have been conducted to determine familial aggregation of hyperactivity disorders or other psychiatric disorders because the closeness of the biological relationship should affect the chance of relatives being affected. Morrison and Stewart (1971) compared the parents of 59 children with ADD with those of 41 control children and found a high prevalence of sociopathy, hysteria and alcoholism in the former. In addition, a significantly greater number of those parents retrospectively reported having ADD as children. Cantwell (1972) compared the parents of 50 children with ADD with those of 50 control children and obtained results similar to those of Morrison and Stewart. Safer (1973) found that full siblings of hyperactive probands were more likely to show behaviour disorders than were their half-siblings. The value of these results is very limited because of methodological difficulties such as different diagnostic criteria, use of retrospective data, and having a psychologically common environment.

Biederman and his co-workers (1986), who compared 22 subjects with ADD and 20 medical controls, found that ADD, oppositional disorder, and major depression were more frequent in the parents and siblings of the ADD subjects than in those of the controls. Furthermore, familial loading for antisocial (including oppositional) disorders has been shown to be confined to subjects with both ADD and oppositional disorder (Biederman, Munir & Knee, 1987). The interpretation of such findings, however, is complicated by the extensive comorbidity seen in the subjects (high rates of conduct disorder, oppositional disorder, major depression, tics and language disorders as well as ADD) and by the non-specificity of the familial loading of psychiatric disorders. These findings allow for no differentiation between genetic and environmental mediation nor between genetic influence on hyperactivity disorders and psychiatric disorder in general (Rutter *et al.*, 1990).

Adoption studies

Safer (1973) reviewed the medical and social service charts of the adopted-away siblings and half-siblings of 17 children with MBD and found that hyperactivity was common. Morrison and Stewart (1971, 1973) and Cantwell (1975) reported that hysteria, sociopathy, alcoholism and a history of hyperactivity in childhood were more common in the biological parents of hyperkinetic children than in the adoptive parents, which suggests genetic transmission of hyperactivity. A number of methodological limitations exist (McMahon, 1980). The biological and adoptee samples were heterogeneous, and the low rate of disorders in the adoptive parents could be no more than the results of selection policies for both the adoptive and biological parents, one of the grounds for the selection of the former being mental health. As for the latter, the findings of parental psychological disorders raises the likelihood of adoption as well as the risk of disorder in the offspring.

Cunningham and his associates (1975) compared the offspring of psychiatrically normal and disturbed parents whose children had been adopted away. Hyperactive disorders were more common in the biological children of disordered parents than in those of normal parents. Bohman and his colleagues (Bohman & Sigvardsson, 1980; Bohman *et al.*, 1982) found that biological children of criminal or alcoholic mothers showed higher levels of activity, inattention, and certain other behaviour problems when brought up in other families. Curiously, the relation between maternal and child behaviour no longer held when the persons lived together.

So far, no firm conclusions can be drawn from the results of adoption studies regarding the genetic transmission of hyperactivity disorders.

Fragile X syndrome

Fragile X syndrome is an X-linked disorder associated with a high prevalence of psychiatric disturbance; in particular, attention deficit disorder and autism. Bregman and his colleagues (1988) conducted a neuropsychiatric evaluation of 14 males with this syndrome and found pervasive hyperactivity, impulsivity, and attentional deficits in all of them. Moreover, 13 met DSM-III criteria for ADD, 10 for ADDH, and 3 for a residual syndrome. Three other studies found that 41 of 50 subjects (82%) had these behavioural characteristics and autistic symptomatology (Finelli *et al.*, 1985; Fryns *et al.*, 1984; Largo & Schinzel, 1985). Further research is needed because the fragile X syndrome is reported more frequently in association with autism than with hyperactivity disorders (Brown *et al.*, 1982; Meryash, Szymanski & Gerald, 1982; August & Lockhart, 1984; Blomquist *et al.*, 1985; De Arce & Kearns, 1984; Gillberg, 1983; Jorgensen *et al.*, 1984; Kerbeshian, Burd & Martsoff, 1984; Levitas *et al.*, 1983; McGillivray *et al.*, 1986; Watson *et al.*, 1984). In short, the information available is insufficient for making conclusions as to a possible role for genetic factors in hyperactivity disorder. Research that surmounts the current methodological limitations is required.

ENVIRONMENTAL TOXINS

Lead affects the brain and causes serious encephalopathy. Moreover, a high concentration of body lead is associated with low IQ and behaviour disturbances (Needleman *et al.*, 1979; Yule *et al.*, 1981; Winneke, 1983). The specificity of the relation between the presence of a high lead concentration and hyperactive behaviour, however, has not been established. Nor has the question been answered of whether lesser degrees of exposure to lead affect cognition and behaviour. David and his co-workers (David, Clarke & Voeller, 1972; David *et al.*, 1977) hypothesised that lead has an aetiological function in hyperactivity on the basis of their findings that children with no other known cause of hyperactivity had higher lead concentrations than the controls. Gittelman and Eskenazi (1983) found no clear-cut relation between lead concentrations and the cognitive performances of hyperactive children and no significant elevation of lead concentrations in hyperactive children. Therefore, the findings of David and his co-workers could not reproduced. Several research groups have used multivariate statistical techniques to examine whether there is a direct relation between lead concentrations and disordered psychological function when environmental factors are taken into consideration. All found that the relation was attenuated by this correction. Some found that it remained statistically significant (Ernhart, Landa & Schell, 1981; Needleman, 1983), others that it did not (Smith *et al.*, 1983; Winneke, 1983). The tentative conclusion is that lead exposure is not the major cause of hyperactivity, that it is neither a necessary nor (except at very high doses) a sufficient cause, and that its weak contributory effect is probably not specific to hyperactivity disorders (Taylor, 1986).

FOOD ADDITIVES

In 1975, Feingold proposed a relation between hyperactivity and such food additives as synthetic colourings, flavourings and preservatives, as well as naturally occurring salicylates in fruits (Feingold, 1975*a,b*). That proposal received widespread publicity without appropriate controlled clinical trials (Rowe, 1988). Subsequent clinical trials that examined the Feingold hypothesis produced inconclusive results (Cook & Woodhill, 1976; Conners *et al.*, 1976; Williams *et al.*, 1978; Harley *et al.*, 1978; Goyette *et al.*, 1978; Weiss *et al.*, 1980; Mattes & Gittelman-Klein, 1978; David, 1987) mainly because the findings have been confounded by logistic and methodological difficulties, the use of varying and imprecise diagnostic criteria for hyperactivity, and the dubious validity and reliability of behavioural outcome measures (Rowe, 1988).

Results from more detailed studies suggest that the non-specific psychological effects of the Feingold diet are likely to be much greater than the specific ones. The outcomes of double-blind trials suggest that specific effects were unusual (Conners *et al.*, 1976; Harley *et al.*, 1978). Egger and his co-workers (1985), however, found that 82% of 76 children with hyperkinetic syndrome of hyperactive behaviour disturbance responded during the open phase of oligoantigentic treatment. Indeed, the parents and paediatricians found that placebo treatment was effective for 80% of 28 responders who participated in the double-blind trial. These results are statistically significant. The subjects were not, however, typical of the hyperkinetic children in the general population, as many had allergic disorders. The rate of atropy in children with hyperkinetic syndrome is about the same as that in the general population (Graham, 1989). Taylor *et al.* (1991) made a random selection of 20 hyperactive and 20 control boys, and obtained answers from 17 of the hyperactives and 19 of the controls. The respondent groups were compared as to medical diagnoses of allergic disorder and the allergic symptoms of red eyes, running nose, wheezing, night cough, mouth ulcers, abdominal bloating, colic, headaches, eczema, excessive thirst, and dark circles under the eyes. The only significant difference found was for excessive thirst. This was mentioned by 7 of the 17 pervasively and persistently hyperactive boys but by only one of the 19 controls. These results fail to support the claim that atopic symptoms are very much more common in hyperactive children (McGee, Stanton & Sears, 1993). There is considerable need to reproduce the results described in the study done by Egger and his group on children who do not show such marked evidence of atopy.

David (1987) investigated 24 children claimed by parents to have definite adverse responses to tartrazine and benzoic acid. No change in behaviour was noted by the parents or nursing staff after the administration of placebos or the active substances. Twenty-two (91.7%) of these children returned to a normal diet without exacerbation. Rowe (1988) subjected 55 heterogeneously hyperactive children to a six-week trial of the Feingold diet. Forty (72.7%) showed improved behaviour and 26 (47.3%) remained improved for 3–6 months after cessation of the diet. A double-blind crossover study was then conducted on 8 of 14 children whose parents claimed that a particular cluster of behaviour was associated with the ingestion of foods containing synthetic colourings. The subjects were kept on a diet free from synthetic additives for 18 weeks and were challenged daily with a placebo or 50 mg of tartrazine or carmoisine. Two significant responders were identified whose behavioural patterns featured extreme irritability, restlessness and sleep disturbance. Rowe has pointed out that the strict criteria followed for inclusion in studies concerned with hyperactivity based on ADD may miss children who show behavioural changes associated with the ingestion of food colourings. Kaplan and his associates (1989) subjected 24 preschool children with ADDH to a controlled trial of their experimental diet. This diet is broader than those used previously in that it eliminates not only artificial colours and flavours but also chocolate, monosodium glutamate, preservatives, caffeine, and any substance that families report might affect a specific child. This diet also is low in simple sugars. More than half the subjects exhibited reliable improvement in behaviour and negligible placebo effects.

The trials run by Egger's and Kaplan's groups probably were based on atypical assemblages of hyperactive children and must be interpreted accordingly (Taylor *et al.*, 1991). Marshall (1989) hypothesised that allergic reactions engender cholinergic/adrenergic activity imbalances in the central nervous system, leading to poorly regulated arousal levels and ADHD behaviour in a small subgroup of children with ADHD; but, it is most unlikely that an allergic mechanism has a major function in the pathogenesis of hyperactivity disorder. Weiss (1982) reviewed the literature and concluded that Feingold, to some extent, is correct. Several well-controlled studies suggest that, in the population of children diagnosed with ADD, there is evidence of behavioural improvement when the Feingold diet is used in perhaps 5-10% of the children (Varley, 1984), and that at least 19 (24%) of 78 hyperactive children on a few foods elimination diet improved in their behaviour, and worsened on the reintroduction of the provoking foods (Carter *et al.*, 1993). It might be likely that particular foods and/or food additives have a certain role in causing hyperactive behaviour in some cases.

CONCLUSION

The aetiology and pathogenesis of hyperactivity disorders have been continuously and intensively investigated by epidemiological, diagnostic, neuropsychological, genetic, sociopsychological and biological approaches. The known results of biological, primarily neurochemical, investigations have been reviewed in this chapter. Now evidence is constantly accumulating but, because of methodological limitations, we still do not have a non-contradictory hypothesis that explains the pathogenesis of hyperactivity disorders. Dysfunction of multi-neurotransmitter systems is the most plausible hypothesis so far. Improvement of the methodology and techniques used to study hyperactivity disorders, and more rigorous research to establish their aetiology and pathogenesis are urgently needed.

REFERENCES

American Psychiatric Association (1980). Diagnostic statistical manual of mental disorders (3rd edn). Washington, DC: American Psychiatric Association.

American Psychiatric Association (1987). Diagnostic statistical manual of mental disorders (3rd edn. revised). Washington, DC: American Psychiatric Association.

Andreasen, N.C. (1988). Brain imaging:application in psychiatry. *Science* **239**, 1381–8.

Arnold, L., Wender, P., McColskey, K. & Synder, S.H. (1972). Levoamphetamine and dextroamphetamine: Comparative efficacy in the hyperkinetic syndrome: assessment by target symptoms. *Archives of General Psychiatry,* **27**, 816–22.

August, G.J. & Lockhart, L.H. (1984). Familial autism and the fragile X chromosome. *Journal of Autism and Developmental Disorders,* **14**, 197–204.

Baraban, J.H. & Aghajanian, G.K. (1981). Noradrenergic innervation of serotoninergic neurones in the dorsal raphe: demonstration by electronmicroscopic autoradiography. *Brain Research,* **204**, 1–11.

Bender, L. (1947). Childhood schizophrenia:a clinical study of 100 schizophrenic children. *American Journal of Orthopsychiatry,* **17**, 40–56.

Bhagauan, H.N., Coleman, M. & Coursina, D.B. (1975). The effect of pyridoxine hydrochloride on blood serotonin and pyridoxal phosphate contents in hyperactive children. *Pediatrics,* **55**, 437–41.

Biederman, J., Gastfriend,D.R. & Jellinek, M.S. (1986). Desipramine in the treatment of children with attention deficit disorder. *Journal of Clinical Psychopharmacology,* **6**, 359–63.

Biederman, J., Munir, K., Knee, D., Habelow, W., Armentano, M., Autor, S., Hoge, S.K. & Waternaux, C. (1986). A family study of patients with attention deficit disorder and normal controls. *Journal of Psychiatric Research,* **20**, 263–74.

Biederman, J., Munir, K. & Knee, D. (1987). Conduct and oppositional disorder in clinically referred children with attention deficit disorder: a controlled family study. *Journal of the American Academy of Child and Adolescent Psychiatry,* **26**, 724–7.

Blier, P., DeMontigny, C. & Chaput, Y. (1987). Modification of the serotonin system by antidepressant treatments: implications for the therapeutic response in major depression. *Journal of Clinical Psychopharmacology,* **7**, 24–35S.

Blomquist, H.K., Bohman, M., Edvinsson,S.O., Gillberg, C., Gustavon, K-H., Holmgren, C. & Wahlstrom, J. (1985). Frequency of the fragile X syndrome in infantile autism: a Swedish multicenter study. *Clinical Genetics,* **27**, 113–17.

Bohman, M. & Sigvardsson, S. (1980). A prospective longitudinal study of children registered for adoption. *Acta Psychiatrica Scandinavica,* **61**, 339–55.

Bohman, M., Cloninger, C.R., Sigvardsson, S. & von Knorring, A.-L. (1982). Predispostion to petty criminality in Swedish adoptees: I. Genetic and environmental heterogeneity. *Archives of General Psychiatry,* **29**, 1233–41.

Bregman, J.D., Leckman, J.F. & Ort,S.I. (1988). Fragile X syndrome: Genetic predisposition to psychopathology. *Journal of Autism and Developmental Disorders,* **18**, 343–54.

Brown, G.L., Ebert, M.H., Hunt, R.D. & Rapoport, J.L. (1981). Urinary 3-methoxy-4-hydroxyphenylglycol and homovanillic acid response to D-amphetamine in hyperactive children. *Biological Psychiatry,* **16**, 779–87.

Brown, G.J., Murphy, D.L., Langer, D.H., Ebert, M.H., Post, R.M. & Bunney, W.E., Jr. (1984). Monoamine enzymes in hyperactivity: response to d-amphetamine. Paper presented at the annual meeting for the American Psychiatric Association, Toronto.

Brown, W.T., Jenkins, E.C., Friedman, E., Brooks, J., Wisniewski, K., Raguthu, S. & French, J. (1982). Autism is associated with the fragile X syndrome. *Journal of Autism and Developmental Disorders,* **12**, 303–8.

Callaway, E., Halliday, R. & Naylor, H. (1983). Hyperactive children's event-related potentials fail to support underarousal and maturational-lag theories. *Archives of General Psychiatry,* **40**, 1243–8.

Cantwell, D. (1972). Psychiatric illness in the families of hyperactive children. *Archives of General Psychiatry,* **27**, 414–17.

Cantwell, D. (1975). Genetic studies of hyperactive children: psychiatric illness in biologic and adopting parents. In, *Genetic Research in Psychiatry*, eds. R. Fieve *et al.*, pp. 273–80. Baltimore: Johns Hopkins University Press.

Caparulo, B., Cohen, D., Rothman, S., Young, G., Katz, N., Shaywitz, S. & Shaywitz, B. (1981). Computed tomographic brain scanning in children with developmental neuropsychiatric disorders. *Journal of the American Academy of Child and Adolescent Psychiatry,* **20**, 338–57.

Carter, C.M., Urbanowicz, M., Hemsley, R., Mantilla, L., Strobel, S., Graham, P.J. & Taylor, E. (1993). Effects of a few food diet in attention deficit disorder. *Archives of Disease in Childhood,* **69**, 564–8.

Church, W.H., Justice, J.B.Jr. & Neill,D.B. (1987). Detecting behaviourally relevant changes in extracellular dopamine with microdialysis. *Brain Research,* **412**, 397–9.

Coleman, M. (1971). Serotonin concentrations in whole blood of hyperactive children. *Journal of Pediatrics,* **78**, 985–90.

Colton, T. (1974). *Statistics in Medicine*. Boston: Little, Brown.

Conners, C.K., Goyette, C.H., Southwick, D.A., Lees, J.M. & Andrulonis, P. (1976). Food additives and hyperkinesis: a controlled double-blind experiment. *Pediatrics,* **58**, 154–66.

Cook, P.S. & Woodhill, J.M. (1976). The Feingold dietary treatment of the hyperkinetic syndrome. *Medical Journal of Australia,* **2**, 85–90.

Cooper, J.R., Bloom, F.E. & Roth, R.H. (1982). The Biochemical Basis of Neuropharmacology, 4th edn. New York: Oxford University Press.

Courchesne, E. (1987). A neurophysiological view of autism. In *Neurobiological Issues in Autism,* eds. E.Schopler & G.B. Mesibov, pp. 285–324. New York: Plenum Press.

Cunningham, C.E. & Barkley, R.A. (1978). The effects of methylphenidate on the mother–child interactions of hyperactive identical twins. *Developmental Medicine and Child Neurology,* **20**, 634–42.

Cunningham, L., Cadoret, R., Loftus, R. & Edwards, J.E. (1975). Studies of adoptees from psychiatrically disturbed biological parents. *British Journal of Psychiatry,* **126**, 534–9.

David, O., Clarke, J. & Voeller, K. (1972). Lead and hyperactivity. *Lancet,* **ii**, 900–3.

David, O.J. Hoffman, S.P. Sverd, J. & Clark, J. (1977). Lead and hyperactivity: lead levels among hyperactive children. *Journal of Abnormal Child Psychology,* **5**, 405–16.

David, T.J. (1987). Reaction to dietary tartrazine. *Archives of Diseases in Childhood,* **62**, 119–22.

Dawson-Sanders, B. & Trapp, R.G. (1990). *Basic and Clinical Biostatistics*. Connecticut: Appleton & Lange.

De Arce, M. & Kearns, A. (1984). The fragile X syndrome: the patients and their chromosomes. *Journal of Medical Genetics,* **21**, 84–91.

Donchin, E., Heffly, E., Hillyard, S.A., Loveless, N., Maltzman, I., Ohman, A., Rosler, F., Ruchkin, D. & Siddle, D. (1984). Cognition and event-related potentials: II. The orienting reflex and P300. In *Brain and Information: Event-related Potentials*, eds. R. Karrer, J. Cohen, & P. Tueting, *Annals of the New York Academy of Science,* **425**, 39–57.

Donnelly, M., Rapoport, J.L., & Ismond, D.R. (1986*a*). Fenfluramine treatment of childhood attention deficit disorder with hyperactivity: a preliminary report. *Psychopharmacology Bulletin,* **22**, 152–4.

Donnelly, M., Zametkin, A.J., Rapoport, J.L., Ismond, D.R., Weingartner, H., Lane, E., Oliver, J., Linnoila, M. & Potter, W. (1986*b*). Treatment of childhood hyperactivity with desipramine: plasma drug concentration, cardiovascular effects, plasma and urinary catecholamine levels, and clinical response. *Clinical Pharmacology and Therapeutics,* **39**, 72–81.

Dray, A., Gonye, T.J., Oakley, N.R. & Tanner, T. (1976). Evidence for the existence of a raphe projection to the substantia nigra in the rat. *Brain Research,* **113**, 45–57.

Dykman, R.A., Holcomb, P.J., Oglesby, D.M. & Ackerman, P.T. (1982). Electrocortical frequencies in hyperactive, learning-disabled, mixed and normal children. *Biological Psychiatry,* **17**, 675–86.

Egger, J., Carter,C.M., Graham, P.J., Gumley, D. & Soothill, J.F. (1985). Controlled trial of oligoantigenic treatment in the hyperkinetic syndrome. *Lancet,* **i**, 540–5.

Elia, J., Gulotta, C., Rose, S.R., Marin, G. & Rapoport, J.L. (1994). Thyroid function and attention-deficit hyperactivity disorder. *Journal of American Academy of Child and Adolescent Psychiatry,* **33**, 169–72.

Ernhart, C.B., Landa, B. & Schell, N.B. (1981). Subclinical levels of lead and developmental deficit – a multivariate follow-up reassessment. *Pediatrics,* **67**, 911–19.

Faull, K.F., Kraemer, H.C., Barchas, J.D. & Berger, P.A. (1981). Clinical application of the probenecid test for measurement of monoamine turnover in the CNS. *Biological Psychiatry,* **16**, 879–99.

Feingold, B.F. (1975*a*). Hyperkinesis and learning disabilities linked to artificial food flavors and colors. *American Journal of Nursing,* **75**, 797–803.

Feingold, B.F. (1975*b*). *Why Your Child is Hyperactive*. New York: Random House.

Ferguson, H.B., Pappas, B.A., Trites, R.L., Peters, D.A.V. & Taub, H. (1981). Plasma free and total tryptophan, blood serotonin, and the hyperactivity syndrome: no evidence for the serotonin deficiency hypothesis. *Biological Psychiatry,* **16**, 231–38.

Ferguson, H.B. & Rapoport, J.L. (1983). Nosological issues and biological validation. In M. Rutter (ed.), *Developmental Neuropsychiatry*, pp. 369–384. New York: Guilford Press.

Finelli, P., Pueschel, S.M., Padre-Mendoza, T. & O'Brien, M. (1985). Neurological findings in patients with the fragile-X syndrome. *Journal of Neurology, Neurosurgery, and Psychiatry,* **48**, 150–3.

Fryns, J.P., Jacobs, J., Kleczkowska, A. & Van den Berghe, H. (1984). The psychological profile of the fragile X syndrome. *Clinical Genetics,* **25**, 131–4.

Fuller, R.W., Perry, K.W., Bymaster, F.P. & Wong, D.T. (1978). Comparative effects of pemoline, amfoelic acid, and amphetamine on dopamine uptake and release in vitro on brain 3,4- dihydroxy-phenylacetic acid concentration on spiperone-treated rats. *Journal of Pharmacy and Pharmacology,* **30**, 197–8.

Garfinkel, B.D., Wender, P.H., Sloman, L., & O'Neill, I. (1983). Tricyclic antidepressant and methylphenidate treatment of attention deficit disorder in children. *Journal of the American Academy of Child and Adolescent Psychiatry,* **22**, 343–8.

Gastfriend, D.R., Biederman, J. & Jellinek, M.S. (1984). Desipramine in the treatment of adolescents with attention deficit disorder. *American Journal of Psychiatry,* **141**, 906–8.

Gillberg, G. (1983). Identical triplets with infantile autism and the fragile X syndrome. *British Journal of Psychiatry,* **143**, 256–60.

Gittelman, R. & Eskenazi, B. (1983). Lead and hyperactivity revisited: an investigation of nondisadavantaged children. *Archives of General Psychiatry,* **40**, 827–33.

Gittleman-Klein, R., Klein, D.F., Katz, S., Saraf, K. & Pollack, E. (1976). Comparative effects of methylphenidate and thioridazine in hyperkinetic children. *Archives of General Psychiatry,* **33**, 1217–31.

Goldberg, L.I., Volkman, P.H. & Kohli, J.D. (1978). A comparison of the vascular dopamine receptor with other dopamine receptors. *Annual Review of Pharmacology and Toxicology,* **18**, 57–79.

Goodman, R. & Stevenson, J. (1989). A twin study of hyperactivity: II. The etiological role of genes, family relationships and perinatal adversity. *Journal of Child Psychology and Psychiatry,* **30**, 691–709.

Goyette, C.H., Conners, C.K., Petti, P.A. & Curtis, L.E. (1978). Effects of artificial colours on hyperactive children: a double-blind challenge study. *Psychopharmacology Bulletin,* **14**, 39–40.

Graham, P.J. (1989). Practical aspects of dietary management of the hyperkinetic syndrome. In *Attention Deficit Disorders: Clinical and Basic Research,* eds. T. Sagvolden & T. Archer, pp. 181–190. Hillsdale: Lawrence Erlbaum Associates.

Greenberg, A.S. & Coleman, M. (1973). Use of blood serotonin levels for the classification and treatment of hyperactive behaviour disorders. *Neurology,* **23**, 428.

Greenberg, A.S. & Coleman, M. (1976). Depressed 5-hydroxyindoleacetic acid levels associated with hyperactive and aggressive behaviour. *Archives of General Psychiatry,* **33**, 331–6.

Grunewald-Zuberbeiter, E., Grunewald, G. & Raske, A. (1975). Hyperactive behaviour and EEG arousal reactions in children. *Electroencephalography and Clinical Neurophysiology,* **38**, 149–59.

Halaris, A.E., Belendiuk, K.T. & Freedman, D.X. (1975). Antidepressant drugs affect dopamine uptake. *Biochemical Pharmacology,* **24**, 1896–8.

Harcherik, D.F., Cohen, D.J., Ort, S., Paul, R., Shaywitz, B.A., Volkmar, F.R., Rothman, S.L.G. & Leckman, J.F. (1985). Computed tomographic brain scanning in four neuropsychiatric disorders of childhood. *American Journal of Psychiatry,* **142**, 731–4.

Harley, J.P., Ray, R.S., Tomasi, L., Eichman, P.L., Matthews, C.G., Chun, R., Cleeland, C.S. & Traisman, E. (1978). Hyperkinesis and food additives: testing the Feingold hypothesis. *Pediatrics,* **61**, 818–28.

Haslam, R.H.A. & Dalby, J.T. (1983). Blood serotonin levels in the attention deficit disorder. *New England Journal of Medicine,* **309**, 1328.

Hauser, P., Zametkin, A.J., Martinez, P., Viliello, B., Matochik, J.A., Mixon, J. & Weintraub, B.D. (1993). Attention deficit hyperactivity disorder in people with generalised resistance to thyroid hormone. *New England Journal of Medicine,* **328**, 997–1001.

Heffron, W.A., Martin, C.A. & Welsh, R.J. (1984). Attention deficit disorder in three pairs of monozygotic twins: a case report. *Journal of the American Academy of Child and Adolescent Psychiatry,* **23**, 299–301.

Holcomb, P.J. & Dykman, R.A. (1983). Late ERP components in ADD, RD, and normal boys. *Psychophysiology,* **20**, 446.

Holcomb, P.J., Ackerman, P.T. & Dykman, R.A. (1986). Auditory event-related potentials in attention and reading disabled boys. *International Journal of Psychophysiology,* **3**, 263–73.

Hynd, G.W., Hern,K.L., Novey, E.S., Eliopulos, D., Marshall, R., Gonzalez, J.J. & Voeller, K.K. (1993). Attention deficit–hyperactivity disorder and asymmetry of the caudate nucleus. *Journal of Child Neurology,* **8**, 339–47.

Ionescu, G., Kiehl, R., Ona, L. & Wichmann-Kunz, F. (1990). Abnormal plasma catecholamines in hyperkinetic children. *Biological Psychiatry,* **28**, 547–50.

Irwin, M., Belendink, K., McCloskay, K. & Freedman, D.X. (1981). Tryptophan metabolism in children with attention deficit disorder. *American Journal of Psychiatry,* **138**, 1082–85.

Jorgensen, O.S., Nielsen, K.B., Isager, T. & Mouridsen, S.E. (1984). Fragile X chromosome among child psychiatric patients with disturbances of language and social relationships. *Acta Psychiatrica Scandinavica,* **70**, 510–14.

Kaplan, B.J., McNicol, J., Conte, R.A. & Moghadam, H.K. (1989). Dietary replacement in preschool-aged hyperactive boys. *Pediatrics,* **83**, 7–17.

Kerbeshian, J., Burd,L. & Martsoff, J. (1984). A family with fragile X syndrome. *Journal of Nervous and Mental Disease,* **172**, 549–51.

Khan, A.U. & DeKirmenjian, H. (1981). Urinary excretion of catecholamine metabolites in hyperkinetic child syndrome. *American Journal of Psychiatry,* **138**, 108–12.

Kuczenski, R. (1983). Biochemical actions of amphetamines and other stimulants. In

Stimulants: Neurochemical Behaviour and Clinical Perspectives, ed. I. Crease, pp. 31–63. New York: Raven Press.

Kuperman, S., Gaffney, G.R., Hamdan-Allen, G., Preston, D.F. & Venkatesh, L. (1990). Neuroimaging in child and adolescent psychiatry. *Journal of the American Academy of Child and Adolescent Psychiatry,* **29**, 159–72.

Langer, D.H., Rapoport, J.L., Brown, G.L., Ebert, M.H. & Bunney, W.E. (1982). Behavioral effects of carbidopa/levodopa in hyperactive boys. *Journal of the American Academy of Child and Adolescent Psychiatry,* **21**, 10–18.

Largo, R.H. & Schinzel, A. (1985). Developmental and behavioural disturbances in 13 boys with Fragile-X syndrome. *European Journal of Pediatrics,* **143**, 269–75.

Lassen, N.A., Henriksen, L. & Paulson, O.B. (1981). Regional blood flow in stroke by ^{133}Xe inhalation and emission tomography. *Stroke,* **12**, 284–8.

Levitas, A., Hagerman, R.J., Braden, M., Rimland, B., McBogg, P. & Matteus, I. (1983). Autism and the fragile X syndrome. *Journal of Developmental and Behavioural Pediatrics,* **3**, 151–8.

Linnoila, M., Guthrie, S., Lane, E.A., Karoum, F., Rudorfer, M. & Potter, W.Z. (1986). Clinical studies on norepinephrine metabolism: how to interpret numbers. *Psychiatry Research,* **17**, 229–39.

Lipton, S.V., McGouth, T.P. & Shaywitz, B.A. (1980). Effects of apomorphine on escape performance and activity in developing rat pups treated with 6-hydroxydopamine. *Pharmacology Biochemistry Behavior*, **13**, 371–7.

Loiselle, D.L., Stamm, J.S., Maitinsky, S. & Whipple, S. (1980). Evoked potential and behavioural signs of attention dysfunctions in hyperactive boys. *Psychophysiology,* **17**, 193–201.

Lopez, R.C. (1965). Hyperactivity in twins. *Canadian Psychiatric Association Journal,* **10**, 421–6.

Lordon, J.F., Rickert, E.J., Dawson, R. & Pellymounter, M.A. (1980). Forebrain norepinephrine and the selective processing of information. *Brain Research,* **199**, 569.

Lou, H.C., Henriksen, L. & Bruhn, P. (1984). Focal cerebral hypoperfusion in children with dysphasia and/or attention deficit disorder. *Archives of Neurology,* **41**, 825–9.

Lou, H.C., Henriksen, L. & Bruhn, P. (1990). Focal cerebral dysfunction in developmental learning disabilities. *Lancet*, **335**, 8–11.

Lou, H.C., Henriksen, L., Bruhn, P., Børner, H. & Nielsen, J.B. (1989). Striatal dysfunction in attention deficit and hyperkinetic disorder. *Archives of Neurology,* **46,** 48–52.

Maas, J.W., Hattox, S.E., Greene, N.M. & Landis, D.H. (1980). Estimate of dopamine and serotonin synthesis by the awake human brain. *Journal of Neurochemistry*, **34**, 1547–49.

Maas, J.W. & Leckman, J.F. (1983). Relationship between central nervous system noradrenergic function and plasma and urinary MHPG and other metabolites. In *MHPG: Basic Mechanisms in Psychopathology*, ed. J.W. Maas, pp. 33–43. New York: Academic Press.

McGee, R., Stanton, W.R. & Sears, M.R. (1993). Allergic disorders and attention deficit disorder in children. *Journal of Abnormal Child Psychology,* **21**, 79–88.

McGillivray, B.C., Herbst, D.S., Dill, F.J., Sandercock, H.J. & Tischler, B. (1986). Infantile autism: An occasional manifestation of fragile(X) mental retardation. *American Journal of Medical Genetics*, **23**, 353–8.

McMahon, R.C. (1980). Genetic etiology in the hyperactive child syndrome: a critical review. *American Journal of Orthopsychiatry,* **50**, 145–50

Magner, J.A., Petrick, P., Menezes-Ferreira, M.M., Stelling, M. & Weintraub, B.D. (1980). Familial generalised resistance to thyroid hormones: report of three kindreds and correlation of patterns of affected tissues with the binding of [^{125}I] triiodo-thyronine to fibroblast nuclei. *Journal of Endocrinological Investigation,* **9**, 459–70.

Mann, C.A., Lubar, J.F., Zimmerman, A.W., Miller, C.A. & Muenchen, R.A. (1992). Quantitative analysis of EEG in boys with attention-deficit-hyperactivity disorder: Controlled study with clinical implications. *Pediatric Neurology,* **8**, 30–6.

Marshall, P. (1989). Attention deficit disorder and allergy: a neurochemical model of the relation between the illnesses. *Psychological Bulletin*, **106**, 434–46.

Mason, S.T. & Fibiger, H.C. (1978). Noradrenaline and spatial memory. *Brain Research,* **156**, 382–6.

Matsui, T. & Hirano, A. (1977). *Brain Anatomy for CT SCAN*. Tokyo: Igaku Shoin.

Mattes, J.A. & Gittelman-Klein, R. (1978). An intensive cross-over study of the affects of artificial food colorings in a hyperkinetic child. *American Journal of Psychiatry*, **135**, 987–8.

Menachem, E.B., Persson, L., Schechter, P.J., Haegle, K.D., Huebert, N. & Hardensberg, J. (1989). Cerebrospinal fluid parameters in healthy volunteers during serial lumbar punctures. *Journal of Neurochemistry*, **52**, 632–5.

Meryash, D.L., Szymanski, L.S. & Gerald, P.S. (1982). Infantile autism associated with the fragile X syndrome. *Journal of Autism and Developmental Disorders*, **12**, 295–301.

Molina, V.A. & Orsingher, O.A. (1981). Effects of Mg-pencoline on the central catecholaminergic system. *Archives International Pharmadynamic*, **251**, 66–79.

Montagu, J.D. (1975). The hyperactive child: a behavioral, electrodermal, and EEG investigation. *Developmental Medicine and Child Neurology*, **17**, 299–305.

Morrison, J.R. & Stewart, M.A. (1971). A family study of the hyperactive child syndrome. *Biological Psychiatry*, **3**, 189–95.

Morrison, J.R. & Stewart, M.A. (1973). The psychiatric status of the legal families of adopted hyperactive children. *Archives of General Psychiatry*, **3**, 189–95.

Naruse, H., Hayashi, T., Takesada, M., Nakane, A. & Yamazaki, K. (1989). Metabolic changes of aromatic amino acids and monoamines in infantile autism and developement of new treatment related to the finding. *No To Hattatsu*, **21**, 181–9.

Nasrallah, H.A., Loney, J., Olson, S.C., McCalley-Whitters, M., Kramer, J. & Jacoby, C.G. (1986). Cortical atrophy in young adults with a history of hyperactivity in childhood. *Psychiatry Research*, **17**, 241–6.

Needleman, H. (1983). The neuropsychological consequences of low level exposure to lead in childhood. In *Lead Versus Health: Sources and Effects of Low Level Lead Exposure*, eds. M. Rutter & R. Russell Jones. Chichester: Wiley.

Needleman, H., Gunnor, C., Leviton, A., Read, R., Peresie, H., Maher, C. & Barrett, P. (1979). Deficits in psychologic and classroom performances of children with elevated dentine lead levels. *New England Journal of Medicine*, **300**, 689–95.

Nemzer, E.D., Arnold, L.E., Votolato, N.A. & McConnel, H. (1986). Amino acid supplementation as therapy for attention deficit disorder. *Journal of the American Academy of Child and Adolescent Psychiatry*, **25**, 509–13.

Nichols, P.L. & Chen, T.C. (1981). *Minimal Brain Dysfunction: A Prospective study.* Hillsdale: Erlbaum.

Nishizawa, K., Maruyama, T., Iwata, T., Furuya, Y. & Hashizume, T. (1981). Estimation of stochastic risk form computed tomographic examination in Japan, 1979: 3. Estimation of population doses and stochastic risks. *Nippon Acta Radiologica,* **41**, 436–41.

Nurse, B., Russell, V.A. & Taljaard, J.J.F. (1985). Effect of chronic desipramine treatment on adrenoceptor modulation of [^{3}H] dopamine release from rat nucleus accumbens slice. *Brain Research,* **334**, 235–42.

Ornitz, E.E. (1978). Biological homogeneity or heterogeneity? In *Autism: A Reappraisal of Concepts and Treatment*, eds. M. Rutter. & E. Schopler, pp. 243–250. New York: Plenum.

Parenti, M., Tirone, F., Olgiati, V.R. & Groppetti, A. (1983). Presence of opiate receptors on striatal serotoninergic nerve terminals. *Brain Research,* **280**, 317–22.

Potter, W.Z., Scheinin, M., Golden, R.N., Rudorfer, M.V., Cowdry, R.W., Calil, H.M, Ross, R.J. & Linnoila, M. (1985). Selective antidepressants and cerebrospinal fluid: lack of specificity on norepinephrine and serotonin metabolite. *Archives of General Psychiatry,* **42**, 1171–81.

Rapoport, J.L, Quinn, P.O., Bradbard, G., Riddle, K.D. & Brooks, E. (1974*a*). Imipramine and methylphenidate treatments of hyperactive boys. *Archives of General Psychiatry,* **30**, 789–93.

Rapoport, J.L., Quinn, P.O., Scribanic, N. & Murphy, D.L. (1974*b*). Platelet serotonin of hyperactive school age boys. *British Journal of Psychiatry,* **125**, 138–40.

Rapoport, J.L., Mikkelsen, E.J., Ebert, M.H., Brown, G.L., Weise, V.L. & Kopin, I.J. (1978). Urinary catecholamine and amphetamine excretion in hyperactive and normal boys. *Journal of Nervous and Mental Disease,* **166**, 731–7.

Rapoport, T.L., Buchsbaum, M.S. & Weingartner, H. (1980). Dextroamphetamine: its cognitive and behavioural effects in normal and hyperactive boys and normal men. *Archives of General Psychiatry,* **37**, 933–43.

Rapoport, J.L., Zametkin, A., Donnelly, M. & Ismond, D. (1985). New drug trials in attention deficit disorder. *Psychopharmacology Bulletin,* **21**, 232–6.

Raskin, L.A., Shaywitz, S.E., Shaywitz, B.A., Anderson, G.M. & Cohen, D.J. (1984). Neurochemical correlates of attention deficit disorder. *Pediatric Clinics of North America,* **31**, 387–96.

Rasmusson, A.M., Riddle, M.A., Leckman, J.F., Anderson, G.M. & Cohen, D.J. (1990). Neurotransmitter assessment in neuropsychiatric disorders of childhood. In *Application of Basic Neuroscience to Child Psychiatry, eds.* S.I. Deutsch, A. Weizman & R. Weizman, R. (pp. 33–59). New York: Plenum Publishing Corporation.

Refetoff, S. (1990). Resistance to thyroid hormone, *Thyroid Today,* **13**, 1–11.

Riddle, M.A., Hardin, M.T., Cho, S.C., Woolston, J.L. & Leckman, J.F. (1988). Desipramine treatment of boys with attention-deficit hyperactivity disorder and tics: preliminary clinical experience. *Journal of the American Academy of Child and Adolescent Psychiatry,* **27**, 811–14.

Riegelman, R.K. & Hirsch, R.P. (1989). *Studying a Study and Testing a Test*, 2nd edn. Boston: Little, Brown and Company.

Rowe, K.S. (1988). Synthetic food colourings and 'hyperactivity': a double-blind crossover study. *Australian Paediatric Journal,* **24**, 143–7.

Rutter, M. (1981). Psychological sequelae of brain damage in children. *American Journal of Psychiatry,* **138**, 1533–44.

Rutter, M. (1989). Attention deficit disorder/hyperkinetic syndrome: conceptual and research issues regarding diagnosis and classification. In *Attention Deficit Disorder: Clinical and Basic Research*, eds. T. Sagvolden & T. Archer, pp. 1–24. Hillsdale: Lawrence Erlbaum Associates.

Rutter, M., Tizard, J. & Whitmore, K. (1970). *Education, Health and Behaviour*. London: Longmans.

Rutter, M., MacDonald, H., Le Couteur, A., Harrington, R., Bolton, O. & Bailey, A. (1990). Genetic factors in child psychiatric disorders. II. Empirical findings. *Journal of Child Psychology and Psychiatry,* **31**, 39–83.

Safer, D.J. (1973). A familial factor in minimal brain dysfunction. *Behaviour Genetics,* **3**, 175–186.

Sagvolden, T. & Archer, T. (1989). *Attention Deficit Disorder: Clinical and Basic Research* pp. 25–29. Hillsdale: Lawrence Erlbaum Associates.

Satterfield, J.H. & Schell, A.M. (1984). Childhood brain function differences in delinquent and non-delinquent hyperactive boys. *Electroencephalography and Clinical Neurology,* **57**, 199–207.

Satterfield, D.H., Lisser, L.I., Sand, R.E. & Cantwell, D.P. (1973). EEG aspects of the diagnosis and treatment of minimal brain dysfunction. *Annals of the New York Academy of Sciences,* **205**, 273–82.

Satterfield, J.H., Schell, A.M. & Backs, R.W. (1987). Longitudinal study of AERPs in hyperactive and normal children: relationship to antisocial behaviour. *Electroencephalography and Clinical Neurophysiology,* **67**, 531–6.

Satterfield, J.H., Schell, A.M., Nicholas, T. & Backs, R.W. (1988). Topographic study of auditory event-related potentials in normal boys and boys with attention deficit disorder with hyperactivity, *Psychophysiology,* **25**, 591–606.

Schachar, R. (1991). Childhood hyperactivity. *Journal of Child Psychology and Psychiatry,* **32**, 155–91.

Shaffer, D., O'Connor, P.A., Shafer, S.Q. & Prupis, S. (1983). Neurological 'soft signs': their origins and significance for behaviour. In *Developmental neuropsychiatry*, ed. M. Rutter, pp. 144–163. New York: Guilford Press.

Shaywitz, B.A., Cohen, D.J. & Bowers, M.B. (1977). CSF monoamine metabolites in children with minimal brain dysfunction: evidence for alteration of brain dopamine. *Journal of Pediatrics,* **90**, 67–71.

Shaywitz, B.A., Klopper, J.H. & Gordon, J.W. (1978). Methylphenidate in 6-hydroxydopamine-treated developing rat pups. *Archives of Neurology,* **35**, 463–9.

Shaywitz, S.E. & Shaywitz, B.A. (1982). Biological influences in attentional disorders. In *Developmental Behavioural Pediatrics*, eds. M.D. Levine, W.B. Carey, A.C. Crocker *et al.*, pp. 746–755. Philadelphia: W.B. Saunders.

Shaywitz, S.E. & Shaywitz, B.A. (1989). Critical issues in attention deficit disorder. In *Attention Deficit Disorder: Clinical and Basic Research*, eds. T. Sagvolden & T. Archer, pp. 53–69. Hillsdale: Lawrence Erlbaum Associates.

Shaywitz, B.A., Shaywitz, S.E. Byrne, T., Cohen, D.J. & Rothman, S. (1983). Attention deficit disorder: quantitative analysis of CT. *Neurology,* **33**, 1500–3.

Shaywitz, B.A., Yager, R.D. & Klopper, J.H. (1976*a*). Selective brain dopamine depletion in developing rats: an experimental model of minimal brain dysfunction. *Science,* **191**, 305–8.

Shaywitz, B.A., Yager, R.D., Klopper, J.H. & Gordon, J.W. (1976*b*). Paradoxical response to amphetamine in developing rats treated with 6-hydroxydopamine. *Nature,* **261**, 153–5.

Shekim, W.O., DeKirmenjian, H. & Chapel, J.L. (1977). Urinary catecholamine metabolites in hyperkinetic boys treated with D-amphetamine. *American Journal of Psychiatry,* **134**, 1276–79.

Shekim, W.O., DeKirmenjian, H. & Chapel, J.L. (1979). Urinary MHPG excretion in minimal brain dysfunction and its modification by D-amphetamine. *American Journal of Psychiatry,* **136**, 667–71.

Shekim, W.O., Davis, L.G., Bylund, D.B., Brunngraber, E., Fikes, L. & Lanham, J. (1982). Platelet MAO in children with attention deficit disorder and hyperactivity: a pilot study. *American Journal of Psychiatry,* **139**, 936–8.

Shekim, W.O., Javaid, J., Davis, J.M. & Bylund, D.B. (1983). Urinary MHPG and HVA excretion in boys with attention deficit disorder and hyperactivity treated with D-amphetamine. *Biological Psychiatry,* **18**, 707–14.

Shetty, T. (1971). Alpha rhythms in the hyperkinetic child. *Nature* (*London*), **234**, 476.

Shetty, T. & Chase, T.N. (1976). Central monamines and hyperactivity of childhood, *Neurology.* **26**, 1000–2.

Simon, H., LeMoal, M., Stinus, L., & Calas, A. (1979). Anatomical relationships between the ventral mesencephalic tegmentum-A10 region and the locus coeruleus as demonstrated by antegrade and retrograde tracing techniques. *Journal of Neural Transmission,* **44**, 77–86.

Singer, H.S., Reiss, A.L., Brown, J.E., Aylward, E.H., Shih, B., Chee, E., Harris, E.L., Reader, M.J., Chase, G.A., Bryan, R.N. & Denckla, M.B. (1993). Volumetric MRI changes in basal ganglia of children with Tourette's syndrome. *Neurology,* **43**, 950–6.

Smith, M., Delves, T., Lansdown, R., Clayton, B. & Graham, P. (1983). The effects of lead exposure on urban children: The Institute of Child Health/Southampton Study. *Developmental Medicine and Child Neurology,* **47**, Suppl., 1–54.

Sokoloff, L. (1981). Localization of functional activity in the central nervous system by measurements of glucose utilisation with radioactive deoxyglucose. *Journal of Cerebral Blood Flow and Metabolism,* **1**, 7–36.

Sutton, S. & Ruchkin, D.S. (1984). The late positive complex: advances and new problems. In *Brain and Information: Event-related Potentials*, eds. R. Karrer, J. Cohen & P. Tueting. *Annals of the New York Academy of Sciences,* **425**, 1–23S.

Swann, A.C., Mass, J.W., Hattox, S.E. & Landis, D.H. (1980). Catecholamine metabolites in human plasma as indices of brain function: effects of debrisoquin. *Life Sciences,* **27**, 1857–61.

Taylor, E.A. (1986). The causes and development of hyperactive behaviour, In*The Overactive Child*, ed. E.A. Taylor, pp. 118–160. London: Spastics International Medical Publications.

Taylor, E., Sandberg, S., Thorley, G. & Giles, S. (1991). *The Epidemiology of Childhood Hyperactivity.* Oxford: Oxford University Press.

Ungerstedt, U. (1984). Measurement of neurotransmitter release by intracranial dialysis. In *Measurement of Neurotransmitter Release In Vivo*, ed. C.A. Marsden, pp. 81–105. New York: Wiley.

Varley, C.K. (1984). Diet and the behaviour of children with attention deficit disorder. *Journal of the American Academy of Child and Adolescent Psychiatry,* **23**, 182–5.

Voeller, K.K.S. (1986). Right-hemisphere deficit syndrome in children. *American Journal of Psychiatry,* **143**, 1004–9.

Watson, M.S., Leckman, J.F., Annex, B., Breg, W.R., Boles, D., Volkmar, F.R., Cohen, D.J. & Carter, C. (1984). Fragile X in a survey of 75 autistic males. *New England Journal of Medicine,* **310**, 1462.

Weiss, B. (1982). Food additives and environmental chemicals as sources of childhood behaviour disorders. *Journal of the American Academy of Child and Adolescent Psychiatry,* **21**, 144–52.

Weiss, B., Williams, J.H., Margen, S., Abrams, B., Cann, B., Cirron, L., Cox, C., Mckibben, J., Ogar, D. & Schultz, S. (1980). Behavioural response to artificial food colours. *Science,* **207**, 1487–89.

Weiss R.E., Stein, M.A., Trommer, B. & Refetoff, S. (1993). Attention-deficit hyperactivity disorder and thyroid function. *Journal of Pediatrics,* **123**, 539–45.

Weizman, A., Weitz, R., Szekely, G.A., Tyano, S. & Belmaker, R.H. (1984). Combination of neuroleptic and stimulant treatment in attention deficit disorder with hyperactivity. *Journal of the American Academy of Child and Adolescent Psychiatry,* **32**, 295–8.

Weizman, R., Weizman, A. & Deutsch, S.I. (1990). Biological studies of attention-deficit disorder. In *Application of Basic Neuroscience to Child Psychiatry*, eds. S.I. Deutsch, A. Weizman & R. Weizman, pp. 231–239. New York: Plenum Publishing Corporation.

Wender, P., Epstein, R.S., Kopin, I.J. & Gordon, E.K. (1971). Urinary monoamine metabolites in children with minimal brain dysfunction. *American Journal of Psychiatry,* **127**, 1411–15.

Werry, J.S., Minde, K., Guzman, A., Weiss, G., Dogan, K. & Hay, E. (1972). Studies on the hyperactive child–VII:neurological status compared with neurotic and normal children. *American Journal of Orthopsychiatry,* **42**, 441–50.

Willerman, L. (1973). Activity level and hyperactivity in twins. *Child Development,* **44,** 288–93.

Williams, J.I., Cram, D.M., Tausig, F.T. & Webster, E. (1978). Relative effects of drugs and diet on hyperactive behaviours: an experimental study. *Pediatrics,* **61**, 811–17.

Winneke, G. (1983). Neurobehavioural and neuropsychological effects of lead. In *Lead Versus Health: Sources and Effects of Low Level Lead Exposure*, eds. M. Rutter & Russel Jones, R. Chichester: Wiley.

Winsberg, B.G. & Yepes, L.E. (1978). Antipsychotics (major tranquilizers, neuroleptics). In *Pediatric Psychopharmacology: The Use of Behaviour Modifying Drugs in Children*, ed. J.S. Werry, pp. 234–273. New York: Brunner/Mazel.

World Health Organisation (1978). International Classification of Diseases, 9th edn. Geneva: World Health Organisation.

World Health Organisation (1988). ICD-10: 1988 Draft of Chapter V. Categories F00-99. *Mental, Behavioural and Developmental Disorders*. Geneva: World Health Organisation.

Young J.G., Cohen, D.J., Waldo, M.C., Feiz, R. & Roth, J.A. (1980). Platelet monoamine oxidase activity in children and adolescents with psychiatric disorders. *Schizophrenia Bulletin*, **6**, 324–33.

Yu-cun, S. & Yu-feng, W. (1984). Urinary 3-methoxy-4-hydroxyphenylglycol sulfate excretion in seventy-three school children with minimal brain dysfunction syndrome. *Biological Psychiatry*, **19**, 861–70.

Yule, W., Lansdown, R., Millar, I.B. & Urbanowicz, M.A. (1981). The relationship between lead concentration, intelligence and attainment in a school population: a pilot study. *Developmental Medicine and Child Neurology*, **23**, 567–76.

Yuwiler, A. & Freedman, D.X. (1987). Neurotransmitter research in autism. In *Neurobiological Issues in Autism*, eds. E. Schopler & G.B. Mesibov, pp. 263–284. New York: Plenum Press.

Zametkin, A.J. Rapoport, J.L. (1987). Neurobiology of attention deficit disorder with hyperactivity: where have we come in 50 years? *Journal of the American Academy of Child and Adolescent Psychiatry*, **26**, 676–86.

Zametkin, A.J., Karoum, F., Linnoila, M., Rapoport, J.L., Brown, G.J., Chuang, L.W. & Wyatt, R.J. (1985*a*). Stimulants, urinary catecholamines, and indoleamines in hyperactivity: a comparison of methylphenidate and dextroamphetamine. *Archives of General Psychiatry*, **42**, 251–5.

Zamekin, A.J., Rapoport, J.L., Murphy, D.L., Linnoila, M. & Ismond, D. (1985*b*). Treatment of hyperactive children with monoamine oxidase inhibitors. I: Clinical efficacy. *Archives of General Psychiatry*, **42**, 962–9.

Zametkin, A.J., Rapoport, J.L., Murphy, D.L., Linnoila, M., Karoum, F., Potter, W.Z. & Ismond, D. (1985*c*). Treatment of hyperactive children with monoamine oxidase inhibitors. II: plasma and urinary monoamine findings after treatment, *Archives of General Psychiatry*, **42**, 969–73.

Zametkin, A.J., Nordhal,T.E., Gross, M., King, A.C., Semple, W.E., Rumsey, J., Hamburger, S. & Cohen, R.M. (1990). Cerebral glucose metabolism in adults with hyperactivity of childhood onset. *New England Journal of Medicine*, **323**, 1361–6.

8

Psychosocial contributions

Seija Sandberg and M. Elena Garralda

INTRODUCTION

Environmental and psychosocial factors such as socio-economic deprivation, intrafamilial adversity and dysfunctional parent child relationships have for long been acknowledged as risk factors for disruptive behaviour disorders in children. Whether the same factors also contribute to the causal processes of one particular subtype of behaviour disorder, namely hyperactivity, continues to remain an open question in spite of an increasing number of studies focusing on the issue lately. A reason that has persistently hampered most attempts to clarify this situation is a failure of the particular studies to distinguish between children suffering from pure hyperactivity on the one hand, and the mixed hyperactivity conduct disorder on the other. This is in spite of clear and consistent research evidence suggesting that these two types of externalising behaviour disorder coexist in the majority of children identified as hyperactive, both in clinic-referred (Sandberg, Rutter & Taylor, 1978) and in general population samples (Sandberg, Wieselberg & Shaffer, 1980; Szatmari, Offord & Boyle, 1989). It is therefore surprising that, in many studies, the issue of comorbidity between hyperactivity and conduct disorder continues to be ignored (e.g. Befera & Barkley, 1985; Cunningham & Siegel, 1987). Accordingly, many presumed psychosocial correlates of hyperactivity may in fact be those of conduct disorder, or even non-specific correlates of psychiatric disturbance in general.

There is one possible exception regarding the specificity of psychosocial risk for hyperactivity. This concerns the role that may be played by severely disrupted early attachments (occurring in the context of maternal depression, for example) in contributing to the cause of hyperactivity disorder – particularly when impaired attentional abilities form an essential part of it (Breznitz & Friedman, 1988; Sameroff, Seifer & Zax, 1982).

In this chapter, the aim is to review and discuss the available evidence for psychosocial contributions to childhood hyperactivity. In doing this, as far as it is reasonably possible, the discussion of associated environmental factors will be separated from that of causal or maintaining functions. This is important in order to disentangle the possible mechanisms involved, as well as in striving to avoid unnecessary polarisation of the issues on the lines of the old debate of nature–nurture divide. The second main task is to delineate the likely differential associations and contributions, in terms of psychosocial background factors, to the development of pure hyperactivity disorder on the one hand and hyperactivity associated with a significant component of conduct disorder, on the other. A further main topic of the chapter will be the evidence for the situational nature of hyperactivity, and the implications this has on the possible role of psychosocial causation.

It is with the last-mentioned issue, i.e. situational nature of hyperactivity, that we shall begin. The second section will deal with the nature of the associated psychosocial factors, and debate the issue of differential contributions to pure hyperactivity and to mixed hyperactivity conduct disorder. The third section will examine possible mechanisms by which psychosocial factors may contibute to the development of hyperactivity.

SITUATIONAL NATURE OF HYPERACTIVITY

It is not a gross exaggeration to note that the apparently situational character of hyperactive behaviour has in the past fuelled some fiery discussion between the exponents of 'belief' and 'disbelief' in the entire existence of hyperactivity disorder. In this respect, the contrast of views has probably been at its sharpest between the veteran authorities such as Wender (1971) on the one hand, and Conrad (1976) on the other. The debate was widened into the popularised arena of 'paperback' discussion by Schrag & Divoky (1975).

A plethora of studies clearly suggest that a child may be hyperactive at home but not at school, or vice versa; or even hyperactive at home and school, but not in some third situation such as a summer camp or clinic testing room, for example (Altepeter & Breen, 1992; Firestone & Martin, 1979; Klein & Gittelman–Klein, 1975; Lambert, Sandoval & Sassone, 1978; Rapoport & Benoit, 1975; Rapoport *et al.*, 1986; Sandberg *et al.*, 1978; Sandberg *et al.*, 1980; Taylor *et al.*, 1991). It is possible that a good deal of the reported difference is more apparent than real, the result of invalid measures, idiosyncratic concepts of what constitutes 'a little' or 'a lot' of hyperactive behaviour as measured by questionnaires, for example; or just different degrees of tolerance of overactive behaviour on the part of particular parents and teachers acting as informants. At the same time, however, the agreements have been so low that a child's 'hyperactivity' may vary a great deal from situation to situation, and therefore largely be 'socially caused' as suggested by Conrad (1976).

Whether or not situational factors are the cause of individual differences in hyperactive behaviour, they are nevertheless likely to play a role in determining how such individual differences are manifested. Furthermore, evidence of strong situational variation in hyperactive behaviour does suggest that environmental factors play a significant role in determining the expression of the disorder.

In an attempt to bridge together the dichotomy suggested by the within-child characteristics on the one hand, and the question of situational specificity on the other, Lambert, *et al.* (1978) put forward an 'interactive systems model' incorporating the issues of identification and labelling of childhood hyperactivity. The model posits that individual differences in the organic and psychological make-up of the child, in the family and in the school environment, all interact to determine whether or not a child is labelled hyperactive.

The Lambert *et al.* (1978) model suggests complex interactions between the child's environment and his/her physical and psychological status. Thus, a child with a given physical constitution may under certain environmental conditions be considered hyperactive, yet a biologically identical child growing up in a different environment may not be so labelled. Likewise, it logically follows that two children with different physical constitutions, growing up in different environments, may both be termed hyperactive. This result may be due to biological and environmental factors balancing each other, or combining in ways that affect the probability that the child will receive the label. The most extreme form of this view, one to which only few would be willing to subscribe, would be that any given child placed in a particular environment will be labelled hyperactive. However, were the same child placed in another environment, he/she may not be called hyperactive.

Most people would be reluctant to accept such an extreme position, because we believe that there exists an unknown number, however small, of children who will almost certainly be identified as hyperactive, regardless of the way they are treated at home or school, for example. However, what may be learnt, or indeed should be learnt, from such apparently exaggerated propositions, is that any examination of the possible associations between the environmental dimensions and hyperactive behaviour must take into account variables potentially contributing to the problem. These may be to do with basic aetiological mechanisms, or as in most cases, may affect the severity of the problems.

There is, however, a further explanation. Hyperactive behaviour may in some cases represent an adaptation to the situation, a conflict within the situation, or a 'comment' on the particular social system. By focusing on 'situational hyperactivity' it may be possible to develop a perspective that returns some meaning to the child's behaviour, in contrast to the one of hyperactivity as purely personal pathology, discounting the situation in which it occurs.

MAINTAINING ROLE OF PSYCHOSOCIAL FACTORS

Social and demographic factors

General population-based surveys have provided conflicting evidence for the extent to which hyperactive children differ from their peers on the basis of fairly straightforward indices of psychosocial background, such as social class, family size, intactness of the family unit, etc. For example, the re-analysis by Schachar, Rutter & Smith (1981), of the Isle of Wight survey data (Rutter, Tizard & Whitmore, 1970) on the behaviour of 10 and 11 year-old children, indicated an association between low social class and 'pervasive hyperactivity' (reported as present by both parent and teacher). Children showing 'situational hyperactivity' (rated hyperactive either by parent or teacher) were also more often from families of low social status compared with non-hyperactive controls, but the association was only half as strong as in the case of pervasively hyperactive children However, a subsequent study by Taylor *et al.* (1991) of a total population of 6 and 7 year-old boys attending 'mainstream' schools in an East London Borough failed to demonstrate a significant association between pervasively hyperactive behaviour and the usual indices of the children's social and demographic background such as social class, family size, etc.

The results of the Dunedin Multidisciplinary Child Development Studies by McGee, Williams & Silva (1984, 1985) also failed to find a correlation between pervasive hyperactivity and social disadvantage. The study by Shekim, *et al.* (1985) similarly ended up with negative results in this respect.

Other epidemiological studies have found low social class, often combined with associated high score on a combined index of social disadvantage, to be associated with the diagnostic definition of attention deficit hyperactivity disorder (ADHD) (American Psychiatric Association, 1980). Of these, the following have been carried out in the last decade: Bird *et al.* (1988); Holborrow & Berry (1986); Kuijper & Hirasing (1986); Satin (1985); Shapiro & Garfinkel

(1986); Shen, Wang & Yang (1985); Szatmari, Offord & Boyle (1989); and Velez, Johnson & Cohen (1989).

The situation appears somewhat different if the focus is shifted specifically to the attention deficit side of hyperactivity disorder. The children of lower social classes have quite consistently been shown to perform more poorly on a variety of tests of attention (Kagan, Reznick & Snidman, 1987; Levy & Hobbs, 1981; Taylor *et al.*, 1991).

However, it is to be noted that factors such as social class and family size can at best be regarded as risk indices, as such they tell us little or nothing about actual mechanisms involved in bringing about the increased risk of a particular disorder. Therefore, it is possible that findings based on mere statistical associations between low social class and attentional problems only reflect the underlying mechanisms in the development of the disorder. One such explanation is that care-takers' actions 'educate', or 'fail to educate', the children's attention and self-control. Furthermore, rather than pointing to wider influences of society at large, these associations are likely to have their origins in the interpersonal interaction patterns between the child and his/her family. It is these intrafamiliar factors as possible risk mechanisms for the maintenance, even if not for causation, of hyperactivity disorder that is our next topic.

Intrafamiliar factors

The stability of the family, the quality of parental relationship, illness in a family member and other chronic intrafamilial stress are all factors that influence the functioning of a family unit. This, in turn, is likely to affect the child rearing conditions, with consequences on the physical and emotional well being of the children growing up in that particular family. It is therefore plausible that such intrafamilial processes exert their influence on the development of hyperactivity, among their other effects. We shall now review the evidence regarding each one of these factors in turn.

Family stability

When compared with 'normal', non-hyperactive, controls hyperactive children appear to have suffered more family instability. However, at least two substantial studies have indicated that such adversity is even more specifically associated with a pattern of behaviour closely akin to what, in the present context, is meant by hyperkinetic disorder (i.e. one which is particularly severe or pervasive). In an epidemiological study involving the total population of 3448 6 year-olds living in the city of Göteborg, a group of 138 children initially selected by Teacher Screening Questionnaires for a variety of problems involving behavioural, attentional, perceptual and speech/language functions, as well as fine and gross motor coordination, were followed up a year later for detailed psychiatric and psychosocial assessment (Gillberg & Rasmussen, 1982). History of family break-up was found to be significantly more common among the 54 children, aged 7 years and diagnosed as suffering from 'minimal brain dysfunction syndrome', with or without concomitant attention deficit disorder, compared with children selected for other behavioural or developmental problems.

Another study, again relying on a large representative sample of 492 children drawn from a population of over 5000, by Hartsough & Lambert (1982), and employing a variety of detailed measures, identified a number of general family variables. According to intensive parent interviews, the 249 pervasively hyperactive children (defined by combined parent, teacher and clinician assessment) had experienced significantly more instability in terms of frequent family moves and school changes than the random controls.

Marital discord

Conflictful relationship between the parents has been shown in some studies to be associated with childhood hyperactivity (e.g. McGee, Williams & Silva, 1984). Two things, however, are important to note here. First, the method of sample selection in most studies does not make it possible for specific associations between childhood hyperactivity and parental marital problems to be unequivocally demonstrated even if they existed. Few studies have, for example, differentiated between children suffering from hyperactivity, conduct disorder, and the common group with features of the two (Schachar, 1991). In studies where this distinction has been made, no differences have been found in the proportions of children from maritally discordant homes (McGee *et al.,* 1984; Reeves *et al.,* 1987; Szatmari *et al.,* 1989; Taylor *et al.,* 1986; Sandberg, Rutter & Taylor, 1978; Marshall *et al.,* 1990); with one exception (Taylor *et al.,* 1991) – and even here the association was in a direction opposite to what might have been expected. The children suffering from hyperkinetic disorder (as defined by the ICD-9 criteria) (World Health Organisation, 1978), significantly less often came from homes characterised by marital problems as compared with a matched group of children diagnosed as conduct disordered.

However, rather than being a direct consequence, the likely mechanisms by which parents' discordant relationship exerts its negative influence on children's emotional development is via a qualitatively altered parent–child interaction (Rutter & Quinton, 1984). This issue will be discussed more fully in the section of 'child-specific family environment' of this chapter.

Psychiatric disorder in a parent

Mental disorder in a parent represents a definite risk factor for psychiatric disturbance in children. However, rather than increasing the risk of one particular type of childhood disorder, the effect is largely non-specific. Similarly, when the risks associated with parental mental disorder and the risks stemming from other forms of psychosocial disturbance are compared, few differences are found with respect to specific forms of the common types of emotional and conduct problems in childhood (Rutter & Quinton, 1984). The implication therefore is that the risk stems from some aspects of family disturbance associated with parental mental disorder rather than from the psychiatric condition in the parent as such.

The role of parental psychiatric disorder as a possible causal influence on childhood hyperactivity has been examined in a number of studies (Barkley *et al.*, 1992; Gillberg & Rasmussen, 1982; Taylor *et al.,* 1991). The findings, though somewhat inconsistent, have pointed towards maternal depression possibly contributing to the cause of hyperactivity in the younger age group. Various routes for this effect to come about have been postulated, all of them primarily operating via the disordered interaction between mother and child, and through this adversely influencing the child's ability to achieve cognitive competence or ability to modulate his/her activity level. These mechanisms will be discussed in more detail further on in this chapter.

However, like the studies examing the psychosocial causes for childhood hyperactivity in general, most of those aimed at teasing out the specific role of parental psychiatric illness have been methodologically inadequate. This is because the studies have either relied on clinical samples or failed to provide independent assessments of child behaviour and parental psychiatric state. The main problem with studies relying on clinical samples is that, given the diversity of factors influencing referral to a specialist service, it is likely that the presence of parental psychiatric disorder in itself increases the chances of a child with an existing problem behaviour, such as hyperactivity, getting referred. This means that the correlations between hyperactivity and parental disorder are probably artifically high in clinic-based studies (Sandberg *et al.,* 1978; Taylor *et al.,* 1986).

The issue of non–independence of measurement of child behaviour and parents' psychiatric problems is pertinent to all studies relying on information obtained by questionnaires completed by parents. The problem of the direction of association was, for example, highlighted in an earlier study by Sandberg *et al.* (1980) of London school children. A very high correlation was found between parent ratings, but not teacher ratings, of child hyperactivity, and the mothers' own perceived distress/psychosomatic complaints as measured by a self-rating scale. Without an independent corroboration of the child behaviour in the home situation, it was, however, impossible to work out what this result meant. The children of depressed/distressed mothers might indeed have been showing hyperactivity especially at home, though not necessarily at school. If this was the case, maternal distress might have been just as well the cause as the consequence of child hyperactivity. However, an equally plausible explanation for the high correlation would be that the distressed mothers perceived more hyperactivity in their children's behaviour than did the non-distressed mothers, i.e. the child behaviour in the two groups might in fact have been very similar.

Two epidemiological studies, carried out a decade apart, and employing complementary measures of child hyperactivity and therefore being methodologically fairly sound, have confirmed that there exists an association between child hyperactivity and maternal mental disorder. In the Göteborg study by Gillberg & Rasmussen (1982) mothers' self–perceived distress and increased number of psychiatric contacts within the previous year significantly differentiated between children classified as suffering from MBD/ADD and their controls. Similarly, in the East London study by Taylor *et al.* (1991) maternal depression, as assessed by the Present State Examination (Cooper *et al.*, 1972), was associated with both teacher and parent interview assessment of the children's hyperactive behaviour. Furthermore, the presence of depressive illness in the mother during the previous year correlated significantly with persistence of such pervasive form of child hyperactivity.

Another substantial study based on a longitudinal design and involving young children whose mothers suffered from schizophrenia, neurotic depression or personality disorder, carried out by Sameroff, *et al.* (1982), reported somewhat different findings. When assessed at 30 months of age, the children whose mothers had been diagnosed as depressed when the child was 4 months old were the most likely to be deviant in behaviour: They were less persistent in their efforts, but they were also less active. However, rather than the diagnosis of the mother's illness *per se*, its severity and chronicity were the most important variables predicting child disturbance. These results can be interpreted as showing that young children's attention is affected by their mother's illness because of the impairment of the relationship between the mother and the child that a psychiatric disorder engenders. This conclusion is also supported by a more recent study by Breznitz & Friedman (1988) to which we shall return later in more detail.

It is to be noted, however, that the psychosocial correlates such as family stability, marital discord or parents' mental health, are primarily features characterising the overall family environment. Therefore, as such they are likely to influence the general child-rearing conditions of the family unit in question. When assessed in terms of being 'present' or 'absent', they have to be viewed as factors exerting a 'shared' environmental influence on all children growing up in that particular family, and it would be hard to claim that they impinge on one child any more than on another. To argue the latter, these factors need to be specifically defined and measured in relation to a particular child.

Child-specific family environment

Parent–child interactions

The role of intrafamilial factors as likely contributors to the maintenance of children's hyperactive behaviour has been extensively reviewed by Barkley (1990), Danforth, Barkley & Stokes (1991), Mash & Johnston (1990), and by Fischer (1990). These accounts have clearly highlighted the many problems hyperactive children have in their relationships with their families, and also often argued that the negative interactions in the first place stem from the hyperactive child, rather than it being the case that the behaviour of other family members brings about hyperactivity in the child. Such evidence predominantly rests on studies that have examined the interactions between hyperactive children and their mothers, often in the context of stimulant medication trials (e.g. Barkley, 1988, 1989; Barkley *et al.*, 1985; Cunningham & Barkley 1978, 1979; Schachar *et al.,* 1987). The interactions of hyperactive children and their fathers, as well as siblings, also show similar patterns of conflict, although to a lesser degree (Tallmadge & Barkley, 1983; Taylor *et al.,* 1991). There is also evidence from several studies suggesting that hyperactive children elicit similar negative, controlling and generally directive behaviours from adults, such as teachers, outside the family (Cunningham & Siegel, 1987; Whalen, Henker & Dotemoto, 1980).

However, at the same time other studies have shown that improvements in the maternal techniques of managing difficult child behaviour, in general, result in their children becoming less hyperactive (Pollard, Ward & Barkley,

1983; Strayhorn & Weidman, 1989; Horn *et al.,* 1987), therefore suggesting that the actual behaviour of the child is not the sole factor influencing the patterns of interaction (Danforth, Barkley & Stokes, 1991; Jacobvitz & Sroufe, 1987; Silverman & Ragusa, 1992).

As the conclusions regarding the nature of parent–child relationship in hyperactivity have traditionally been based on observational studies of mother–child interaction, it is only relatively recently that the role of fathers and siblings has been considered. Accordingly, this review will first deal with qualities of the relationship between hyperactive children and their mothers.

Bee (1967) carried out a seminal study of parent–child interaction and child distractibility by using the combined method of laboratory tests of distractibility and selective attention, and home-based observations of mother–child interaction. The results showed that the key differences between distractible and non-distractible children were not to do with the amount of parent–child interaction, but with the patterns of the interaction. Parents of distractible children tended to make specific, rather than general, remarks and seldom offer the child positive encouragement. The mothers of non-distractible children made an equal number of remarks, but they contained fewer specific suggestions. These mothers also encouraged persistence and provided answers only when the child requested them. The results of Bee's study would therefore suggest that it is a parent listening to the child in decision-making interactions, rather than talking the least, that promotes independence and a non-distractible cognitive approach in the child.

A less straightforward pattern of mother–child interactions is suggested by a study of hyperactive pre-schoolers by Campbell *et al.* (1977). While the mothers of hyperactive children gave more specific suggestions regarding the child's impulse control, the children themselves made more comments about the task and requested more feedback from the mother. However, the characteristic that was most notably differentiating the behaviour of the mothers of hyperactive children, as opposed to the mothers of normal children, was their tendency to show less 'give and take' in their interactions with the children. A very similar picture emerged in the detailed observational studies of Cox and his colleagues of depressed mothers interacting with their pre-school-age children (Cox *et al.,* 1987; Puckering, 1989). This research will be discussed later in detail under 'Psychiatric disorder in the parent'.

Another study examining the interactions between mothers and their young children, and fortunate enough to benefit from complementary measures of child behaviour, is that by Prior, Leonard & Wood (1983). The child's hyperactivity as rated by the mother, researcher and pre-school teacher, correlated highly with observed negative interactions between the mother and the child in the home setting. The key characteristics of the interactions were higher number of 'mother-instigated behaviour changes', 'lack of persistence' and higher rates of 'withdrawal behaviour' on the part of the child. The nature of the data does not, however, allow any definite conclusions to be drawn of the directions of the behaviours, i.e. whether the maternal behaviour was the result or the cause of the child's hyperactivity.

The pattern of mutually negative attitudes, and less readiness to respond, especially on the part of mothers, was also characterising the mother–child interactions in a survey by Mash & Johnston (1982) involving two groups of hyper-active children – one of pre-school-age and another aged 8 years, with normal children as controls for both groups. The observers rated the mothers of hyperactive children as more directive and negative in attitude during play sessions. These mothers were also less responsive to child-initiated interactions. Compared with the controls, the hyperactive children asked more questions and were more negative and less compliant with their mothers. They also engaged in less independent activity when mothers were not actively involved in interactions with them. All these behaviours were more marked in the younger hyperactive children. When moving into structured task–situations, the behaviour of the mothers of hyperactive children stood out even more. Compared with the control mothers, they were more directive and negative, and less prepared to interact with the child. Furthermore, their responses to their children were less approving even when the children were interacting appropriately with them. We shall now focus more closely on the issue of child-specific interactions within the context of the social and family factors discussed above, and deal specifically with i) affective content of parent–child relationship; ii) parental psychiatric illness; iii) marital discord; iv) styles of parenting, as well as discuss, v) the effect of drug therapy on the relationship between hyperactive children and their parents.

Affective content of parent–child relationship

The epidemiological study by Taylor *et al.* (1991) referred to above, showed that mothers of pervasively hyperactive boys were more often rated as lacking of warmth, but expressing high levels of criticism towards the child, than the mothers of any of the comparison group children (i.e. boys showing conduct problems without hyperactivity, or inattentiveness without hyperactivity, or the random community controls). The higher levels of criticism also held for the fathers of hyperactive boys. In addition, mother's coping skills with child's challenging behaviour and 'emotional upsets' were significantly poorer in the pervasively hyperactive groups (regardless of whether hyperactivity occurred on its own or in combination with other behaviour problems).

Psychiatric illness in the parent

Parental psychiatric illness as a contributory factor to difficult parent–child interactions has been highlighted in numerous studies. It is maternal depression, in particular, that has received a great deal of attention (for reviews see Beardslee *et al.,* 1983; Puckering, 1989). Depressed mothers have been shown to be more critical, disapproving, aversive and less positive in their interactions with their children than mothers who are not depressed (Hops *et al.,* 1987; Cox *et al.,* 1987; Webster–Stratton, 1988; Weissman *et al.,* 1984). More specifically, depressed mothers are more likely to initiate hostile behaviours towards their children in an indiscriminative manner, which frequently is not contingent on the immediately preceding child behaviour (Mash & Johnston, 1982).

The Cox *et al.* (1987) study demonstrated that depressed mothers tend to respond to child initiations in an inconsistent manner, often only reacting to the escalation of child negative behaviour while ignoring the preceding positive bids from the child. Depressed mothers also play less with their children and find it particularly hard to adopt mutual patterns of play in which their responses would be contingent upon child behaviour (Jouriles, Murphy & O'Leary, 1989).

The implications of these observations are that, with depressed mothers, the child has to get attention by high intensity of demand. However, there is also a matching unfavourable response from the child: even if the depressed mother succeeds in picking up the child's 'cue', though possibly in a less finely tuned manner, the child response in turn is less likely to be contingent, either in tone or content, on the mother's response. The end result of this interactional pattern is a poorer 'meshing' of parent–child responses, with both parties frequently failing to sustain interaction and effectively meet each other's approaches.

Furthermore, certain child characteristics are far more likely to predict unsatisfactory 'linking' of mother–child responses when the mother is depressed; these are existing emotional or behavioural disturbance and poor expressive language skills (Cox *et al.,* 1987). Both of these factors are relevant here. Hyperactive children, when younger, frequently have less well developed language skills and show difficult temperamental characteristics, easily perceived as 'bad behaviour' (Taylor *et al.,* 1991).

The available evidence therefore suggests that the effect of parental depression or distress on child behaviour is likely to be via the interactions between the parent and child. However, after allowing for a psychiatric disorder in a parent, the qualities of the child are important in determining which child, and to what extent, becomes the recipient of negative parental behaviour and attitudes. A temperamentally difficult or demanding child, or one who has a problem in communicating, is more likely to become the target of parental anger and irritation than a more placid child with a more 'easy-going' disposition.

A note of caution, however, is called for in this context. When interpreting research findings, the possibility that depressed mothers will have a tendency to rate their children's behaviour as more deviant than objective assessments of behaviour warrant needs to be kept in mind. This is an issue especially pertinent to interpreting questionnaire-based research of child behaviour (Sandberg *et al.,* 1980). Such parental tendency is likely to be at least partly rooted in a disturbed perception and cognitive distortion due to depressed affect, and also due to reduced tolerance for child misconduct in a depressed parent (Brody & Forehand, 1986; Webster-Stratton & Hammond, 1988).

In summary, data on the possible associations between maternal depression and child behaviour suggest that depressed mothers have altered perceptions on child misconduct and perhaps less tolerance of child behaviour in general. In addition, and in common with parents of hyperactive children, depressed mothers also use excessive disapproval, irritability and aversiveness, and less approval and less positive behaviour in their interactions with their children than non-depressed mothers would to the same behaviours. However, the children of depressed mothers also display more aversion in their interactions with their mothers, as well as behave more aggressively towards them.

Marital discord

Marital discord may function in a similar manner to depression in altering parental perceptions and styles of management of child behaviour (Jouriles, Barling & O'Leary, 1987). The combination of maternal depression and marital discord results in even higher rates of perceived child deviance and actual parent–child conflict, as well as child aggression, than the presence of these two factors in isolation (Hops *et al.,* 1987; Webster–Stratton, 1988). Furthermore, there tends to be high correlation between maternal depression and marital discord in any given family (Cox *et al.,* 1987). It has also been shown that rates of aversive mother–child interaction are even further increased in families where depressed mothers themselves experience greater degree of negative interaction with other adults, such as spouses or relatives (e.g. Dumas, 1986).

It is therefore highly likely that marital discord, maternal depression, paternal antisocial behaviour and marital aggression are significantly interrelated in the families of some hyperactive children. It is this subgroup of hyperactive children with multiple features of family dsyfunction who, in turn, are at a particular risk for developing additional conduct disorder (Taylor *et al.,* 1991). The psychosocial risk factors for hyperactivity associated with significant component of conduct disorder will be examined in more detail in the next section of this chapter.

Styles of parenting

Findings common to two epidemiological studies, one carried out in Göteborg (Gillberg & Rasmussen, 1982), and one in East London (Taylor *et al.,* 1991), indicate a significant association between inconsistent parenting styles and childhood hyperactivity. The feature highlighted by both surveys is parental disagreement in how to handle challenging child behaviour – and in some cases a near complete *laissez faire* attitude of the parents.

Further characteristics of parenting that have been shown to correlate highly with child hyperactive behaviour are lowered parental aspirations regarding the child's academic achievement, less parental involvement and interest in the child's early learning, and less opportunities and encouragement offered to the child (Gillberg & Rasmussen, 1982; Hartsough & Lambert, 1982).

Another indicator of severe child-specific psychosocial stress of possible relevance has been highlighted by Famularo, Kinscherff & Fenton (1992), which draws attention to excessively punitive child rearing practices as a possible contributor to hyperactivity. A group of 61 maltreated children, aged 5–10 years and drawn from the attenders to a juvenile court, were compared with 35 control children. The two groups were compared on diagnoses based on a structured psychiatric interview carried out separately with child and the parent. In terms of the clinical diagnoses of DSM-III-R (American Psychiatric Association, 1987), the children who had suffered maltreatment exhibited significantly greater indices of ADHD (as well as conduct disorder and post-traumatic stress disorder), than controls. Whether physical child maltreatment was a characteristic of parenting even prior to the children showing signs of hyperactivity, or whether it resulted from an inappropriate style of parental control brought about by the child's difficult behaviour in the first place, cannot be ascertained on the basis of data provided. However, there is further suggestive evidence from a study by Hartsough & Lambert (1982) indicating that the parents of hyperactive children are inclined to use more discipline, and particularly resort to physical methods of discipling the child even when compared with behaviour problem controls.

Effect of medication on parent–child relationship

A number of studies have demonstrated that methylphenidate given to hyperactive children results in significant reductions in child negative and off–task behaviour, as well as increase in both contingent and sustained compliance (Barkley, 1988, 1989; Barkley *et al.,* 1985). Furthermore, the study by Schachar *et al.* (1987) showed that methylphenidate increased expressed maternal warmth and decreased maternal criticism. However, medication did not change family cohesion, efficiency of parental coping, or the pattern of interpersonal family interaction.

There is a need for caution against interpreting the results of methyl-phenidate studies in an unduly optimistic light. On the surface, the early mother–child interaction studies by Barkley and his colleagues (e.g. Barkley & Cunningham, 1979; Cunningham & Barkley, 1978), have showed significant increase in child compliance and decrease in mother directiveness and intrusiveness when the hyperactive child is placed on psychostimulant medication. However, at the same time other changes have also been noted taking place: while on the active drug the children tend to become less sociable, which means that they initiate fewer interactions with the mother and generally become less responsive. Thus, instead of actively interacting with their environment, the children tend to engage in solitary play (Barkley & Cunningham, 1979; Cunningham & Barkley, 1978). The way the results are presented in these studies, does not allow the question of whether there has been an actual increase in the amount of positive interaction and attitudes to be examined, because the maternal responses have been rated as 'conditional' to child behaviour. It is therefore possible that the apparent increase in maternal positive attitudes, as displayed in the mothers' interactions with their children, is at least partly a reflection of the children simply demanding/requiring less attention and interaction when placed on methylphenydate. Thus, one might argue, albeit somewhat speculatively, that in a situation analogous to that involving depressed mothers and their children, the child 'keeping to itself' is welcomed by the mother because it 'leaves her alone'. Thus negative interaction is largely replaced by lack of interaction – a fact that might easily get overlooked when interpreting findings of such studies.

This explanation is particularly suggested by another study of the same team (Cunningham & Barkley, 1979), in which the quantity and quality of interactions between hyperactive and normal children with their mothers was assessed during free play and structured tasks. Compared with their normal peers, hyperactive children were significantly more active, less persistent in their tasks and less compliant. The mothers of hyperactive children differed from the mothers of normal children by imposing more structure and control on their children's play and social interactions. In addition, they were also less likely to respond positively to interaction bids from their hyperactive children even when these bids were positive in nature. At the same time, the mothers gave less attention to the child when the child was engaged in solitary play or responding with compliance to the tasks presented to him. It therefore can be questioned whether the controlling and intrusive behaviour on the part of the mothers is, besides a response to the child's overactive behaviour, also contributing to the child's behavioural difficulties in the first place. This possibility is highlighted by the lack of a balancing positive response on the part of the mother to child compliance, as succintly demonstrated by a recent observation study of a group of pre-school-age children with teacher-acknowledged behaviour problems (Gardner, 1994). The study showed the mothers of problem children to be particularly ready to respond with criticism and intrusiveness when the child does something wrong, but at the same time slow to offer positive comments and praise when the child behaves well.

DISTINCTION OF HYPERACTIVITY FROM CONDUCT DISORDER ON THE BASIS OF PSYCHOSOCIAL VARIABLES

One important criterion of whether two separate disorders are independent diagnostic entities is whether or not they can be shown to have distinctly separate aetiologies. In relation to hyperactivity the key questions here have been: Is hyperactivity disorder a valid diagnostic entity, separate from conduct disorder, and can this distinction be made on the basis of the psychosocial correlates of likely aetiological importance?

The early studies approached this question by allocating children into the two problem groups on the basis of parent and/or teacher questionnaire scores, and more or less assumed that the two forms of behavioural disturbance occurred independent of one another, and in different children. However, subsequent studies based on more adequate diagnostic definitions have clearly demonstrated that this is not the case: although, hyperactivity/attention deficit disorder without a concomitant conduct disorder does occur at a reasonable rate, the reverse is not true, i.e. conduct disorder without hyperactivity is a relatively rare phenomenon (Reeves *et al.,* 1987; Taylor *et al.,* 1991). (For extended discussion on this, see Chapter 6 in this volume). Therefore, the key question, as set out above, can be further articulated as follows. Does the combined hyperactivity/conduct disorder differ from pure hyperactivity disorder (and from pure conduct disorder) in terms of its psychosocial correlates of likely aetiological importance? In the light of the findings from a handful of relevant studies (based on general population samples and making the adequate diagnostic distinctions), it appears that, although the two groups largely resemble each other, the addition of conduct disorder tends to bring greater social disability and more adverse family environments (Luk, Leung & Yuen, 1991; Reeves *et al.*, 1987; McGee *et al.*, 1984).

A number of psychosocial factors characterised the mixed hyperactive–conduct disordered group in a study by Luk, Leung & Yuen (1991) who examined 61 clinic-referred boys, aged 6–12 years, all meeting the DSM-III-R criteria for ADHD, and the ICD-9 criteria for hyperkinetic syndrome. A concomitant conduct disorder was present in 34 of the boys, while 27 did not show this co-morbidity. The mixed group and the group with pure hyperactivity differed from each other on a number of indices of psychosocial stress and intrafamiliar relationships. For example, the quality of father–child relationship was less optimal in the mixed group, with lower levels of parental expressed warmth towards the child and poorer coping with the child's challenging behaviour and emotional upsets. (The differences for the mothers were in the same direction but failed to reach statistical significance.) Also, the parents of the mixed group reported their marriage as more discordant and generally less satisfactory. Apart from the problems in the child–parent relationship, the hyperactive boys with a concomitant conduct disorder were also reported as having more negative interactions with their siblings, compared with those showing pure hyperactivity.

The results of the Taylor *et al.* (1991) survey, involving a general population sample of boys, were in many ways very similar. High score on expressed criticism towards the child, as measured separately for mothers and fathers, was significantly more common in the group showing both hyperactivity and conduct disorder. However, the parents of boys with pure hyperactivity were almost as critical as those with the mixed disorder, whereas both the mothers and fathers of the boys selected for conduct problems alone expressed far lower levels of criticism towards the child. It would therefore appear that hyperactivity, rather than conduct disorder, played the more important role in determining the level of parental criticism.

The same study also showed that poor maternal coping skills in dealing with the child's problem behaviour and emotional upsets were particularly characteristic of the hyperactive boys' group, regardless of whether conduct disorder featured in the problems or not. (The shortfall in the mothers' ability to cope was not matched by that of fathers, but assessing this parental quality for fathers was less reliable than for mothers.)

Other aspects of dysfunctional family life that distinguished the boys with a mixed hyperactivity–conduct disorder from the other two problem groups, i.e. pure hyperactivity or pure conduct disorder, were the presence of depressive symptoms experienced by the others over the past year. (These symptoms were often not serious or pervasive enough to warrant the diagnosis of depressive illness.) The mixed group also stood out from the rest by a significantly higher composite score of family relationship problems.

In contrast to the group differences in relation to measures examining either the quality of the relationship between the index child and his parents, or the quality of intersperonal interaction in the family, none of the indices of the overall social status of family, such as social class, number of children, parental employment or past family break-up differentiated between the groups of children showing hyperactivity or conduct disorder on their own, or in combination – nor did they distinguish between these problem groups and the controls.

Reeves *et al.* (1987) compared 88 clinic-referred and 21 community control children on a number of background variables. The clinic group was further divided into three diagnostic groups: 'pure hyperactivity/attention deficit disorder', 'hyperactivity plus conduct disorder with/without oppositional disorder', and 'anxiety disorder'. With one exception, the commonly employed psychosocial background variables failed to differentiate the individual diagnostic groups – though they did differentiate the clinic-referred group as a whole from the control group. The only factors that stood out were alcoholism and antisocial personality disorder which were by far most common in the fathers of the children showing the mixed form of hyperactivity and conduct disorder. In contrast, several, other studies, have indicated that negative mother child interactions are more predictive of conduct disorder than of hyperactivity (Campbell *et al.,* 1986; Campbell & Ewing, 1990; Campbell *et al.,* 1990; Gomez & Sanson, 1994). The same conclusion has been reached in studies of hyperactive adolescents (Barkley *et al.,* 1991, 1992).

The Dunedin multidisciplinary child development study (McGee *et al.,* 1984), involving 489 boys at the age of 7 years, also compared psychosocial backgrounds of children with the following diagnostic distinctions: aggressive conduct disorder, hyperactivity, mixed aggression and hyperactivity disorder, and normal controls. Only a few differences emerged: children with the diagnosis of aggressive conduct disorder were more likely than the other groups to have experienced parental separation. Presence of maternal depression and somatic complaints, as measured by the Malaise inventory, were more common in all problem groups as compared with the controls, whereas 'problematic family relationships' significantly more often characterised the home situations of the children with pure hyperactivity disorder, and of those with pure aggression compared with the controls – or the group with mixed hyperactivity and conduct disorder. The latter finding is surprising and difficult to explain. All in all, the results of this study are somewhat inconsistent and inconclusive, though suggestive of possible aetiological or maintaining role of suboptimal parenting skills, poor maternal mental health, parental separations and discordant family relationship, for both hyperactivity and conduct disorder – on their own, or in combination.

Hyperactivity a risk factor for conduct disorder

There is a strong suggestion, deriving from separate lines of research, that a link exists between childhood hyperactivity, family adversity (stemming from factors such as parental psychopathology or marital discord, for example), and the development of childhood conduct disorder. According to such a model, childhood hyperactivity acts as a vulnerability factor, while intrafamilial adversity operates as a mediating factor for the risk of conduct disorder. The individual components of intrafamilial adversity mediate the risk in their unique ways, with the immediate risk stemming from suboptimal quality of parent–child interaction, both from the point of view of the development and maintance of conduct problems in hyperactive children (Gomez & Sanson, 1994; Samson *et al.*, 1993; Silverman & Ragusa, 1992).

In the course of the East London study by Taylor *et al.* (1991), a short-term longitudinal design was employed by utilising the results of the initial screening with parent and teacher questionnaires, and the subsequent detailed interview measures 9 months later. It was found that the presence of pervasive hyperactivity tended to influence the short-term development of overall behavioural disturbance. The presence of disruptive behaviour, in the form of hyperactivity, conduct disorder, or mixture of the both, at follow-up was significantly predicted by the membership of the screening group. Among the children rated as high on the mixed hyperactivity conduct disorder at screening stage the overall rate of any disorder at follow-up was 81%, compared with 51% in the pure hyperactivity group, 28% in pure conduct disorder group, and 16%, in the controls. The types of succeeding disorders were also different according to the screening groups: membership of the conduct disorder group initially was only a risk factor for subsequent conduct disorder; but membership of the hyperactivity group carried risks for all three, i.e. conduct disorder, hyperactivity and the mixture of the two, 9 months later. These results would suggest that hyperactivity appears to lead to conduct disorder; not vice versa.

In the same Taylor *et al.* (1991) study, two-thirds of the 85 boys showing pervasive hyperactivity at screening still met the criteria for psychiatric disorder 9 months later. The 54 boys with persisting disorder, were compared with the 31 whose high hyperactivity scores had been transient and who did not show disorder at follow-up. Out of the screening questionnaire scores of hyperactivity, conduct problems, and emotional problems, only conduct disorder predicted persistence of problems. In addition to the presenting behaviour at the screening stage, a number of psychosocial background factors were associated with persistence of disorder. This was the case for a high overall score on negative family relationships, for the presence of depression in the mother in the past year, for a history of parental marriage break-up (at any time in the child's life), and for high levels of expressed criticism by mother towards the child. Therefore, the persistence of hyperactivity was associated with conduct disorder symptoms and adverse family life; but these two factors were themselves intercorrelated.

In an attempt to disentangle the relative contribution of the two, analysis of covariance was employed. When conduct disorder symptoms derived from the parent and teacher rating scales at screening were both co-varied, adverse family life still remained associated with persistence of hyperactivity. Conversely, when family relationship index was used as a covariate, persistence of hyper-activity was still associated with initial teacher and parent ratings of conduct disorder.

The findings of the Taylor *et al.* (1991) survey thus indicate that unhappy family life, representing itself in angry, inconsistent parental reactions and high levels of depressive symptoms in the mothers, is likely to negatively affect the outcome of children with an early onset of hyperactivity. However, the significance of the dysfunctional patterns of family relationships may not be so much in themselves acting as a specific cause of hyperactivity, but rather as factors strongly associated with persistence of the disorder. Furthermore, this prediction is considerably strengthened if the early hyperactivity is accompanied by defiant child behaviour.

Striving now to get beyond the apparently amorphous mass of correlations, the following observations regarding the role of maternal depression and parental marital conflict appear relevant as pointers to the possible aetiological mechanisms determining the likely sequence of early hyperactivity leading to conduct disorder in the context of adverse psychosocial conditions. A number of studies have, for example, indicated, that maternal depression, or distress, gives rise to inconsistent and non-contingent management of fairly 'normal' child non-compliance, which in turn increases the likelihood of further child misbehaviour. Such evidence is obviously less strong when stemming from studies that have relied on maternal perceptions (Brody & Forehand, 1986; Dumas & Wahler, 1985; Webster-Stratton, 1988), rather than objective assessments of child behaviour. However, a few recent investigations have demonstrated evidence of actual observed maternal behaviours, such as expressed criticism or aversiveness, as being characteristic features of interactions between depressed mothers and their young children (Jouriles *et al.,* 1989; Webster-Stratton & Hammond, 1988). Of the other forms of intrafamilial stress, marital discord has been shown to be associated with episodes of child aggression and defiance during observed parent–child interaction sequences.

A prospective study by Campbell & Ewing (1990) suggested that maternal depression and marital discord interact in unique ways, depending on the measure examined. Each factor occurring separately increased maternal defensive and complaining behaviour during conflict discussions, but when both were present, complaining occurred less than when marital discord existed without depression. These factors also predicted less use of maternal facilitative behaviour towards the child and less use of remarks helping the child to solve specific problems, all of which could contribute to the development of antisocial behaviour, particularly in vulnerable hyperactive children. Furthermore, the study also indicated that maternal perceptions of child misconduct, and actual maternal controlling behaviour in early childhood, are more predictive of conduct problems later in childhood and in adolescence, than is actual child behaviour during the earlier years.

The relevance of these same intrafamilial adversities throughout the age-span of childhood was demonstrated by Barkley *et al.* (1991) in a study of adolescents which showed that both maternal depression and marital discord were separately associated with mother's verbal insults and put-downs directed at the adolescent, and with reduction in mother's facilitative behaviour.

In this context it is worth noting that nearly two decades ago, Paternite, Loney & Langhorne (1976) articulated a theoretical model positioning the role of hyperactivity as a 'vulnerability' factor for conduct disorder in the face of adverse psychosocial situations and suboptimal child-rearing practices. The authors were led to their conclusion by the results of their detailed follow-up study of 135 boys with hyperkinetic syndrome/minimal brain dysfunction, all attending a specialist clinic. They showed that parental inconsistency, or *laissez faire* attitude, parental modelling of hostility and short-temperedness, accompanied by overall family stress predicted secondary symptoms such as aggression, deficits in impulse control and low self-esteem. On the basis of their results the authors also noted that these parental behaviours were unlikely to be solely the result of frustrations with a constitutionally difficult child, since the parental behaviours expressed themselves differentially depending on the socio-economic status of the family, whereas the primary child behaviours of hyperactivity did not.

When the same sample of 135 boys, aged 4–14 years, was examined 4 to 6 years later it was found that those whose initial problems involved both hyperactivity and aggression tended to show most severe problems at follow-up (again involving both aggression and hyperactivity). This was especially so for boys from the lower social classes. Parental behaviours, such as 'high control' and hostility towards the child, also contributed significantly to the negative child outcome (Loney *et al.,* 1980). In a contemporary review Loney (1980) did indeed conclude that treatment of hyperactive children should be directed at reducing aggressive behaviour and ameliorating adverse environmental circumstances associated with aggression. The latter include family pathology, problems with the parent–child relationship and environmental disadvantage.

An alternative model, involving two independent routes, one via child aggressiveness and one via negative family climate, to determine the long-term course of hyperactivity was suggested by Marshall *et al.* (1990), on the basis of a longitudinal study of 29 families with a hyperactive son. Direct observations of parent–child interaction, standardised assessments of expressed emotion (EE) and ratings of child aggressiveness were used to determine the relative importance of each one of these factors for the long-term course of ADHD. Parental EE turned out to predict parental behaviour towards the child in observed interactions, whereas child aggressiveness failed to do so. The child's behaviour towards parents, however, was highly correlated with observed child aggressiveness, but not with child EE.

The Marshall *et al.* (1990) findings are supported by a contemporaneous longitudinal study by the Loney team. Paternite & Loney (1980) carried out a 5-year follow-up of 99 boys with an established diagnosis of hyperkinetic syndrome, and entered into a pharmachological treatment programme at the age of 7 years. A number of home environment variables correlated significantly with hyperactivity at follow-up. These included overall socio–economic stress, problematic interparental relationship, personality disorder and social deviance in a parent, and lack of time spent with the child. Child aggression at follow-up, however, was best predicted by child aggression at referral.

Barkley (1990) has summarised his views regarding the possible links between hyperactivity and conduct disorder as follows: 'Hyperactivity disorder (ADHD) is a developmental disorder of behavioral disinhibition associated with neuromaturational immaturity and having a strong hereditary predisposition. Conduct disorder is likely to arise with, and be maintained by, family characteristics, particularly parental psychiatric problems and conditions of social adversity, family discord etc. Parental beliefs, attitudes, psychological distress, family's deficient communication and conflict resolution skills also contribute to the development of conduct disorder in hyperactive children.'

Closely referring to Patterson's model, Barkley (1990) articulated a theoretical explanation for the progression of hyperactivity disorder into conduct disorder via the mechanisms of intrafamilial adversity: parent's psychiatric symptoms –> parents' unfavourable mood –> altered perception of child behaviour in terms of exaggerating deviance of behaviour in their hyperactive child –> increase in parental negative behaviour towards the child and decrease in positive statements and general social interactions with the child –> increase in child negative behaviour and decrease in child compliance via coercive exchanges –> escalation of child's deviant behaviour through parental negative reinforcement.

PSYCHOSOCIAL CAUSES OF HYPERACTIVITY

Role of motivation and mediating factors

Up to this point, the concern has been largely with psychosocial correlates of hyperactivity disorder, dealing predominantly with cross-sectional studies, and therefore in a reasonable position to inspect psychosocial factors in terms of their associational and maintaining, rather than causative role. In this latter section of the chapter, attempts are made to take on board the more demanding task of examining the extent to which it is possible to claim that psychosocial factors may be responsible for the cause of hyperactivity disorder. A start is made by focusing on motivation as a factor likely to mediate these associations.

Most attempts at understanding the underlying deficits in hyperactivity have concentrated on the study of attentional processes. However, in order to explain the way in which social and, more particularly, family and other interactions may contribute to hyperactivity, it seems important to also consider motivational aspects. This in turn needs to be guided by the presence or absence of co-morbidity, because the family and social associations of hyperactivity, as discussed before, may vary according to whether there are associated disorders such as conduct disorder, for example. It is well established that, more often than not, overactivity and poor attention span are associated symptoms of conditions other than pure hyperkinetic or attention deficit disorders. The most common ones of these are cognitive anomalies and conduct disorder, while associations with emotional disorder occur less frequently. As with other symptoms such as depression, the symptom of hyperactivity is far more ubiquitous than the syndrome. Furthermore, it is possible that, depending on co-morbidity, different mechanisms determine the way in which psychosocial influences contribute to the maintenance, and possibly even to the cause of hyperactivity disorder. Thus, the associated symptomatology may give clues as to the pre-eminence of different motivational factors in the process.

In striving to understand the role of motivation as an essential contributor to hyperactivity, it is helpful to consider the issue of purpose. Hyperactivity may be defined as a behavioural style characterised by persistent, marked motor activity which is excessive in relation to what most people would regard as necessary for any particular purpose. A possible reason for such surplus activity is that it serves a purpose which is different from the obvious task at hand, or reflects motivations of which the subject need not be aware.

Overactivity, whether motor, cognitive or emotionally expressed, could be construed as a search for the gratification of unmet personal needs for stimulation and exploration, or for a sense of physical and emotional well-being, and safety. It may result from a difficulty in integrating psychological functions in the achievement of a special aim. This formulation of overactivity is congruent with that outlined by Olson in Chapter 5 of this volume.

Olson describes hyperactivity as a disorder of self-regulation with problems in flexibly adapting to life situations that call for differing standards of conduct. The general deficit is in rule-governed behaviour which in itself is under the control of immediately occurring contingencies. She regards this as a deficit in self-regulation, involving a generalised difficulty in integrating the cognitive/affective/motor functions in response to varying situational demands. A hypothesis is put forward indicating that certain experiences at crucial stages in the child's development contribute by altering the regulation of activities aimed at achieving self-control. It is proposed that the quality of the caregiver–infant interaction, via its effect on the development of cognitive/affective schemata, mediates the emergence of basic attentional, motivational and problem-solving skills.

In addition to the above formulation, the possibility is considered that overactivity, or motor activity which is excessive for what is required for a particular purpose, may arise from:

(a) An inherent personality style characterised by redundant motor and mental energy expenditure in relation to the average required for the same specific purposes by most individuals. Family genetic influences are probably important in the transmission of overactive diathesis (Goodman & Stevenson, 1989);
(b) Inefficient modulation and integration by the child of motor, cognitive and emotional activity in the pursuance of an aim, stemming either from intrinsic problems within the area of mental or emotional functioning, or resulting from the environment lacking in the provision of experiences that may effectively facilitate such integration;
(c) In children a further explanation has to be considered, namely spurious overactivity. By this it is meant that the level of the child's activity is only excessive in relation to a particularly inadequate physical environment, or abnormal parental expectations. The latter may be due to ignorance of what constitutes 'normal' given the child's age, or they may be reflecting distortions caused by problems such as debilitating physical illness or depression in a parent, or they may be brought about by constraints placed by the family's inadequate or

> unsuitable living conditions. Due to these reasons the parents may simply be 'out-of-touch', or impeded in coping, with the high levels of energy characteristic of early childhood. Some of these issues have already been discussed earlier in this chapter (section on parental depression and perception of abnormality) and are also noted in Chapter 3 in relation to clinical assessment. Child's overactivity and restlessness are perceived as troublesome by many parents and this is reflected in these being relatively common complaints among the small group of parents whose children though referred to psychiatric clinics, eventually fail to qualify for a clinically confirmed psychiatric disorder (Garralda & Bailey, 1988).

If persistent motor overactivity is a result of a failure in learning to integrate cognitive/affective/motor function in relation to situational demands, the underlying mental deficits, or the contributory environmental factors, are likely to have been present in the first few years of the child's life.

The young child's way of understanding the world, as well as of making sense of his/her internal experiences, is predominantly through sensorimotor means. Thus, in the early years of the development the child's ability to modulate and integrate cognitive, social and emotional schemata will be mediated by sensorimotor activity. Ill-regulated motor activity may therefore be a likely way for the young child to express psychological dysfunction, before and while the child is developing other competencies to control his environment as well as his thinking, his drives and emotions.

Over and above an intrinsic tendency to redundant physical and mental activity in the child, a variety of mechanisms (to be described later in more detail), could lead to difficulties in the child's ability to regulate his activity levels. They all presuppose that the following conditions exist: firstly, that the child has well developed motor skills; secondly, that any associated deficits, or lacks, occur persistently during the first 3 to 4 years of the child's life; and thirdly, that the resulting anomalies evolve from the relative inter-play of intrinsic factors in the child and environmental contributions. These mechanisms may be further subdivided into cognitive and emotional, with the latter involving concepts such as a sense of physical and emotional safety and well-being.

Contributing cognitive factors

A major driving force already apparent in a young child is the search for mental and intellectual stimulation and active exploration of the environment.

Cognitive limitations, including poor language skills, therefore, interfere with the child's ability to effectively engage in activities where intellectual and verbally mediated demands dominate. Such activities will rapidly become devoid of purpose for the child; they will fail to hold his interest and attention, and may result in restless search for more satisfying mental stimulation through overactivity.

The existing evidence supports the central and primary role of cognitive anomalies for the development of overactivity. Regardless of whether studies have been based on clinical or epidemiological samples, decreased IQ levels and communication problems have consistently been found to be associated with pervasive and severe hyperactivity (Sandberg, Rutter & Taylor, 1978; Gillberg & Gillberg, 1989; Taylor *et al.,* 1991). Furthermore, this association seems to be of special relevance in situations where overactivity and distractibility are unaccompanied by other clinical features of psychopatholgy; in other words, in the absence of psychiatric co-morbidity (Taylor *et al.,* 1986).

Though an intrinsic feature of the child, cognitive deficit may well be closely linked to suboptimal environment during the early years of development. Thus, an impoverished or unsettled environment, which fails to provide sufficient and consistent intellectual stimulation, may contribute to both cognitive deficits and overactivity in the child. It is, therefore, somewhat surprising that descriptions of the effects of extreme environmental deprivation on children have not singled out overactivity as a main consequence. This may mean that overactivity was present in these children but that it was not mentioned because of being regarded as an expected consequence of delayed development. Alternatively, it is possible that overactivity is not a consequence when, as appears to be the case, severe deprivation is linked to physical neglect and reduced opportunities for physical activity (Skuse, 1984).

In children growing up in less extreme circumstances, demographic factors and patterns of family interactions have been shown to be related to cognitive and language development. This is evidenced by family size and birth order, institutional rearing, changes in family structure, and quality of the mother/child relationship being associated with intellectual levels in children (Hinde & Stevenson–Hinde, 1987). More specifically, Taylor *et al.* (1991) have highlighted the fact that, in some cases, low socio-economic status correlates with malattentiveness, thus suggesting that an environment lacking in stimulation may contribute both to a slowing of intellectual development and to overactivity (as discussed earlier in this chapter in relation to decreased parental aspirations and involvement). Up to now, the issue of what precise environmental and family factors may affect hyperactivity through their effects on cognitive stimulation has not been addressed directly, or with any consistency.

Contributing emotional factors

In some children, overactivity may be conceived of as resulting from a fault in the child's inner sense that the environment or important others will be able to provide for his needs for physical and psychological well-being and safety. Such a situation would arise either because of exaggerated basic physical or psychological needs in the child, or because of the evironment's insufficient responsiveness to the child's needs. As a result, the child would seek for alternative experiences in an aimless–seeming manner in order to achieve the missing sense of safety and well-being. The purpose of the child's activity thus becomes a fruitless, stereotyped search for experiences to satisfy unmet emotional needs. This may lead to suboptimal patterns of interaction which in themselves perpetuate the dysfunctional activity style. Drawing on the results of psychophysiological studies carried out by one of the authors, as well as by other investigators, the role of these emotional motivational factors will now be discussed in relation to the issue of co-morbidity, on the one hand, and the contributing of environmental stressors, on the other. (For a more general account of recent research on the neurophysiological aspects of the hyperactivity disorder, see Chapter 7 in this Volume.)

Physical and emotional well-being (reward orientation, sensation seeking)

Deficiencies in the child's ability to regulate his motor and mental activities may be a result of the child growing up in an environment which repeatedly frus-trates his wish to have the needs for basic well-being, either physical or psychological, met. This may be through abuse, neglect, or markedly and persistently negative attitudes towards the child. Their effect would be further aggravated by parenting styles which fail to provide sufficient controls and discipline to help the child contain the wish for immediate gratification of need. The result could be a behavioural style involving an impulsive and compulsively incessant search for compensatory rewarding experiences which will persist regardless of the likely negative consequences. In such circumstances the child's own behaviour may begin to gather elements of antisocial or conduct disorder.

Hypersensitivity to reward

The concept of hypersensitivity to reward has long been put forward as a main characteristic of human disinhibition in adults with psychopathic disorder (Gorenstein & Newman, 1980). In children there is evidence from experimental research supporting the notion of increased sensation seeking or reward orientation being present in ADDH (Douglas, 1983), and when overactivity is part of conduct disorder (Garralda, Connell & Taylor, 1991). Douglas (1983) reported unusually high impulsive and psychophysiological arousal responses (skin conductance level) accompanying the administration of rewards in overactive children. She was led to hypothesise that the observed increase in impulsive responses in hyperactive children is due to the influence of arousal and performance (Firestone & Douglas, 1975). Within this formulation, psychophysiological arousal may be seen as a measurable indicator of motivational factors.

Increased reactivity to positive experiences

In terms of arousal, antisocial behaviour is regarded as a result of excessive reactivity to rewards, and as an extreme form of stimulation seeking behaviour, stemming from an unpleasant affective state created by a low reactivity to arousal and rapid adaptation to sensory input. This conclusion is supported by findings of low autonomic nervous system reactivity to simple and meaningless auditory stimuli in antisocial children (Borkovec, 1970). The results of a study of physiological arousal responses by Garralda, Connell & Taylor (1991) suggest the possibility that both reward seeking and sensation seeking operate in children whose hyperactive behaviour is part of a conduct disorder. An increased autonomic nervous system reactivity to experiences with positively rewarding connotations was found in children with conduct disorder, many of whom also had significant symptoms of hyperactivity. These children also showed a failure to lower their arousal levels during periods of silence, suggesting problems in the modulation of arousal, which in turn may be a possible mechanism underlying the sensation–seeking behaviour. The concept of 'excessive search for sensation' is consistent with findings from experimental work suggesting that the impulsiveness underlying the children's hyperactive behaviour is related to 'delay aversion', with the main difficulty being the hyperactive child's inability to wait for a delayed reward (Sonuga–Barke, Taylor & Heptinstall, 1992); with the immediacy rather than the size of reward being of importance.

Theories of motivation

Understanding the difficulties of hyperactive children within such a framework may benefit from a brief outline of current theories on motivational factors. Bozarth (1991) has summarised the conceptual models of motivation encompassing the energising and directional mechanisms that govern behaviour. Two main explanatory models were outlined: one based on drive reduction theory and the other one on incentive motivational theory. The drive reduction theory postulates that organisms are motivated by drives that push the animal towards the goal object, the behavioural objective being the reduction of the drive. The incentive motivational theory, in turn, stipulates that organisms are motivated by the incentive value of various stimuli which pull the animal towards the goal object, motivation being generated by the expectancy of reward: the primary motivation is not to reduce the drive but to increase and maintain contact with the incentive stimuli. The evidence discussed above would suggest that in the case of hyperactive children, both drive reduction shown by the combination of delay aversion and sensation seeking, and an incentive orientation (reward orientation), operate together.

Bozarth (1991) has further described the role of the hypothalamus as a possible centre for motivational effects on the grounds that electrical stimulation through electrode placements along the medial forebrain bundle (extending from the lateral hypothalamus to the ventral segmental areas) produce the strongest intrinsically rewarding effects. Dopamine is regarded as playing an important role in the rewarding effects of electrical brain stimulation, with the role of noradrenaline being less well supported. Therefore, changes in dopamine function may underlie some of the incentive-based motivations discussed above.

Glow & Glow (1979) argued that the reason for hyperactive children's high reward orientation is that they are relatively insensitive to reinforcement and that it is the lack of perceived rewards that leads them to disobedience, problems in socialisation, poor self control and poor ability to delay gratification. By implication, this could also lead to increased sensation seeking or 'delay aversion', and would therefore suggest that drive reduction is the main motivation. Glow & Glow (1979) hypothesised that the fundamental deficit is a delay in the development of a feedback system whereby the child sees his physical and social environment as chaotic and one where attending to the relationship between his responses and the environmental events is very difficult. Glow & Glow (1979) further suggest that stimulant medication helps the hyperactive child to attend to such feedback. Other means of helping the child to counteract his difficulty would be through encouragement to attend to the effects of his own actions and stick to an activity longer than he normally would. Presumably this would first reduce sensation seeking, and then increase the likelihood of the child being in the position to respond to reinforcement, thus reducing his excessive tendency for reward seeking.

Psychosocial contributors to excessive sensation seeking and reward orientation.

Earlier on in this chapter, attention has already been drawn to an increased likelihood that children suffering from the combination of hyperactivity and conduct disorder have undergone adverse life experiences disposing them to be deprived of a sense of personal well-being. These include psychiatric disorder, particularly antisocial behaviour and alcoholism, in a parent (Schachar & Wachsmuth, 1990). It is further to be noted that parental psychiatric disorder, especially personality disorder and depressive illness, is often associated with multiple family adversities which impede the parents' ability to provide a secure and stable loving environment devoid of major strains in family relationships, adequate care and consistent discipline (Rutter & Quinton, 1984).

The presence of a hostile and unhappy family environment, often accompanied by poor exercising of control for the child's behaviour, seems of special relevance when hyperactivity is associated with defiant and antisocial behaviour (Taylor *et al.*, 1991). Angry, inconsistent parental reactions and high levels of maternal depression contribute to a hostile atmosphere of poor coping with frequent criticising of the child. The combination of these factors is also a powerful predictor for the persistence of hyperactivity regardless of whether there is accompanying conduct disorder. The work of Olson, Bates & Bayles (1990) offers further empirical support for the role of maternal attitudes for the development of children's cognitive style and reward seeking. In their follow-up study of pre-school children, it was found that responsive, cognitively stimulating parent–toddler interactions in the second year modestly predicted cognitive non-impulsivity and ability to delay gratification at school entry.

The development of a positive view of oneself and favourable self concept are regarded as essential for a person's good psychological adjustment. Persistent negative feedback, whether the result of the child's overactivity or not, will reduce the chances that the child's needs for socially rewarding experiences are met. If this occurs at a crucial time in the child's development, when he or she is learning to integrate motor and mental activity, it could lead to increased motor restlessness, overactivity and disruptive behaviour in the futile search for satisfactory and rewarding experiences. Thus, Glow & Glow (1979) postulated that a chaotic and unrewarding environment, situations of particularly low responsiveness to the child (as might be found in depressed mothers), parental inconsistency, disagreements about child-rearing practices and/or marked discontinuities of caretaking, could lead in the child to a sense of inability to control his environment, 'learned helplessness' and to hyperkinetic impulse disorder, with 'insensitivity to reinforcement'.

Excessive sensation- rather than reward-seeking may in itself be a factor determining continuation of disturbed behaviour into adulthood, and even predicting future parenting difficulties in the next generation. Cloninger, Sigvardson & Bohman (1988) studied a high risk sample of offspring of criminal and alcoholic parents, with some of the children fostered, some adopted, and some returned to their parents. On the basis of research records collected at the age of 11 years, the children's behaviour was rated for novelty seeking, harm avoidance, and reward dependence. When these ratings were used to predict behaviour at follow-up, low harm avoidance and high novelty seeking were associated with raised rate of alcoholism in the children when grown up.

However, is reward/sensation-seeking of specific relevance for children with the combined conduct disorder and hyperactivity, or is it simply a feature of conduct disorder *per se*? How important is it that anomalies necessarily be present in the pre-school period, thus handicapping the development of self-regulation? Are both reward and sensation seeking necessary for the symptoms of hyperactivity to develop? What is the relative importance of intrinsic temperamental features in the child, or of environmental factors, for their continuation? Do these intrinsic and environmental characteristics persist alongside the clinical disorders? What are the treatment implications of reward and sensation seeking having a primary mediating role? These are critical questions to settle for reward/sensation-seeking to be shown to have clinical relevance for our understanding of conduct disorder and hyperactivity – individually and in combination.

Safety: Threat and fear

Changes in motor and mental activity levels are commonly known to be a feature of states of anxiety and fear (Marks, 1987). Such changes, however, may be in either direction; towards over- or under-activity. Thus, depending on the nature of the anxiety-inducing stimulus, the temperamental and behavioural style of the individual, and the 'restrictive' or 'open' nature of the physical and emotional environment, a person in a state of anxiety or fear may show restlessness and agitation; or just as well 'freezing' and inactivity.

It is possible that anxiety-related overactivity in a young child is a manifestation of certain extreme deviations and shortfalls in the child's immediate caretaking environment. This may, for example, be the case with a temperamentally active and agile child whose physical or emotional integrity is exposed to severe threat at the time when the child is striving for self-regulation and mastery. Such threat may stem from being abused or abandoned, for example. Likewise, young children who are living in environments where adults fail to master fear (e.g. through parent suffering from phobic panic state), or where parents fail to shelter the child from anxiety-provoking situations, or are unable to help him to contain normal childhood fears, may develop a persistent style of anxiety- and fear- proneness expressing itself as excessive restlessness. Given such scenarios, clinical hyperactivity would best be seen as part of an anxiety disorder, accompanied by restless search for emotional security in order to be relieved of an 'uncomfortable' emotional state of anxiety.

There does exist evidence from epidemiologically based studies to suggest that in some children hyperactivity is part of an anxiety disorder, though the link is far less strong than with conduct disorder or with cognitive deficits (Taylor *et al.*, 1991; Biederman *et al.*, 1992). Relating to what was postulated above, it is likely that specific underlying psychological and biological factors operate in such cases. Thus, it has, for example, been shown that children whose hyperactivity/attention deficit is linked to anxiety disorder exhibit lesser degrees of impulsivity and motor overactivity, and fewer antisocial symptoms than hyperactive children without the underlying anxiety disorder (Pliszka, 1992). Furthermore, the presence of both hyperactivity and anxiety decreases the likelihood of the child's symptoms responding favourably to stimulant medication (Taylor *et al.*, 1987).

As discussed earlier, findings from physiological studies of arousal may serve as evidence that motivational factors are of relevance in hyperactivity accompanied by anxiety. Children suffering from emotional disorders, a number of whom also exhibit high levels of motor activity, have been shown to differ from children with conduct disorder and from healthy controls, in terms of background arousal levels, as measured by skin conductance and heart rate, as well as in their electrophysiological responses to stimulation. Thus, emotionally disturbed children have been documented as showing excessive autonomic nervous system responses to the anticipation of potentially stressful or unpleasant experiences (Garralda *et al.,* 1991). In addition, those children whose emotional symptoms are particularly severe also exhibit high resting heart rate levels and reduced responses to neutral stimuli (Garralda, Connell & Taylor, 1989).

A picture therefore emerges of the hyperactive anxious child as one with increased adrenergic autonomic baseline activity, with decreased general reactivity to overall 'neutral' environmental stimulation, but hypersensitivity to negative and potentially threatening life situations. In children with a proneness to overactive motor behaviour this might well lead to a characteristic tendency to fidgetiness, and in a search for safety, to anxious 'running away' from environmental changes or demands, perceived as threatening.

An important question arising from this formulation is why anxiety is linked to overactivity in some children and not in others. It is possible that the presence of temperamental overactivity in the child is pre-requisite for this. The experience of a sheltered or specially overprotective environment, as often described in children with anxiety disorder, may reduce the risk of an overactive response. Alteratively, anxious hyperactivity may be a result of especially stressful experiences of loss, or threat of loss, early on in childhood. It may also be further compounded by exposure to parental anxiety since increased rates of anxiety disorder have been noted in the families of children with attention deficit hyperactivity disorder (Biederman *et al.,* 1991). It is therefore possible that children model their behaviour on anxious–restless overactivity in their parents. In such situations overactive behaviour may also allow the child to create some physical distance in order to reduce the burden of anxiety fuelled by parental psychiatric disorder.

Safety: Disrupted attachments

A further child psychiatric condition of which hyperactivity can be a major feature, and environmental factors also play an important role, are attachment disorders. This issue is also discussed in Chapter 5 by Olson.

Attachment has been understood as a safety-regulating and stimulation-promoting mechanism, as an expression of a biological propensity in the child to behave in ways which promote proximity and contact with the mother figure (Bowlby, 1971). Motor activity and exploration of the environment are intrinsic aspects of this process, the child using the mother as a base to explore the environment by advancing away from her to progressively more distant targets. Attachments develop as a consequence of parental responsiveness to such innate proximity-regulating behaviours in the child during a sensitive period of the first 3 years of life. This period is therefore important, not just for social and emotional development, but also for the development of the regulation of motoric and attentional behaviours, as will be discussed later. Lack of adequate availability for the child of mother, or main care-taker, at this crucial time, would result in persisting dysfunction in the child's ability to regulate attention and motor activity. This is likely to be due to the failure to experience the required sense of security drawn from the predictability of the mother's presence.

Olson (see Chapter 5) has reviewed the evidence regarding attachment anomalies and overactivity. Although not entirely unequivocal, the available studies offer evidence that the security of the mother–child attachment is related to a toddler's willingness to comply with the mother's request and engage in constructive problem solving, as well as to 'on-task' behaviour. Thus, securely attached children are on the whole more compliant, enthusiastic and attentive to maternal suggestions than insecurely attached children. Security of mother–infant attachments has also been found to predict cognitive non-impulsivity and ability to delay gratification at the time the child enters school (Olson *et al.,* 1990). Conversely, insecurity of early mother–child attachments has been shown to be related to teacher ratings of behavioural impulsivity and interpersonal hostility in pre-school age.

However, this work, which has been based on laboratory ratings of attachment anomalies using the classical Ainsworth's experimental situation method, has failed to demonstrate a consistent link between laboratory ratings of attachment anomalies during infancy and the later development of psychiatric disorders in children. Consequently, the extent and precise nature by which these anomalies contribute to the development of clinical hyperactivity/attention deficit disorders remains unclear.

There does, however, exist empirical evidence suggesting that the experience of seriously disrupted attachments during the early years has a significant effect on the child's motoric and attentional regulation. Taylor *et al.* (1986) found that classroom hyperactivity in 6-year-olds had only one significant psychosocial association: a lengthy previous episode of institutional care. Tizard & Hodges (1978) have outlined evidence that disruptive early experiences, such as institutional rearing and parenting breakdown, are associated with overactivity and attentional problems in a school-aged child. Furthermore, these behavioural patterns are slow to remit and have been shown to persist even years after successful fostering or adoption (Deutsch *et al.*, 1982).

The association between disrupted parenting and hyperactivity appears to apply especially when disrupted parenting occurs before the age of 3 years, suggesting that there is a sensitive attachment period when certain cognitive as well as social skills are acquired (Tizard & Hodges, 1978; Deutsch *et al.*, 1982; Wolkind & Rutter, 1985; Hersov, 1990). Disrupting this developmentally vital process would lead to continuing parallel problems of overactivity and poor social relationships.

Haddad & Garralda (1992) have described school-age children presenting to child psychiatric clinics with a combination of hyperkinetic syndrome and severely disrupted early experiences. In children with such life histories hyperactivity was unaccompanied by biological indicators, the problem behaviour had an onset in early childhood and had persisted in spite of children having lived for years in stable substitute families. Another characteristic of such children was that their hyperactivity was associated with other features of attachment disorders such as attention-seeking behaviour, indiscriminate friendliness, poorly modulated peer interactions, and in some children hoarding of food. The authors argued that early deprivation would have resulted in difficulties by the children in developing enduring attachments and an inner sense of emotional security, and led to problems in controlling and regulating attention and activity levels.

It is, however, unclear whether the emotional insecurity and poor sense of safety and consequent disrupted attachments are the crucial factor leading to hyperactivity in the children who have experienced major early disruptions. An alternative route may be via anomalous development of sensation and reward-seeking mechanisms described above in connection with co-morbid hyperactivity and conduct disorder. This is possible since the behaviour of the children who have experienced early disruptions frequently has accompanying antisocial features. It would be of theoretical and practical interest to clarify this in future work.

Other environmental factors

As discussed earlier in this chapter, a number of environmental factors have been suggested as playing a causal role in hyperactivity disorders. These include maternal depression and interparental discord. Because of their known associations, both these factors may lead to overactivity via any of the mechanisms described above. Thus, maternal depression has been shown to be associated with suboptimal parenting and poor parent–child relationship, with delayed cognitive development in young children, with behavioural and with attachment disorders. Furthermore, parental discord is commonly found in association with maternal depression, parenting disruption and the presence of personality disorder in the father.

We may therefore conclude that there exists some theoretical, clinical and empirical support for the possibility that the mechanisms described above mediate the links between family and environmental factors and the causation of childhood hyperactivity. However, much of the evidence is indirect, and the relative validity and specificity of these mechanisms in relation to different types of co-morbidity can only be ascertained by future clinical observations and carefully targeted research.

Constitutional vs. environmental determinants of hyperactivity disorder

Keeping in mind the empirical evidence reviewed above, we shall now consider further the possible mechanisms by which a hyperactivity disorder may develop in individual children and the ways in which interpersonal and other psychosocial adversities may mediate this process. Given that the evidence to date is by no means complete to construct an entirely satisfactory model, some of the discussion that follows is bound to be speculative. In doing so, we shall refer to existing theoretical propositions which have been put forward. In brief, conceptual models explaining the cause of hyperactivity can in broad terms be assigned to four principal approaches.

First, there is the symptom-based model, also known as a biological/constitutional model (represented, e.g. by Wender, 1971). Within this approach, report of (hyperactive) behaviour is considered evidence of a symptom equal to a finding on a medical laboratory test, for example. Prevalence of the disorder (illness) is determined by estimating the number of persons showing the required number of symptoms. The symptoms are not viewed in terms of their environmental contingencies, but are assumed to be by-products of the child's constitutional state. In fact, because symptoms are seen as reflections of an internal condition they are not regarded as behaviours *per se*. The majority of earlier prevalence studies have approached hyperactivity disorder from such a basis by failing to take into account neither the source of the report nor the context of the behaviour.

A second model, one that incorporates a sociological and anthropological perspective, has been referred to as the 'social systems model' (represented, e.g. by Minuchin *et al.*, 1975). This model entails that hyperactive behaviour is defined by the child's social environment, including the child's role in a particular situation such as the family, or the school, for example. Within the social systems framework, very little emphasis is based on the constitutional make-up of the child, or on individual temperamental differences in children. Instead, hyperactivity is regarded as an 'achieved status', it is a role played by those assigned the status. Such a status exists within, and is specific to, the social system in which it occurs.

A third model, initially put forward by Lambert, Sandoval & Sassone (1978), is defined as a 'single interactive system model', incorporating both the social and the child-centred perspectives. According to this multidimensional model, the individual differences in both the make-up (organic and psychological) of the child, and in the environment (family and school, for example), are likely to contribute to whether or not a particular child is identified as hyperactive. The model posits a complex interaction between the child's environment and his/her physical and psychological status.

An issue closely related to how different environments are likely to increase or decrease the likelihood of a child being identified as hyperactive is that of situation-specificity of hyperactive behaviour. Main effect models, following a nature–nurture dichotomy, postulate independent effects of constitutional and environmental factors on the development of behavioural deviance. However, the majority of longitudinal studies have shown that the early biological risk factors account for only a small proportion of the behavioural variance beyond the first two years or so. It, therefore, has to be concluded that main effect models are applicable only in very extreme conditions.

Studies based on models that postulate an interaction between constitutional and environmental influences have demonstrated statistically significant relationships between biological complications early in the individual's life, and behavioural deviance at a later age. However, even though representing some advancements over the main effect models, the interactional models are still too static to detect the possible developmental mechanisms involved. Sameroff & Chandler's (1975) 'transactional model' aimed to meet this need. They argued that from an early age children actively organise and structure their environment, and that development involves a continuing mutual influence between the organism and its surroundings. The model also assumes that there are no inherently stable characteristics of either individuals or their circumstances (Sameroff, Seifer & Zax, 1982).

The notion that young children and their care-takers mutually shape each other's behaviour forms the basis of many recent longitudinal studies of temperament. The basic concept is that there are inter-individual differences in biologically rooted styles of behaviour. Such differences in turn affect children's interactions with their environment.

Taken to the context of childhood hyperactivity, it is postulated that characteristics such as high activity level, short attention span, and impulsivity are 'temperamental' expressions of biological risk which in some environmental conditions will contribute to the development of the clinical syndrome of hyperactivity. Thus even genetic aetiology is likely to be multifactorial and due to underlying neurochemical factors. The inheritance is polygenic with the liability being influenced by sex hormonal factors and/or very early social influences, which both will increase the liability of hyperactivity in boys.

Kalverboer (1988) has examined the development of hyperactivity in the theoretical framework of 'learned helplessness', the concept originally developed by Seligman (1974). The state of learned helplessness would be likely to arise if the child lived in situations in which no consistent relationships could be perceived between his behaviours and their effects. Such children in turn would have a higher chance of finding themselves in situations where their behaviour, because of being rather unstable due, for example, to early neurological disorders, would elicit suboptimal responsiveness, or inappropriate responses, from the care-taking environment. The same factors can also negatively affect the development of attachment relationships and competence.

This chain of developments has its origins in the early days of the person's life. In a young child, the temporal organisation of behaviour appears to be a powerful determinant of social reactions from the environment. (A healthy newborn has a characteristic organisation of sleep and wake states; other vital functions such as sucking and crying also have a periodic character.) This temporal organisation of the baby's behaviour in turn allows the care-taker to make use of it in interaction processes and to adapt her/his behaviour to fluctuations in the child's state and orientation. It has been suggested that this pattern of alternation presents a precursor for the later process of role-talking (Kaye, 1977). Thus, if the organisation of child's behavioural states is upset, that can have repercussions for the ability of the care-taker to respond appropriately to the child. This in turn may have effects on the child's cognitive processes.

Another theoretical proposition of hyperactivity disorder, also based on the transactional model, is that put forward by Glow & Glow (1979). They described hyperactivity as a 'developmental defect of motivation' arising from the foundation of 'learned ineffectiveness'; the latter being a basic mechanism by which children raised in chaotic environments develop learning difficulties. A parallel process applies to the development of hyperactivity disorder. Through their biological vulnerabilities, such as brain damage or genetic predisposition, for example, children may have fundamental deficiencies in processing feedback from the environment. This in turn makes the child's transactions with the environment less rewarding, and the child will lose the motivation to try. Thus, to the hyperactive child even a normally organised environment may appear chaotic because he would not be able to process the feedback. This also would make it hard for such a child ever to be aware of himself contributing to the less rewarding interaction.

This theory is compatible with the existence of multiple causes for hyperactivity: it focuses on biological/constitutional susceptibility on the one hand, and on environmental predisposing factors such as parental inconsistency, discordant child-rearing practices and discontinuities in care-taking, on the other. Furthermore, it leads one to look for the role of unfavourable early experiences in children displaying hyperactive behaviour, and particularly for the importance of inadequate environmental responsiveness to the child as might be found in a parent who is emotionally 'unavailable' due to depressive illness, marital conflict etc. Another question requiring further study is that of disrupted early attachment relationships as possible causal agents for childhood hyperactivity disorder.

CONCLUSIONS

The situational nature of hyperactivity behaviour suggests that environmental, social and family factors may be of primary importance for the development of a clinically relevant disorder of hyperkinesis. However, it seems likely that rather than directly causing it, the environment mainly influences the expression of overactivity, acting as a stressor or trigger mechanism in pre-disposed vulnerable children.

A number of environmental factors have been shown to be associated with hyperactivity in children. These include overall social disadvantage, which is particularly linked to attention deficits, family instability and marital discord, as well as psychiatric disorder in parents, especially maternal depression. In addition, particular styles of family relationships have been described: with mothers being more directive and negative in their attitudes towards the child, with more inconsistent parenting and interparental disagreement on child rearing. Due to the predominantly cross–sectional nature of the studies so far available, it is difficult to be sure to what extent these factors are the result of, rather than contributory to the child's hyperactivity. Moreover, family interactions, particularly those between mothers and children, appear to be partly reversed by drug therapies which reduce overactivity in the child. However, it seems plausible that, as discussed in the section on causal mechanisms, an environment which does not provide sufficient cognitive stimulation, rewarding experiences or social stability in the early pre-school years, will have an adverse effect on the child's ability to modulate levels and organisation of motor and attentional activity. These effects may be further magnified by negative parent–child interactions.

The high co-morbidity reported between hyperactivity and other disorders of conduct is in line with the fact that the two conditions share a number of adverse social and family-associated factors. The indications are that the combination of these disorders is linked with more psychosocial disadvantage than the presence of any one of these disorders alone; and that it carries a worse prognosis. The combined presence of high levels of social disadvantage and adverse family environment may therefore be especially psychopathogenic.

Regarding the direction, the balance of evidence suggests that rather than conduct disorder leading to hyperactivity, the reverse is true; with overactivity being a precursor of conduct disorder in a number of children. In these cases conduct disorder is likely to arise from and be maintained by family adversity, deficient communication and conflict resolution skills.

We have discussed the conceptual models which explain hyperactivity in terms of four principal approaches: (i) A symptom-based or biological–constitutional model whereby the symptoms are assumed to be byproducts of the child's constitutional state; (ii) a model that incorporates a sociological and anthropological perspective, or social systems model of hyperactivity, where this is regarded as an achievement status, in other words, as a role played by those assigned this status. Hyperactive behaviour is defined by the child's social environment, including the child's role in a particular situation, such as the family or the school. (iii) The third model is known as the single interactive systems model which incorporates both previous models; individual differences in the make-up of the child and the environment will contribute to whether or not a particular child is identified as hyperactive.

(iv) in a more developed version of the interactive systems framework using transactional analysis, hyperactivity is understood as resulting from the continuing mutual influence between the organism and its surroundings. It may be an expression of a temperamental or biological risk for high activity levels, short attention span and impulsivity, complicated by a state of learned helplessness, and arising when the child lives in situations in which no consistent relationships can be perceived between his behaviour and its effects. Up to a point this may result from the child's overactive behaviour. This chain of developments would have its origin in the early days of the individual's life, as in a young child the temporal organisation of behaviour appears to be a powerful determinant of social reactions from the environment.

Hyperactivity disorder can be regarded in part as a developmental defect of motivation, arising from the foundation of learned ineffectiveness, whereby the child's difficulty makes transactions with the environment less rewarding and the child loses the motivation to try. This notion is compatible with the existence of multiple causes for over-activity and explains the role of unfavourable early experiences in children displaying hyperactive behaviour, particularly the importance of inadequate environmental responsiveness to the child as might be found in parents who are emotionally unavailable due to depressive illness or marital conflict.

Specific contributory motivational factors are further discussed in the light of co-morbidity of hyperactivity with other disorders, especially conduct disorder. Hyperactivity may be defined as a behavioural style of persistent increased motor activity which is devoid of an obvious purpose. This may result: (i) from constitutional over-activity in the absence of co-morbidity; (ii) from cognitive limitations sometimes consequent in a poorly stimulating environment; (iii) from a particularly sensation-seeking and reward-orientated style of searching behaviour, in children with associated conduct disorders; (iv) when anxiety disorders are the main comorbid feature, overactivity may be understood as the result of restless anxiety and aim at achieving safety by increasing distance and escaping from threatening situations, and (v) in children with severely disrupted attachments, hyperactivity may be viewed as an excessive or disorganised search for emotional security stemming from insufficient parental responsiveness to the child's innate proximity-regulating behaviours at the sensitive attachment periods in the child's life. The existing literature on associated psychosocial factors suggests ways in which these mechanisms might be operating. However, much of the evidence is indirect and the validity and specificity in relation to different types of co-morbidity can only be ascertained by future research.

REFERENCES

Altepeter, T.S. & Breen, M.J. (1992). Situational variation in problem behaviour at home and school in attention deficit disorder with hyperactivity: a factor analytic study. *Journal of Child Psychology and Psychiatry,* **33**, 741–8.

Amado, H. & Lustman, P.J. (1982). Attention deficit disorders persisting in adulthood: a review. *Comprehensive Psychiatry,* **23**, 3–14.

American Psychiatric Association (1980). *Diagnostic and Statistical Manual of Mental Disorders. Third edition.* Washington, DC:APA.

American Psychiatric Association (1987). *Diagnostic and Statistical Manual of Mental Disorders. Third edition – Revised.* Washington, DC:APA.

Barkley, R.A. (1988). The effects of methylphenidate on the interactions of preschool ADHD children with their mothers. *Journal of the American Academy of Child and Adolescent Psychiatry,* **27**, 336–41.

Barkley, R.A. (1989). Hyperactive girls and boys. Stimulant drug effects on mother–child interactions. *Journal of Child Psychology and Psychiatry,* **30**, 379–90.

Barkley, R.A. (1990). The families of ADHD children. *In Attention Deficit Hyperactivity Disorder: A Handbook for Diagnosis and Treatment,* ed. R.A. Barkley, pp. 130–68. New York: The Guilford Press.

Barkley, R.A. & Cunningham, C.E. (1979). The effects of methylphenidate on the mother–child interactions of hyperactive children. *Archives of General Psychiatry,* **36**, 201–8.

Barkley, R.A., Karlsson, J., Pollard, S. & Murphy, J.V. (1985). Developmental changes in the mother–child interactions of hyperactive boys: effects of two dose levels of Ritalin. *Journal of Child Psychology and Psychiatry,* **26**, 705–15.

Barkley, R.A., Fischer, M., Edelbrock, C.S. & Smallish, L. (1991). The adolescent outcome of hyperactive children diagnosed by research criteria: III. Mother–child interactions, family conflicts and maternal psychopathology. *Journal of Child Psychology and Psychiatry,* **32**, 233–5.

Barkley, R.A., Anastopoulos, A.D., Guevremont, D.C. & Fletcher, K.E. (1992). Adolescents with attention deficit hyperactivity disorder: mother–child interactions, family beliefs and conflicts, and maternal psychopathology. *Journal of Abnormal Psychology,* **20**, 263–88.

Barkley, R.A., Karlsson, J., Strzelecki, E. & Murphy, J. (1984). Effects of age and Ritalin dosage on the mother–child interactions of hyperactive children. *Journal of Consulting and Clinical Psychology,* **52**, 750–8.

Bee, H. (1967). Parent–child interaction and distractibility in 9 year old children. *Merril–Palmer Quarterly,* **13**, *175–90.*

Beardslee, W. R., Bemporad, J., Keller, M.B. & Klermean, G.L. (1983). Children of parents with major affective disorder: a review. *American Journal of Psychiatry,* **140**, 825–32.

Befera, M.S. & Barkley, R.A. (1985). Hyperactive and normal girls and boys: Mother–child interaction, parents' psychiatric status and child psychopathology. *Journal of Child Psychology and Psychiatry,* **26**, 439–52.

Biederman, J., Munir, K. & Knee, D. (1987). Attention deficit disorder with and without conduct and oppositional disorder: a controlled family study. *Journal of the American Academy of Child and Adolescent Psychiatry,* **26**, 724–7.

Biederman, J., Newcorn, J. & Sprich, S. (1991). Comorbidity of attention deficit hyperactivity disorder with conduct, depressive, anxiety and other disorders. *American Journal of Psychiatry,* **148**, 564–77.

Biederman, J., Faraone, S.V., Keenan, K., Steingard, R. & Tsuang, M.T. (1991). Familial association between attention deficit disorder and anxiety disorders. *American Journal of Psychiatry,* **148**, 251–6.

Biederman J, Faraone S. V., Keenan, K., Benjamin J., Krifcher B., Moore C., Sprich–Buckminster S., Ugaglia K., Jellinek M. S., Steingard R., Spencer T. Norman D., Kolodny R., Kraus I., Perrin J., Keller M.B. & Tsuang M. T., (1992). Further evidence for family–genetic risk factors in attention deficit hyperactivity disorder. *Archives of General Psychiatry,* **49**, 728–38.

Bird, H.R., Canino, G., Rubio–Stipec, M., Gould, M.S., Ribera, J., Sesman, M., Woodbury, M., Huertas–Goldman, S., Pagain, A., Sanchez–Lacay, A. & Moscoso, M. (1988). Estimates of the prevalence of childhood maladjustment in a community survey in Puerto Rico: the use of combined measures. *Archives of General Psychiatry,* **45**, 1120–6.

Borkovec T. D. (1970). Autonomic reactivity to sensory stimulation in psychopathic, neurotic and normal juvenile delinquents. *Journal of Consulting and Clinical Psychology,* **35**(2), 217–22.

Bowlby, J. (1971). *Attachment and Loss, Vol. 1, Attachment.* Harmondsworth: Penguin Books.

Bozarth M. A. (1991). The Mesolimbic Dopamine System as a Model Reward System. In

The Mesolimbic Dopamine System: From Motivation to Action, eds. P. Willner & J. Scheel–Kruger. New York: John Wiley.

Breznitz, F. & Friedman, S.L. (1988). Toddlers' concentration: does maternal depression make a difference? *Journal of Child Psychology and Psychiatry,* **29**, 267–79.

Brody, G.H. & Forehand, R. (1986). Maternal perceptions of child maladjustment as a function of the combined influence of child behaviour and maternal depression. *Journal of Consulting and Clinical Psychology,* **54**, 237–40.

Campbell, S.B. & Ewing, L.J. (1990). Follow-up of hard to manage preschoolers: Adjustment at age 9 and predictors of continuing symptoms. *Journal of Child Psychology and Psychiatry,* **31**, 871–89.

Campbell, S.B., Schleifer, M., Weiss, G. & Perlman, T. (1977). A two-year follow-up of hyperactive preschoolers. *American Journal of Orthopsychiatry,* **47**, 149–62.

Campbell, S.B., Ewing, L.J., Breaux, A.M. & Szumowski, E.K. (1986). Parent–referred problem three-year-olds: follow-up at school entry. *Journal of Child Psychology and Psychiatry,* **27**, 473–88.

Campbell S.B. Ewing, Pierce, E.W., March, C. & Ewing , L. (1990). Non–compliant behaviour, overactivity, and family stress as predictors of negative maternal control in preschool children. *Development and Psychopathology*, **3**, 175–90.

Cloninger C. R., Sigvardsson S. & Bohman M. (1988). Childhood personality predictors of alcohol abuse in young adults. *Alcoholism,* **12**, 494–505.

Conrad, P. (1976). *Identifying Hyperactive Children. The Medicalisation of Deviant Behavior.* Massachusetts: Lexington Books.

Cooper, J.E., Kendall, R.E., Gurland, B.J., Sharpe, L., Copeland, J.R.M. & Simon, R. (1972). *Psychiatric Diagnosis in New York and London. Institute of Psychiatry, Maudsley Monograph 20.* London: Oxford University Press.

Cox, A.D., Puckering, C., Pound, A. & Mills, M. (1987). The impact of maternal depression in young children. *Journal of Child Psychology and Psychiatry*, **28**, 917–28.

Cunningham, C.E. & Barkley, R.A. (1978). The effects of methylphenidate on the mother–child interactions of hyperactive identical twins. *Developmental Medicine and Child Neurology,* **20**, 634–42.

Cunningham, C.E. & Barkley, R.A. (1979). The interactions of normal and hyperactive children with their mothers in free play and structured tasks. *Child Development*, **50**, 217–24.

Cunningham, C.E. & Siegel, L.S. (1987). Peer interactions of normal and attention-deficit-disordered boys during free-play co-operative task, and simulated classroom situation. *Journal of Abnormal Child Psychology,* **15**, 247–68.

Cunningham, C.E., Siegel, L.S. & Offord, D.R. (1985). A developmental dose response analysis of the effects of methylphenidate on the peer interactions of attention deficit disordered boys. *Journal of Child Psychology and Psychiatry,* **26**, 955–71.

Dalby, J.T., Fox, S.L. & Haslam, R.H.A. (1982). Adoption and foster care rates in pediatric disorders. *Developmental and Behavioral Pediatrics,* **3**, 61–4.

Danforth, J.S., Barkley, R.A. & Stokes, T.F. (1991). Observations of interactions between parents and their hyperactive children: an analysis of reciprocal influence. *Clinical Psychology Review,* **11**, 703–27.

Deutsch, C.K. (1989). Adoption and attention deficit disorder. In *Attention Deficit Disorder, IV Current Concepts of Emerging Tends in Attentional and Behavioural Disorders of childhood*, eds. L.M. Bloomingdale & J.M. Swanson, pp. 67–79. Oxford: Pergamon Press.

Deutsch, C.K., Swanson, J.M., Bruell, J.H., Cantwell, D.P., Weinberg, F. & Baren, M. (1982). Over representation of adoptees in children with the attention deficit disorder. *Behavior Genetics,* **12**, 231–8.

Douglas, V.I. (1983). Attention and cognitive problems. In *Developmental Neuropsychiatry*, ed. M. Rutter, pp. 280–329. New York: Guildford Press.

Douglas, V.I. (1985). The response of ADD children to reinforcement: theoretical and clinical implications. In *Attention Deficit Disorder: Identification, Course And Treatment Rationale,* ed. L.M. Bloomingdale, pp. 49–66, New York: Spectrum.

Douglas, V.I. (1988). Cognitive deficits in children with attention deficit disorder with hyperactivity. In *Attention Deficit Disorder: Criteria, Cognition, and Intervention,* eds. L.M. Bloomingdale & J. Sergeant, pp. 65–82. New York: Pergamon Press.

Dumas, J.E. (1986). Indirect influences of maternal social contacts on mother–child interactions: A setting event analysis. *Journal of Abnormal Child Psychology,* **14**, 203–16.

Dumas, J.E. & Wahler, R.G. (1985). Indiscriminate mothering as a contextual factor in aggressive–opposition child behaviour: "Damned if you do and damned if you don't". *Journal of Abnormal Child Psychology,* **13**, 1–17.

Famularo, R., Kinscherff, R. & Fenton, T. (1992). Psychiatric diagnoses of maltreated children: preliminary findings. *Journal of the American Academy of Child and Adolescent Psychiatry,* **31**, 863–7.

Firestone, P. & Douglas, V. (1975). The effects of reward and punishment on reaction times and autonomic activity in hyperactive and normal children. *Journal of Abnormal Child Psychology,* **3**, 201–16.

Firestone, P. & Martin, J.E. (1979). An analysis of the hyperactive syndrome: a comparison of hyperactive, behavior problem, asthmatic and normal children. *Journal of Abnormal Child Psychology,* **7**, 261–73.

Fischer, M. (1990). Parenting stress and the child with attention deficit hyperactivity disorder. *Journal of Clinical Child Psychology,* **19**, 337–46.

Gardner, F.E. (1994). The quality of joint activity between mothers and their children with behaviour problems. *Journal of Child Psychiatry and Psychiatry,* **35**, 935–48.

Garralda M. E., & Bailey D. (1988). Child and parental factors related to the referral of children to child psychiatry. *British Journal of Psychiatry,* **153**, 81–9.

Garralda M. E., Connell J., & Taylor D.C. (1989). Peripheral psychophysiological changes in children with conduct and emotional disorders: basal levels and reactivity to sounds. *Behavioural Neurology,* **2**, 125–33.

Garralda M. E., Connell J., & Taylor D. (1991). Psychophysiological anomalies in children with conduct and emotional disorders. *Psychological Medicine,* **21**, 947–57.

Gillberg, C. & Rasmussen, P. (1982). Perceptual, motor and attentional deficits in seven–year–old chidren: background factors. *Developmental Medicine and Child Neurology,* **24**, 752–70.

Gillberg, I.C. & Gillberg, C. (1989). Six year–old children with perceptual, motor and attention defecits: outcome in the 6–year perspective. In *Attention Deficit Disorder and Hyperkinetic Syndrome*, eds. T. Sagvolden and T. Archer, pp. 93–103. Hilsdale N.: Erlbaun Assoc.

Glow, P.H. & Glow, R.A. (1979). Hyperkinetic impulse disorder: a developmental deficit of motivation. *Genetic Psychology Monographs,* **100**, 159–231.

Gomez, R. & Sanson, A.V. (1994). Mother–child interactions and noncompliance in hyperactive boys with and without conduct problems. *Journal of Child Psychology and Psychiatry,* **35**, 477–90.

Goodman, R. & Stevenson, J. (1989). A twin study of hyperactivity–II. The aetiological role of genes, family relationships and perinatal adversity. *Journal of Child Psychology and Psychiatry,* **30**, 691–709.

Gorenstein E. E., & Newman J. P., (1980). Disinhibitory psychopathology: a new perspective and a model for research. *Psychology Review,* **87**, 301–15.

Haddad, P.H. & Garralda, M.E. (1992). Hyperkinetic syndrome and disruptive early experiences. *British Journal of Psychiatry,* **161**, 700–3.

Hartsough, C.S. & Lambert, N.M. (1982). Some environmental and familial correlates and antecedents of hyperactivity. *American Journal of Orthopsychiatry,* **52**, 272–87.

Hersov, L. (1990). Aspects of adoption: the seventh Jack Tizard memorial lecture. *Journal of Child Psychology and Psychiatry,* **31**, 493–510.

Hinde R. A. (1980). Family influences. In *Developmental Psychiatry,* ed. M. Rutter. London: Heinemann.

Hinde, R.P. & Stevenson–Hinde, J. (1987). Interpersonal relationships and child development. *Developmental Review,* **7**, 1–21.

Hodges, J. & Tizard, B. (1989). IQ and behavioural adjustment of ex-institutional adolescents. *Journal of Child Psychology and Psychiatry,* **30**, 53–75.

Holborrow, P.L. & Berry, P.S. (1986). Hyperactivity and learning difficulties. *Journal of Learning Disabilities,* **19**, 426–31.

Hops, H., Biglan, A., Sherman, L., Arthur, J., Friedman, L. & Osteen, V. (1987). Home observations of family interactions of depressed women. *Journal of Consulting and Clinical Psychology,* **55**, 341–6.

Horn, W.R, Ialongo, N., Popovich, S. & Peradotto, D. (1987). Behavioural parent training and self-control therapy with ADD-H children: comparative and combined effects. *Journal of Clinical Child Psychology,* **16**, 57–68.

Jacobvitz, D. & Sroufe, L.A. (1987). The early caregiver–child relationship and attention deficit disorder with hyperactivity in kindergarten: a prospective study. *Child Development,* **58**, 1496–504.

Jenkins, J.M. & Smith, M.A. (1991). Marital disharmony and children's behaviour problems: aspects of a poor marriage that affect children adversely. *Journal of Child Psychology and Psychiatry,* **32**, 793–810.

Jouriles, E.N., Barling, J. & O'Leary, K.D. (1987). Predicting child behavior problems in maritally violent families. *Journal of Abnormal Child Psychology,* **15**, 165–73.

Jouriles, E.N., Murphy, C.M. & O'Leary, K.D. (1989). Effects of maternal mood on mother–son interaction patterns. *Journal of Abnormal Child Psychology,* **17**, 513–26.

Kagan, J., Reznick, J.S. & Snidman, N. (1987). The physiology and psychology of behavioural inhibition in children. *Child Development,* **58**, 1459–73.

Kalverboer, A.F. (1988). Follow-up of biological high-risk groups. In *Studies of Psychosocial Risk: The Power of Longitudinal Data,* ed. M. Rutter, pp. 114–137. Cambridge: Cambridge University Press.

Klein, D.F. & Gittelman-Klein, R. (1975). Problems in the diagnosis of minimal brain dysfunction and the hyperkinetic syndrome. *International Journal of Mental Health,* **4**, 45–60.

Kuijper, A. & Hirasing, R.A. (1986). Prevalentie van hyperactief gedrag bij vijf–jarigen (Prevalence of hyperactivity in five-year old children). *Tijdschrift voor Orthopedagiek, Kinderpsychiatrie en Kinderpsychologie,* **11**, 120–30.

Lambert, N.M., Sandoval, J. & Sassone, D. (1978). Prevalence of hyperactivity in elementary school children as a function of social system definers. *American Journal of Orthopsychiatry,* **48**, 446–62.

Loney, J. (1980). Hyperkinesis comes of age: what do we know and where should we go? *American Journal of Orthopsychiatry,* **50**, 28–42.

Levy, R., & Hobbs, G., (1981). The diagnosis of attention deficit disorder (hyperkineses) in children. *Journal of the American Academy of Child Psychiatry,* **20**, 376–84.

Loney, J., Langhorne, J.E.Jr., Paternite, C.E., Whalemklahn, M.A., Blair–Brocker, C.T. & Hacker, M. (1980). The Iowa habit: hyperkinetic/aggressive boys in treatment. In *Human Functioning in Longitudinal Perceptive: Studies of Normal and Psychopathinic population,* eds. S.B. Sells, R Randall, M. Roff, J.S. Strauss & W. Pollin. Baltimore: Williams & Wilkins.

Luk, S.L., Leung, P.W.L. & Yuen, J. (1991). Clinic observations in the assessment of pervasiveness of childhood hyperactivity. *Journal of Child Psychology and Psychiatry,* **32**, 833–50.

McGee, R., Williams, S. & Silva, P.A. (1984). Background characteristics of aggressive, hyperactive and aggressive-hyperactive boys. *Journal of the American Academy of Child and Adolescent Psychiatry,* **23**, 280–4.

McGee, R., Williams, S. & Silva, P.A. (1985). Factor structure and correlates of ratings of inattention, hyperactivity and antisocial behavior in a large sample of 9-year old children from the general population. *Journal of Consulting and Clinical Psychology,* **53**, 480–90.

Manuzza, S., Klein, R.G, Bonagura, N., Malloy, P., Giampino, T.L. & Addalli, K.A. (1991). Hyperactive boys almost grown up. 10. Replication of psychiatric status. *Archives of General Psychiatry,* **48**, 77–83.

Marks, I.M. (1987). The development of normal fear: a review. *Journal of Child Psychology and Psychiatry,* **28**, 667–97.

Marshall, V.G., Longwell, L., Goldstein, M.J. & Swanson, J.M. (1990). Family factors associated with aggressive symptomatology in boys with attention deficit hyperactivity disorder: a research note. *Journal of Child Psychology and Psychiatry,* **31**, 629–36.

Mash, E.J. & Johnston, C. (1982). A comparison of the mother–child interactions of younger and older hyperactive and normal children. *Child Development,* **53**, 1371–81.

Mash, E.J. & Johnson, C. (1990). Determinants of parenting stress: Illustrations from families of hyperactive children and families of physically abused children. *Journal of Clinical Child Psychology,* **19**, 331–8.

Minuchin, S., Baker, L., Rosman, B.L., Liebman, R., Milman, L. & Todd, T.C. (1975). A conceptual model of psychosomatic illness in children. *Archives of General Psychiatry,* **32**, 1031–8.

Moffitt, T.E. (1990). Juvenile delinquency and attention deficit disorder: boys' developmental trajectories from age 3 to age 15. *Child Development,* **61**, 893–910.

Olson, S.L., Bates, J.E. & Bayles, K. (1990). Early antecedents of childhood impulsivity. The role of parent–child interaction, cognitive competence, and temperament. *Journal of Abnormal Child Psychology,* **18**, 317–34.

Paternite, C. & Loney, J. (1980). Childhood hyperkinesis: relationships between symptomatology and home environment. In *Hyperactive Children: The Social Ecology of Identification and Treatment*, eds. C.K. Whalen & B. Henker, pp. 105–41. New York: Academic Press.

Paternite, C.E., Loney, J. & Langhorne, J.E. (1976). Relationships between symptomatology and SES-related factors in hyperkinetic/MBD boys. *American Journal of Orthopsychiatry,* **46**, 291–301.

Pliszka S. R. (1992). Comorbidity of attention–deficit hyperactivity disorder and overanxious disorder. *Journal of the American Academy of Child and Adolescent Psychiatry,* **31**, 197–203.

Pollard, S., Ward, H.A. & Barkley, R.A. (1983). The effects of parent training and Ritalin on parent–child interactions of hyperactive boys. *Child and Family Behavior Therapy,* **5**, 51–68.

Porter, B. & O'Leary, K.D. (1980). Marital discord and childhood behavior problems. *Journal of Abnormal Child Psychology,* **8**, 287–95.

Prior, M., Leonard, A. & Wood, G. (1983). A comparison study of preschool children diagnosed as hyperactive. *Journal of Pediatric Psychology,* **8**, 191–207.

Prinz, R.J., Connor, P.A. & Wilson, C.C. (1981). Hyperactive and aggressive behaviour in childhood: Intertwined dimensions. *Journal of Abnormal Child Psychology,* **9**, 191–202.

Prinz, R.J., Myers, D., Holden, E., Tarnowski, K. & Roberts, W. (1983). Marital disturbance and child problems: a cautionary note regarding hyperactive children. *Journal of Abnormal Child Psychology,* **11**, 393–9.

Puckering, C. (1989). Annotation: Maternal depression. *Journal of Child Psychology and Psychiatry,* **30**, 807–17.

Rapoport, J. L. & Benoit, M. (1975). The relation of direct home observations to the clinic evaluation of hyperactive school age boys. *Journal of Child Psychology and Psychiatry,* **16**, 141–7.

Rapoport, J.L., Donnelly, M., Zametkin, A. & Carroucher, J. (1986). Situational hyperactivity in a US clinical setting. *Journal of Child Psychology and Psychiatry,* **27**, 639–46.

Reeves, J.C., Werry, J.S., Elkind, G.S. & Zametkin, A. (1987). Attention deficit, conduct, oppositional and anxiety disorders in children: II. Clinical characteristics. *Journal of the American Academy of Child and Adolescent Psychiatry,* **26**, 144–55.

Richman, N., Stevenson, J. & Graham, P. (1982). *Pre-school to School: A Behavioural Study.* London: Academic Press.

Rogeness, G.A., Hoppe, S.K., Macedo, C.A., Fisher, C. & Harris, W.R. (1988). Psychopathology in hospitalised adopted children. *Journal of the American Academy of Child and Adolescent Psychiatry,* **27**, 628–31.

Rutter, M. & Quinton, D. (1984). Parental psychiatric disorders: effects on children. *Psychological Medicine,* **14**, 853–80.

Rutter, M., Tizard, J. & Whitmore, K. (eds.) (1970). *Education Health and Behaviour.* London: Longmans.

Sameroff, A.J. & Chandler, M.J. (1975). Reproductive risk and the continuum of caretaking casualty. In *Review of Child Development Research,,* Vol 4, ed. F.D. Horowitz, pp. 187–244. Chicago: University of Chicago Press.

Sameroff, A.J., Seifer, R. & Zax, M. (1982). Early development of children at risk for emotional disorders. *Monographs of the Society for Research in Child Development, 199, Vol. 47, No. 7.* Chicago: University of Chicago.

Samson, A., Smart, D., Prior, M. & Oberklaid, F. (1993). Precursors of hyperactivity and aggression. *Journal of the American Academy of Child and Adolescent Psychiatry,* **32**, 1207–16.

Sandberg, S.T., Rutter, M. & Taylor, E. (1978). Hyperkinetic disorder in clinic attenders. *Developmental Medicine and Child Neurology,* **20**, 279–99.

Sandberg, S.T., Wieselberg, M. & Shaffer, D. (1980). Hyperkinetic and conduct problem children in a primary school population: Some epidemiological considerations. *Journal of Child Psychology and Psychiatry,* **21**, 293–311.

Schachar, R.J. (1991). Childhood hyperactivity. *Journal of Child Psychology and Psychiatry,* **32**, 155–91.

Schachar, R. & Wachsmuth, R. (1990). Hyperactivity and parental psychopathology. *Journal of Child Psychology and Psychiatry,* **31**, 381–92.

Schachar, R.J. & Wachsmuth, R. (1991). Family dysfunction and psychosocial adversity: comparison of attention deficit disorder, conduct disorder, normal and clinical controls. *Canadian Journal of Behavioral Science,* **23**, 332–48.

Schachar, R.J., Rutter, M. & Smith, A. (1981). The characteristics of situationally and pervasively hyperactive children: implications for syndrome definition. *Journal of Child Psychology and Psychiatry,* **22**, 375–92.

Schachar, R.J., Taylor, E., Wieselberg, M., Thorley, G. & Rutter, M. (1987). Changes in family function and relationships in children who respond to methylphenidate. *Journal of the American Academy of Child and Adolescent Psychiatry,* **26**, 728–32.

Schrag, P. & Divoky, D. (1975). *Myth of the Hyperactive Child.* New York: Pantheon.

Seligman, M.E.P. (1974). Depression and learned helplessness. In *The Psychology of Depression,* eds. R.J. Friedman & M.M. Katz, pp. 83–125. Washington, DC: Winston.

Shapiro, S.K. & Garfinkel, B.D. (1986). The occurrence of behavior disorder in children: the interdependence of attention deficit disorder and conduct disorder. *Journal of the American Academy of Child and Adolescent Psychiatry,* **25**, 809–19.

Shekim, W.O., Kashani, J., Beck, N., Cantwell, D., Martin, J., Rosenberg, J. & Costello, A. (1985). The prevalence of attention deficit disorders in a rural mid-western community sample of nine-year-old children. *Journal of the American Academy of Child and Adolescent Psychiatry,* **24**, 765–70.

Shen, Y–C., Wang, Y–F. & Yang, X–L. (1985). An epidemiological investigation of minimal brain dysfunction in six elementary schools in Beijing. *Journal of Child Psychology and Psychiatry,* **26**, 777–87.

Silverman, I.W. & Ragusa, D.M. (1992). A short–term longitudinal study of the early development of self–regulation. *Journal of Abnormal Psychology,* **20**, 415–35.

Skuse, D. (1984). Extreme deprivation in early childhood. – I. Diverse outcomes for three siblings from an extraordinary family. *Journal of Child Psycholology and Psychiatry,* **25**, 523–41.

Sonuga–Barke, E.J., Taylor, E. & Heptinstall, E. (1992). Hyperactivity and delay aversion: II. The effect of self versus externally imposed stimulus presentation periods on memory. *Journal of Child Psychology and Psychiatry,* **33**, 399–409.

Strayhorn, J.M. & Weidman, C.S. (1989). Reduction of attention deficit and internalizing symptoms in pre-schoolers through parent–child interaction training. *Journal of the American Academy of Child and Adolescent Psychiatry,* **28**, 888–97.

Szatmari, P., Offord, D.R. & Boyle, M.H. (1989). Correlates, associated impairments and patterns of service utilization of children with attention deficit disorder: findings from the Ontario Child Health Study. *Journal of Child Psychology and Psychiatry,* **30**, 205–17.

Tallmadge, J. & Barkley, R.A. (1983). The interactions of hyperactive and normal boys with their mothers and fathers. *Journal of Abnormal Child Psychology,* **11**, 565–79.

Taylor, E., Sandberg, S., Thorley, G. & Giles, S. (1991). *The Epidemiology of Childhood Hyperactivity. Maudsley Monographs,* **33**. Oxford: Oxford University Press.

Taylor, E., Schachar, R., Thornley, G. & Wieselberg, M. (1986). Conduct disorder and hyperactivity: separation of hyperactivity and antisocial conduct in British child psychiatric patients. *British Journal of Psychiatry,* **149**, 760–7.

Taylor, E., Schachar, R., Thorley, G., Wieselberg, H.M., Everitt, B. & Rutter, M. (1987). Which boys respond to stimulant medication? A controlled trial of methylphenidate in boys with disruptive behaviour. *Psychological Medicine,* **17**, 121–43.

Tizard, B. & Hodges, J. (1978). The effect of early institutional rearing on the development of eight-year-old children. *Journal of Child Psychology and Psychiatry,* **19**, 99–118.

Velez, N., Johnson, J. & Cohen, P. (1989). A longitudinal analysis of selected risk factors for childhood psychopatholoy. *Journal of the American Academy of Child and Adolescent Psychiatry,* **28**, 861–4.

Verhulst, F.C., Althaus, M. & Vershus-den Bieman, H.J. (1990). Problem behaviour in international adoptees: I. An epidemiological study. *Journal of the American Academy of Child and Adolescent Psychiatry,* **29**, 94–103.

Webster–Stratton, C. (1988). Mothers' and fathers' perceptions of child deviance: roles of parent and child behaviours and parents adjustment. *Journal of Consulting and Clinical Psychology,* **56**, 909–15.

Webster–Stratton, C. & Hammond, M. (1988). Maternal depression and its relationship to life stress, perceptions of child behavior problems, parenting behaviours, and child conduct problems. *Journal of Abnormal Child Psychology,* **16**, 299–315.

Weissman, M., Prusoff, B., Gammon, G.D., Merikangas, K., Leckman, J. & Kidd, K. (1984). Psychopathology in the children (ages 6–18) of depressed and normal parents. *Journal of the American Academy of Child and Adolescent Psychiatry,* **23**, 78–84.

Weissman, M.M., Gammon, G.D., John, K., Merikangas, K.R., Warner, V., Prusoff, B.A. & Sholomkas, D. (1987). Psychopathology in the children of depressed and normal parents: direct interview studies. *Archives of General Psychiatry,* **44**, 847–53.

Wender, P. (1971). *Minimal Brain Dysfunction In Children.* New York: Wiley.

Werry, J.S., Reeves, J.C. & Elkind, G.S. (1987). Attention deficit, conduct, oppositional, and anxiety disorders in children: I. A review of research on differentiating characteristics. *Journal of the American Academy of Child and Adolescent Psychiatry,* **26**, 1333–43.

Whalen, C.K., Henker, B. & Dotemoto, S. (1980). Methylphenidate and hyperactivity: effects on teacher behaviors. *Science,* **208**, 1280–2.

Wolkind, S. & Rutter, M. (1985). Separation, loss and family relationships. In *Child and Adolescent Psychiatry: Modern Approaches,* 2nd edn., ed. M. Rutter & L. Hersov. Oxford: Blackwell Scientific.

World Health Organisation (WHO). (1978). *International Classification of Diseases,* 9th edn. Geneva: WHO.

9

Sex differences and their significance

Ellen Heptinstall and Eric Taylor

INTRODUCTION

The literature on hyperactivity may give the impression that it is solely a problem of males, since study after study is confined to boys. Such a strategy may well be justified. There is little doubt that a male predominance is one of the most consistent findings about hyperactivity and this must raise the possibility that affected females are in some way different. The research approach of studying the sexes separately has much to be said for it, but unfortunately the process usually seems to stop with the investigation of boys. As a result, clinicians have little scientific guidance about how to proceed in the many instances when a girl with hyperactivity is referred. Furthermore, the opportunity of studying sex differences which could help to understand the causes has been neglected.

The main theme of this chapter is that the sex differences in hyperactivity are important and carry clues about the nature of the disorder. Any conclusion has to be provisional because there is too little research to allow for replicated conclusions. The most basic point of all remains unanswered: whether to use the same grounds for defining a case in females as in males. The empirical findings that are available so far will be described before going on to consider issues about the nature and possible aetiology of the sex differences. Most of all, it is hoped to stimulate more clinical debate and research enquiry into hyperactivity in girls.

EMPIRICAL STUDIES OF SEX DIFFERENCES

Sex differences in prevalence

The most consistent finding in studies of hyperactivity has been the unequal representation of the sexes. Still (1902) first noted that in clinic-referred children problem behaviour or 'moral deficiency' as it was then termed, was more common in boys than in girls. Since then, many studies have reported an over-representation of boys in hyperactivity. In Britain, Thorley (1984) and James & Taylor (1990) found a ratio of 3 boys to 1 girl in samples of clinically diagnosed hyperkinetic children. In the United States, Ross & Ross (1982), reviewing several studies of clinic-referred samples, found a ratio of 5 boys to 1 girl with ADDH. More recent studies of clinically diagnosed hyperactive children carried out in the United States reported ratios of 3 boys to 1 girl (Berry, Shaywitz & Shaywitz, 1985) and 2 boys to 1 girl (Ackerman, Dykman & Oglesby, 1983). This male predominance also appeared in samples of children with neurological problems. Ingram (1956) found that brain-damaged boys were almost twice as likely to show hyperactive behaviour than similarly affected girls. In a study of 830 epileptic children, Ounsted (1955) found hyperkinesis in 55 boys and 15 girls, giving a ratio of almost 4 :1.

Population based studies of hyperactivity have reported similar sex differences. Using the Conners Teacher Rating Scale as a screening measure, Trites *et al.*(1979) found hyperactivity at a ratio of 3 boys to 1 girl in a sample of 14 000 elementary school children. Other studies using the Conners Teacher Rating Scale have reported ratios of 5 boys to 1 girl (Campbell & Redfering, 1979) and 4 boys to 1 girl (Glow, 1980). Using the Rutter B Scale for teachers only, McGee *et al.* (1985) found a ratio of 8 boys to 1 girl in a study of 940 children aged 7 in New Zealand. A study using both the Rutter A and B Scales (for parents and teachers, respectively) reported a ratio of almost 3 boys to 1 girl (Schachar, Rutter & Smith, 1981). The Ontario Child Health Study, relying on the Achenbach Child Behavior Checklist to screen a large number of children aged 4 to 16, found an overall sex ratio of 3 boys to 1 girl (Szatmari, Offord & Boyle, 1989*b*). Studies using other screening measures reported boy–girl ratios varying from 2:1 (Werry & Quay, 1971; Shekim *et al.,* 1985) to 4:1 (Hartsough & Lambert, 1982) and 6:1 (Lambert, Sandoval & Sassone, 1978). The variations in sex ratios in these studies are likely to be influenced by differences in measurements and sampling characteristics. Studies using teacher questionnaire ratings only (Campbell & Redfering, 1979, McGee *et al.,* 1985) reported a higher proportion of boys than studies using both parent and teacher ratings

(Schachar *et al.,* 1981, Szatmari *et al.,* 1989b). Variations in age may also have contributed to higher or lower sex ratios, but the consistent reports of an over-representation of boys means that the presence of sex differences in prevalence is not in doubt. Unfortunately, this finding has frequently been the conclusion rather than the starting point of a discussion.

This chapter will attempt to determine from the scientific evidence what implications these differences in prevalence between the sexes may have. This will involve a comparison of hyperactive boys with hyperactive girls in order to examine whether they share the same problem and whether the same explanatory structure applies. For this reason, the published studies will be reviewed to establish whether a consensus exists. However, one of the studies to be included in this review is at the present moment published only in report form (Taylor, 1991). This study represents an investigation carried out together with colleagues Seija Sandberg, Edmund Sonuga-Barke and Jo Bowyer. It was designed as a two-stage epidemiological survey of 6- to 8-year old girls attending schools in a London borough. It used the same methods as a study of boys of the same ages, living in the same area (Taylor *et al.,* 1991). The first stage consisted of a screen of the whole population. Out of the 2285 girls registered in schools in the assigned area, full teacher ratings were obtained for 2033 girls and full parent ratings for 1687 girls. The instruments used were the Rutter A (2) and B (2) rating scales, as well as an abbreviated version of the Conners scale. Girls were characterised as 'hyperactive' or 'conduct disordered' if they scored above the cutoffs for those scales that had been established for boys (Taylor *et al.,* 1991). Girls were less likely to show either problem than boys; the ratio was 1:2.5 for hyperactivity and 1:2.1 for conduct disorder. However, the sex ratio for emotional disorder was 1:1.

The second stage constituted a more detailed observational, interview and experimental study of selected groups of girls, defined by their scores on the screening questionnaires. All the hyperactive girls were included into this stage and divided into two groups: one with and one without conduct disorder. Other selected groups comprised conduct disordered girls without hyperactivity and a random sample of control children who did not meet criteria for either hyperactivity or conduct disorder. All subjects were studied using a standardised investigator-based parent interview, a structured and standardised teacher interview, observation during a testing session, a neurological examination, reading tests, IQ tests and attention tests. The parent interview also covered details about family relationships and histories of disorder in other family members.

One of the analyses compared the deviant girls with the deviant boys. The hyperactive girls were unequivocally less active than the hyperactive boys when their movements were measured physically, directly observed or recorded through the detailed behavioural interviews. It was therefore clear that under-recognition by teachers and parents could not account for the lower prevalence in girls.

Sex differences in behaviour characteristics

Core symptoms

Hyperactive behaviour is characterised by overactivity, inattentiveness and impulsiveness. Much of the research providing evidence for the presence of these behaviour characteristics in hyperactive children has concentrated on boys. The few studies which included both sexes have emphasized that, like hyperactive boys, hyperactive girls are more overactive, more inattentive and more impulsive than non-hyperactive children (Kashani *et al.,* 1979; deHaas & Young, 1984; deHaas, 1986; Breen, 1989). Several studies relying on teacher reports found higher levels of this hyperactive behaviour in boys than in girls. The majority of these studies used the Conners Teacher Rating Scale to identify hyperactive children (Werry, Sprague & Cohen, 1975; Werry & Hawthorne, 1976; Taylor & Sandberg, 1984; deHaas, 1986). Using the Rutter B Scale for teachers, McGee *et al.* (1985) also found that boys were rated as significantly more hyperactive than girls. These results were taken to indicate that teachers identify problematic behaviour more readily in boys than in girls. This possibility was supported by a study using both parent and teacher reports of behaviour (Breen & Altepeter, 1990). In a group of clinically diagnosed hyperactive children, teachers regarded boys as having more severe behaviour problems than girls. In contrast, parents reported similar problems for both sexes.

A number of studies including both sexes have used measures avoiding possible reporting bias. Amongst the most frequently used measures were the Matching Familiar Figures Test for impulsiveness and the Continuous Performance Test or the Stroop Colour–Word Test for inattentiveness. The findings of these studies showed few differences in the behaviour of referred boys and girls. Ackerman *et al.* (1983) reported that hyperactive girls were slightly more impulsive than hyperactive boys, but the differences were not statistically significant. Horn, Wagner & Ialongo (1989) found striking similarities in impulsive and inattentive behaviour in clinically diagnosed hyperactive boys and girls aged 6 to 11. Observations of behaviour also failed to find sex differences. Breen (1989) found no differences in off-task, out-of-seat or fidgety behaviour in a sample of referred boys and girls. Using similar playroom observation measures, Befera & Barkley (1985) also reported an absence of differences in behaviour between referred boys and girls.

Few population studies using psychometric measures included both sexes, but most which did have reported different levels of hyperactive behaviour in boys and girls, with the exception of one small sample study. A group of 13 boys and 13 girls who had been identified as hyperactive by their teachers showed no significant differences in impulsive or inattentive behaviour (deHaas, 1986). The direct comparison of hyperactive boys and hyperactive girls meant that teachers may have identified only girls who presented behaviour problems similar to those of hyperactive boys. The population study, described above, attempted to reduce stereotyped reports by studying boys and girls separately and found a number of sex differences in psychometric measures. Although hyperactive girls were less active during testing than hyperactive boys, they showed more inattentive behaviour. A population study that included observations was the Fels longitudinal study, following up children from birth (Battle & Lacey, 1972). Hyperactivity was defined as an excess of motor activity as observed at home, at school and in summer camp. At the ages of 6 to 10, boys were found to have significantly higher hyperactivity scores than girls. However, impulsive and inattentive behaviour were not measured.

Thus, referral or identification bias may contribute to an absence of sex differences in certain studies. Although the available evidence is scant, population studies using observational or test measures have reported some, but not particularly striking, sex differences in hyperactive behaviour.

The overlap with conduct disorder

Studies of hyperactivity have frequently reported an overlap with conduct disordered behaviour such as disobedience, destructiveness and aggressiveness (Sandberg, Rutter & Taylor, 1978; Werry, Reeves & Elkind, 1987). Stewart *et al.* (1981) found that, in a group of 175 clinically diagnosed children, 61% of hyperactives also showed conduct disorder, while 67% of conduct disorder children showed definite hyperactivity. Loney & Milich (1982) found an even higher proportion of co-morbidity in a sample of boys (75%) despite attempts to maximise the separation of both disorders. In British clinics, where any diagnosis related to hyperactivity is rare, most children diagnosed as conduct disordered meet DSM-III criteria for ADDH (Taylor *et al.,* 1986). It is possible that referral bias increases the likelihood of overlap in clinic cases. Children showing both hyperactive and conduct-disordered behaviour may present particularly severe management problems which would make referral more likely.

McGee, Williams & Silva (1984) found that aggressive hyperactive boys were referred almost four times as often as non-aggressive hyperactive boys. In population studies the degree of overlap varied according to the screening measures used. Relying on the Conners Teacher Rating Scale, Trites & Laprade (1983) found 64% of hyperactive children to be conduct disordered and 65% of conduct-disordered children to be hyperactive. In the Ontario Child Health study using the Achenbach Child Behaviour Check list, roughly 40% of ADDH children and adolescents aged 4 to 16 also had conduct disorder (Szatmari *et al.*, 1989*b*). In a population study of boys identified as having behaviour problems by Rutter A and B Scales, conduct disorder was found in 22% of hyperactive children (Taylor *et al.*, 1991).

Few studies examining the overlap of hyperactivity and conduct disorder either included girls or analysed the sexes separately. One clinic-based study found a mixture of hyperactive and 'unsocialised aggressive' (USA) behaviour in 39% of boys and 49% of girls (Stewart *et al.*, 1981). USA behaviour was defined as aggressive, non-compliant, destructive or hostile. Hyperactive behaviour was characterised by an abnormally high activity level, difficulty in attention or concentration and difficulty in finishing tasks. Population studies found similar excesses of overlap in girls as compared to boys. Pelham *et al.* (1989) reported the presence of oppositional/defiant behaviour in 39% of inattentive/overactive boys and 44% of inattentive/overactive girls. The study (see the section on differences in prevalence) found conduct disorder in 58% of hyperactive boys and 61% of hyperactive girls. Szatmari, Boyle & Offord (1989*a*) found more conduct disorder in hyperactive girls (50%) than in hyperactive boys (44%) aged 12 to 16. In the younger age group (4 to 11) the overlap was slightly lower in girls (36%) than in boys (42%).

More important than the figures for overlap are those for relative risk which are substantially greater for girls than for boys. Szatmari *et al.* (1989*a*) found that ADDH girls were 40 times more likely to have conduct disorder than non-hyperactive girls, while ADDH boys were 14 times more likely to have conduct disorder than non-hyperactive boys.

Intellectual ability and academic performance

Hyperactive behaviour has frequently been linked with poor educational achievement. Lambert & Sandoval (1980) have suggested that approximately 50% of hyperactive children have learning difficulties, while Safer & Allen (1976) estimated the overlap to apply to as much as 80% of hyperactives. However, the nature of these learning difficulties is not clear. In a review of studies Keogh (1971) found that reported deficits in hyperactive children varied from overall low academic achievement to specific reading problems or visual motor dysfunction. Nevertheless, reports of a relationship between hyperactivity and learning problems have been consistent.

As is the case in other areas of hyperactivity, little distinction has been made between hyperactive girls and hyperactive boys with learning problems. The few studies to examine sex differences in this area have been contradictory in their findings. Berry, Shaywitz & Shaywitz (1985) claimed that referred hyperactive girls showed more prominent cognitive deficits than referred hyperactive boys. In particular, girls showed more severe language impairment than boys. In addition, hyperactive girls had a lower mean IQ than hyperactive boys. These findings correspond with those reported on a group of referred hyperkinetic children (James & Taylor, 1990). Language problems were found in 26% of boys and 66% of girls. Boys had a mean IQ of 77, while the mean IQ of girls was 67. In contrast, other studies of referred hyperactive children found no sex differences in learning problems and academic performance (Horn *et al.,* 1989; Breen, 1989). There is some indication that the choice of measures may have contributed to the inconsistency in findings. Studies reporting greater cognitive impairment in girls (Berry *et al.,* 1985; James & Taylor, 1990) estimated IQ from several subtests of a standard test battery, while two studies reporting an absence of sex differences (Horn *et al.,* 1989; Breen, 1989) based their results only on the Peabody Picture Vocabulary Test.

Very few population-based studies have examined sex differences in intellectual ability and academic performance. Szatmari *et al.* (1989*b*) collected data on a variety of impairments such as poor relationships and low competence in skills. School performance was included but not separately analysed. Levels of impairment did not differentiate the sexes. Our own studies, mentioned above, showed that 'pure hyperactive' girls had a lower mean IQ (92.0) than pure hyperactive boys (101.0). Mixed hyperactive/conduct-disordered girls also showed a lower mean IQ (89.5) than their male counterparts (95.0).

Peer relationships

A large body of literature has suggested that hyperactive children have more negative relationships with their peers and fewer friends than non-hyperactive children (Klein & Young, 1979; Milich & Landau, 1982; Pelham & Bender, 1982). The concern about the effect of poor peer relationships on hyperactive children is reflected by the unusually large number of studies examining both sexes. The majority of these studies, using a variety of measures, reported similarities in boys and girls. Parents', teachers' and peers' reports of hyperactive children showed similar problems. Both hyperactive boys and girls were described as more negative towards their peers and more disruptive in group play (Johnston, Pelham & Murphy, 1985; Berry *et al.,* 1985; deHaas, 1986; Horn *et al.,* 1989). An observational study reported similar difficulties (Battle & Lacey, 1972). Only two studies reported differences in the severity of the problems in boys and girls. In a referred sample, girls were found to suffer more peer rejection, while boys were more dominating and physically aggressive towards their peers (Berry *et al.,* 1985). In a sample of 607 school children, hyperactive boys were found to be more withdrawn as well as more aggressive towards their peers than hyperactive girls (Johnston *et al.,* 1985). However, it appeared that generally the difficulties in peer relationships applied to both sexes.

The parent–child relationship

Unlike studies of peer relationships in hyperactive children, studies examining the parent–child relationship have mostly concentrated on boys. A number of studies, all based on playroom observations, found mothers of hyperactive boys more encouraging but also more disapproving and more directive in structured tasks compared to mothers of non-hyperactive boys, while in free play they were less responsive and more controlling (Campbell, 1973; Campbell, 1975; Cunningham & Barkley, 1979; Mash & Johnston, 1982). The only study to include fathers as well as mothers reported no inter-parental differences in behaviour (Tallmadge & Barkley, 1983). The inclusion of non-hyperactive brothers in the interaction enabled Tarver-Behring, Barkley & Karisson (1985) to demonstrate that mothers were more directive and less responsive towards hyperactive sons than towards non-hyperactive sons.

Few studies included both sexes and examined possible differences in the parent-child relationship. In a referred sample, Befera & Barkley (1985) found mothers of hyperactive boys more negative and less responsive than mothers of hyperactive girls. Similar sex differences were observed in a population sample (Battle & Lacey, 1972). It appeared therefore from the limited evidence available that parents tend to react more negatively towards hyperactive boys than towards hyperactive girls.

Adolescent and adult outcome

The outcome of hyperactive girls is particularly poorly researched. This is not surprising since the majority of original studies concentrated on boys. One study of 123 hyperactive children followed up over eight years included a small number of girls (12) but they were not analysed separately from the boys (Fischer *et al.,* 1993). The adolescent outcome of hyperactive boys is very well documented, while less is known about how they fared as adults. From their review of follow-up studies Klein & Mannuzza (1991) concluded that, in adolescence, hyperactive boys retain significant levels of restlessness and poor attention, showed a greater rate of school failure and more frequently engaged in antisocial activities than non-hyperactive adolescent boys. Lilienfeld & Waldman (1990) came to similar conclusions, but argued that the reported persistence of antisocial behaviour may be an artefact of the overlap between hyperactivity and conduct disorder.

As will be discussed in a later section, some biological theories of the aetiology of hyperactivity lead to the expectation of a worse outcome for girls. The only study to date which compared hyperactive adolescent boys and girls reported an opposite finding; 42% of boys and 25% of girls were diagnosed as hyperactive at follow-up (Mannuzza & Gittelman, 1984). However, the small number of hyperactive girls (12) makes it hard to draw firm conclusions. In addition, this study did not report on the educational achievement and the social adjustment of the hyperactive subjects. More follow-up studies including girls are therefore required to determine how far their outcome differs from that of hyperactive boys.

THE NATURE OF THE SEX DIFFERENCES

The preceding review of differences in prevalence and associations of hyperactivity between the sexes has shown a number of contradictions. This is not surprising since population and clinic-referred samples are likely to differ in their characteristics. Furthermore, questionnaire scores in the general population and DSM clinical diagnosis in referred populations may be difficult to compare. Inconsistency is therefore to be expected and for this reason a meta-analysis of studies has not been attempted. The major conclusion has to be that more research is needed with improved classificatory concepts and methods of identification. Until this happens, it is difficult to disentangle genetic, physical and social contribution to the differences. Other conclusions must also be tentative.

First, it must be asked whether the sex differences could be entirely due to rater bias. Some rater bias is likely to derive from differential adult attitudes to affected boys and girls, but can this account entirely for the differences? If parents and teachers systematically underestimate the restlessness and inattentiveness of girls, one would expect to find that when using objective test measures, girls scoring above a cut-off on their caregivers' ratings would be more overactive than boys scoring above the same cut-off.

In fact, the opposite seems to be the case. Girls identified as hyperactive in a population screen were less hyperactive than boys when directly observed (Taylor, 1991). This finding suggests that caregivers tend to over-rate hyperactivity in girls. The true difference between the sexes is therefore likely to be greater than that estimated by screening measures and rating scales.

The factors determining the identification of children as hyperactive are crucial both for scientific understanding of identified groups and for adequate care provision, and need to be more thoroughly researched. The effects of caregivers' attitudes appear to be complex. On the one hand, parents and teachers seem to overestimate the hyperactivity level of girls. On the other hand, they do not seem to regard high levels of hyperactivity in girls as a problem (Taylor, 1991) which means that specialist treatment may not be sought as often as could be expected. Findings that hyperactive boys are more frequently referred to clinics than hyperactive girls do not mean very much without detailed information about the comparability of the sexes in terms of developmental level and degree of hyperactivity. Future research will need to be systematic in describing prevalence and severity of symptoms for the sexes at different levels of community identification. Caregivers might, of course, be correct in applying different standards to boys and girls. Nevertheless, even if this is the case, it would not contradict the conclusion that male predominance cannot be explained by rater effects on the recognition of hyperactivity.

The second question that needs to be addressed is whether the male predominance can be attributed to other conditions. Males certainly show higher levels of aggression (Block, 1983) or other antisocial conditions (Stewart *et al.,* 1981) and hyperactivity is so much more common in children with conduct disorder (Stewart *et al.,* 1981; Loney & Milich, 1982) that the sex difference in the prevalence of hyperactivity might simply be a consequence of that for antisocial behaviour. However, this assumption is refuted by the fact that the sex ratio for 'pure' hyperactivity (i.e. without either conduct disorder or emotional disorder) is similar to that for mixed disorders (Taylor, 1991). In theory, some other disorder might be responsible for the sex difference, but it is not clear what it could be. Learning disorders are unlikely to explain the male predominance since they are more common in hyperactive girls (Berry *et al.,* 1985; James & Taylor, 1990).

A third way of explaining the sex difference involves the definition of hyperactivity. It has frequently been pointed out that diagnostic criteria and rating scales for conduct disorder heavily emphasise 'male' behaviours such as fighting rather than 'female' ones such as verbal cruelty and sexual precocity. As yet, there is no evidence of a specifically female pattern of hyperactivity which differs from the usual pattern of inattentiveness and restlessness. However, this matter could be examined more fully by establishing whether inattentiveness in psychological testing has different correlates in boys and girls.

Provisionally, therefore, it is concluded that the sex differences in hyperactivity are not an artefact of rater or instrument effects and are not secondary to differences in other disorders. This leaves the question whether girls are protected against disorders in general or specific disorders involving hyperactivity in particular. The simplest way to answer this question would be to exclude all cases of disorder in a population (e.g. all those scoring above a cut-off) and to determine whether a sex difference still exists. This study looked specifically at this possibility and found a sex difference amongst the controls, with boys scoring higher than girls. This makes it likely that hyperactivity is less common in girls because of a general protection enjoyed by the whole population of females, and not because discrete disorders involving hyperactivity are less often present in girls. This protection could either be a decreased variability in girls, or a resistance to hyperactivity. An examination of sex effects on very high levels of attentiveness and self-control would be needed to distinguish between he two types of protection.

Unfortunately, this way of considering the dimensional or categorical nature of the sex difference is not wholly reliable. It assumes that it is known where a cut-off or a category should be placed. Since the distribution of hyperactivity appears to be continuous in the population, and the level constituting a risk is not yet defined by epidemiologically based longitudinal studies, any cut-off remains arbitrary. This reservation applies just as much to DSM-IV and ICD-10 criteria as to questionnaire scores, because they are based on committee decisions and field studies of current diagnostic practice which fail to give scientific answers to the level of definition that is required. Since the cut-off or diagnosis is arbitrary, it could be wrong. If it is wrong, it could lead to a misleading answer to an important distinction.

At a much higher level of definition – that giving the older ICD-9 category of hyperkinetic syndrome – sex differences remain much the same. However, the mixture theory analysis applied by James & Taylor (1990) provided support for the hypothesis that more than one condition was involved. A 'non-developmental' disorder, not characterised by a lower IQ or language delay, seemed scarcely to exist in referred hyperactive girls. On the other hand, the boy–girl ratio for 'developmental' hyperkinesis associated with a lower IQ was relatively low. Latent class analyses could now be applied to epidemiological data to test the possibility of a female protection which is of fundamental importance to understanding the nosology of the disorders. The conclusion seems to be that there is a general protective effect for females and that the possibility of a more specific protection against a subtype of disorder needs more study.

If, as has been concluded, girls' behaviour generally differs from that of boys, the question whether to apply separate standards for the sexes becomes crucial. At present, nearly all clinical practice and research apply absolute thresholds although rater effects imply that some uncontrolled relative scaling may occur. The desirability of separate standards for the sexes would be best answered by considering outcome. If, with a lower level of hyperactivity, girls showed the same psychological adjustment problems as hyperactive boys, it would be necessary to apply a relative threshold for clinical diagnosis, rather than an absolute one. So far, the existing literature has only shown that hyperactive girls are less likely to remain affected in adolescence than hyperactive boys (Mannuzza & Gittelman, 1984). Proponents of a relativistic approach to diagnosis would argue that an equal hyperactivity score for a girl and a boy at follow-up implies that the girl is more impaired because she is more deviant from the norm for her sex. Therefore, outcome needs to be assessed in terms of social adjustment rather than merely the continuation of original symptoms. As has been pointed out earlier, this type of research is, as yet, not available for girls. It follows that, for the moment, we have to be content with considering surrogate measures of severity. Are the complications of hyperactivity (aggression, poor peer relationships, educational failure) more salient in girls scoring above the same level as affected boys? Are neurodevelopmental problems greater? Does a relativistically defined group of girls have the same associations as a group of boys with disorders involving hyperactivity? The clearest answer to these questions comes from associations with other forms of neurodevelopmental delay. The London and New Zealand epidemiological studies agree that girls with hyperactivity show more developmental problems, for example, in language and cognition, than hyperactive boys (McGee *et al.*, 1984; Taylor, 1991). Furthermore, girls who are identified on the basis of their relative deviance from the female mean for hyperactivity show similar developmental problems as boys. The point is not fully established and studies are not unanimous, but the strongest evidence must come from studies based on representative populations and using standardised scales for identifying hyperactivity rather than clinical diagnosis. However, the meaning of the finding needs further consideration. If developmental delays are a result of hyperactivity, it would be legitimate to take them as an index of the severity of the condition of hyperkinesis and conclude with McGee *et al.* (1984) that equal numbers of boys and girls ought to be diagnosed. However, this is by no means accepted as the reason for the association between hyperkinesis and developmental disorders. If hyperkinesis results from developmental delays, one would expect hyperkinetic girls to be more developmentally delayed because a larger dose of the aetiological factor was required to overcome the female protection. If this is the correct explanation, or if, as suggested, the frequency of delays in females is a consequence of their relative invulnerability to an alternative causal pathway, it would still be appropriate to apply the same measures and thresholds of recognition to boys as to girls. On the current evidence, hyperactive boys and hyperactive girls score similarly on impairment of relationships and co-morbid aggression.

In summary, girls are protected against the development of hyperactivity, and in particular against hyperactivity without signs of neurodevelopmental delay. The full extent of the protection is obscured by adults' tendency to identify girls as hyperactive on weaker behavioural grounds. Once they have reached caseness, they show behaviour which is similar to that of hyperactive boys. Thus, there is a true sex difference that theories of aetiology must explain.

THE AETIOLOGY OF SEX DIFFERENCES

Several explanations regarding the cause of the difference in prevalence between the sexes have been offered. They do not refer exclusively to hyperactivity but apply to all major categories of childhood behaviour disorders (Eme,1979). Theories regarding the aetiology of childhood psychopathology can be divided into three broad categories: environmental, biological and genetic. This section will briefly describe the different factors and discuss their applicability to hyperactive behaviour.

Environmental factors

Differential socialisation practices have been regarded as a cause for the greater prevalence of boys in most types of behaviour problems, but there is disagreement over their true effect. Block (1983) has argued that socialisation practices favour the cognitive development of boys by providing them with more opportunity for independent problem solving in a variety of contexts.

However, although boys have consistently been found to be more aggressive, more active and more impulsive than girls from an early age (Maccoby & Jacklin, 1980; Block, 1983), there is no clear evidence that differential socialisation practices precipitate hyperactive behaviour in boys. One should not exaggerate the size of the sex differences in behaviour. In a meta-analysis of aggression, Hyde (1984) concluded that only 5% of the variance is due to sex differences, while the other 95% are accounted for by within-sex variations and errors of measurement. This conclusion is particularly important since greater aggression in boys has been the most consistent finding in the literature of sex differences (Block, 1983). In a meta-analysis of sex differences in behaviour in general, Lytton & Romney (1991) claimed that parents reinforce biological differences. This claim corresponds with a report by Hyde (1984) that more recent studies have shown a decline in the sex differences in aggression. The author hypothesised that this decline may be due to changing socialisation practices as well as changing observers' perceptions.

Another environmental influence on greater male psychopathology has been said to be a greater male vulnerability to psychological stress. In a study of families in which one parent was a psychiatric patient, Rutter (1970) found that discord and disruption in the home were consistently and strongly associated with antisocial behaviour in boys but not in girls. Maccoby & Jacklin (1974) found several studies showing that boys became more distressed when separated from their parents than girls. These findings of a stronger link between psychological stress and disturbed behaviour in boys have not been shown to apply to hyperactive behaviour. The studies described previously found no marked differences in marital discord and maternal depression in the families of hyperactive boys and girls. In any case, substantial improvements in the family relationships of children whose hyperactive behaviour had declined by treatment with drugs (Schachar *et al.*, 1987) have suggested that hyperactivity is a cause rather than a consequence of family dysfunction.

Biological factors

Explanations of a biological cause for sex differences in behaviour disorders can be traced back to the theory of a greater male immaturity. Girls have been seen to be more mature than boys at all stages of development. At birth, boys are described as several weeks behind girls in maturity. The difference increases to one year at the time of starting school and widens to two years at puberty (Garai & Scheinfeld, 1968; Rutter, 1970). The sex differences in maturity have been attributed to factors on the Y chromosome, namely that males have 4 to 5% less chromosomal material than females (Childs, 1965; Gualtieri & Hicks, 1985). It has frequently been suggested that this relative male immaturity is at least partly responsible for a greater male susceptibility to almost any kind of physical problem because it exposes them to a greater risk of damage (Taylor & Ounsted, 1972). Boys have more pregnancy and birth complications (Ounsted, 1972), they are more likely to suffer from infectious diseases (Taylor & Ounsted, 1972) and more frequently show neurodevelopmental abnormalities (Gualtieri & Hicks, 1985). The theory that this 'selective male affliction' can be attributed to a maternal immunoreactivity to the male foetus has been put forward by Gualtieri & Hicks (1985), but has met with some scepticism (Adinolfi, Polani & Crolla, 1985). There is widespread agreement that, although boys are more frequently afflicted with many diseases and neurodevelopmental disorders, affected girls develop a more severe form. Studies have shown a greater overall prevalence of males in mental retardation, but at the lowest levels of IQ the proportion of females is higher (Taylor & Ounsted, 1972). In a population study of early childhood psychoses, Wing (1981) found less impairment of comprehension, communication and imaginative play in girls, but those who were impaired were more likely to be mentally retarded than boys. Taylor & Ounsted (1972) have explained this phenomenon by arguing that, because girls mature faster, they will have acquired a relatively greater degree of divergence from their norm when they cross the threshold into the pathological area and will therefore be worse affected than boys. However, the finding that hyperkinetic girls show more developmental delays than hyperkinetic boys (see above) does not provide strong support for the theory of a general greater male susceptibility to disease. Girls may be socially and psychologically protected from the development of hyperkinesis, and a greater concentration of pathogenetic factors may be required to break down this protection.

Genetic factors

Genetic explanations for the excess of males do not include X-linked inheritance in the face of father–son transmission. A two-threshold model is possible: females need a 'higher dose' of the relevant genes in order to display the same pathology as males. Such a theory suggests that affected females would have a larger number of relatives suffering from the relevant disorder than males. Evidence for this has been found in Tourette syndrome (Baron *et al.*, 1981), stuttering (Kidd, Reich & Kessle, 1973), pyloric stenosis (Kidd & Spence, 1976) as well as antisocial behaviour and criminality (Cloninger *et al.*,

1978). Kashani *et al.* (1979) claimed that the two-threshold model applied to hyperactivity after finding a significantly higher prevalence of psychiatric disorder amongst the parents of hyperactive girls than amongst the parents of hyperactive boys. However, although the two-threshold model would predict a greater prevalence of hyperactivity in the relatives of hyperactive girls, this would not necessarily apply to psychiatric disorders in general. Other studies of hyperactivity failed to support the two-threshold model. Mannuzza & Gittelman (1984) found a greater prevalence of ADDH in the parents of hyperactive boys than in the parents of hyperactive girls. A similar finding was reported by James & Taylor (1990) and by Faraone *et al.* (1991). All three studies showed similar methodological limitations rendering the findings inconclusive. The numbers of girls were relatively small (12, 18 and 20, respectively) and all three studies relied on retrospective recall of parents' or first-degree relatives' childhood hyperactivity. In addition, the use of clinic-referred samples could have confounded the findings because of possible differential referral biases for boys and girls.

In an attempt to settle the uncertainty regarding the applicability of the two-threshold model to hyperactivity, Goodman & Stevenson (1989*b*) employed a population twin study. The authors argued that the two-threshold model predicted that twin brothers of hyperactive girls would be more frequently hyperactive than twin brothers of hyperactive boys. This prediction was not confirmed; siblings were not significantly more likely to be hyperactive if they had an affected twin sister than if they had an affected twin brother. The strength of the study's design casts doubt on the importance of genetic factors in causing sex differences in hyperactivity. However, the age of the twins in this study (13) was rather higher than would be desirable when studying a condition such as hyperactivity which develops at an early age and alters over time in response to external stressors.

In summary, sex differences have provided evidence for the presence of a biological aetiology to hyperactivity, but they have not demonstrated that the differences between the sexes is in itself based upon biological factors.

IMPLICATIONS FOR FUTURE RESEARCH

It is clear that the sex differences in hyperactivity are scientifically interesting and may well give clues to the aetiology of the disorder. For this reason alone it would be well worthwhile to conduct further research in order to test the various explanatory theories reviewed above. From the evidence available so far, a few points are particularly intriguing. First, the sex differences have pointed at the possibility that there are in fact two types of hyperkinesis: one with and one without cognitive impairment. This deserves study with other strategies as well as sex comparisons. Secondly, there is substantial evidence against an over-representation of hyperactivity in the families of hyperactive girls. This is a puzzling finding, given the general view that genetic factors enter into the aetiology. Of course, the evidence is most unsatisfactory. The criteria for recognising affected family members may even be invalid. Genetic studies need to be carried out for many other reasons, and they will probably contribute to understanding the nature of the heterogeneity in syndromes of overactivity and attention deficit.

Another outstanding matter is the lack of satisfactory knowledge of the determinants of social adjustment in hyperactive girls. They may or may not be similar to those in boys. The different psychological meaning of puberty for boys and girls might entail a difference in course in adolescence, as might the altered reactions of teachers, parents and peers. Current knowledge suggests that mild degrees of hyperactivity either protect girls against educational failure or enhance the risk compared to boys. This leaves a great uncertainty about how to proceed clinically, when to intervene and what prognosis to give.

Cautious clinical practice can be based on a reading of the research evidence reviewed in this chapter. The clinician following this line will not be quick to diagnose hyperactivity in a girl, but will maintain the same criteria for inattentiveness, restlessness and impulsiveness that would be applied for boys. Once diagnosed, girls will be expected to be at risk of psychological maladjustment and treatment is therefore necessary. Behavioural modification, personal counselling and stimulant medication will all have helpful short-term effects, but the use of treatments to promote psychological adjustment in the longer term will have to be based on an individual judgement about the strengths and weaknesses of a girl's development and environment. Milder degrees of hyperactive behaviour should not be given undue weight in a diagnostic formulation because the appearance of antisocial behaviour, peer relationship impairment and educational failure are likely to be more important determinants of outcome and more rewarding targets for therapy.

REFERENCES

Ackerman, P.T., Dykman, R.A. & Oglesby, D.M. (1983). Sex and group differences in reading and attention disordered children with and without hyperkinesis. *Journal of Learning Disabilities,* **16**, 407–15.

Adinolfi, M., Polani, P.E. & Crolla, J.A. (1985). Is the sex ratio at birth affected by immune selection? *Experimental and Clinical Immunogenetics,* **2**, 54–64.

Baron, M., Shapiro, E., Shapiro, A. & Rainer, J.D. (1981). Genetic analysis of Tourette syndrome suggesting major gene effect. *American Journal of Human Genetics,* **33**, 767–75.

Battle, E.S. & Lacey, B. (1972). A context for hyperactivity in children over time. *Child Development,* **43**, 757–73.

Befera, M.S. & Barkley, R.A. (1985). Hyperactive and normal girls and boys: mother–child interactions, parent psychiatric status and child psychopathology. *Journal of Child Psychology and Psychiatry,* **26**, 439–52.

Berry, C.A., Shaywitz, S.E. & Shaywitz B.A. (1985). Girls with attention deficit disorder: A silent minority? A report on behavioral and cognitive characteristics. *Pediatrics,* **76**, 801–9.

Block, J.H. (1983). Differential premises arising from differential socialisation of the sexes: some conjectures. *Child Development,* **54**, 1335–54.

Breen, M.J. (1989). Cognitive and behavioral differences in ADDH boys and girls. *Journal of Child Psychology and Psychiatry,* **30**, 711–17.

Breen, M.J. & Altepeter, T.S. (1990). Situational variability in boys and girls identified as ADHD. *Journal of Clinical Psychology,* **46**, 486–90

Campbell, S.B. (1973). Mother–child interaction in reflective, impulsive and hyperactive children. *Journal of Developmental Psychology,* **8**, 341–347.

Campbell, S.B. (1975). Mother–child interaction: a comparison of hyperactive, learning disabled and normal boys. *American Journal of Orthopsychiatry,* **45**, 51–7.

Campbell, E.S. & Redfering, D.L. (1979). Relationships among environmental and demographic variables and teacher-rated hyperactivity. *Journal of Abnormal Child Psychology,* **7**, 77–81.

Childs, B. (1965). Genetic origin of some sex differences among human beings. *Pediatrics,* **35**, 798.

Cloninger, C.R., Christiansen, K.O., Reich, T. & Gottesman, I.I. (1978). Implications of sex differences in the prevalences of antisocial personality, alcoholism and criminality for familial transmission. *Archives of General Psychiatry,* **35**, 941–51.

Cunningham, C.E. & Barkley, R.A. (1979). The interaction of normal and hyperactive children with their mothers in free play and structured tasks. *Child Development,* **50**, 217–24.

Eme, R.F. (1979). Sex differences in childhood psychopathology: a review. *Psychological Bulletin,* **86**, 574–95.

Faraone, S.V., Biederman, J., Keenan, K. & Ming, T.T. (1991). A family-genetic study of girls with DSM-III attention deficit disorder. *American Journal of Psychiatry,* **148**, 112–17.

Fischer, M., Barkley, R.A., Fletcher, K.E. & Smallish L. (1993). The adolescent outcome of hyperactive children: predictors of psychiatric, academic, social and emotional adjustment. *Journal of the American Academy of Child and Adolescent Psychiatry,* **32**, 324–32.

Garai, J. & Scheinfeld, A. (1968). Sex differences in mental and behavioral traits. *Genetic Psychology Monographs,* **77**, 169–299.

Glow, R.A. (1980). A validation of Conners teacher questionnaire and a cross-cultural comparison of prevalence of hyperactivity in children. In *Advances in Human Psychopharmacology,* eds. G.D. Burrows & J.S. Werry, Vol. **1**, pp. 302–320. Greenwich CT: JAI Press.

Goodman, R. & Stevenson, J. (1989*a*). A twin study of hyperactivity -I. An examination of hyperactivity scores and categories derived from Rutter teacher and parent questionnaire. *Journal of Child Psychology and Psychiatry,* **30**, 671–90.

Goodman, R. & Stevenson, J. (1989*b*). A twin study of hyperactivity-II. The aetiological role of genes, family relationships and perinatal adversity. *Journal of Child Psychology and Psychiatry,* **30**, 691–709.

Gualtieri, T. & Hicks, R.E. (1985). An immunoreactive theory of selective male affliction. *The Behavioral and Brain Sciences,* **8**, 427–41.

deHaas, P.A. (1986). Attention styles and peer relationships of hyperactive and normal boys and girls. *Journal of Abnormal Child Psychology,* **14**, 457–67.

deHaas, P.A. & Young, R.D. (1984). Attention styles of hyperactive and normal girls. *Journal of Abnormal Child Psychology,* **12**, 531–46.

Hartsough, C. & Lambert, N. (1982). Some environmental and familial correlates and antecedents of hyperactivity. *American Journal of Orthopsychiatry,* **52**, 272–87.

Horn, W.F., Wagner, A.E. & Ialongo, N. (1989). Sex differences in school-aged children with pervasive attention deficit hyperactivity disorder. *Journal of Abnormal Child Psychology,* **17**, 109–25.

Hyde, S.J. (1984). How large are gender differences in aggression? A developmental meta-analysis. *Developmental Psychology,* **20**, 722–36.

Ingram, T.T. (1956). Characteristic form of overactive behaviour in brain-damaged children. *Journal of Mental Science,* **102**, 550-8.

James, A. & Taylor, E.A. (1990). Sex differences in the hyperkinetic syndrome of childhood. *Journal of Child Psychology and Psychiatry,* **31**, 437–46.

Johnston, C., Pelham, W.E. & Murphy, H.A. (1985). Peer relationships in ADDH and normal children: a developmental analysis of peer and teacher ratings. *Journal of Abnormal Child Psychology,* **13**, 89–100.

Kashani, J., Chapel, J.L., Ellis, J. & Shekim, W.O. (1979). Hyperactive girls. *Journal of Operational Psychiatry,* **10**, 145–8.

Keogh, B. (1971). Hyperactivity and learning disorders: Review and speculation. *Exceptional Children,* **38**, 101–9.

Kidd, K.K. & Spence, M.A. (1976). Genetic analyses of pyloric stenosis suggesting a specific maternal effect. *Journal of Medical Genetics,* **13**, 290-4.

Kidd, K.K., Reich, T. & Kessle, R.S. (1973). A genetic analysis of stuttering suggesting a single major locus. *Genetics,* **74**, 137.

Klein, A.R. & Young, R.D. (1979). Hyperactive boys in their classroom. Assessment of teacher and peer perceptions, interactions and classroom behaviours. *Journal of Abnormal Child Psychology,* **7**, 425–42.

Klein, R.G. & Mannuzza, S. (1991). Long-term outcome of hyperactive children: A review. *Journal of the American Academy of Child and Adolescent Psychiatry,* **30**, 383–7.

Lambert, N.M. & Sandoval, J. (1980). The prevalence of learning disabilities in a sample of children considered hyperactive. *Journal of Abnormal Child Psychology,* **8**, 33–50.

Lambert, N.M., Sandoval, J. & Sassone, E. (1978). Prevalence of hyperactivity in elementary school children as a function of social system definers. *American Journal of Orthopsychiatry*, **48**, 446–63.

Lilienfeld, S. & Waldman, I.D. (1990). The relationship between childhood attention-deficit hyperactivity disorder and adult antisocial behavior reexamined: the problem of heterogeneity. *Clinical Psychology Review,* **10**, 699–725.

Loney, J. & Milich, R. (1982). Hyperactivity, inattention and aggression in clinical practice. In *Advances in Developmental Behavioral Pediatrics,* eds. M. Wolraich, & D.K. Routh, vol. 3. Greenwich, Connecticut: JAI Press.

Lytton, H. & Romney, D.M. (1991). Parents' differential socialization of boys and girls: a meta-analysis. *Psychological Bulletin,* **109**, 267–96.

Maccoby, E.E. & Jacklin, C.N. (1980). Sex differences in aggression: a rejoinder and reprise. *Child Development,* **51**, 964–80.

McGee, R., Williams, S. & Silva, A. (1984). Behavioral and developmental characteristics of aggressive, hyperactive and aggressive–hyperactive boys. *Journal of the American Academy of Child and Adolescent Psychiatry,* **23**, 270-9.

McGee, R., Williams, S., Bradshaw, J., Chapel, J.L., Robins, A. & Silva, P.A. (1985). The Rutter Scale for completion by teachers: factor structure and relationships with cognitive abilities and family adversity for a sample of New Zealand children. *Journal of Child Psychology and Psychiatry,* **26**, 727–40.

Mannuzza, S. & Gittelman, R. (1984). The adolescent outcome of hyperactive girls. *Psychiatry Research,* **13**, 19–29.

Mash, E.J. & Johnston, C.A. (1982). A comparison of the mother–child interactions of younger and older hyperactive and normal children. *Child Development,* **53**, 1371–81.

Milich, R. & Landau, S. (1982). Socialization and peer relations in the hyperactive child. In *Advances in Learning and Behavioral Disabilities*, eds. K. Gadow and I. Bialer, Vol. 1. Greenwich, Connecticut: JAI Press.

Ounsted, C. (1955). The hyperkinetic syndrome in epileptic children. *Lancet,* **ii**, 303–11.

Ounsted, M. (1972). Gender and intrauterine growth. In *Gender Differences: Their Ontogeny and Significance*, eds. C. Ounsted & D.C. Taylor. Edinburgh: Churchill Livingstone.

Pelham, W.E. & Bender, M.E. (1982). Peer relationships in hyperactive children: description and treatment. In *Advances in Learning and Behavioral Disabilities*, vol. 1, K. Gadow & I. Bialer, Greenwich, Connecticut: JAI Press.

Pelham, W.E., Milich, R., Murphy, D.A. & Murphy, H.A. (1989). Normative data on the IOWA Conners Teacher rating scale. *Journal of Clinical Child Psychology,* **18**, 259–62.

Ross, D.M. & Ross, S.A. (1982). *Hyperactivity: Current Issues, Research and Theory.* Wiley: New York.

Rutter, M. (1970). Sex differences in children's response to family stress. In *The Child in his Family*, eds. E.J. Anthony & C. Koupernik. New York: Wiley.

Safer, D.J. & Allen, R.P. (1976). *Hyperactive Children: Diagnosis and Management.* Baltimore: University Park Press.

Sandberg, S.T., Rutter, M. & Taylor, E. (1978). Hyperkinetic disorder in psychiatric clinic attenders. *Developmental Medicine and Child Neurology,* **20**, 279–99.

Schachar, R., Rutter, M. & Smith, A. (1981). The characteristics of situationally and pervasively hyperactive children. *Journal of Child Psychology and Psychiatry,* **22**, 375–92.

Schachar, R., Taylor, E., Wieselberg, M., Thorley, G. & Rutter, M. (1987). Changes in family functioning and relationships in children who respond to methylphenidate. *Journal of the American Academy of Child and Adolescent Psychiatry,* **26**, 728–32.

Serbin, L.A., O'Leary, K.D., Kent, R.N. & Tanick, I.J. (1973). A comparison of teacher response to the pre-academic and problem behaviour of boys and girls. *Child Development,* **44**, 796–804.

Shekim, W.O., Kashani, J., Beck, N., Cantwell, D., Martin, J., Rosenberg, J. & Costello A. (1985). The prevalence of attention deficit disorders in a rural midwestern community sample of 9-year old children. *Journal of the American Academy of Child and Adolescent Psychiatry*, **24**, 765–70.

Shepherd, M., Oppenheim, B. & Mitchell, S. (1966). Childhood behaviour disorders and the child guidance clinic: an epidemiology study. *Journal of Child Psychology and Psychiatry,* **7**, 39–52.

Stewart, M.A., Cummings, C., Singer, S. & DeBlois, C.S. (1981). The overlap between hyperactive and unsocialized aggressive children. *Journal of Child Psychology and Psychiatry,* **22**, 35–46.

Still, G.F. (1902). The Coulstonian lectures on some abnormal psychical conditions in children. *Lancet,* **i**, 1008–12, 1077–82, 1163–68.

Szatmari, P., Boyle, M. & Offord, D.R. (1989a). ADDH and conduct disorder: degree of diagnostic overlap and differences among correlates. *Journal of the American Academy of Child and Adolescent Psychiatry,* **28**, 865–72.

Szatmari, P., Offord, D.R. & Boyle, M.H. (1989*b*). Ontario Child Health Study: prevalence of attention deficit disorder with hyperactivity. *Journal of the American Academy of Child and Adolescent Psychiatry,* **30**, 219–30.

Tallmadge, J. & Barkley, R.A. (1983). The interactions of hyperactive and normal boys with their fathers and mothers. *Journal of Abnormal Child Psychology,* **11**, 565–80.

Tarver-Behring, S., Barkley, R.A. & Karisson, J. (1985). The mother–child interactions of hyperactive boys and their normal siblings. *American Journal of Orthopsychiatry,* **55**, 202–9.

Taylor, D.C. & Ounsted, C. (1972). The nature of gender differences explored through ontogenetic analyses of sex ratios in disease. In *Gender Differences: Their Ontogeny and Significance,* eds. C. Ounsted & D.C. Taylor. Edinburgh: Churchill Livingstone.

Taylor, E. (1991). An epidemiological study of hyperactivity in girls. *Report to Wellcome Trust.*

Taylor, E. & Sandberg, S. (1984). Hyperactive behavior in English school children: a questionnaire survey. *Journal of Abnormal Child Psychology,* **12**, 43–56.

Taylor, E., Everitt, B., Thorley, G., Schachar, R., Rutter, M. & Wieselberg, M. (1986). Conduct disorder and hyperactivity II. A cluster analytic approach to the identification of a behavioural syndrome. *British Journal of Psychiatry,* **149**, 768–77.

Taylor, E., Sandberg, S., Thorley, G. & Giles, S. (1991). *The Epidemiology of Childhood Hyperactivity*. Maudsley Monographs, No. 33. Oxford: Oxford University Press.

Thorley, G. (1984). Hyperkinetic syndrome of childhood: clinical characteristics. *British Journal of Psychiatry,* **144**, 16–24.

Trites, R.L. & Laprade, K. (1983). Evidence for an independent syndrome of hyperactivity. *Journal of Child Psychology and Psychiatry,* **24**, 573–86.

Trites, R.L., Dugas, E., Lynch, G. & Ferguson, B.H. (1979). Prevalence of hyperactivity. *Journal of Paediatric Psychology,* **4**, 179–88.

Werry, J.S. & Hawthorne, D. (1976). Conners' teacher questionnaire – norms and validity. *Australia and New Zealand Journal of Psychiatry,* **10**, 257–62.

Werry, J.S. & Quay, H.C. (1971). The prevalence of behaviour symptoms in younger elementary school children. *American Journal of Orthopsychiatry,* **41**, 136–43.

Werry, J.S., Sprague, R.L. & Cohen, M.N. (1975). Conners' teacher rating scale for use in drug studies with children – an empirical study. *Journal of Abnormal Child Psychology,* **3**, 217–29.

Werry, J.S., Reeves, J.C. & Elkind, G.S. (1987). Attention deficit, conduct, oppositional and anxiety disorders in children:I – A review of research on differentiating characteristics; II – Clinical characteristics. *Journal of the American Academy of Child and Adolescent Psychiatry,* **26**, 133–55.

Wing, L. (1981). Sex ratio in early childhood autism and related conditions. *Psychiatry Research,* **5**, 129–37.

10

Cross-cultural aspects

Siu-Luen Luk

INTRODUCTION

Cross-cultural study of childhood psychopathology is an exciting and rapidly developing field. Its primary concern is how cultural factors influence the aetiology, expression, course, out-come, and epidemiology of childhood mental disorders. The magnitude of the cultural influence is related to the nature of the disorder. If the disorder is a developmentally inappropriate increase of behaviour with no organic cause, then the variability across cultures is expected to be high. However, even in the most severe neurological diseases or disorders, cultural influence still occurs since cultural factors affect how an individual and family experience, interpret, and respond to the disorder and how the society at large respond to the person's behaviour.

There are many definitions of culture (Brislin, 1983). Marsella (1988) defined it as 'shared learned behaviour which is transmitted from one generation to another for purposes of individual and societal growth, adjustment and adaptation; culture is represented externally as artifacts, roles, and institutions, and it is represented internally as values, beliefs, attitudes, epistemology, consciousness, and biological functioning'. This definition is very comprehensive and illustrates several important points. First, within a culture, people share learned behaviour. Secondly, a distinction should be made between external and internal representation of culture. Thirdly, culture goes deeper than the belief system; it may affect the biological functioning of individuals.

Cross-cultural comparison of the rates of occurrence of a disorder is a powerful approach in epidemiological study. One is interested in both similarities and differences. Similarity across culture would suggest that there is a biological basis for the disorder, and that this basis is largely unaffected by cultural processes. The more exciting result is to discover significant differences across cultures suggesting differences in aetiological factors. Even if there is no difference in the basic rate of occurrence, cultural factors may affect the manifestations of the disorder in terms of variations in the clustering of the symptoms, occurrence of associated symptoms and how the symptoms are dealt with by the others.

Hyperactivity means an enduring style of behaving in an overactive, inattentive and impulsive fashion (Taylor, 1986). It is a broad behavioural description of children's behaviour and as such does not carry any aetiological implications. Depending on the aetiology, the influence of cultural factors will vary. It is important to remember that hyperactivity is a concept developed in the western culture based on clinical observation. This concept may be entirely unheard of in other cultures. Thus, for the purpose of cross-cultural comparison, the best way to start is to begin with the description of individual behaviours. They are overactivity, inattentiveness and impulsivity.

Overactivity will mean simply a quantitative excess of movement, often described as restless, cannot sit still; inattentive behaviours are usually described as not paying attention, short concentration span, not able to finish work in time, changing too quickly from one subject to another; impulsive behaviours refer to quick response, inappropriate for the demands of the situation, or behaving without thinking about the consequences.

CROSS-CULTURAL COMPARISON

The observation of children behaving in an overactive and inattentive manner, which requires the clinician's attention, was first reported at the turn of this century (Schachar, 1986; see also Chapter 1). Since then, the phenomenon has been reported in different societies in different parts of the world. Apart from North America and Europe, it has certainly been reported in Africa and Asia (Minde & Cohen, 1978; Shen, Wang & Yang, 1985). Thus, hyperactive behaviour does not appear to be a culture-bound feature.

The most popular way to measure hyperactive behaviour has been by the use of self-report questionnaires for parents and teachers. In a cross-cultural comparison, an identical instrument should be used for all assessments. This often means applying a measure developed in one society to another, and therefore its reliability and validity need to be established separately for each society. This is particularly true in the case of questionnaires.

The Teacher Rating Scale (CTRS), developed by Conners (1969, 1973), has become the most commonly used instrument for the measurement of hyperactivity. Good psychometric properties have been demonstrated when it is used in different cultures. Table 10.1 demonstrates the comparison of individual items of hyperactive behaviour across different cultures.

Table 10.1 shows that hyperactive behaviours have been reported in different

Table 10.1[a]. *Cross-cultural comparison of overactive, inattentive and impulsive behaviour items in the Conners' teacher rating scale*

Behaviour	Australia (Holborow *et al.* 1984)		New Zealand (Werry & Hawthorne 1976)		Germany (Sprague *et al.* 1977)		USA (Werry *et al.* 1975)		Hong Kong (Luk *et al.* 1988*b*)	
Behaviour	(2)	(3)	(2)	(3)	(2)	(3)	(2)	(3)	(2)	(3)
Restless, overactive	13.0	5.0	12.0	7.9	14.3	3.2	4.8	2.1	15.3	7.1
Constantly fidgeting	13.6	4.8	21.8	7.4	9.9	2.9	11.3	2.1	20.2	9.6
Fails to finish, short attention span	10.5	7.0	16.0	9.6	17.2	5.5	8.3	2.8	19.4	6.4
Inattentive, distractible	13.6	7.2	21.8	13.4	19.9	6.9	11.4	3.8	27.5	11.9
Excitable, impulsive	13.9	5.5	16.0	7.7	12.4	3.1	6.2	2.1	16.0	5.6
Disturbing other children	12.0	5.4	16.3	8.9	11.3	3.2	6.9	2.1	11.3	5.0

a: numbers are percentages, (2) = pretty much (3) = very much.

societies with a range from 2.1% to 7.9% for definite overactivity, from 3.8% to 13.4% for definite inattentive behaviour, and from 2.1% to 7.7% for definite 'impulsivity'. In addition, some studies have showed consistently higher ratings on all the three behaviour items.

The Child Behavior Check List (CBCL) (Achenbach & Edelbrock, 1978), has also been employed to study children's behaviour across cultures. These studies have satisfied the criteria of careful translation, good reliability, and the use of randomly selected community samples. So far, results from USA, Netherlands, Thailand and Australia have been reported (Achenbach *et al.*, 1987*a*, 1990; Weisz *et al.*, 1987*a*, 1989). The comparison of the individual items of hyperactive behaviour is shown in Table 10.2.

The results indicate a lot of differences across cultures. Parents in the Netherlands and Sydney (Australia), but not in Thailand, made significantly higher ratings when compared with parents in the USA. Teachers in Thailand, on the other hand, gave much higher ratings when compared with teachers in the USA. Taken at face value, these results may indicate the possibility of considerable cultural differences in both the parents' and the teachers' reports of hyperactive behaviours in children.

FACTOR ANALYTICAL STUDIES OF BEHAVIOUR RATING SCALES ACROSS CULTURES

Although individual hyperactive behaviours are reported in much the same frequencies across cultures, they may nevertheless cluster differently in separate societies. It is therefore important to test whether the same patterns of behaviour occur in different cultures. Factor analytical studies of behaviour rating scales have been carried out to examine this issue (Conners, 1969; Taylor & Sandberg, 1984; Werry & Hawthorne, 1976; Glow, 1981; Trites, Blouin & Laprade, 1982; Luk, Leung & Lee, 1988*a*). Results of studies using the CTRS are summarised in Table 10.3.

The first finding is that items pertaining to hyperactivity and conduct problems, or some combination of the two, emerge as the first factor and account for the greatest variance. Secondly, in some studies hyperactivity could be seen to form a separate factor from that of inattention. Thirdly, although hyperactivity and conduct problem items were divided into separate factors in a proportion of studies, there nevertheless was always a strong overlap of items between the two clusters.

Factor analytical studies have also been carried out with other behaviour rating scales. Achenbach and his colleagues reported findings of factor analysis of the CBCL across cultures. The results showed a separation of two broad factors, 'overcontrolled' and 'undercontrolled'. Hyperactive behaviour and conduct problems clustered together to form the main part of the factor of 'undercontrolled' factor. Second-order factor analysis showed a partial separation of conduct and hyperactivity with only some overlap (Achenbach & Edelbrock, 1978; Achenbach *et al.*, 1987*c*). Schachar, Rutter & Smith (1981) reported the results of factor analysis of the Rutter teacher and parent rating scales as employed in the Isle of Wight epidemiological study. There was a factor of three items indicating behaviour commonly attributed to hyperactivity: very restless, fidgety, and cannot settle to anything for more than a few moments. Similar findings were obtained in a recent epidemiological study on hyperactivity in Hong Kong Chinese children (Ho, personal communication).

A separate line of evidence obtained by clinical observations also supported the strong clustering of hyperactive behaviours. In a clinical study of 64 boys

Table 10.2. *Comparison of North American with Dutch, Thai and Australian children on the hyperactive behaviour items of the CBCL*

Item		Parent				Teacher			
		Nationality[a]	Sex[b]	Age[c]	SES[d]	Nationality[a]	Sex[b]	Age[c]	SES[d]
(8)	Cannot concentrate								
	USA/Dutch	(2)[D]	(1)[m]	(1)NL	(<1)[L]	N.S.	(3)m	N.S.	(1)[L]
	USA/Thai	N.S.	(2)[m]	N.S.	/	(6)T	(4)[m]	N.S.	/
	USA/Sydney	(2)[S]	(2)m	N.S.	/	/	/	/	/
(10)	Hyperactive								
	USA/Dutch	(4)[D]	(1)[m]	(2)[y]	(1)[L]	N.S.	(4)[m]	N.S.	(<1)[L]
	USA/Thai	N.S.	(1<)[m]	N.S.	/	(5)[T]	(6)[m]	N.S.	/
	USA/Sydney	(<1)[S]	(<1)[me]	N.S.	/	/	/	/	
(41)	Impulsive								
	USA/Dutch	N.S.	(<1)[m]	N.S.	N.S.	N.S.	(4)[m]	N.S.	(1)[L]
	USA/Thai	N.S.	(2)[m]	N.S.	/	(3)[T]	(4)[m]	N.S.	/
	USA/Sydney	(3)[S]	(<1)[m]	(<1)[NLe]	/	/	/	/	/

NOTE: items are designated with the CBCL item numbers. Numbers in the body of the table indicate the percent of variance in items scores accounted for by each independent variable and covariate, where the effect was significant at $p<.01$.
a = D = Dutch; T = Thailand, S = Sydney scoring higher than USA.
b = M = males scored higher.
c = NL = non-linear age effect, Y = younger children scored higher.
d = l = lower SES children scored higher.
e = not significant when corrected for the number of analyses.

Table 10.3. *Comparison of factor analyses in different studies*

Item	Conners (1969)	Luk *et al.* (1988*b*)	Taylor *et al.* (1991)	Werry *et al.* (1975)	Glow (1981)	Trites *et al.* (1982)
12	C	/	C	C	C	C
15	C	C-H	C	C	C	C
17	C	C-H	C	H	C	H-I
21	C	C-H	C	C	C	C
25	C	/	/	C	C	C
31	C	C-H	C	C	C	C
32	C	C-H	C	C	C	C
36	C	C-H	C	C	C	C
38	C	C-H	C	C	C	C
18	C	C-H	A	C	A	C
19	C	/	A	C	A	C
20	C	C-H	A	C	A	C
1	H	C-H	H-I	H	H-I	H-I
2	H	C-H	H-I	H	H-I	H-I
5	H	C-H	H-I	H	H-I	H-I
6	H	C-H	C	H	H-I	H-I
14	H	C-H	H-I	H	H-I	H-I
29	H	C-H	C	/	C	H-I
4	I	/	H-I	/	/	H-I
7	I	I	H-I	H	H-I	H-I
8	I	I	H-I	I	H-I	H-I
11	I	I	/	I	/	/
24	I	/	/	I	/	/
26	I	/	/	/	/	/

NOTE:
C = conduct problem. H = hyperactivity. I = attentive-passive.
A = antisocial. H-I = combined factor of hyperactivity and inattentiveness.
C-H = combined factor of hyperactivity and conduct problem.
/ = items not loaded in factor of conduct problem or hyperactivity or inattention.

referred to the Children's Department of the Maudsley Hospital, London, interviews were carried out with children in the standard format described by Rutter & Graham (1968). This yielded a number of interviewer ratings of psychiatric symptoms. Factor analysis of the interview instrument has indicated that the first factor to emerge was made up chiefly by the items of overactivity, short attention span, distractibility, fidgetiness and social disinhibition (Taylor *et al.*, 1986). In another clinical study of 61 Chinese boys referred to the child unit, Department of Psychiatry, University of Hong Kong, using the same interview format, a similar factor of hyperactivity was obtained (Luk, Leung & Yuen, 1991).

These findings suggest that the hyperactive behaviours do indeed cluster in similar ways across cultures which supports the idea that a behaviour pattern characterised by motor overactivity, inattention and impulsiveness exists regardless of the nature of the society it is measured in. However, the findings also raise two further issues. First, the strong correlations between hyperactivity and conduct problem items question the usefulness of the concept of hyperactivity as distinct from conduct problems. Secondly, the separation of hyperactivity into overactivity/impulsivity and inattention factors suggests that it may be important to subdivide hyperactivity into three subgroups, i.e. pure overactivity/impulsiveness, pure inattention, and a combination of the three.

SEPARATION OF THE DIMENSIONS OF HYPERACTIVITY AND CONDUCT PROBLEMS

The separation of the hyperactivity dimension and the antisocial conduct dimension has been demonstrated by Taylor *et al.* (1986) in the study referred to above. Two subscales of hyperactivity and defiance were obtained from both the parent interview (Parental Account of Children's Symptoms, PACS), and the Teacher Rating Scale (CTRS). The two scales were tested against laboratory and clinical measures of activity, attention, cognitive performance, psychosocial background including family relationships. The hyperactivity scale was associated with greater motor activity, younger age, poorer cognitive performance and more minor neurological deficits. The defiance scale was associated with impairment of family relationships and adverse social factors. To test whether this is true across different cultures, a comparable study, using the same instruments was carried out on Hong Kong Chinese children (Luk et al., unpublished data). The results replicated the separation of the hyperactivity and the antisocial conduct dimensions.

CROSS-CULTURAL COMPARISON OF CHILDHOOD HYPERACTIVITY USING BEHAVIOUR RATING SCALE RESULTS

The data from cross-cultural comparisons, referred to above, support a pattern of behaviour with overactivity, inattention and impulsiveness, which is distinct from the general cluster of behaviour problems universally detected in comparable questionnaire surveys. However, from the findings discussed so far, it is not certain whether we are dealing with a dimension of hyperactivity which is continuously distributed in the general population, or whether we are dealing with a disorder which is discontinuous and a gold standard can be set up

Table 10.4. *Cross national findings on Conners' teacher rating scale scores*

	S.London (Taylor & Sandberg) (1984) (*N* = 437) Mean	S.D.	Mid West USA (Werry *et al.*) (1975) (*N* = 291) Mean	S.D.	New Zealand (Werry & Hawthorne) (1976) (*N* = 418) Mean	S.D.	Hong Kong (Luk *et al.*) (1988) (*N* = 914) Mean	S.D.	Canada (Trites *et al.*) (1979) (*N* =14 083) Mean	S.D.
Conduct problem										
Boys	0.39	/	0.21	0.93	0.60	0.53	0.42	0.47	0.25	0.44
Girls	0.20	/	0.08	0.30	0.42	0.47	0.18	0.30	0.15	0.31
Inattentive-passive										
Boys	0.70	/	0.60	0.58	0.96	0.60	1.01	0.58	0.63	0.66
Girls	0.51	/	0.43	0.55	0.71	0.58	0.72	0.52	0.40	0.55
Tension anxiety										
Boys	0.52	/	0.29	0.29	0.61	0.46	0.55	0.38	0.48	0.52
Girls	0.52	/	0.35	0.35	0.73	0.56	0.66	0.44	0.56	0.56
Hyperactivity										
Boys	0.84	/	0.56	0.56	1.07	0.73	1.03	0.78	0.65	0.76
Girls	0.46	/	0.25	0.25	0.58	0.65	0.40	0.51	0.30	0.53

applicable to all cultures, or maybe a combination of both. Using the results of behaviour rating scale studies, it is possible to carry out cross-cultural comparisons based on both concepts.

Based on Conners' original factor structure, the factor scores of the CTRS as applied in different countries are compared and shown in Table 10.4.

As can be seen from Table 10.4, the Hong Kong Chinese children and the New Zealand children, mainly from European descent, received the highest ratings on the factor of overactivity/impulsiveness, inattention and conduct problems. In contrast, very little difference is seen in the tension/anxiety factor scores.

The prevalence rate of a disorder can be obtained by using cut-off points on the rating scale. If an absolute magnitude is used, the lowest cut-off score employed so far is that of 1.5 applied to the mean on the abbreviated version of the CTRS (ATRS) (Holborow & Berry, 1986; Goyette, Conners & Ulrich, 1978). The score of 1.5 was deduced from the original study by Werry *et al.* (1975), and it was equivalent to about 2SD above the mean. Studies carried out in other countries have different means and SDs. Barkley (1982), for example, has recommended that the cut-off should be set at 2SD above the mean. Table 10.5 summarises the results of a number of epidemiological investigations and demonstrates the rates of 'hyperactivity' when based on the 1.5 and 2SD above the mean cut-offs on the ATRS in such cross-cultural comparisons.

Table 10.5 clearly indicates that if 2SD above the mean is used as the cut-off,

Table 10.5 *Percentage of children identified as 'hyperactive' in different countries according to cut–off selected on the abbreviated Conners' teacher rating scale*

	Boys %	Girls %
Cut–off > 1.5		
USA (*n*=291) (Werry *et al.*, 1975)	9	2
New Zealand (*n*=418) (Werry & Hawthorne, 1976)	22	9
Germany (*n*=5357) (Sprague *et al.*, 1977)	12	5
Canada (*n*=14 083) (Trites *et al.*, 1979)	21	8
Australia (*n*=1759) (Holborow *et al.*, 1984)	18	5
Italy (*n*=344) (O'Leary & Vivian, 1985)	19.9	2.6
Hong Kong (*n*=914) (Luk *et al.*, 1988*b*)	17.7	5.6
Cut-off > 2 S.D.		
USA (>1.5)	9	2
New Zealand (>2.1)	5	4
Germany (>1.8)	6	3
Canada (>2.1)	7	2
Australia (>1.9)	8.8	2.4
*Italy (> 2)	7.5	1.3
Hong Kong (> 1.95)	7.1	0.5

NOTE: * The actual mean + 2 S.D. was 1.87.

then the prevalence rate of the disorder of hyperactivity is fairly similar across cultures. However, the results also reveal other important issues. All the studies showed a skewing of the distribution curve to the right, and therefore the percentage of children above 2SD is more than that predicted by a normal distribution curve. In addition, there is a consistent sex difference with males having a higher rate than females. Significant differences are also found when the children's socio-economic backgrounds are considered. Some studies have found an increase in the rate of hyperactivity in urban areas as compared with rural areas (Luk *et al.*, 1988*a*; Schachar *et al.*, 1981; Goodman & Stevenson, 1989; Offord *et al.*, 1987). However, when there is a marked difference in the degree of poverty between the rural and urban areas, then the poor rural area has come up with a higher rate (Shen *et al.*, 1985; Weisz *et al.*, 1987*a*; Glow, 1981). It is also of interest to note that the findings in Hong Kong and China have turned out to be contrary to those expected. The earlier literature suggested that hyperactivity is uncommon in the Chinese population (Ho, 1981), but this clearly is not the case.

CROSS-CULTURAL COMPARISON OF DIAGNOSTIC DIFFERENCE IN CHILDHOOD HYPERACTIVITY

There are very substantial differences especially in the frequency by which the clinical diagnosis of childhood hyperactivity disorder between the UK and the USA is applied. Taylor (1985) compared the diagnostic rate across the Atlantic by examining data from clinical records including, drug prescription records, case registries, and epidemiological studies. He came up with an estimate of the diagnosis being about 20 times higher in the USA compared with the UK.

This particular difference is better described as cross-national rather than cross-cultural as the two countries would be considered as rather similar if all the countries in the world are rank-ordered according to main cultural differences. Data from teacher rating scale studies (as shown in Tables 10.4 and 10.5) also fail to support such a great cross-national difference. The reasons for this large apparent difference regarding the clinical diagnosis have been further explored by a joint UK and USA project (Prendergast *et al.*, 1988). Case histories of 6–11 year-old boys were evaluated by British and American research teams, as well as British and American clinical panels, using both the ICD-9 and DSM-III diagnostic guidelines. There was very little difference between the two specially trained research teams in terms of the diagnosis of hyperkinetic syndrome in the ICD-9, and attention deficit disorder in the DSM-III. However, the ICD-9 generated much fewer diagnoses of the disorder as a whole than did the DSM-III. The difference was even greater for UK clinicians compared with their American colleagues. The authors concluded that the format of the diagnostic scheme, as well as the clinical training, contributed to the difference in the reported rates.

The term attention deficit disorder was used in the DSM-III for the diagnosis of childhood hyperactivity. As such, it is a broader concept than the ICD-9 diagnosis of hyperkinetic syndrome. The guidelines also advised that teachers reports of hyperactivity should be given primary consideration over those by parents. Pervasiveness across various situations, or the child's behaviour in the clinic, were not essential diagnostic criteria.

Within the ICD-9 classification system, pervasive hyperactivity was regarded as of paramount important. It was defined as hyperactivity occurring both at home and at school. In a number of studies pervasive hyperactivity has been found to differ from situational hyperactivity by being associated with different cognitive style, poorer prognosis, more attention defect, more reading difficulties and stronger association with overall emotional/behavioural disturbance (Bordreault *et al.*, 1988; Campbell, Endman & Bernfield 1977; Schachar *et al.*, 1981; Schleifer *et al.*, 1975).

S.-L. Luk

CULTURAL INFLUENCE ON THE CONCEPT OF PERVASIVENESS

The difference between pervasive hyperactivity and situational hyperactivity was first emphasised by Schachar *et al.* (1981). In this study, pervasiveness was defined as hyperactivity scores being above cut–off points on both the parent and teacher rating scales.

Taylor *et al.* (1991) also studied the criteria of pervasiveness by using a semi-structured interview (PACS)(Taylor *et al.*, 1986) with the parents to obtain detailed accounts of the individual components of hyperactivity. Using this, he was able to reduce the number of children meeting the pervasiveness criteria by 80%. In fact, the direct observation data turned out to be redundant for the definition of pervasiveness (Taylor *et al.*, 1991).

Schachar and his colleagues demonstrated in two separate studies that pervasive hyperactivity, but not situational hyperactivity, is associated with a specific deficit in the executive process of inhibitory control (Chee *et al.*, 1989; Schachar & Logan, 1990). Like Taylor *et al.* (1991), they used a semi-structured interview with the parents, and a rating scale for teachers to assess hyperactivity. Direct observation data were not required.

The author's clinical experience, while working in Hong Kong, had suggested that some of the children reported by both parents and teachers to be hyperactive also displayed hyperactive behaviour under direct clinical observation, while others did not. A systematic clinical study was subsequently set up to compare these two groups of children (Luk, Leung & Yuen 1991). This study will now be described here in some detail in order to illustrate the cultural influence on the concept of pervasiveness.

Sixty-one boys, aged 6–12 years, were specially selected from children referred to the child psychiatric clinic, Queen Mary Hospital, University of Hong Kong. The selection criteria were that they were described by both school and parents as showing a pattern of restless and inattentive behaviour, and a clinical interview with the mother confirmed those complaints to a degree that supported a diagnosis if hyperkinetic syndrome according to the ICD-9, or ADHD on the DSM-III-R criteria. All the subjects were living in a family home, attended normal schools and had an IQ over 70 on WISC. None of the children suffered overt neurological disease, or psychotic illness; nor had any psychotropic drugs prescribed in the preceding 6 months.

The measures included (1) Rutter's questionnaire for parents (RPS) (Rutter, Tizard & Whitmore, 1970); (2) Conners' teacher rating scale (CTRS) (Conners, 1973); (3) parental account of childhood symptoms (PACS) (Taylor et al., 1986); (4) psychiatric interview with the child as described by Rutter &

Graham (1968); (5) measurement of activity level using modified actomoters (Schulman & Reisman, 1959); (6) social background factors and family relationships assessed in the course of the parent interview; (7) assessment of minor neurological deficit (Sandberg, Rutter & Taylor, 1978); (8) assessment of clumsiness (Gubbay, 1975); (9) Psychometric tests including the Wechsler intelligence scale for children, standardised for use in Hong Kong (HK–WISC) (Lee, Priester & Yung, 1983); cancellation of rapidly recurring target figures tests (CRRTFT) (Gardner, 1980); continuous performance test (CPT) (Erlenmeyer-Kimling & Cornblatt, 1978); Porteus' maze test (Porteus, 1947), and matching Familiar Figures Test for impulsivity (MFFT) (Cairns & Crammock, 1978).

In the case of all the subjects, clinical interviews were carried out with the parents. A full clinical history was taken, followed by a psychiatric interview with the child. School information was obtained from the parents, including school reports. Diagnoses were then made according to the ICD-9 and DSM-III-R criteria. The above procedures were carried out by either a child psychiatrist or a clinical psychologist experienced in working with children, both of whom had been trained in Britain, and with evidence of good inter-rater reliability (Luk & Leung, 1989). On the basis of the clinical observations, a decision was made on whether the child exhibited hyperactivity in the clinic situation. In most cases, this would mean that the child was overactive, leaving his seat at least once during the psychiatric interview without being asked to. Hyperactivity was also noted if the child was very restless, and fidgety even if he/she remained seated throughout. A research assistant, blind to the previous information, was trained to carry out the remaining assessments, including PACS, demographic data, family relationships, minor neurological deficits, clumsiness test, and the other psychological tests. Movement during the IQ test and CPT were recorded by actometers.

Out of the 61 subjects, 43 exhibited hyperactive behaviour during the clinical interview (G1), while 18 did not do so (G2). The behaviour ratings of the two groups according to CTRS, RPS, PACS, actometer and the observation during the clinical interview are compared in Table 10.6.

The results presented in Table 10.6 indicate that the two groups of children (G1 and G2) were indistinguishable from one another on measures of reported behaviour, including hyperactivity. However, the groups differed significantly from one another in the degree of hyperactivity as directly observed during the clinical interview.

In contrast to the differences according to behaviour, the two groups did not differ from one another on any of the social indices, apart from a trend of G1 children being somewhat younger. The area of greatest inter-group differences

Table 10.6. *Results of behaviour ratings between 'clinic observable' and 'reported' hyperactivity*

	G1 n=43 Mean (SD)	G2 n=18 Mean (SD)	P values (t-test)
CTRS			
Total score	48.4 (17.2	42.5 (14.0)	0.17
Conduct problem	1.02 (0.62)	0.87 (0.50)	0.33
Inattention/passive	1.51 (0.58)	1.38 (0.39)	0.35
Anxiety/tension	0.66 (0.45)	0.38 (0.23)	0.02
Hyperactivity	1.97 (0.79)	1.93 (0.67)	0.83
Sociability	0.67 (0.59)	0.59 (0.46)	0.59
Rutter parents' questionnaire			
Total score	19.8 (7.9)	18.7 (5.9)	0.54
Neurotic score	1.50 (1.67)	1.44 (1.42)	0.83
Conduct score	4.16 (2.56)	4.67 (1.88)	0.40
Hyperactivity score	4.95 (1.23)	4.67 (1.72)	0.53
PACS			
Emotion scale	0.44 (0.33)	0.42 (0.32)	0.86
Conduct scale	0.95 (0.57)	0.96 (0.49)	0.93
Hyperactive scale	1.17 (0.55)	0.90 (0.60)	0.11
Hyperactivity at clinic interview	7.30 (2.64)	2.33 (1.24)	0.00
*Actometer reading in IQ test**			
Hand	43.9 (31.2)	27.7 (9.4)	0.03
Leg	30.4 (24.1)	14.1 (17.6)	0.05
*Actometer reading in CPT**			
Hand	16.1 (12.5)	9.0 (7.8)	0.06
Leg	17.7 (11.3)	8.1 (9.4)	0.03

G1: Children with both reported and clinic-observable hyperactivity.
G2: Children with reported hyperactivity only.
* G1 (n = 24), G2 (n = 9) because actometers were not available in the beginning.

was that of neuropsychological tests: the G1 children scored lower on IQ, had more minor neurological deficits, including clumsiness, and scored lower on psychometric tests of attention in terms of making more errors, missing responses, and having a longer and more fluctuating reaction time. To partial out the age and IQ effects, an analysis of variance was carried out. Controlling for age and IQ tended to attenuate the differences, although the differences remained statistically significant for activity level, overall attention score, and minor neurological deficits regardless of that.

The results of this study therefore suggest that in the assessment of pervasiveness of hyperactivity in the Hong Kong Chinese children, direct observa-

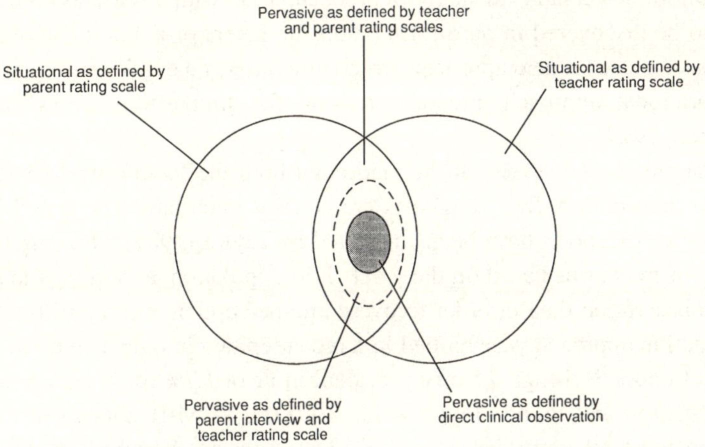

Fig. 10.1 Different ways of defining a disorder of childhood hyperactivity in the Hong Kong studies.

tions are crucially important. In this particular study, the information obtained by semi-structured interview with the parent did not make much impact on the selection of pervasive subjects, whereas the data based on direct observations proved to be essential. It may therefore be concluded that the assessment of pervasiveness of hyperactivity requires a different approach in different cultures. Figure 10.1 summaries the various ways the disorder of childhood hyperactivity in Hong Kong may be defined along the dimension of pervasiveness.

THE CULTURE-FREE AND THE NON-CULTURE-FREE DIAGNOSIS

As discussed in the previous section, there is much controversy about how broadly the disorder of hyperactivity should be defined. The obvious question that follows is whether it is possible to establish diagnostic criteria for a disorder of hyperactivity which are 'culture free'? Were those to be established, it would enable epidemiological studies to be carried out across cultures in order to compare the prevalence of hyperactivity. Such approach would also be similar to the line of investigation on schizophrenia carried out by the World Health Organisation (1973).

This proposition has, however, been strongly criticised by medical anthropologists (e.g. Kleinman, 1987). Kleinman has coined the term 'traditional transcultural psychiatry' meaning 'a preoccupation with disease as an entity, a thing to be discovered in pure form under the layers of cultural camouflage'. He has suggested a new approach which emphasises the differences, whereas the traditional approach attempts to look for similarities across cultures (Kleiman, 1977).

An argument, however, can be made that both the 'culture-free' diagnosis and the 'non-culture-free' diagnosis are equally important. The criteria for a culture-free diagnosis have been suggested by Taylor (1986) who emphasised the use of the norms based on the local child population, as well as the use of direct observation data in order to overcome perception and report bias. This combination approach was applied in a recent epidemiological study based in an East London Borough where a prevalence rate of 1.7% for hyperkinetic disorder (ICD-9) was found (Taylor *et al.*, 1991). If DSM-III diagnostic criteria had been used, the prevalence rate would have been much higher. The DSM-III criteria are fairly similar to the application of a cut off point on the Teacher Rating Scale as shown in Table 10.5. Although the DSM-III diagnosis has been criticised as over-inclusive (Sandberg, 1981), some studies have demonstrated that it has some validity (Porrino *et al.*, 1983; Rapoport & Benoit, 1975; Rapoport *et al.*, 1986; Szatmari, Boyle & Offord, 1989). In the final analysis, these children have been considered by their parents or teachers as having a number of hyperactive symptoms and their development are likely to be affected. The fact that they also need help is important to recognise.

The concern is to study the relationship between the cultural factors and the 'culture-free' diagnosis on one hand, and in relation to the 'non-culture-free' criteria on the other. The latter tends to produce a much larger 'fuzzy' group, with the word fuzzy being used because of its uncertain boundaries.

In looking for cultural differences, there are three main approaches. The first one is to study the differences in the rate of prevalence of the 'culture-free' diagnosis. Any difference found will offer a valuable opportunity to study the aetiology of the condition. The second approach involves examining the ways culture influences the 'culture-free' diagnosis in terms of the perception, reporting and recognition of symptoms as well as the processes of referral, diagnosis and management. Even if there turned out to be no differences in the aetiology and the rates of the disease, the possible variation in the personal, familial and social responses to it, and their interaction with the disease, are likely to be illuminating. Thirdly, there is a need to study the 'non-culture-free' diagnosis. It is expected that the rates of such diagnosis would vary greatly across cultures. It is also likely that such diagnostic criteria would yield a very heterogeneous group with different aetiological factors. Some of the problems might also be very mild and the reason they would be considered as 'hyperactivity' would be purely because of perception bias. It would nevertheless be important to include such mild 'hyperactivity' as it would possibly generate important knowledge from the point of cross-cultural comparison.

THE LABELLING OF THE HYPERACTIVE PHENOMENON

Apart from how to define a disorder, it is also important to consider how the phenomenon is labelled. ADDH (DSM-III) is a category constructed in the USA to label a broad group of children described as hyperactive. Other labels are also employed, such as 'learning disorder' which is a term often used in the education literature. In Prendergast *et al.*'s (1988) study, it appeared that conduct disorder is the term preferred by British child psychiatrists instead of ADDH. Labelling has two important effects. First, it has heuristic value. ADDH emphasises the attention deficits of hyperactive children, and has led to much valuable research in this important area. The term learning disorder on the other hand, would focus on the specific learning difficulties in reading, writing and mathematics. Secondly, labelling implies a certain treatment approach. The term ADDH in the USA tended to lead to a pharmacological treatment approach, whereas the term conduct disorder in the UK tended to focus the treatment on the children's familial, social and psychological difficulties. A label of 'reward dysfunction disorder' might also be relevant in another culture, and would draw our attention on the hyperactive child's abnormal response to reward and punishment (Henlein & Caul, 1987).

It is also possible to imagine that in cultures where the concept of hyperactivity is unheard of, the process of labelling may be very different; for example, a lot of these children would just be labelled as 'naughty'. The advantages and disadvantages of labelling are complex. Some studies have shown that the labelling of hyperactivity relieves the parents and teachers of feelings of guilt and inadequacy, which would in turn enable them to better accept the child in question. Also, labelling may enable a child and the family to obtain the extra funding required for the child's special needs and for psychosocial support of the family.

CULTURAL INFLUENCE ON THE AETIOLOGY

Assuming it is possible to establish a culture-free diagnostic scheme, and to apply reliable and valid measures of child behaviour across very divergent cultures, finding significant differences between them in the rate of childhood hyperactivity would raise the obvious question about the role of aetiological factors accounting for the discrepancy in rate. The first step could be to establish a biological marker capable of validating the diagnosis. One illuminating example of such a procedure is the study by Zametkin *et al.* (1990). The authors carried out a study using positron emission tomography in adults who had been hyperactive in their childhood, as well as having a positive family history. Compared with normal controls the ex-hyperactive groups showed a significant abnormality of glucose metabolic rate in the superior frontal and pre-motor cortex region. Due to its radiological hazards this technique, unfortunately, is not applicable to children at present. Also, studies of brain biochemistry have so far failed to produce conclusive results. One promising line of research may be the study of the evoked potentials of the brain (Courchesne & Yeung-Courchesne, 1988).

The multiplicity of causes for hyperactivity has been summarised by Taylor (1986). These include genetic factors, birth injury, brain trauma and infection, food allergy and intolerance, toxin poisoning, psychosocial factors and maternal alcohol consumption during pregnancy. (See also, Chapters 7 and 8 for reviews of causal mechanisms.) The prevalence of all these factors can vary considerably across different societies. Thus, it would not be surprising if future studies produce different prevalence rates for 'the culture-free diagnosis'.

Studies on infant temperament suggest that there may indeed be some racial differences in the temperament of infants. Bronson (1972) noted less motor reactivity to novel stimuli among infants of Asian ancestry compared with those of Caucasian origin. Freedman & Freedman (1969) and Ko (1988) reported Chinese infants to be more easily habituated, calmed and consoled than infants of Caucasian origin. The link between these allegedly inborn constitutional characteristics and the later behavioural symptoms is yet to be explored.

CULTURAL INFLUENCE ON THE PRESENTATION OF SYMPTOMS

In adult psychiatry, cross-cultural comparisons of major psychiatric disorders have indicated differences in symptom presentation. Studies of depressive disorders have, for example, demonstrated that among non-Western samples of depressed patients, there is an increase of somatisation, and a decrease in depressive affect and cognition compared with patients similarly diagnosed in the Western countries (Jablensky *et al.*, 1981; Kleinman, 1982). Likewise, a study by WHO of first-contact cases of schizophrenia found that the symptoms of patients from developing countries were more often characterised by voices speaking to the subject, and by visual hallucinations, while patients from developed countries more often suffered from systematised delusions, primary delusions, delusional mood, and thought insertion (Sartorius *et al.*, 1986). In the light of these observations it would be surprising if there were no differences in the presentation of symptoms across cultures for childhood hyperactivity.

The presentation of the hyperactive symptoms is likely to be a product of the interaction between the child's constitutional characteristics and the environment. In terms of cultural influences, two main factors should be considered; child rearing practices and the school environment. The 'problem suppression–facilitation' model described by Weisz *et al.* (1987*b*) would appear relevant for this discussion. It suggests that cultural factors may specifically suppress the development of certain child problems and facilitate the development of certain other problems.

There exists a good deal of evidence to suggest that there are considerable differences in the child-rearing practices between different societies. In order to illustrate some of the salient issues, the differences between the Western developed countries and the Chinese culture are compared. Several themes emerge which are likely to be relevant to hyperactivity. First, Chinese parents appear more concerned about the expressions of physical aggression in their children (Ekblad, 1986; Ho, 1986). Secondly, Chinese parents tend to foster dependency, whereas assertiveness and independent behaviour are encouraged by Western parents (Ho, 1986). Thirdly, academic achievement is strongly emphasised by Chinese parents. To sit down and concentrate on academic work is a very important part of the training (Chen & Stevenson, 1989). If these child-rearing practices have an impact on the behaviour of children, then it would be reasonable to hypothesise that there would be a suppressing effect on the hyperactive symptoms.

The school environment is also different. For example, in the primary schools of Hong Kong, the classes are generally more structured. Children are expected to sit still and concentrate on their assigned tasks. Also, they are usually forbidden to leave their seat. The classroom routines in the first few years of primary school in countries like the UK or New Zealand tend to be very different. For example, in most lessons children are allowed to move around in the classroom. They are encouraged to carry out tasks they are interested in at their own pace. Considering the problem suppression–facilitation model, it is reasonable to hypothesise that the classroom situation in Hong Kong is likely to suppress hyperactive behaviour whereas in UK and New Zealand, hyperactive behaviour might in fact be facilitated.

The author has carried out two clinical studies of hyperactive children, one in the UK and one in Hong Kong (Luk, Thorley & Taylor, 1987; Luk *et al.*, 1991). In both studies, actometers modified from calendar wrist watches (Schulman & Reisman, 1959), were employed to quantitatively measure the activity level of the child during the psychometric test situation. Both groups of children had been rated grossly hyperactive, i.e. showing hyperactive symptoms in the home, school and clinical situations. The psychological tests used in both studies were similar. Although there were some differences in the duration of the tests, the results were considered comparable because the scores related to minutes of elapsed time. The actometers employed in the two studies were made from two different brands. This obstacle was overcome by a calibration experiment carried out by a colleague experienced in the use of this device (Taylor, personal communication).

Four actometers were mounted on a rigid rod which was in turn strapped to the non-dominant leg of the 15 children involved for a period of approximately an hour with the readings taken immediately at the end of the period. It was found that the correlations between the pairs of actometers used on the same study were high. However, the mean values differed greatly between the UK and Hong Kong instruments. Accordingly, regressions were plotted and readings of the actometers used in one country can be translated to compare those used in the other country. There were 12 boys in the UK study with the mean age was 133 months (SD 13.6). The Hong Kong study involved 43 boys with the mean age of 95.6 months (SD 19.3). It might have been expected that the younger age in the Hong Kong sample would have favoured them having a higher activity level. However, this expectation was not borne out by the results: the mean score on the wrist actometer was 43.9, (SD 31.2) for the Hong Kong, and 152.1 (SD 66.5) for the UK groups. For the ankle actometers the scores were 30.4 (SD 24.1) in Hong Kong, and 180.4 (SD 120.3) in the UK (two tail Student's tests were 4.5, $p<.001$ and 3.9, $p<.001$ respectively). The results therefore support the hypothesis that Hong Kong Chinese children have a lower activity level. This is in line with the author's clinical experience after having observed hyperactive children both in the UK and in Hong Kong.

If activity level is much affected by cultural factors, then it could be argued that it is not a core feature of hyperactivity, and that the definition of the syndrome should not require an absolute level of activity as the cut-off for a disorder. Apart from activity level, attention level could of course be similarly affected by child rearing practices or school environments. At present there are no cross-cultural comparison data available on measurements of attention.

In considering the 'problem suppression-facilitation model' several ways of interaction can occur. One can assume some very severe cases of hyperactivity described, 'as driven by motor', which occur after severe head injury or encephalopathy. In such situations cultural influence is likely to be minimal as far as symptom presentation in concerned. For cases with pervasive hyperactivity arising from a genetic cause, suppression and facilitation can occur as discussed in the previous paragraphs. When the non-pervasive form of hyperactivity is considered, cultural factors may be able to suppress or facilitate the symptoms to the extent of producing or not producing a disorder.

The 'problem suppression-facilitation model' is supported by a series of studies carried out by Weisz and his colleagues in Thailand examining two broad-band behaviour problem dimensions; characterised by overcontrolled behaviour (e.g. fearfulness, worrying, somaticising) on the one hand and under-controlled behaviours on the other (e.g. disobedience, fighting, arguing) as derived from factor analytic studies of children's behaviour (Achenbach & Edelbrock, 1978). Thailand is a Buddhist country where children's aggression and other forms of under-controlled behaviour are disapproved, and discouraged and their inhibition and other over-controlled behaviours are likely to be condoned and even encouraged. Weisz and his colleagues compared the problem behaviours of the Thai children with US children with the hypothesis that Thai children will have more problems involving overcontrolled behaviour and fewer problems involving undercontrolled behaviour.

In their first study (Weisz *et al.*, 1987*b*), based on a sample of 760 clinic-referred children, 376 from Thailand and 384 from the US, behaviour problems as reported by the parents were recorded. The results showed that overcontrolled problems were reported much more often in the Thai than the US children; undercontrolled problems on the other hand, were reported much more frequently in the US children than in the Thai children. In the second study (Weisz *et al.*, 1987*a*), the Child Behavior Checklist, CBCL (Achenbach & Edelbrock, 1978), a parent report form, was used to study 960 children (360 from Thailand and 600 from the US), aged 6 to 11 years. It was found that the Thai children were rated much higher on items indicating overcontrolled behaviour compared with the US children. In contrast no differences between the two cultures were found for the undercontrolled behaviour problems. In addition, the Thai children had significantly higher overall problem scores than the US children. In the third study (Weisz *et al.*, 1989), the Child Behavior Checklist Teacher's Report Form was applied to representative samples of 359 Thai children and 586 children from the US, both aged 6 to 11 years. The Thai children had a significantly higher scores on both over-controlled and on undercontrolled behaviour compared with the American children.

Furthermore, the scores for overcontrolled behaviour were significantly higher than the scores for uncontrolled behaviour among the Thai children, whereas within the US sample the reverse was true.

The results of these studies support the above hypothesis that cultural factors in Thailand facilitate the occurrence of overcontrolled behaviour problems. In addition, the Thai children were rated much higher than the US children especially according to teacher reports. Weisz *et al.* (1988) proposed 'an adult distress threshold model' to explain this finding suggesting that the Thai adults have a lower threshold for recognising children's problem behaviour than their US counterparts.

CULTURAL INFLUENCE ON THE RECOGNITION OF AND HELP-SEEKING FOR HYPERACTIVITY

The 'adult distress threshold model' suggests that culturally mediated adult attitudes may help to determine which particular child behaviours are considered to be a problem and which will reach the adult threshold for distress, and therefore results in a referral for help.

The author and his colleagues carried out a study on teacher ratings of children's behaviour problems and referral patterns (Luk *et al.*, 1988*a*, *b*) in Hong Kong. The results of it are relevant to the above model. The teachers of a representative sample of 914 children, ranging in age from 6 to 12 years, and attending primary schools in Hong Kong, were asked to fill in the Conners' teacher rating scale (CTRS). Two months later, they were asked to decide which ones of the children had behavioural or emotional problems meriting a referral to professionals for help, assuming that resources were unlimited. Out of the total of 240 teachers, 222 responded, giving a final sample of 874 children, representing 95.6% of the original one. Several interesting results emerged. First, as shown in Table 10.4, teachers in Hong Kong rated the children higher on the subscales of conduct problems, hyperactivity and inattention, but not on the one of tension/anxiety when compared with results from similar studies carried out in other countries. This would suggest that teachers in Hong Kong may have a lower threshold for the recognition of hyperactivity or conduct problems.

Secondly, a total of 55 students were considered as requiring referral to a specialist child mental health service, giving a referral rate of 6.3%. The referred group and the non-referred group are compared in Table 10.7. The referred group had significantly higher mean scores on conduct and hyperactivity problems, but not on anxiety/tension problems, compared with the

Table 10.7. *Comparison of referred and non-referred students*

	Referred n = 55		Non–referred n = 819		
	Mean	SD	Mean	SD	p[a]
CTRS scores:					
Total score	0.80	.42	0.56	.38	0.000
CTRS factor scores:					
Factor 1 (conduct)	0.59	.56	0.29	.40	0.000
Factor 2 (inattentive/passive)	1.23	.56	0.86	.56	0.000
Factor 3 (anxiety/tension)	0.60	.36	0.59	.42	0.94
Factor 4 (hyperactivity)	1.06	.89	0.73	.73	0.008

[a] P value according to t-test or χ^2 -test.

children who were not referred. This suggests that teachers in Hong Kong are more likely to refer children with conduct problems or hyperactivity for help, as compared with children whose psychological problems are predominantly of the internalising type.

The validity of the CTRS in Hong Kong children was examined in a previous study (Luk & Leung, 1989). In the course of this study the estimate of sensitivity and specificity of CTRS for detection of conduct disorder and hyperactivity were established. For 100% specificity and 100% sensitivity the CTRS total scores were 44 and 12, respectively. A score of 36 on the CTRS gave an optimal specificity of 88%, and sensitivity of 83%. These CTRS scores were then used to study the validity of the referrals ‘hypothetically’ made by the teachers. Table 10.8 summarises the results.

There was a significant difference in the distributions of the referred and non-referred groups. This supports the validity of the teacher referrals. Seventy-five cases which were above the CTRS total score of 44 (specificity 100%) were not referred. The probability that these 75 students would require professional help was very high. This represents 86.2% of the cases above the cut-off of 44. These results therefore suggest that teachers in Hong Kong may have a lower threshold for the recognition of hyperactivity and conduct problems, but they tend to refer children with problems of undercontrolled behaviour more readily than children with overcontrolled behaviour. However, in general they tend to have high threshold for making a referral for help. Thus, if one is studying a clinic population, the various tendencies in the adult distress model may work against one another, creating a complicated and possibly biased composition of a clinical population.

Table 10.8. *Distribution According to Different CTRS Scores*

CTRS total score	Referred $n = 50$	Non–referred $n = 783$	χ^2 test P value
>36	20	147	0.01
<36	30	636	
>44	12	75	0.001
<44	38	710	

NOTE: CTRS total score >36, specificity =88%, sensitivity = 82.9%, >44, specificity = 100%.

CULTURAL INFLUENCE ON THE CO-MORBIDITY OF HYPERACTIVITY

Childhood hyperactivity disorders are frequently associated with co-morbid conditions. The commonest one is conduct disorder. Children in whom hyperactivity and conduct disorder occur together tend as a group to have more severe symptoms and worse prognosis (Szatmari *et al.*, 1989; Barkley *et al.*, 1990). Factors which are known to contribute in an important way to the aetiology of conduct disorder vary across cultures. This is true, for example of broken homes, large family size and parents' mental health problems. Therefore variation of these factors in the society will affect the degree of co-morbidity of conduct disorder and hyperactivity. Other co-morbidities that need further investigation across cultures include the occurrence of anxiety disorder and depression.

CULTURAL INFLUENCE ON THE MANAGEMENT

Clinicians moving their clinical practices from one culture to another should always study and bear in mind the various cultural factors that may influence how mental health problems should be managed. Cultural influences may, for example, help to protect or aggravate the problem, and they may interact differently with different characteristics of the problem. Therefore clinical practices may require modification so that children and the families obtain the optimal benefit from the management of their problems. These issues will be discussed in the light of the author's personal experience of working in Hong Kong, London, UK, and Dunedin, New Zealand.

One of the important factor is the availability of services for child mental health problems. In the developing countries child psychiatry as a discipline still remains relatively underdeveloped. This is likely to contribute to childhood hyperactivity being under-referred and underdiagnosed. Hyperactive children are probably considered as simply naughty, and managed accordingly.

The acceptance of drug treatment is another issue. In North America, the diagnosis of hyperactivity is often followed by administration of drug treatment (Safer & Krager, 1988), whereas in the UK, drugs are seldom prescribed (Taylor, 1985). In Hong Kong, parents are quite willing to accept the doctor's authority and the treatment of children's problems by drugs if the doctor decides to prescribe them. In New Zealand, where the author worked for some time in the recent past, the general ethos is against using psychotropic medication for children's behaviour problems. This is also reflected by the fact that methylphenidate is on restricted prescription there.

The meaning of the concept of a child psychiatric disorder, as interpreted by the various cultures is of some interest. In New Zealand, for example, the tendency appears to be to avoid any labelling. Hence all children, irrespective of their handicap, are mainstreamed into the normal school system.

The school environment also makes a lot of difference. The Hong Kong schools tend to have a high student/staff ratio with often more than 40 pupils per class. Teachers usually adopt a structured approach to teaching, and the pupils are expected to follow the pace of the teacher. They are also exposed to much competition. On the whole, these school characteristics put considerable demands especially on hyperactive children. Consequently, their difficulties are often exposed early on in primary school, as they are expected to fit in with the routine instead of the school being in the position to provide a more individualised programme for them. This often makes the management of the child's hyperactivity at school extremely difficult.

In New Zealand, on the contrary, the schools allow a good deal more individual freedom. It is also common to provide an individualised programme for each child. The children are judged on their own progress, and not in competition with others, until they enter secondary school. There is also a strong trend against testing of the children. The pupil/staff ratio is low and there is more project-oriented study so that the children can work at their own pace. This also means that there is a higher tolerance of hyperactive behaviour in the school. In addition, it is often feasible to arrange teaching in a small remedial class, and to have teaching aides to help the child in the classroom, as well as in the playground.

The following are two case histories illustrating some of the differences in management of hyperactive children in different cultures.

A 6-year-old Chinese boy in Hong Kong presented with pervasive overactivity, inattention and impulsiveness with onset at the age of three. He was very poor in fine motor skills which affected his handwriting. Intellectual assessment showed an above average IQ; however, the subscore coding on WISC was very low. The level of family functioning was within normal limits. The parents accepted the diagnosis of a hyperkinetic syndrome and were happy with drug treatment. As a result of this the boy's behaviour improved substantially both at home and at school. Other forms of treatment included helping the parents to appreciate the child's strengths and weaknesses, supportive individual psychotherapy with the child, liaison with the school, helping the parents and school to develop a behavioural programme focusing on the child's desirable behaviour and building up his confidence, and occupational therapy to improve his motor skills. The improvement at home was well maintained, but the child's behaviour at school deteriorated again after a period of time. The school complained that the child did not complete his homework. It transpired that the child had a good verbal performance, but did poorly whenever he had to write down the answers. He was therefore very reluctant to do copying exercises which constitute most of the daily homework for primary school children in Hong Kong. The relationship between the child and the teacher deteriorated rapidly to the extent that the child refused to do any class or home work, handed in blank examination answer sheets and became very disobedient and disruptive at school. Further liaison work was carried out with the school which was unsuccessful because the school insisted that written work was essential in the assessment of a pupil's performance.

A 7-year-old boy of a European origin in New Zealand presented to the child psychiatry clinic because the school teacher was concerned that he was more restless and inattentive than other children in the classroom. The parents had also noticed this at home but they did not think it was a problem. The clinical examination, confirmed that the boy did indeed have pervasive overactivity, inattention and impulsiveness with onset around the age of three. He had started primary school at the age of five. For the first two years in school the teachers had not mentioned any problems to the child's parents, and therefore the parents were quite surprised by the subsequent complaints by the school teacher. When the term hyperactivity was mentioned, the parents felt unhappy about such a label, although they agreed that their child did need help. Both the school and the parents were reluctant to even consider the possibility of drug treatment. They were, however, very willing to receive advice on classroom management on how to improve his self-esteem and peer relationships and to implement an individual behavioural programme in the child. A school meeting was held and the school decided to seek extra teaching hours for the child both in the classroom and on the playground. He was also granted individualised remedial help in a small class on some subjects.

CULTURAL INFLUENCE ON THE OUTCOME OF HYPERACTIVITY

Several long term follow-up studies, most being carried out in the US have clearly showed that childhood hyperactivity leads to poor prognosis (Barkley *et al.*, 1990). Similarly, McGee *et al.* (1991) in Dunedin, New Zealand, followed up a community-based sample of preschool-age hyperactive children 12 years after the initial assessment, and found that they have a much worse prognosis than groups of children with pure language problems or normal controls.

In adult psychiatry, it has been shown that schizophrenia, especially schizophrenia in female patients, has a better prognosis in the developing countries compared with the developed ones (Leff, 1988). The findings have also suggested that for a schizophrenic patient, finding a role in the family and the community that is optimal for his/her functioning is very important in determining the prognosis of the illness. In the developing countries, there is a higher chance for this to happen. It is an open question whether anything comparable might apply to the problem of childhood hyperactivity. Up to now, outcome studies have not been carried out in developing countries.

A MODEL FOR CROSS-CULTURAL ASPECTS OF HYPERACTIVITY

Figure 10.2 summarises the points raised above. The Chinese population in Hong Kong will be used as the basis for discussion here. There is a possibility that constitutionally, Chinese children have a lower vulnerability to hyperactivity. The Chinese child rearing practices, school environment, and social expectations tend to suppress gross motor activity and facilitate inhibition. On the other hand, Chinese adults tend to have a lower tolerance for hyperactivity and conduct problems in children. Therefore, reports of parents and teachers tend to produce very high ratings of hyperactivity and conduct problems, despite the possibility that in absolute terms, such problems may exist to a lesser degree in Hong Kong than in Western countries. The concept of hyperactivity is unfamiliar to Chinese adults. In parental ratings, hyperactivity symptoms tend to be mixed up with conduct problems. The threshold for referring children for help is generally high among the Chinese population. Thus, in any given clinic population of child psychiatry patients, only the severe cases may be referred. Depending on the diagnostic scheme employed in a particular study, the prevalence rate will vary, although this is more of a problem between

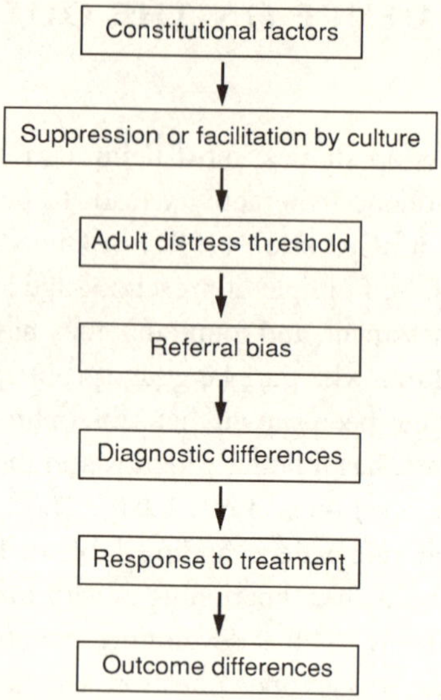

Fig. 10.2 A model for the cross-cultural aspects of childhood hyperactivity.

the ICD and DSM classification systems and not a problem arising from the Chinese population as such. The present hypothesis is that there is no difference in the rate of culture-free diagnosis of hyperactivity, although the presentation of symptoms may be different. The rate of the non-culture-free diagnosis may be high, but the boundaries of these types of problems are unclear. Chinese adults tend to accept a medical practitioner's opinion including prescriptions of medication for treatment of hyperactivity. However, there are many difficulties in helping the child to adjust to the school system. At present there is no data on the long-term outcome of the hyperactivity disorder in Chinese children.

FINAL COMMENTS

Childhood hyperactivity is a behavioural syndrome affected by cultural factors in terms of how it is manifested, perceived, tolerated, referred and managed. There is much controversy about how broadly the disorder of hyperactivity should be defined. Establishing diagnostic criteria for a disorder of hyperactivity which can be applied across cultures will facilitate the comparison of prevalence. However, children who are considered as hyperactive but do not meet the above culture-free diagnostic criteria should also be included in future investigations. Both approaches would be useful in our effort to understand the influence of cultures and its relationship with childhood hyperactivity. The former approach emphasises the similarities and the latter attempts to look for differences.

REFERENCES

Achenbach, T.M. & Edelbrock, E.S. (1978). The classification of child psychopathology: a review and analysis of empirical efforts. *Psychological Bulletin,* **85**, 1275–1301.

Achenbach, T.M., Verhulst, F.C., Baron, G.D. & Akkerhuis, G.W., (1987a). Epidemiological comparisons of American and Dutch children: I. Behavioural/emotional problems and competencies reported by parents for ages 4 to 16. *Journal of American Academy of Child and Adolescent Psychiatry,* **26**, 317–325.

Achenbach, T.M., Verhulst, F.C., Edelbrock, C., Baron, G.P. & Akkerhuis, G.W. (1987b). Epidemiological comparisons of American and Dutch children: II. Behavioural/emotional problems reported by teachers for ages 6 to 11. *Journal of American Academy Child and Adolescent Psychiatry,* **26**, 326–32.

Achenbach, T.M., Verhulst, F.C., Baron, G.D. & Althans, M. (1987c). A comparison of syndromes derived from the child behavioural checklist for American and Dutch boys aged 6–11 and 12–16. *Journal of Child Psychology and Psychiatry,* **28**, 437–54.

Achenbach, T.M., Hensley, V.R., Phares, V. & Grayson, D. (1990). Problems and competencies reported by parents of Australian and American children. *Journal of Child Psychology and Psychiatry,* **31**, 265–86.

Barkley, R.A. (1982). Defining hyperactivity/ADD: a working set of reference. *Advances in Clinical Child Psychology,* **5**, 153–80.

Barkley, R.A., Fischer, M., Edelbrock, C.S. & Smallish, L. (1990). The adolescent outcome of hyperactive children diagnosed by research criteria: I. An 8-year prospective follow-up study. *Journal of American Academy of Child Adolescent Psychiatry,* **29**, 546–57.

Bordreault, M., Thiverge, J., Cote, R., Boutin, P., Julien, Y. & Bergeron, S. (1988) Cognitive development and reading achievement in pervasive-ADD situational-ADD and control children. *Journal of Child Psychology and Psychiatry,* **29**, 611–19.

Brislin, (1983). Cross-cultural research in psychology. *Annual Review of Psychology,* **34**,363–400.

Bronson, G.W. (1972). Infants' reactions to unfamiliar persons and novel objects. *Monographs of the Society for Research in Child Development,* Vol. 37, No. 3, Serial No. 148.

Cairns, E. & Crammock, T. (1978). Development of a more reliable version of the matching families figures test. *Developmental Psychology,* **14**, 555–60.

Campbell, S.B., Endman, M.W. & Bernfield, G. (1977). A three-year follow-up of hyperactive pre-schoolers into elementary school. *Journal of Child Psychology and Psychiatry,* **18**, 239–49.

Chee, P., Logan, G., Schachar, R., Lindsay, P. & Wachsmuth, R. (1989). Effects of event rate and display time on sustained attention in hyperactive, normal, and control children. *Journal of Abnormal Child Psychology,* **17**, 371–91.

Chen, C.S. & Stevenson, H.W. (1989). Housework: a cross-cultural examination. *Child Development,* **60**, 551–61.

Conners, C.K. (1969), A teacher's rating scale for use in drug studies with children. *American Journal of Psychiatry,* **126**, 884–8.

Conners, C.K. (1973). Rating scales for use in drug studies in children. *Pharmacological Bulletin Special Issue – Pharmacotherapy of Children.*

Courchesne, E. & Yeung–Courchesne, R., (1988). Event-related brain potentials. In *Assessment and Diagnosis in Child Psychopathology,* eds. M. Rutter, A.H. Tuma & I.S. Lann, pp. 264–299. London: Guilford Press.

Ekblad, S. (1986). Social determinants of aggression in a sample of Chinese primary school children. *Acta Psychiatrica Scandinavica,* **73**, 515–23.

Erlenmeyer–Kimling, L. & Cornblatt, B. (1978). Attentional measures in a study of children at high-risk for schizophrenia. *Journal of Psychiatric Research,* **14**,93–8.

Freedman, D.G. & Freedman, N.C. (1969). Behavioural differences between Chinese–American and European–American newborns. *Nature, London* **224**, 1227–

Gardner, R.A. (1980). *The Objective Diagnosis of Minimal Brain Dysfunction*. pp. 68–70. New York: Jason Aronson.

Glow, R.A. (1981). Cross-validity and normative data on the Conner's Parent and Teacher Rating Scales. In *The Psychosocial Aspects of Drug Treatment for Hyperactivity,* eds. K.D. Gadow & J. Loney, pp. 107–150. Boulder, Colorado: Westview Press.

Goodman, R. & Stevenson, J. (1989). A twin–study of hyperactivity – I. An examination of hyperactivity scores and categories derived from Rutter teacher and parent questionnaires. *Journal of Child Psychology and Psychiatry,* **30**, 671–89.

Goyette, C., Conners, C.K. & Ulrich, R.F. (1978). Normative data on revised Conners parent and teacher rating scales. *Journal of Abnormal Child Psychology,* **6**, 221–36.

Gubbay, S.S. (1975). The clumsy child. *A Study of Developmental Apraxia and Agnosic Ataxia.* London: Saunders.

Henlein, M. & Caul, W.F. (1987). Attention deficit disorder with hyperactivity: a specific hypothesis of reward dysfunction. *American Journal of Child and Adolescent Psychiatry,* **26**, 356–62.

Ho, Y.F., (1981). Childhood psychopathology: a dialogue with special reference to Chinese and American cultures. In *Normal and Abnormal Behaviour in Chinese culture,* eds. A. Kleinman & T.Y. Lin, pp. 137–156. D. Reidel City.

Ho, Y.F., (1986). Chinese patterns of socialisation: A critical review. In *The Psychology of the Chinese People,* ed. M.H. Bond, pp. 1 – 35. Hong Kong: Oxford University Press.

Holborow, P., & Berry, P. (1986). A multinational, cross-cultural perspective on hyperactivity. *American Journal of Orthopsychiatry,* **56**, 320–22.

Holborow, P., Berry, P. & Elkins, J. (1984). Prevalence of hyperkinesis: a comparison of 3 rating scales. *Journal of Learning Disabilities,* **17**, 411–15.

Jablensky, A., Sartorius, N., Giulbinat, W. & Ernberg, G. (1981). Characteristics of depressive patients contacting psychiatric services in four cultures. *Acta Psychiatric Scandinavica,* **63**, 308–18.

Kleinman, A. (1977). Culture, depression and the 'new' cross-cultural psychiatry. *Social Science and Medicine,* 11, 3–11.

Kleinman, A. (1982). Depression and neurasthenia in the People's Republic of China. *Culture, Medicine and Psychiatry,* **6**, 1–80.

Kleinman, A. (1987). Anthropology and psychiatry: the role of culture in cross-cultural research on illness. *British Journal of Psychiatry,* **151**, 447–54.

Ko, L. (1988). Psychological assessment of new born babies and cultural differences. Paper presented at the First Conference on Hong Kong's Young Children organised by the Hong Kong Council of Early Childhood Education and Services.

Lee, P.L.M., Priester, H.J. & Yung, G.Y.M. (1983). Factor analysis and construct validity of the Hong Kong–Weschler Intelligence Scale for Children (HK–WISC). Unpublished manuscript.

Leff, J. (1988). *Psychiatry Around the Globe, a Transcultural View.* 2nd edn. London: Gaskell.

Luk, S.L. & Leung, P.W.L. (1989). Conner's teacher's rating scale – a validity study in Hong Kong. *Journal of Child Psychology and Psychiatry,* **30**, 785–93.

Luk, S.L., Thorley, G. & Taylor, E. (1987). Gross overactivity – a study by direct observation. *Journal of Psychopathology and Behavioural Assessment,* **9**, 173–82.

Luk, S.L., Leung, P.W.L. & Lee, P.L.M. (1988*a*). Conner's teacher rating scale in Chinese children in Hong Kong. *Journal of Child Psychology and Psychiatry,* **29**, 165–74.

Luk, S.L., Leung, P.W.L., Lee, P. & Lieh–Mak, F. (1988*b*). Teacher's referral of children with mental health problems – a study of primary schools in Hong Kong. *Psychology in Schools,* **25**, 121–29.

Luk, S.L., Leung, P.W.L. & Yuen, J. (1991). Clinic observations in the assessment of pervasiveness of childhood hyperactivity. *Journal of Child Psychology and Psychiatry* (in press).

McGee, R., Partridge, F., Williams, S. & Silva, P.A. (1991). A twelve-year follow-up of preschool hyperactive children. *Journal of American Academy of Child and Adolescent Psychiatry,* **30**, 224–32.

Marsella, A.J. (1988). Cross-cultural research on severe mental disorders: issues and findings. *Acta Psychiatrica Scandinavica Supplement,* **344**, 7–22.

Minde, K.K. & Cohen, N.J. (1978). Hyperactive children in Canada and Uganda: a comparative evaluation. *Journal of the American Academy of Child Psychiatry,* **17**, 76–487.

Offord, D.R., Boyle, M.H., Szatmani, P., Ree–Grant, N.L., Links, P.S., Cadman, D.T., Byles, J.A., Crawford, J.W., Blum, H.M., Byrne, C., Thomas, H. & Woodward, C.A. (1987). Ontario Child Health Study: II. Six-month prevalence of disorder and rates of service utilization. *Archives of General Psychiatry,* **44**, 832–6.

O'Leary, & Vivian (1985). Hyperactivity in Italy. *Journal of Abnormal Child Psychology,* **13**, 485–500.

Porrino, L., Rapoport, J.L., Ismond, D., Sceery, W., Behar, D. & Bunney, W. (1983). Twenty-four hour motor activity in hyperactive children and controls. *Archives of General Psychiatry,* 40**,** 681–7.

Porteus, S. (1947). *The Porteus Maze Test Manual*. London: Harrap.

Prendergast, M., Taylor, E., Rapoport, J.L., Bartko, J., Donnelly, M., Zametkin, A., Ahearn, M., Dunn, G. & Wieselberg, H.M. (1988). The diagnosis of childhood hyperactivity: a US – UK cross-national study of DSM-III and ICD-9. *Journal of Child Psychology and Psychiatry,* **29**, 289–300.

Rapoport, J.L. & Benoit, M. (1975). The relation of direct home observations to the clinic evaluation of hyperactive school age boys. *Journal of Child Psychology and Psychiatry,* **16**, 141–7.

Rapoport, J.L., Donnelly, M., Zametkin, A. & Carroughan, J. (1986). Situational hyperactivity in a US setting. *Journal of Child Psychology and Psychiatry,* **27**, 639–46.

Rutter, M., & Graham, P. (1968). The reliability and validity of the psychiatric assessment of the child. I. Interview with the child. *British Journal of Psychiatry,* **114**, 563–79.

Rutter, M., Tizard, J. & Whitmore, K. (1970). *Education, Health and Behaviour*. London: Longman.

Safer, D.J. & Krager, J.M. (1988). A survey of medication treatment for hyperactive/inattentive students. *Journal of American Medical Association,* **260**, 2256–8.

Sandberg, S.T. (1981). 'The overinclusiveness of the diagnosis of hyperkinetic syndrome'. In *Strategic Intervention for Hyperactive Children,* ed. R. Gittelman. New York: M.E. Sharpe.

Sandberg, G.T., Rutter, M. & Taylor, E. (1978). Hyperkinetic disorder in psychiatric clinic attenders. *Developmental Medicine and Child Neurology,* **20**, 279–99.

Sartorius, N., Jablensky, A., Korten, A., Kernberg, G., Anker, M., Cooper, J.E. & Day, R. (1986). Early manifestations and first contact incidence of schizophrenia in different cultures. *Psychological Medicine,* **16**, 909–28.

Schachar, R.J. (1986). Hyperkinetic syndrome: historical development of the concept. In *The Overactive Child,* ed. E. Taylor, pp. 19–40. Oxford: Blackwell.

Schachar, R. & Logan, G.D. (1990). Impulsivity and inhibitory control in development and psychopathology. *Developmental Psychology,* **26**, 710–20.

Schachar, R.J., Rutter, M. & Smith, A. (1981). The characteristics of situationally and pervasively hyperactive children: implications for syndrome definition. *Journal of Child Psychology and Psychiatry,* **22**, 373–92.

Schleifer, M., Weiss, G., Cohen, N., Elman, M., Cvejic, H. & Kruger, E. (1975). Hyperactivity in preschoolers and the effect of methylphenidate. *American Journal of Orthopsychiatry,* **45**, 38–50.

Schulman, J.L. & Reisman, J.M. (1959). An objective measure of hyperactivity. *American Journal of Mental Deficiency,* **64**, 455–6.

Shen, Y.C., Wang, Y.F., & Yang, X.L. (1985). An epidemiological investigation of minimal brain dysfunction in six elementary schools in Beijing. *Journal of Child Psychology and Psychiatry,* **26**, 777–88.

Sprague, R., Vohen, M., Eichelseder, W. (1977). Are there hyperactive children in Europe and the South Pacific? *Presented to the American Psychological Association, San Francisco.*

Szatmari, P., Boyle, M. & Offord, D.R. (1989). ADDH and conduct disorder: degree of diagnostic overlap and differences among correlates. *Journal of American Academy of Child and Adolescent Psychiatry,* **28**, 865–72.

Taylor, E. (1985). Syndrome of overactivity anfd attention deficit. In *Child and Adolescent Psychiatry, Modern Approaches,* 2nd edn, eds. M. Rutter, & L. Hersov, pp. 424–443. Oxford: Blackwell.

Taylor, E. (1986). Childhood hyperactivity. *British Journal of Psychiatry,* **149**,562–73.

Taylor, E. & Sandberg, S. (1984). Hyperactive behaviour in English school children: a questionnaire survey. *Journal of Abnormal Child Psychology,* **12**, 143–56.

Taylor, E., Schachar, R., Thorley, G. & Wieselberg, M. (1986). Conduct disorder and hyperactivity I: separation and hyperactivity of antisocial conduct in British child psychiatric patients. *British Journal of Psychiatry,* **149**, 760–7.

Taylor, E., Sandberg, S., Thorley, G. & Giles, S. (1991). The epidemiology of childhood hyperactivity. *Institute of Psychiatric Maudsley Monograph.* London: Oxford University Press (in press).

Trites, R.L., Blouin, A.G.A. & Laprade, K. (1982). Factor analysis of the Conner's teacher rating scale. Based on a large normative sample. *Journal of Consulting and Clinical Psychology,* **50**, 615–23.

Trites, R.L., Dugas, E., Lynch, G. & Ferguson, H.B. (1979). Prevalence of hyperactivity. *Journal of Paediatric Psychology,* **4**, 179–88.

Weisz, J.R., Suwanlert, S. Chaiyasit, W., Weiss, B., Achenbach, T.M. & Walter, B.R. (1987*a*). Epidemiology of behavioural and emotional problems among Thai and American children: parent reports for ages 6 to 11. *Journal of American Academy of Child and Adolescent Psychiatry,* **26**, 890–7.

Weisz, J.R., Suwanlert, S., Chaiyasit, W., & Walter, B.R. (1987*b*). Over and under controlled referral problems among children and adolescents from Thailand and the United States: the Wat and Wai of cultural differences. *Journal of Consulting and Clinical Psychology,* **55**, 719–26.

Weisz, J.R., Suwanlert, S., Chaiyasit, W., Weiss, B., Walter, B.R. & Anderson, W.W. (1988). Thai and American perspectives on over and undercontrolled child behaviour problems: exploring the threshold model among parents, teachers and psychologists. *Journal of Consulting and Clinical Psychology,* **56**, 601–9.

Weisz, J.R., Suwanlert, S., Chaiyasutm W., Weiss, B., Achenbach, T.M. & Trevanthan, D. (1989). Epidemiology of behavioural and emotional problems among Thai and American children: Teacher reports for aged 6–11. *Journal of Child Psychology and Psychiatry,* **30**,471–84.

Werry, J.S. & Hawthorne, D. (1976). Conner's teacher questionnaire – norms and validity. *Australian and New Zealand Journal of Psychiatry,* **10**, 257–62.

Werry, J.S., Sprague, R.L. & Cohen, M.N. (1975). Conners' Teacher rating scale for use in drug studies with children – an empirical study. *Journal of Abnormal Child Psychology,* **3**, 217–29.

World Health Organisation (1973). *International Pilot Study of Schizophrenia.* Geneva. WHO.

Zametkin, A.J., Nordahl, T.E., Gross, M., King, A.C., Semple, W.E., Rumsey, J., Hamburger, S. & Cohen, R.M. (1990). Cerebral glucose metabolism in adults with hyperactivity of childhood onset. *New England Journal of Medicine,* **323**, 1361–6.

11

Hyperactivity, reading disability and schooling

Jim Stevenson

INTRODUCTION

Hyperactivity is a behavioural dimension along which children vary from those showing well-organised, calm behaviour to those showing restlessness and inattention that produces chaotic and disorganised behaviour Taylor (1986*a*,*b*). The topic of this chapter is the extent to which variation along this hyper-activity dimension is related to educational difficulties for the child. These educational difficulties will include both problematic behaviour at school and learning disabilities, specifically reading disability. A third aspect of behaviour, antisocial behaviour or conduct disorder, is often associated with both hyperactivity and with reading disability. In order to understand the possible links between hyperactivity and reading disability, it is essential to take account of this common association with conduct disorder.

Of the learning disabilities, reading disability will be the main focus in this chapter. It is the most pervasive learning disability both in terms of the number of children affected and the range of educational experiences that are affected. Reading disability has also been the subject of most of the major studies of learning disability in children with hyperactivity.

Taylor's (1986) formulation of hyperactivity as a behavioural dimension centred on the degree of inattentive restlessness explicitly excludes impulsivity. This is justified by the finding that impulsivity as either a cognitive or behavioural phenomenon is not distinctively associated with hyperactivity; it is just as common in conduct disorder (Taylor *et al*., 1991). A second feature of hyperactivity is that it can be either situationally specific (usually behaviour shown at home only or at school only) or pervasive (shown both at school and at home). It is generally accepted that pervasive hyperactivity is the potentially most handicapping of these conditions and of the greatest educational significance (Goodman & Stevenson, 1989*a*).

Unfortunately much of the relevant research on educational aspects of hyperactivity has been undertaken in the USA and uses subjects classified under the DSM-III-R nomenclature of ADHD or the earlier DSM-III version attention deficit disorder (ADD). In both these classificatory schemes impulsivity is one of a number of symptoms contributing to the designation of a case. Additionally, under the DSM classifications, the child's dysfunctional behaviour can be situational or pervasive. As a consequence, extreme hyperactivity is not synonymous with attention deficit hyperactivity disorder (ADHD) as formulated within DSM-III-R (American Psychiatric Association, 1987) and consequently different prevalence is obtained (Taylor *et al.*, 1991).

When hyperactivity is being referred to, it will be taken to refer to children who are at the extreme on a dimension of behavioural inattention and restlessness and who show this behaviour pervasively. This is not the same as the hyperkinetic disorder as defined in ICD-10 (WHO, 1988), which has a number of more stringent requirements for the diagnosis to be made and applies a number of explicit exclusion criteria. However, it will be necessary to cover the American research, and where studies have been based upon DSM classifications the terms ADDH and ADHD are used.

The inconsistencies between studies in the definition of hyperactivity inevitably makes integrating findings across studies more difficult. A further source of confusion concerns whether the association between hyperactivity and reading disability is based upon a continuous measure of each or upon extreme groups only. If a cut-off point has been used to designate a group at the extreme of this continuum, a further confound concerns variation in the placement of this cut-off.

The following definitions will be used in the chapter.

Hyperactivity: HA – children with extreme pervasive hyperactivity (when situational hyperactivity is the subject of the study it will be specified), ADD – attention deficit disorder with no hyperactivity, ADDH – attention deficit disorder with hyperactivity (DSM-III), ADHD – attention deficit hyperactivity disorder (DSM-III-R).

Reading disability: RD – poor reading achievement. Reading age is significantly below chronological age (i.e. reading backwardness) or reading age significantly below that expected on the basis of chronological age and IQ (i.e. specific reading retardation). There are a number of studies that use broader indicators of academic or school performance. Reading is highly correlated with general attainment and conclusions from studies using a broader definition of learning disability have been subsumed under the RD heading.

Conduct disorder (DSM-III/DSM-III-R, ICD-10): CD – here includes children showing extreme degrees of antisocial behaviour.

The co-morbidity of hyperactivity, reading disability and conduct disorder will be the major issue addressed in this chapter. The overlap can be extensive as found in a study of clinic referrals by Barkley *et al.* (1991) who reported that 68% of children with ADHD also had oppositional defiant disorder and 39% had conduct disorder. A similar extent of co-morbidity is found in epidemiological samples (e.g. Taylor *et al.*, 1991). It has become clear that inattentiveness and restlessness constitute a separate disorder from that typified by antisocial, defiant behaviours. They show a double dissociation, i.e. each has their own distinctive set of correlates. For example, Taylor *et al.* (1986) demonstrated that hyperactivity was associated with poorer cognitive performance and neuropsychological abnormalities, whereas antisocial behaviour is associated with impaired family relationships and adverse social circumstances. Reading disability has been thought to show distinctive associations with both hyperactivity (e.g. Hynd *et al.*, 1991) and with antisocial behaviour (Rutter & Yule, 1975) which again points to the need to consider hyperactivity, conduct disorder and reading disability jointly.

There have been a number of recent review articles on the associations between the three. The summary of research in this chapter will not attempt to review again the literature covered by Schachar (1991), Shaywitz and Shaywitz (1991) and Hinshaw (1992*a*,*b*). Instead, the conclusions from these reviews will be used, and in the main, reference will be made only to specific studies published since these reviews. Where necessary, certain earlier studies will be returned to where they add distinctively to the argument being developed.

Hinshaw (1992*b*) highlights an important issue when he suggests that 'in childhood, inattention and hyperactivity are stronger correlates of academic problems than is aggression; by adolescence, however, antisocial behaviour and delinquency are clearly associated with underachievement'. This developmental perspective is crucial when considering the mechanisms producing the associations between the three. Depending on the age group being studied and the time period over which any follow-up is conducted so the strength and nature of the associations found will vary. However, most studies include subjects from a wide age range and this may mask a developmental progression.

Furthermore, Hinshaw (1992*b*) observes that when more stringent definitions of externalising disorders (including hyperactivity) and IQ-discrepant definitions of achievement deficits (especially reading) have been adopted, about 20% of children with externalising disorders show achievement deficits and a similar percentage of children with achievement deficits have externalising disorders. This figure will vary depending on the stringency with which each condition is defined (Semrud-Clikeman *et al.*, 1992). Nevertheless, this indicates a partial independence of HA and RD, i.e. they are not synonymous nor does developing one necessarily entail the later onset of the other.

The significance of hyperactivity as a contributor to failure at school has been repeatedly emphasised (Cantwell & Baker, 1991; Levy, Harper & Weinberg, 1992). Sometimes these difficulties are thought to arise as a result of neurological deficits of some kind which disrupt the normal learning process (Hynd *et al.*, 1991). Others such as Carey (1992) have interpreted the school difficulties as stemming from temperamental characteristics or behavioural style that does not fit in with 'the demands of the modern school environment'. Here we see the origins of conflicts over whether the educational difficulties of the hyperactive child are primarily focused within the child or whether the problems are seen to arise from the interaction between the child and the school system. The former view leads to interventions that are child focused (e.g. behavioural programme or drug treatment); the latter leads to interventions based on changes of classroom organisation and on the task demand placed upon children.

It has been observed on a number of occasions that many of the studies in this field are of questionable methodological adequacy (Lie, 1992). It is beyond the scope of this chapter to consider these methodological issues. The excellent reviews by Hinshaw (1992*b*) and Rowe and Rowe (1992*a*) provide such a critique.

The chapter is organised along the following lines. The first section reviews the evidence on the nature of the behavioural difficulties shown by the hyperactive child at school. The second and the main section of the chapter is an extended review of the inter-relationships between hyperactivity, reading disability and conduct disorder. This review follows the structure of a model of the influences on these conditions and culminates in a suggestion of the possible mechanisms involved. The last section briefly describes some of the interventions designed to alleviate the schooling difficulties experienced by hyperactive children.

BEHAVIOUR AT SCHOOL

Situational and pervasive hyperactivity

It has been found that children can be usefully divided into those showing situational and those showing pervasive hyperactivity (Goodman & Stevenson,

1989*a*). Many studies fail to indicate whether they are dealing with situational or pervasive hyperactivity. However, as Goodman and Stevenson (1989*a*) argue, children with school only situational hyperactivity are very similar to pervasively hyperactive children. With this in mind, it is likely that most of the studies reviewed here are of children with school based or pervasive hyperactivity.

The prevalence of ADDH has been found to be 9% for boys and 3% for girls (Szatmari, Offord & Boyle, 1989*a*,*b*). The following prevalences were obtained when the children in this Canadian epidemiological study were divided into pervasive ADDH (0.5%), home situational ADDH (1.5%) and school situational ADDH (3.8%). There are consistent cross-cultural variations in the prevalence rate obtained for ADDH and hyperactivity which cannot be explained away simply by differences in sampling (Taylor, 1987). However, much of the seeming variation in prevalence is attributable to definitional differences between different studies which is exacerbated by the use of arbitrary cutting points to identify extreme hyperactivity.

The significance of the pervasive/situational distinction has been challenged by Costello, Loeber and Stouthamer-Loeber (1991). They suggest that the supposedly more extreme form of pervasive hyperactivity is largely attributable to differences in the person reporting the children's behavioural symptoms. They concluded that, when the source of information was independent of parents' or teachers' judgments, no differences were found between situationally and pervasively hyperactive, impulsive and inattentive children. However, as van der Meere, Wekking and Sergeant (1991) have shown, for example, there are indications that pervasively hyperactive children do show difficulties in behavioural organisation that can be demonstrated on experimental tasks that are independent of any rating biases.

It has been argued that school is the best setting for the systematic evaluation of children with attention deficit hyperactivity disorder (Atkins & Pelham, 1991). Children can be rated by independent observers on a range of learning and social tasks. Such assessments include teacher rating measures, direct observations in classrooms and on playgrounds, peer rating and sociometric measures, and academic performance. Altepeter and Breen (1992) have taken further the assessment of school and home based situational hyperactivity. They used the home/school situations questionnaires (HSQ/SSQ) developed by Barkley. For the HSQ, four factors emerged (non-family transactions, custodial transactions, task-performance transactions and isolate play) accounting for 61% of variance. For the SSQ, three factors emerged (unsupervised settings, task performance and special events), accounting for 68% of variance in these assessments. It appears that the structure of the behaviour of hyperactive children may be differently organised at home and at school but that instruments with known factor structures are available to make the appropriate assessments.

Children who show hyperactivity in school are very much at risk of showing the same characteristics as pervasively hyperactive children. This means that their behaviour cannot be attributed solely to some feature of the school setting or to the interaction between an aspect of experience at school and some characteristic of the child. It is very likely that the consequences for the child's education are serious and are not restricted to the school situation alone. For example, Beck, Young and Tarnowski (1990) used reports from mothers and teachers to designate 30 boys aged 6 to 9 years as pervasively hyperactive, situationally hyperactive, or not hyperactive at home or school. Mothers of pervasive hyperactive boys reported significantly more overall stress in their relationship with their child. Mothers of pervasive hyperactive boys also rated themselves as more depressed, less competent, more restricted, and frustrated compared to control mothers.

It can be expected that school-based hyperactivity will occur in approximately 5% of the population of school children. These children are likely to show a variety of disruptive behaviours both at school and elsewhere. They are also likely to be experiencing other difficulties, including fraught relationships with their parents.

Preschool setting

The first systematic epidemiological survey of preschool behaviour problems was that undertaken by Richman, Stevenson and Graham (1982). They found that in 3 year-olds overactivity or restlessness presented a marked difficulty in 12.9% of children and inattention in 5.7%. These particular behaviours were strongly related to language delays during the preschool period and to the risk of children showing behaviour problems 5 years later.

There are indications that these prevalence figures and the characteristics of children with components of hyperactivity are found across cultures. For example, Luk *et al.* (1991) studied 3 year-old Chinese children in Hong Kong attending preschool facilities. The preschool behaviour checklist (PBCL) was completed by preschool teachers. The factor structure of the PBCL was very similar to that obtained from its original British study (McGuire & Richman, 1986). As in studies in other cultures, boys had more hyperactive, conduct, and speech problems. Luk *et al.* (1991) conclude that the results suggest a certain degree of universality of symptomatology for children at the preschool level.

The findings of continuing risk into school age for preschool children who show pervasive hyperactivity was extended by McGee *et al.* (1991). A group of hyperactive children was identified which constituted 2% of a population sample of preschool children. When followed-up at the age of 15, 75% of these children showed significant disabilities associated with hyperactivity and poor academic performance. Campbell and Ewing (1990) also found that children with stable problems during the preschool period were at risk for showing externalising problems at age 9 years and that ADHD showed the greatest persistence of problems from the age of three years.

It has been found that attention problems amongst children with developmental disorders can be accurately identified at the time of school entry. Korkman and Peltomaa (1991) used a neuropsychological test profile to predict attention problems at school. On the basis of a longitudinal study of 46 children with mild developmental disorders, they identified a subgroup with problems in impulse control, sustained attention, and selective attention. These children were found to show classroom-based attention deficits during the first year of school.

It is clear then that hyperactive behaviour is discernible before school entry and can be a significant feature of children's behaviour in preschool settings. Indeed, children who show inattentive, restless behaviour at this early age are particularly at risk for persisting behaviour problems at least through the years of primary education. This re-emphasises that it is unlikely that school-based situational factors account for the behaviour since the pattern is well established before school entry in many children. However, for other children, school entry may represent the first context in which hyperactive behaviour is expressed.

Other children

It has often been reported that children and adolescents with hyperactivity show a deficit in social competence (e.g. Barkley *et al.*, 1991) and this is likely to affect adversely their relationship with other children (Pelham & Bender, 1982). The children themselves can become acutely aware of the extent to which their behaviour is disruptive. For example, Barkley *et al.* (1991) found that adolescents themselves agreed with parents and teachers that they were more likely than control subjects to show antisocial acts.

Such lack of social competence and excess of disruptive behaviour can lead to rejection by peers. Sociometry is one of the most sensitive indicators of children's peer relationships. The procedure of classmate nominations of children who are 'liked best' and 'liked least' can be used to place children into the following categories: popular (many 'liked best' nominations), rejected (many 'liked least' nominations), neglected (few nominations), controversial (rated both 'liked best' and 'liked least' by different children) and average (an intermediate mix of ratings).

Using this procedure Schaughency *et al.* (1992) found that in a sample of 110 school children from Buenos Aires aged 6 to 11 years, these sociometric status groups had significantly different mean teachers' ratings of the children's behaviour. Surprisingly, both rejected and popular children were more likely to be rated as inattentive. However, motor hyperactivity, impulsivity, and aggression were not related to sociometric status.

To understand why the behaviour of hyperactive children should suffer such negative peer evaluation, Madan-Swain and Zentall (1990) studied 25 hyperactive 8 year-old children (10 'liked' by peers and 15 'disliked'). Their social interactions with a normal control were contrasted with that in pairs of non-hyperactive children. When with a disliked hyperactive partner the normal children tended to become more negative and active, were less talkative and cooperative than when with a control child. The disliked hyperactive children themselves were more likely to make negative statements than other children. Unfortunately the design of the study did not include disliked non-hyperactive children, so it cannot be concluded that there is anything specific to the behaviour of ADHD children that is linked to their sociometric status.

The social status of ADHD boys was investigated by Flicek (1992) using a variety of sociometric and teacher ratings. It was found that the combination of ADHD and learning disability was particular associated with peer rejection, low peer popularity and disruptive social behaviour. This study indicates that attention deficit and learning disability show a marked interaction in their relationship to social status. Flicek (1992) suggests that this is due to the greater aggression or withdrawal shown by children with attention deficit hyperactivity disorder + learning disability. These results are of particular relevance to the management of hyperactive children in the classroom, where the social difficulties experienced by attention deficit disorder + learning disability children need to be taken into account in providing complementary work on social skills alongside those concentrating on attention control or remediation of reading.

Hyperactive children's disorganised and inattentive behaviour can lead to social isolation within the child's peer group. The rejection experienced by the hyperactive child as a consequence of a lack of social skills and their disruptive behaviour can thereby lead to a further lowering of self-esteem and an increased risk of conduct disorder.

To summarise, this first section has identified that hyperactive children show a range of disruptive and inattentive behaviours at school. These behaviours are likely to be shown at home as well. Hyperactivity is likely to have been apparent in these children before school entry and is often associated with language delays. The children with early onset HA are more at risk both for fraught family relationships and for later behaviour problems. At school children with hyperactivity are likely to be rejected especially if they show learning disabilities in addition. It is the association between hyperactivity and these learning disabilities and particularly reading disability that is the subject of the next section.

READING

Before considering the detailed studies of hyperactivity and reading disabilities, the specificity of this association needs to be considered. Is it possible that hyperactivity and reading disability are associated simply as part of a general high rate of other disturbances in some hyperactive children? Livingston, Dykman and Ackerman (1991) investigated the co-diagnoses of children with attention deficit disorder. Over 40% of the children showed reading disability or were slow learners but they had no higher rate of psychiatric diagnoses than those attention deficit disorder children who read adequately. This suggests that, when attention deficit disorder and reading disability co-occur, this is not simply part of a more widespread or more severe pathology in these children.

Two recently published epidemiological studies on the validity of alternative classifications of hyperactivity have reached contrasting conclusions about the significance of the association with reading disability. Both studies used large samples of the population, i.e. 1490 7 to 11 year-old American children (August & Garfinkel, 1993) and 3215 6 and 7 year-old British boys (Taylor *et al.*, 1991). The studies also used a two stage design using screening questionnaires, i.e. August and Garfinkel: Child Behaviour Checklist – Teacher Report Form (Achenbach & Edelbrock, 1986) and Taylor *et al.*: Rutter Teacher and Rutter Parent Scales augmented by additional hyperactivity items (see Taylor & Sandberg, 1984 for details). At the second stage, August and Garfinkel used the DICA-R (Reich *et al.*, 1987) to confirm a DSM-III-R diagnoses and Taylor *et al.* used the PACS (Taylor *et al.*, 1986) for diagnostic purposes.

August and Garfinkel (1993) divided their sample in a number of ways: pervasive vs. situational ADHD, severe vs. mild ADHD, ADHD vs. ADD/WO (i.e. attention deficit without hyperactivity). Comparison within these sets and against a 'subclinical' control group (i.e. high scorers on the CBCL who did not meet the criteria for ADHD) failed to identify any differences in mean reading scores. They therefore conclude that reading disability is not an important correlate of any of the subcategories of hyperactivity.

By contrast Taylor *et al.* (1991) found that children with ADD alone had markedly lower reading scores as did a co-morbid hyperactive/conduct disorder group. However in both cases the low reading scores were not significantly below that expected from the IQs of the children in these groups. A more parsimonious explanation is that the ADD children were experiencing more general intellectual delays of which lower reading scores were a secondary consequence.

The results of Taylor *et al.* (1991) are supported by Hynd *et al.* (1991). They differentiate between children with ADD alone and those with ADD plus hyperactivity. A large proportion (60%) of the ADDnoH children had a co-diagnosis of a developmental reading or arithmetic disorder while none of the ADDH children received such a co-diagnosis.

One difference between the findings from August and Garfinkel (1993) and Taylor *et al.* (1991) was the much lower mean IQ for the ADD-only group in the British (88) than in the American study (106). However, in both studies, hyperactive children were seen to be at risk for emotional disorders (co-morbid anxiety disorder in the USA and high emotional disorder scores in the UK).

Some of the differences between these studies could be attributed to sampling differences (only boys in UK, both sexes in USA; 55% response rate from parents in USA, 80% in UK). However the use of the DSM-III and DSM-III-R criteria by August and Garfinkel (1993) allows impulsivity to contribute to the required number of symptoms for case identification. As Taylor *et al.* (1991) have demonstrated the inclusion of impulsivity symptoms clouds the picture by increasing the number of children identified and by reducing the distinction between hyperactivity and other conditions especially conduct disorder.

Whether subtypes of ADHD children can be found which have different strengths of association with reading difficulties was also investigated by Bauermeister *et al.* (1992). On the basis of factor analysis and cluster analysis they found a number of subtypes: pure hyperactivity, pure inattention and hyperactivity plus inattention. Although these groups could be distinguished in terms of their behavioural profiles and on a number of external validating criteria (SES and pregnancy complications) they did not differ significantly from each other in school performance, although they all performed less well than control children.

Similar findings were reported by Cantwell and Baker (1992) who tested the validity of the distinction between ADD with or without hyperactivity in a

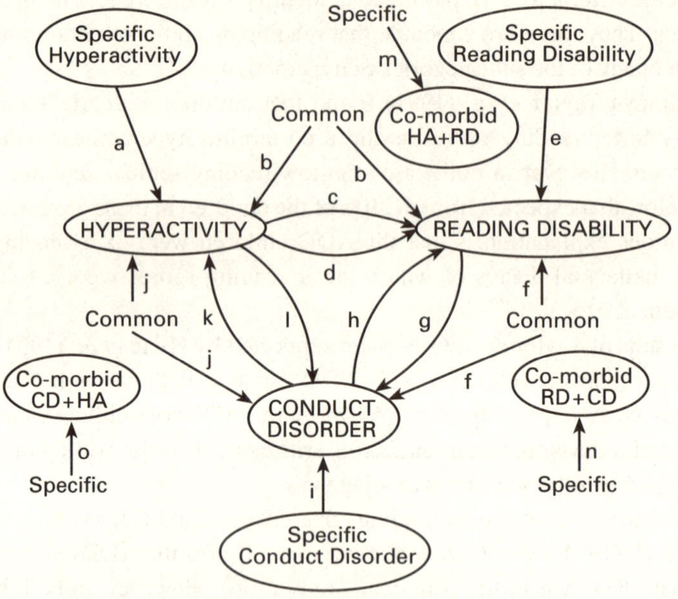

Fig. 11.1 A model of the possible relationships between conduct disorder, reading disability and hyperactivity.

sample of children referred to a speech/language clinic. Although these groups could be differentiated on a number of external criteria, there were no marked differences in the level of learning disorders in the two groups.

In order to provide a systematic framework for discussing the diverse literature on hyperactivity and reading disability, a model is presented in Fig. 11.1. This sets out the possible routes through which reading disability and hyperactivity could become associated. The potential importance of associations mediated via conduct disorder is recognised by explicitly adding conduct disorder to the model.

Each condition (hyperactivity, reading disability and conduct disorder) could be subject to the following influences: specific influences that are not shared with the other two conditions, common influences which they share with another condition and direct influences from one of the other conditions. These latter effects can be unidirectional or reciprocal. In their discussion of the possible causal models for co-morbidity Caron and Rutter (1991) identify three further mechanisms.

First, the two co-morbid conditions could actually be the same basic nosological category. In the present case this is unlikely given the extensive range of distinct specific influences on each condition.

Secondly, two conditions could have distinct but correlated causes. This possibility cannot be logically differentiated from the common influence formulation. At root any correlation will be seen to be the result of the action of some shared cause. The uncertainties over which formulation to adopt hinge on whether or not the source of this shared influence has been established and how long the causal chain has to be before the common and the correlated cause model can be sensibly distinguished. This can be illustrated by considering Hinshaw's (1992*b*) conclusion that inattention and hyperactivity are linked with academic problems as a result of common antecedent variables. Some of these he identifies as lying within the child's developmental history, e.g. subaverage IQ, language deficits and neurodevelopmental problems. Others belong to the wider social context of the family, e.g. family adversity. By mixing proximal and distal causes in this way the distinction between common and correlated causal formulations becomes blurred. For this reason, both mechanisms are subsumed under the notion of common causes.

Third, it is possible that co-morbid cases represent an aetiologically distinct group. This possibility has been recognised in the model by specific co-morbid influences.

Using the framework in Fig. 11.1 the research literature has been summarised in Table 11.1. To avoid having to review an unmanageable number of studies, the reviews of Schachar (1991) and Hinshaw (1992*b*) have been taken as starting points for evaluating the significance of paths in the model. Particular weight has been given to studies that have contrasted the association between hyperactivity, conduct disorder and reading disability within the same data set. This is highly desirable if differences in associated characteristics are to be identified. Each path in Figure 11.1 will be considered in turn and the influences involved identified.

Specific influences on hyperactivity

The evidence that hyperactivity does constitute a distinct diagnostic group within the broad range of externalising disorders is overwhelming. For example Schachar (1991) identifies hyperactivity as associated with low IQ, abnormal neurological features and the beneficial effects of central nervous system stimulants as distinctive features of hyperactivity.

There have been a number of studies that have found specific effects on HA of disrupted early parenting. Verhulst, Althaus and Versluis-den Bieman (1990) found that boys from a variety of countries adopted by Dutch parents were twice as likely as non-adopted boys to show behaviour problems. This excess

Table 11.1. *Summary of empirical studies testing for components of model in Fig. 11.1 on the influences on hyperactivity (HA), reading disability (RD) and conduct disorder (CD).*

Path	Study	Nature of influence
(a) Specific influences on HA		
	Schachar (1991)	Low IQ Abnormal neurological features Positive response to stimulants
	Hodges & Tizard (1989)	Early institutional care
	Schachar & Wachsmuth (1991)	Disrupted care
	Verhulst *et al.* (1990)	
	Taylor *et al.* (1991)	Poor cognition Neuropsychological abnormalities
	Pennington *et al.* (1993)	Executive function deficits
	Goodman & Stevenson (1989*b*)	Genetic differences
	Gillis *et al.* (1992)	
	Stevenson (1992)	
(b) Common influences on HA and RD		
	Hinshaw (1992*b*)	Maternal depression Low IQ Language deficits Neurodevelopmental delay
	McGee *et al.* (1991)	Early language delay
	Stevenson *et al.* (1993)	Genetic differences
(c) Influence of HA on RD		
	Hynd *et al.* (1991)	Present for ADDnoH only
	Fergusson & Horwood (1992)	Effect present (and no path 'd')
	Rowe & Rowe (1992)	Effect present and also path 'd'
	Douglas & Benezra (1990)	Executive function deficits can lead to RD

Table 11.1. *(cont.)*

Path	Study	Nature of influence
(d) Influence of RD on HA		
	Rowe & Rowe (1992*a*,*b*)	Effect present
	Pennington, Grossier & Welsh (1993)	Phenocopy hypothesis
	McGee & Share (1988)	Late onset ADD
	McGee, Williams & Feehan (1992)	
(e) Specific influences on RD		
	Ackerman, Dykman & Gardner (1990)	Phonological deficit
	Pennington *et al.* (1993)	
(f) Common influences on RD and CD		
	Sturge (1982)	Social disadvantage
	Olweus (1983)	
(g) Influence of RD on CD		
	Olweus (1983)	Present
(h) Influence of CD on RD		
	Patterson, DeBaryshe & Ramsey (1989)	Effects of coercive extend from home to classroom
(i) Specific influences on CD		
	Schachar (1991)	Psychosocial adversity Poor parental coping Interparental inconsistency for discipline
	Miller *et al.* (1993)	Parental psychopathology Poor marital relationship
	Lahey *et al.* (1988)	Parental psychopathology
(j) Common influences on CD and HA		
	Schachar (1991)	Low socio-economic status
	Moffitt (1990)	Family dysfunction Overcrowding Poverty
	Cadoret & Stewart (1991)	Genetic
	Szatmari *et al.* (1990)	Neurocognitive impairment

Table 11.1. *(cont.)*

Path	Study	Nature of influence
(k) Influence of CD on HA		
	None	
(l) Influence of HA on CD		
	Hynd *et al.* (1991)	Present especially for ADDH (less for ADD)
	Richman, Stevenson & Graham (1982) Campbell & Ewing (1990)	Preschool HA leads to later CD
(m) Specific influence on HA+RD		
	NONE	
(n) Specific influence on RD+CD		
	Szatmari, Reitsma-Street & Offord (1986)	Pregnancy and birth complications
(o) Specific influence on CD+HA		
	Taylor *et al.* (1991)	Poor family relationships Maternal depression
	McGee *et al.* (1992)	Present especially when ADD associated with early language delay
	Moffitt (1990) Forness *et al.* (1992)	Worse than ADHD and CD alone on many measures including reading

was particularly marked for hyperactivity. A study of formerly institutionalised children has shown that children with disrupted early care are particularly at risk of showing hyperactivity as at eight years of age (Tizard & Hodges, 1978) and that this is still a distinctive feature of their behaviour in adolescence (Hodges & Tizard, 1989). Schachar and Wachsmuth (1991) found repeated parent–child separations to be associated with ADDH, and Haddad and Garralda (1992) found severe disruption of early care to be a common feature in case studies of five children with hyperkinetic syndrome.

Disrupted early parenting seems to be one of the most distinctive correlates of hyperactivity. Plausible mechanisms can be suggested whereby the insecurity consequent upon disrupted early parenting leads to anxiety. This anxious arousal may, in turn, induce restlessness and disorganised behaviour. This mechanism may also contribute to the co-morbidity between hyperactivity and anxiety disorders. All influences on hyperactivity have to take into account the specific cognitive and neuropsychological deficits shown by hyperactive children (Pennington *et al.*, 1993; Taylor, 1991). There is evidence to suggest that genetic differences between children might explain a significant proportion of the variance in hyperactive behaviour (Goodman & Stevenson, 1989*b*; Gillis *et al.*,1992; Stevenson, 1992). As will be discussed below it has yet to be established whether genetic effects on hyperactivity are specific or whether they are shared with RD.

Common influences on hyperactivity and reading disability

Hinshaw (1992*b*) concludes that the literature is consistent with underlying mechanisms in both directions whereby hyperactivity/inattention can lead to reading deficits (e.g. Jorm *et al.*, 1986; McGee *et al.*, 1986; McGee *et al.*, 1986), antisocial behaviour can cause later academic failure (Patterson *et al.*, 1989; Huesmann, Eron & Yarmel, 1987) and reading failure can lead to later delinquency (Maughan, Gray & Rutter, 1985).

However, Hinshaw (1992*a,b*) suggests that the evidence is most consistent with a shared common aetiology for externalising disorders and academic underachievement. This approach compounds the effects associated with hyperactivity and those with conduct disorder. However, as Hinshaw (1987) showed earlier, hyperactivity and conduct disorder have distinct factors associated with each of them and these factors themselves tend to be correlated. This means that the common influences on hyperactivity and reading disability can be separated from those on conduct disorder and reading disability.

One strong candidate for a common cause here is maternal depression–

anxiety which can lead to reading difficulties not explained by low IQ (Richman *et al.*, 1982) and to inattention (Breznitz & Friedman, 1988). Both these associations have been replicated in one longitudinal study (Estrada *et al.*, 1987). Other possible common factors are below average IQ, language deficits and neurodevelopmental delay (Hinshaw, 1992*b*).

For example, McGee *et al.* (1991) found evidence that, in an epidemiological sample of preschoolers, children with pervasive hyperactivity were more likely to be in families with high levels of social adversity. These children were very much at risk for poor academic achievement including reading disability. One striking finding from this study was that only 25% of the children who were pervasively hyperactive were deemed to have recovered by the age of 15 years. One postulated common cause creating hyperactivity and poor reading could then be the social adversity in the family backgrounds of the children, with delayed language development a more proximal common cause.

The mechanisms whereby initial language deficits lead through to later HA have not been tested. However, the plausible common links between language delay and RD have been established. One component of language disability, i.e. phonological processing deficits, are seen to be the basis of many reading disabilities (Wagner & Torgeson, 1987). Although it should be noted that others have emphasised the link between syntactic deficits in language disordered children and later reading difficulties either specifically (Bishop & Adams, 1990) or alongside phonological deficits (Scarborough, 1991). It has also been shown that language plays a crucial role in the self-regulation of behaviour and thereby affects externalising behaviour including hyperactivity (Hogan & Quay, 1984; Rutter, 1987). There are other associations, however, in that language delays are commonly found to be related to later internalising disorders (Stevenson, Richman & Graham, 1985) as well as to ADD (Beitchman, Hood, Rochon & Peterson, 1989). To summarise, Hinshaw (1992*b*) provides a careful evaluation of the quality of the evidence for unidirectional and bidirectional effects between externalising disorders and academic underachievement. The weight of evidence indicates that, in addition to plausible effects in both directions, i.e. hyperactivity leading to reading disability and vice versa, there are strong common influences on both conditions.

There is increasing evidence that both reading disabilities and hyperactivity are subject to genetic influences. Apart from a small twin study by Willerman (1973), the first systematic analysis of genetic influences on hyperactivity using well-validated measures was that undertaken by Goodman and Stevenson (1989*a*,*b*). This showed that, once potential rating biases had been taken into account, about 40% of the variance in hyperactivity scores in 13 year-old children could be attributed to genetic differences. A separate analysis of the genetic effects on extreme hyperactivity scores (Stevenson, 1992) found that genetic effects were even stronger. It has become common practice in behaviour genetic analyses to differentiate between individual heritability (h^2) and group heritability (h^2_g). Group heritability estimates the extent to which a condition construed as the extreme of a continuum (such as hyperactivity) is determined by genetic differences between children. Individual heritability, on the other hand, is an estimate of the contribution of genetic variation to individual differences across the entire continuum. Stevenson (1992) obtained a value for h^2_g of 0.81 $\pm$0.51 for hyperactivity. Hyperactivity appears to be a condition where h^2_g is somewhat greater than h^2; this is not the case with reading disability where the two heritabilities are quite similar.

These indications of strong genetic effects on hyperactivity have been replicated. Gillis *et al.* (1992) estimated h^2_g for ADHD scores from the Diagnostic Interview for Children and Adolescents (Reich *et al.*, 1987) for 37 identical and 37 fraternal twin pairs. They obtained a value for h^2_g of 0.98 $\pm$0.26. These group heritabilities for hyperactivity were obtained from the London and Colorado twin reading studies. Parallel analyses suggested that reading and especially spelling abilities were similarly influenced by genetic differences between children (DeFries, Fulker & LaBuda, 1987; Stevenson, 1991). This raises the possibility that since both hyperactivity and literacy have genetic aetiologies could it be that their co-occurrence might be due to the same genetic factors influencing both disabilities.

The first attempt to undertake such an analysis was that of Gilger, Pennington and DeFries (1992). They used the Colorado twin reading study sample of monozygotic and dizygotic twin pairs, in which at least one member of each pair is reading disabled. Both members of the twin pair were assessed for attention-deficit hyperactivity disorder (ADHD). Within pair cross-concordances of the reading disability and ADHD for monozygotic twins were larger than for dizygotic twins but not significantly so. They concluded that 'in some cases reading disability and ADHD may occur together because of a shared genetic aetiology and that a genetically mediated co-morbid subtype may exist.' This initial analysis may have failed to detect significant zygosity difference in the cross-concordances through a lack of power. To overcome this problems Stevenson *et al.* (1993) used an enlarged sample of Colorado twins and jointly analysed data from the London Twin Reading Studies as well. Power was increased by both employing larger sample sizes and by using a bivariate extension of the multiple regression procedure developed by DeFries and Fulker (1985, 1988) for the estimation of h^2_g. Stevenson *et al.* (1993) found that 75% of the tendency of hyperactivity and spelling disability to co-occur could be attributed to shared genetic factors. If this result can be replicated, it would have profound implications for our models of the origins of school-based difficulties in hyperactive children. It suggests that the mechanisms producing the learning disabilities of hyperactive children are largely a consequence of genetic effects.

This finding has a number of puzzling features. It has been shown that the genetic effects on reading are almost exclusively mediated by deficits in phonological processing (Olson *et al.*, 1989; Stevenson, 1991). It is difficult to see why genetic influences on phonological processing should also influence inattention and restlessness. Indeed cognitive theory identifies attentional control and phonological processing as distinct functions within models of working memory (Baddeley, 1992). Furthermore, it is not sufficient to postulate a general attention mechanism that if deficient will also adversely affect phonological processing. If that were to be the case, it would be expected that other aspects of the reading process would be similarly effected. Olson *et al.* (1989) and Stevenson (1991) have shown that orthographic abilities are not affected by genetic differences between children. It should be borne in mind that shared genetic aetiology could arise by genetic factors influencing one condition which, in turn, leads to the second condition. This possibility will be returned to in the discussion of the effects of reading disability on hyperactivity.

One possibility is that the reading disabilities of hyperactive children are different from those of non-hyperactive children. In hyperactive children it may be that genetic effects on reading are rather more extensive than in non-hyperactive children. To test this possibility the London twin reading study results were re-analysed to estimate the heritability of spelling ability in non-hyperactive and hyperactive children. The heritability of spelling ability for non-hyperactive children was 0.54 and 0.24 for hyperactive children; this is a non-significant difference in the opposite direction to that predicted above and therefore is consistent with reading disability in hyperactivity being similar to that in other children. Rather better evidence that reading disability associated with hyperactivity is the same as reading disability occurring alone comes from the studies of Ackerman *et al.* (1990) and Pennington *et al.* (1993) which are discussed below.

There is some indirect evidence of a genetic mechanism underlying the association between hyperactivity and school attainment. When a condition is influenced by genetic factors and at the same time shows gender difference in prevalence, then the less frequently affected gender usually has a stronger family history and/or is more severely affected (Rutter *et al.*, 1990). There is one report (Brown, Madan-Swain & Baldwin, 1991) that indicates that hyperactive girls (the gender with the lowest prevalence rate of hyperactivity and reading disability) have poorer academic achievement. Indeed, over time, this effect was found to become more marked with ADHD girls showing more severe deficits than ADHD boys in school attainment, cognitive functioning and with peer relationships.

There is a consistent finding that girls with hyperactivity are underidentified within the school system (Berry, Shaywitz & Shaywitz, 1985). McGee, Williams & Silva (1987) showed that, by using same-sex distributions for the identification of inattentive boys and girls, groups with very similar characteristics can be identified in the two sexes. They suggest that, once the contaminating effects of teacher expectations about higher levels of aggressive behaviour in boys have been taken into account, the true prevalence rate of handicapping conditions with an inattentive component is very similar for boys and girls.

The relationship between activity level and impulsivity is complex, not least in terms of there being marked sex differences. Victor, Halverson and Montague (1985) showed that activity level predicted impulsive behaviour in boys but not in girls. Therefore, it cannot be assumed that sex differences in prevalence rates of hyperactivity obtained from epidemiological samples (e.g. Szatmari, Offord & Boyle, 1989*a*,*b*) can be explained away simply in terms of sex bias in behavioural ratings (see also Goodman & Stevenson, 1989*a* for sex differences in non-referred samples on experimental tests of attention).

Levy and Hobbes (1989) present findings on the association between ADDH and conduct disorder and the relationship between reading and hyperactivity. They found evidence from scores on reading, spelling and attention tasks that ADDH and conduct disorder could be differentiated from more severe forms of ADDH by the latter's low scores on a vigilance factor but not on a factor concerned with reading. The second intriguing suggestion from this study is that phonetic spelling ability (i.e. the ability to produce a phonetically correct spelling for a target word) loads on the attention factor rather than the reading factor in 5.9 to 11.9 year-olds.

The finding of Stevenson *et al.* (1993) that spelling and hyperactivity share a common genetic loading might be thought to relate to this. To test whether this finding could be replicated, similar measures from the London twin reading study were subjected to a parallel factor analysis. The measures are not directly comparable but do cover the same domains, i.e. reading, spelling, attention and intelligence. The analysis was restricted to boys in this sample of 13 year-olds. Using principal components to extract factors with a subsequent varimax rotation it was found that spelling did load (.88) with the reading scores (.93, .91) on a the first factor which also loaded on IQ (.84). The second factor was an attention factor on which a sustained attention measure loaded (.97), whilst spelling (.09) and the reading measures did not. This factor analysis of the

London twin study has failed to replicate the Levy and Hobbes (1989) result. It has to be left open as to what extent phonetic spelling ability is more strongly related to attention abilities than other aspects of literacy.

To summarise, there is considerable evidence in support of the notion that hyperactivity and reading disability share some common causes. Some of these are social in origin, e.g. maternal depression. Others may result from shared genetic aetiology.

Influence of hyperactivity on reading disability

In trying to evaluate the evidence for the effects of hyperactivity on reading disability as distinct from the effects of reading disability on hyperactivity, longitudinal data are highly desirable. It allows the direction of effects to be potentially unconfounded by using the logic that early factors can cause later ones and not vice versa.

One of the most sophisticated examinations of the putative causal relationships between reading and attention deficits using this methodology was that conducted by Fergusson and Horwood (1992). They used latent variable analysis (Loehlin, 1987) to test a model of the possible reciprocal relationships between attention deficit and reading achievement. The model concerns the changes in attention abilities and reading seen in 10 to 12 year-old children. Using data from a subsample of a birth cohort of 777 children they found that the most parsimonious model suggests that at the age of 12 years the predominant direction of causality is that attention deficits influence reading achievement. Within their data there was no indication that reading achievement influenced attention ability. An effect of hyperactivity on reading was also found by Rowe and Rowe (1992*b*); this study will be discussed in more detail in the next section.

A feature of the Fergusson and Horwood study that distinguishes it from the majority of those reported in the chapter is that it concerned individual differences in attention and reading abilities across the entire range in the population at age 10 and 12 years (see the discussion of Rowe and Rowe, 1992*a* below for the effects of age on this relationship). For the total population at this age it may be that any effects of reading disability on attention are slight. However, for those with marked reading disability and who are experiencing educational failure, the effects on attention, impulsivity and activity levels may be more marked.

Douglas and Benezra (1990) assessed memory problems associated with attention deficit disorder with hyperactivity (ADDH) and reading disability of boys aged 7 to 12 years. Across all verbal tasks, deficits became most apparent in ADDH boys on measures requiring organised, deliberate rehearsal strategies, sustained strategic effort, and careful consideration of response alternatives. This pattern suggests impaired self-regulatory or 'executive' processes. Children with reading disability showed more generalised deficits across the verbal measures, suggesting problems with verbal processing. They concluded that in children with both attention deficit disorders with hyperactivity and reading disability, the reading difficulties arise from the underlying executive function deficits associated with the attention deficits. Such results therefore support the hypothesis that when co-morbidity occurs the reading disability is a secondary consequence of the more primary attention deficit. These results are just the reverse of those reported by Pennington, Grossier & Welsh (1993).

It would appear obvious that attention deficits would adversely effect many learning situations including learning to read. However, as Taylor *et al.* (1991) have emphasised, the attention deficits in hyperactive children do not simply comprise poor selective attention. Evidence that hyperactivity affects reading is not prolific, but a number of studies do suggest such an effect.

Influence of reading disability on hyperactivity

It was reported above that Fergusson and Horwood (1992) did not find evidence of an effect of poor reading attainment on attention. Rowe and Rowe (1992*a*,*b*) also used latent variable analysis to study the relationship between inattentiveness in the classroom and reading achievement. They had a large sample but from a wider age than Fergusson and Horwood (5–14 years). Independent of family socio-economic status, age, and gender, students' inattentiveness had strong negative effects on their achievement. However, in addition 'the findings indicated strong reciprocal effects, suggesting that whereas inattentive behaviours lead to reduced achievement, reading achievement – mediated by attitudes and reading activity at home – leads to increased attentiveness in the classroom'. This conclusion is somewhat different to that reached by Fergusson and Horwood.

Rowe and Rowe fitted a number of alternative models to their data. The analysis that most closely parallels that of Fergusson and Horwood is that based upon a non-recursive model. This considers the concurrent reciprocal impact of reading attainment and inattention on each other. The path coefficient for the standardised solution for inattention on reading found by Rowe and Rowe (1992*b*) was –0.96 in the 12–14 year-old children. The equivalent coefficient obtained by Fergusson and Horwood was –0.12. The reverse path for the effect of reading on inattention was –0.88 for Rowe and Rowe and a non-significant –0.02 for Fergusson and Horwood. The effects in both directions show little difference across age group in the Rowe and Rowe study.

The inconsistency cannot be explained readily by reference to differences in the measures used in the two studies. In both cases teacher ratings were used for attention deficits and reading comprehension. The New Zealand study did have an additional measure on word recognition and the Australian study used teacher ratings on criterion-based profiles of reading in addition to testing to gain an overall index of reading attainment. The resolution of the differences between these two studies will have to rely on additional replications.

Pennington *et al.* (1993) used a full 2×2 design to test the cognitive characteristics of children with and without ADHD and reading disability. They used a test for 'double dissociation' to establish whether there was evidence that ADHD lead to reading disability or vice versa. This approach aims to establish the independent origin of two conditions by demonstrating that cases with each condition have a distinct set of deficits and do not show the deficits associated with the other condition. In the case of ADHD only Pennington *et al.* (1993) predicted that executive functions (i.e. planning, set-shift ability, impulse control and sustained attention) would be deficient. These executive function tests are thought to reflect processes within the frontal lobes. By contrast for reading disability, only phonological processing would be deficient. They went further to predict that co-morbid ADHD+reading disability cases would be deficient in phonological processing. This would indicate that the ADHD characteristics of these children were a secondary consequence of the primary reading disability condition.

The results of the Pennington, Grossier & Welsh (1993) study confirmed the double dissociation of executive function and phonological processing deficits consistent with each having a separate origin and also supported the hypothesis that ADHD deficits can arise as a 'phenocopy' produced by reading disability i.e. the ADHD+reading disability co-morbid group can have the same behavioural characteristics as ADHD alone but that, at the neurocognitive level, their characteristics are of reading disability children.

August and Garfinkel (1990) found that 39% of a sample of ADHD boys also demonstrated a specific reading disability. They compared boys with ADHD only with mixed ADHD + reading disability and normal controls on a range of cognitive and attention measures. Both ADHD subgroups performed significantly worse than controls on measures of executive function. Only ADHD + reading disability boys differed from controls on measures or rapid word naming and vocabulary. These results suggest that ADHD and reading disability have separate cognitive bases.

Ackerman *et al.* (1990) found that children with attention deficit disorder (ADD) and dyslexia (n = 82) made significantly more errors than normally reading children with ADD (n = 83) on a simple auditory test of phonological sensitivity to rhyme and alliteration (Bradley, 1984). This suggests that reading disability in ADD plus reading disability children stems from the same causes as in non-ADD children, namely phonological processing deficits.

The notion that reading disability and hyperacitivty have distinct neuropsychological bases receives support at the electrophysiological level (Harter, Diering & Wood, 1988). They found that evoked potentials in boys with ADD and with reading disability were different. Furthermore at the neurophysiological level, it has been reported that children with reading disability alone were no different from children with reading disability associated with ADD (Duffy & McAnulty, 1990). This suggests that in the co-morbid children, ADD arises as a secondary consequence of reading disability. However, Duncan *et al.* (1994) have evidence that, in terms of event-related evoked potential, adults with reading disability who have a history of ADHD had specific abnormalities in the late (P300) phase of visual evoked potentials that were different form those with RD alone. This is more consistent with the notion of co-morbid reading disability plus ADHD having a distinct neurological basis.

Pennington *et al.* (1993) acknowledge that previous studies have failed to demonstrate a distinctive deficit for ADHD children in executive functions or the pattern of results consistent with the phenocopy hypothesis (e.g. Felton *et al.*, 1987; Felton & Wood, 1989; Kupietz, 1990; McGee *et al.*, 1989). Schachar (1991) has also concluded that much of the experimental work by Sergeant and his colleagues has failed to establish executive function deficits in hyperactive children (e.g. Sergeant & Scholten, 1985).

Barkley, Grodzinsky and DuPaul (1992) reviewed 22 studies on frontal lobe dysfunction in ADD subjects. They concluded that there were very inconsistent results across studies and that confounds such as age, other co-morbid conditions and variations in the definitions of ADD contribute to the lack of clarity in the findings. They also conducted a study of their own. However, the findings of Barkley *et al.* (1992) cannot be used to test the double dissociation hypothesis for ADHD and reading disability put forward by Pennington *et al.* (1993) since they did not have the full 2×2 design. However their own findings did not support the notion that executive function deficits *per se* were specifically associated with ADD. In their admittedly small samples the learning disorder only children often also had low scores on executive function tests. They also failed to find consistent differences on these tests between clinically referred groups of ADD+H and ADD-H children.

The reasons put forward by Pennington *et al.* (1993) for the differences between their results and those of previous studies are (a) they had clearly specified a priori the double dissociation they expected for the deficits in ADHD and in reading disability, and (b) by not relying on clinic referrals alone for their sample they included proportionately more mild cases of ADHD+reading disability, where the onset of ADHD as a consequence of reading disability is more likely to be present.

This raises the important issue that it is unlikely that all co-morbid cases of ADHD and reading disability result from the same processes. Pennington *et al.* (1993) clearly argue that ADHD can arise as a phenocopy from a more basic reading disability deficit, however, they acknowledge that other ADHD+reading disability subtypes may include cases where both executive function and phonological processing deficits are found. This position is similar to that taken by August and Garfinkel (1989) who suggests that perhaps 20% of ADHD children constitute a distinct group with the basic cognitive deficits of reading disabled children.

The importance of the experimental design adopted by Pennington *et al.* (1993) has been recognised previously. In responding to a critique (Share, 1988) of their earlier study (Tarnowski, Prinz, & Nay, 1986) Tarnowski, Prinz and Nay (1988) concluded that they 'strongly recommend that future research on attention performance in ADDH and learning disorder populations subdivide samples on each dimension in order to avoid masking potentially meaningful group differences'.

Further significant support for the notion that there is a distinct form of ADD that can arise as a secondary consequence of reading disability has come from the Dunedin study (McGee & Share, 1988; McGee, Williams & Feehan, 1992). They reconstructed the developmental histories of children showing age of onset of ADD at preschool (3 years), at school entry (5–6 years) and at age 7 years. The late onset cases, i.e. only showing ADD from age 7 years onward, were only distinguished from non-ADD children by their low reading scores. McGee *et al.* (1992) propose that ADD in this group arises as a consequence of their reading difficulties. By contrast the ADD subjects in the early onset groups had more pervasive and long-lasting deficits including a marked tendency for co-morbidity with conduct or oppositional disorders at ages 11 and 15 years. It is this group that are thought to show 'truly pervasive, inattentive' ADD.

It should be noted that Fergusson and Horwood (1992) measured the behavioural features of ADHD and only the net effects of reading in word recognition and comprehension. Using the approach advocated by Pennington *et al.* (1993), it would be of considerable interest to repeat the model testing approach with longitudinal data adopted by Fergusson and Horwood but using measures of executive function and phonological processing.

Until recently the mechanisms whereby hyperactivity could lead to reading disability were better understood than those leading from reading disability to hyperactivity. There is now an increasing amount of evidence that reading disability may lead to a form of hyperactivity. There is conflicting evidence for the role of executive function deficits in ADD. However, the findings of Pennington *et al.* (1993) represent an important development and their phenocopy hypothesis needs to be tested further and their findings replicated. The possibility that reading disability leads to hyperactivity raises the issue that subtypes of hyperactivity can be identified with similar behavioural characteristics but with distinct underlying cognitive deficits.

Specific influences on reading disability

There is a strong consensus that the distinctive feature of reading disability is that at core there is a deficit in phonological processing (Wagner & Torgesen, 1987). In reading these are shown by difficulties in associating strings of letters with their sound properties and this deficit has its origins in children's ability to process phonological information in spoken language (Bradley & Bryant, 1985). As was discussed above, a major influence on individual differences in phonological processing is genetic differences between children.

In the context of the present review, the key question is whether phonological processing deficits are found in children with hyperactivity and whether they are also found in co-morbid hyperactivity and reading disability children. The two studies that were discussed above that have tested these effects directly are those by Ackerman *et al.* (1990) and Pennington *et al.* (1993). Both these studies showed that children with reading disability and hyperactivity had phonological deficits and that phonological deficits were restricted to children with reading disability and were not part of the general cognitive deficits of hyperactive children. Hence phonological deficits clearly meet the logical requirements of specific influence on reading disability. Specific distal causes of reading disability are more difficult to identify. Stevenson and Fredman (1990) concluded that family size was one of the few characteristics influencing reading ability that was not similarly related to general intelligence.

Common influences on reading disability and conduct disorder

A major landmark study identifying the co-occurrence of conduct disorder and reading disability was that undertaken on the Isle of Wight by Rutter, Tizard and Whitmore (1970). They established a specific association between specific reading retardation (i.e. reading attainment below that expected on the basis of IQ) and antisocial behaviour/conduct disorder. In reviewing the subsequent epidemiological studies Hinshaw (1992*a*) concludes that this putative association has not been replicated. Indeed, there are findings to suggest that reading disability is associated with neurotic disturbance and that behavioural disturbance is often as common in reading backward children as it is children with specific reading retardation.

One of the few studies to suggest a possible association between conduct disorder and reading disability on the basis of correlated background factors is that of Sturge (1982) which was undertaken as part of the inner London follow-up to the original Isle of Wight study. She specifically postulates a correlation between a biological predisposition to language and reading problems which might be correlated with social disadvantage and family discord. The latter are factors which increase the risk of conduct disorder.

Olweus (1983) was able to explore the possibility that common factors were contributing to the co-occurrence of reading disability and conduct disorder. Using a large sample of boys followed through their early adolescence, he found that once antecedent variables, i.e. background factors such as social class, parental divorce and parity, were controlled there was no residual impact of early aggression on poor school grades or the other way round. It would appear within this data set that the common background factors broadly associated with social disadvantage accounted for the association between grades at school and aggressive behaviour.

There is evidence that goes against the idea that conduct disorder and hyperactivity might share a common genetic aetiology. Stevenson and Graham (1993) analysed data from a sample of 13 year-old twins. They used the bivariate extension of the group heritability method (see above). The two conditions in this study were extreme antisocial behaviour as measured on the Rutter scales and spelling disability. Unlike the findings for hyperactivity and spelling, there was no evidence for common genetic influences on conduct disorder and spelling disability.

There is therefore only weak evidence for common causes for reading disability and conduct disorder and those that have been identified tend to be distal and are associated with social disadvantage.

Influence of reading disability on conduct disorder

In the course of the review by Hinshaw (1992*a*,*b*) it is cogently argued that many of the studies claiming to have identified unidirectional (and indeed bi-directional) effects between conduct disorder and reading disability have failed to include the minimal requirements of such a study. In particular, the analysis has to consider both the contemporaneous correlations between the two conditions as well as the within and between condition correlations over time.

Of the studies meeting these requirements, only one (by Shonfeld *et al.*, 1988) suggested an effect of verbal ability on conduct disorder. It should be noted that this study did not use reading ability as a predictor but verbal IQ. The only other study to meet Hinshaw's requirements is that of Olweus (1983), which showed that aggressivity became more marked in those adolescents who had poor school attainment.

Influence of conduct disorder on reading disability

In his review Hinshaw (1992*b*) suggests that although plausible, the case made by Patterson *et al.* (1989) for the adverse impact of anti-social behaviour on academic attainment has not been adequately tested. He cites Huesmann *et al.* (1987) as providing one of the few sets of findings where early antisocial behaviour has been shown to relate to later low achievement when the effects of early achievement and IQ are controlled.

Specific influences on conduct disorder

In reviewing the literature on the differentiation of conduct disorder from HA Schachar (1991) concluded that conduct disorder was specifically associated with psychosocial adversity, poor parental coping and inter-parental inconsistency in maintaining discipline within the home. However, in a report of two complementary studies of families with a 3 year-old and with 9 to 13 year-old children, Miller *et al.* (1993) argue that the origins of antisocial behaviour do not lie just in parenting style. The individual's adjustment, e.g. depression, and the quality of the marital relationship have a powerful influence on their relationships with their children and may be a better focus for intervention in such families.

In identifying the specific influences on conduct disorder it has become apparent that different individuals may develop conduct disorder through a number of different routes (Moffitt, 1990). The subtle effects that can be present are illustrated by the study of Caspi *et al.* (1993). They showed that the emergence of delinquency in girls could take place via two routes; the route taken by a particular girl was likely to depend on her past history of externalising behaviours. For those girls with no previous history an early age of onset of the menarche was crucial in exposing the girls to a delinquent peer group. This in turn increased the risk of her showing antisocial behaviour. By contrast, for girls with a previous history of externalising problems, age at menarche was not related to exposure to a delinquent peer group but rather age of menarche was more directly related to antisocial behaviour ('norm-violations'). In both cases, the net effect of age at menarche and familiarity with delinquent peers was to explain approximately half the variance in antisocial behaviour.

Other studies of family histories of ADD and conduct disorder have found more specific associations across generations which suggest that ADD and conduct disorder are distinct conditions (Frick *et al.*, 1991). Lahey *et al.* (1989) studied the personality profiles on the MMPI of mothers of ADD and conduct disorder children. They found that conduct disorder is linked to maternal personality disorder, but ADD/H is not. Lahey *et al.* (1988) found that conduct disorder is linked to parental psychopathology but ADD/H is not.

There is also psychometric evidence that HA and CD are distinct. On the basis of factor analyses of behavioural symptoms Blouin *et al.* (1989) concluded that independent orthogonal factors of HA and CD are reliably detectable. Similar findings of factorial independence were reported by Hinshaw *et al.* (1987).

Therefore, notwithstanding effects of hyperactivity and conduct disorder on each other, there are a number of specific influences on conduct disorder *per se*. These particular influences on conduct disorder lie largely within characteristics of the parents and the family.

Common influences on conduct disorder and hyperctivity

A range of adversities were suggested by Schachar (1991) to typify the families of children with conduct disorder + hyperactivity. These include low SES, over-crowding and poverty. These findings are well illustrated by Moffitt (1990) in a longitudinal analysis of the behaviour of a birth cohort of 435 boys. At age 13, the following groups were identified: ADD + delinquent, ADD only, delinquent only, and non-disordered. The ADD + delinquent boys consistently fared the worst on the assessments of family adversity, verbal intelligence, and reading. Their antisocial behaviour began before school age, escalated at school entry, and persisted into adolescence. The ADD-only boys had normal family characteristics and intelligence and reading scores, and showed only mild antisocial behaviour in middle childhood. The delinquent-only boys showed no early risk from family, low intelligence, or reading deficit, and remained relatively free of conduct problems until they initiated delinquency at age 13. On the basis of these findings Moffitt (1990) predicted that the ADD + delinquent boys especially would continue to show criminal behaviour into adulthood. It should be noted that some other groups of conduct disordered children are also highly at risk of continuing difficulties into adulthood, such as those experiencing residential care (Zoccolillo *et al.*, 1992).

An adoption study by Cadoret and Stewart (1991) suggests that 'aggressivity' and hyperactivity might share the same genetic risk. They found that delinquency in the biological parent was associated with an increased risk of ADHD and adult antisocial personality in the adopted-away sons. Within the adoptees ADHD predicted later aggressivity. These findings suggest that genetic factors contribute to the onset of ADHD which in turn may lead to aggressivity and conduct disorder. A more parsimonious but perhaps less plausible account would be that the same genetic factors independently increased the risk of both ADHD and conduct disorder. Faraone *et al.* (1991) conducted a study of the 457 first degree relatives of children and adolescents referred to a clinic for ADD and conduct disorder. They found an incidence of familiality which was consistent with common risk factors for ADD and conduct disorder.

Szatmari *et al.* (1990) studied what they called 'neurocognitive impairments (NCI)' among children with psychiatric disorders who had been referred to a clinic. They found that NCI were more strongly associated with externalising rather than internalising disorders especially when shown at school. They found that children with ADDH did not show more NCI than conduct disorder children. This is surprising given the conclusions reached by Schachar (1991) in his review of previous neurocognitive studies. He suggests that hyperactivity is much more frequently found to have associated neurological and cognitive deficits than are children with conduct disorder. The construct of NCI that was used was a very wide one including IQ, rapid automatised naming, visual perceptual and visual motor and facial recognition amongst others. Unfortunately, the paper does not provide separate mean scores for conduct disorder and ADDH children, and so it cannot be determined whether the ADDH and conduct disorder children might have been different on a subset of the neuropsychological battery they used.

One factor that conduct disorder and ADD children tend to have in common is low verbal IQ. When IQ differences were controlled for (along with age and sex) Werry, Elkind and Reeves (1987) found few residual differences between

ADD and conduct disorder children. This finding along with that of Szatmari *et al.* (1990) tends to suggest a lack of differentiation between conduct disorder and hyperactivity at a cognitive level. However, the major trend in the literature is for hyperactivity and not conduct disorder to have associated cognitive deficits.

Influence of conduct disorder on hyperactivity

There have been no reliable findings supporting the notion that conduct disorder affects hyperactivity (Taylor, 1986).

Influence of hyperactivity on conduct disorder

It has been suggested that children with ADD and hyperactivity are more likely to show conduct disorder. In contrast to ADDnoH children, those classified as ADDH tended to have a co-diagnosis of conduct disorder (40%) (Hynd *et al.*, 1991). However, this does not imply that hyperactivity is causing conduct disorder.

Rather better evidence for an effect of hyperactivity on conduct disorder comes from the longitudinal studies such as those starting during the preschool period. These have been introduced in the preschool section above. The studies of Richman *et al.* (1982), McGee *et al.* (1991), and Campbell and Ewing (1990) all indicate that early developing hyperactivity places the child at a much increased risk of developing externalising disorders including conduct disorder at a later age. McGee *et al.* (1992) have suggested that hyperactivity leading to conduct disorder is a distinctive feature of early onset hyperactivity but argue that this is evidence for hyperactivity + conduct disorder being a separate syndrome since it is uniquely associated with delayed early language development. There is a need for detailed studies of the processes mediating these associations where aspects of family responses to early behaviour and child characteristics such as self-esteem are likely to be particularly pertinent.

Specific influence on hyperactivity+reading disability

There is no substantial evidence that hyperactivity+reading disability constitute a syndrome that is qualitatively distinct from either hyperactivity or reading disability alone. Instead, different studies have found hyper-activity+reading disability children to share the characteristics of both HA alone and RD alone children or a mix of the two. There is no evidence for a distinct cause for hyperactivity+reading disability.

Specific influence on reading disability+conduct disorder

In a study of the pregnancy and birth complication associated with anti-social behaviour Szatmari, Reitsma-Street and Offord (1986) found that those antisocial adolescents with such a history were more likely to have reading disability. They suggest that conduct disorder + reading disability may then represent a distinct subgroup of conduct disorder adolescents. This finding has not been replicated.

Specific influence on conduct disorder+hyperactivity

Lie (1992) reviewed follow-up studies to test the hypothesis that the ADHD is a precursor of later criminality and abuse of alcohol and illicit drugs. Hyperactivity without conduct problems did not lead to an increased frequency of delinquency. In subjects with ADHD as well as conduct problems in childhood the outcome was poor and worse than for those with CD without ADHD.

However, before concluding that hyperactivity+conduct disorder is a separate condition, the possibility has to be considered that the worse outcome for these co-morbid adolescents could be due either to their having a more severe form of one of the disorders or that the risk factors are acting simply additively. An example of the co-morbid group simply being a more severely affected subgroup is the finding that, when conduct disorder co-occurs with ADD, a more severely aggressive form of the disorder is shown (Walker *et al.*, 1987). An additive risk mechanism is the most parsimonious explanation for the findings of Schachar and Wachsmuth (1991). In a sample of just over 100 boys aged between 7 and 11 years, they found that conduct disorder was associated with high levels of parent–child dysfunction and adverse psychosocial factors. ADDH was associated with moderate levels of adversity only and particularly prolonged parent–child separations. When the co-morbid group was examined both sets of risk factors were present.

A more convincing case for a separate aetiology for hyperactivity+conduct disorder was made by Taylor *et al.* (1991). They found that poor family relationships and maternal depression were distinctive features of the families of children in the hyperactivity+conduct disorder group. These characteristics are also found in families of children with language delay, which is a characteristic of hyperactivity+conduct disorder children identified by McGee *et al.* (1992). The latter concluded that co-morbid ADD+conduct disorder children may be different from other ADD children (a suggestion first made by August & Stewart, 1982). The co-morbid ADD+conduct disorder children were more likely to show onset of ADD by age 3 years and this group had a tendency to have the poorest early language development. This suggests that in these children ADD and CD arise from a common origin which is perhaps marked by particularly delayed early language development.

The possible distinctiveness of an ADD+conduct disorder co-morbid group was found by Forness *et al.* (1992*a*,*b*). This group had lower reading scores than ADD alone. A similar picture emerged from the New Zealand data analysed by Moffitt (1990). This raises the intriguing possibility that children with the conjunction of hyperactivity, reading disability and conduct disorder might constitute a distinct group. To test this notion a study would be required that had sufficient cases to allow the associated characteristics of this three-way co-morbid group to be compared to the characteristics of each of the twofold co-morbid groups, i.e. hyperactivity+reading disability, reading disability+conduct disorder, conduct disorder+hyperactivity.

Conclusions concerning the association between hyperactivity, reading disability and conduct disorder

This overview of the recent research on the associations between hyperactivity, reading disability and conduct disorder shows there to be both certain areas of consensus and other aspects that still need further clarification. The influences where there is some degree of general agreement between a wide variety of studies have been summarised in Figure 11.2. Both hyperactivity and reading disorder are thought to result from some basic cognitive deficit. In the case of reading disability, the nature of this deficit has been clearly identified as involving phonological processing. However, for hyperactivity there is less agreement. The effect of the deficit is to affect performance adversely on attention tasks but it may be that more general cognitive deficits (e.g. in executive functions) are involved rather than simple attention processes *per se*. There is evidence that the cognitive deficits in hyperactivity and reading disability are influenced by genetic factors. The evidence for direct genetic effects on phonological disability is strong. As far as the genetic effects on hyperactivity are concerned, these could be via direct genetic influences on underlying cognitive

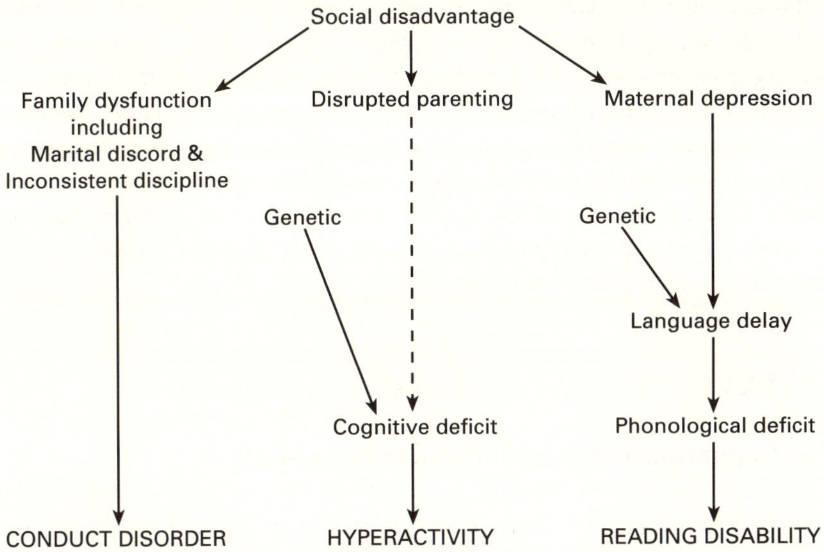

Fig. 11.2 The final model of the most significant influences on conduct disorder, reading disability and hyperactivity (solid line=good consistent evidence, broken line=some replicated evidence but significance uncertain).

deficits or by the impact of RD on HA. That is genetic influences on phonological ability may produce reading disability. This may in turn produce, through processes that are as yet not understood, a form of hyperactivity which is a phenocopy of the hyperactivity that arises directly from cognitive deficits. In this way what appears to be common genetic effect on hyperactivity and reading disability is in fact mediated via genetic influences on reading disability alone.

By contrast, there is no replicated evidence for a cognitive deficit underlying conduct disorder nor is there evidence in children and adolescents for a genetic effect on conduct disorder. Instead, conduct disorder is most consistently associated with family characteristics. These distal causal factors for conduct disorder may be mediated by more proximal influences on the child such as the coercive family processes described by Patterson and his colleagues (Patterson *et al.*, 1989). The associations that arise between conduct disorder and hyperactivity and reading disability are then seen to be due to associations between distal causal factors of conduct disorder on the one hand and the distal causal factors for hyperactivity and reading disability on the other, e.g. maternal depression or disrupted parenting. A second mechanism involves the developmental progression from hyperactivity to conduct disorder.

Within the summary in Fig. 11.2 maternal depression has a potentially crucial role as the most clearly demonstrated distal influence that reading disorder and hyperactivity have in common. Further associations between hyperactivity, conduct disorder and reading disability may be created by common associations of disrupted parenting, maternal depression and family dysfunction with social disadvantage. If these background factors are allied with genetic differences that are also acting to predispose the child towards phonological deficits, synergic effects may be present to produce children showing all three disabilities which may then be particularly resistant to treatment and vulnerable to long-term adverse outcomes.

INTERVENTION AT SCHOOL

Psychopharmacology and school-based changes

Although stimulants have been widely adopted in the USA as a treatment for difficult classroom behaviour, including hyperactivity, there is even in the USA a widespread ignorance about these drugs and their effects on children (Kasten, Coury & Heron, 1992). A major weakness in the literature on drug effects on hyperactivity has been the lack of information on classroom-based effects. There have been many studies such as de Sonneville, Njiokiktjien and Hilhorst (1991) which have shown quite specific effects (in this case on vigilance during sustained attention). What is unclear is whether such effects make educationally significant differences in the classroom.

One of the first studies to address the issue of ecological validity was that of Douglas *et al.* (1986). They were able to demonstrate educationally significant improvements in a variety of classroom-based assessments as a result of the administration of methylphenidate.

It has been argued that the mechanisms whereby methylphenidate has beneficial effect on academic performance are through a general impact on information processing. Balthazor, Wagner and Pelham (1991) used a variety of general and specific information processing tasks on a group of attention deficit disorder children who had been shown to respond to methylphenidate with improved reading comprehension. The tasks included letter-matching and phonological processing which were used to indicate the effects of stimulant medication on specific information processing abilities. They found that there was no evidence of a beneficial effect on any of the specific measures.

A further issue in the detection of significant benefits of stimulant medication is whether the children with attention deficit disorder with hyperactivity respond better to methylphenidate than those with attention deficit alone.

Barkley, DuPaul and McMurray (1991) investigated this issue using ratings of academic performance in addition to other measures. More children with attention deficit disorder alone were clinically judged as having no clinical response (24%), whereas most of attention deficit disorder with hyperactivity children were judged to be positive responders (95%).

Dykman and Ackerman (1991) examined children with a DSM-III diagnosis of attention deficit disorder. They were divided into those showing ADD with hyperactivity (ADDH), ADD with hyperactivity and aggressivity (ADDHA), and ADD alone. Over half the sample (n = 94) were poor readers, with 82 meeting discrepancy criteria for specific reading disability. The behavioural subgroups did not differ significantly in IQ or reading attainment. Both groups with and without reading disability could be differentiated from a control group on laboratory measures of sustained attention and impulse control. In this study, stimulant medication did not differentially benefit any particular subgroup of hyperactive children and its impact did not vary according to which cognitive disabilities are present.

As well as having an impact on information processing *per se*, there is concern to know whether the child with hyperactivity will show a more adaptive behavioural style as result of stimulant medication. Evans and Pelham (1991) evaluated the effects of two doses of psychostimulants on nine ADHD students' performance in an experimental classroom. Double-blind, placebo-controlled assessment revealed significant and clinically important effects of psychostimulants for two thirds of the subjects. Improvements in attention and behaviour during lectures, and noted by observers and by teachers were identified.

Gadow *et al.* (1990) investigated the effect of methylphenidate on the aggressive behaviour of hyperactive children. They found that methylphenidate suppressed non-physical aggression in the classroom, and could decrease physical aggression and verbal aggression in the playground. It should be noted that these effects were identified by teachers but not by parents using parallel instruments and therefore may be situationally specific.

Although there may be evidence that cognitive processing and behaviour are enhanced by medication, the demonstration of improvements in academic attainment and particularly reading scores may be more difficult to achieve. The significance of stimulant treatment for reading performance is still unresolved. It is suggested that this is due in part to difficulties in separating out the confounding effects of conduct disorder. In a double-blind, placebo controlled trial of methylphenidate (Forness *et al.*, 1991, 1992*a*,*b*), the subjects were divided into those with ADHD but no conduct disorder and those with a comorbid diagnosis of ADHD and conduct disorder. There were no significant effects of methylphenidate on the reading of the ADHD only group. Significant effects were found for reading comprehension in the ADHD + conduct disorder group.

Therefore there is no convincing and well-replicated finding that methylphenidate can improve the reading attainment of hyperactive children. The issue of treating children with both ADHD and reading disability was given particular attention by Hinshaw (1992*b*). He argues persuasively that treatment for each facet of the child's problems should be planned separately. This will entail specific educational remediation for the reading disability and a combination of behavioral, psychosocial and pharmacological interventions for the ADHD. Hinshaw suggests that the involvement of parents and teachers is highly desirable since child-based behavioural interventions are rarely successful. There is some evidence that enhanced academic attainment can have beneficial effects on classroom behaviour (Coie & Krebbiel, 1984) but cannot be expected to have significant effects on behaviour in other contexts.

Behavioural and cognitive–behavioural approaches

In reviewing the literature Abikoff and Klein (1992) conclude that behaviour treatments have little demonstrated utility in ADHD. Where gains have been demonstrated, they have often not generalised beyond the clinical setting (e.g. Pisterman *et al.*, 1989). Furthermore, studies that have been adequately designed to test the comparative effects of behaviour therapy and stimulant treatment indicate that behaviour therapy alone is less effective than stimulant treatment alone (Abikoff & Klein, 1992). When administered together there is no additional effect produced over and above that resulting from the medication treatment itself. This is an extreme position. Yule (1986) has identified behavioural-based methods that can make substantial improvements in hyperactive children's behaviour including that shown in the classroom.

Cognitive–behaviour therapy has also been seen as a potentially beneficial approach to ADHD. However when subjected to controlled trials it has not been shown to be effective either alone or in enhancing the effects of stimulant treatment (Abikoff, 1987). The use of cognitive therapy with or without behavioural treatment with children showing impulsivity was reviewed by Baer and Nietzel (1991). A wide range of treatment modalities were examined including self-statement modification, reinforcement contingencies, modelling, strategy training, problem-solving training, and plus various combinations of treatments. Baer and Nietzel (1991) suggest that interventions for impulsivity can produce an improvement equivalent to a third to three-quarters of a standard deviation relative to untreated control subjects.

It may be that behavioural and cognitive techniques can aid impulsivity but as was discussed earlier, impulsivity is neither distinctive nor central to the hyperactive child's difficulties. Clearly, there is no consensus over the utility of behavioural or cognitive approaches and there is a real difficulty in demonstrating effectiveness outside the clinical setting.

Family treatments

There is a good case to be made that, for some HA children, a treatment that involves a wide range of family members is likely to be particularly beneficial. There is no shortage of proposals for what such a treatment regime may comprise (e.g. Ziegler & Holden, 1988). It is more difficult to identify an adequately evaluated treatment programme.

An exception is the study by Barkley *et al.* (1992). They conducted a randomised controlled trial of three alternative forms of family treatment for hyperactive children aged between 12 and 18 years. The three treatments were: behaviour management training, problem-solving and communication training, and structural family therapy. Families were assessed at pre- and post-treatment and at a 3-month follow-up. There were significant gains for all treatments including reductions in negative communication, conflicts, and anger during conflicts and improved ratings of school adjustment.

However, Barkley *et al.* (1992) suggest that although the group mean scores may have shown significant changes, the number of children showing reliable recovery as a result of the treatments was from 5 to 20%. Clearly, what this study has shown is that improvements in behaviour can be achieved using family treatment and that these improvements can generalise to the classroom, but that the majority of children will remain hyperactive. In this sense, family treatments can ameliorate some of the behavioural symptoms of hyperactivity but do not address the basic causes of the condition. It should also be recognised that improvements in family relationships can be brought about by stimulant treatments alone (Barkley, 1988).

Pedagogical technique

A recent controversy has arisen concerning the educational needs of ADHD children. In particular Silver (1990) has questioned the need to use novel pedagogic methods with these children. He argues that, once their attention deficits have been treated using medication and specific behavioural management techniques, they do not require specific learning experiences.

The strategy should be to bring ADHD children to a situation where they can benefit from the educational experiences provided to all children. These he has detailed in a guide to clinical management of ADHD (Silver, 1992) and includes classroom organisation (placing the child near to the teacher and reducing extraneous distracters) and behavioural management (providing the child with good role models form other pupils, setting and maintaining limits, the use of positive comments to enhance self-esteem). In these terms, Silver (1990) argues that ADHD should not be treated as a learning disability.

This argument has been contested (Murphy & Hicks-Stewart, 1991; McBurnett & Pfiffner, 1991; Stolzenberg & Cherkes-Julkowski, 1991) but largely on theoretical grounds. There is a need for empirical studies that can test the effectiveness of alternative pedagogic methods with hyperactive children. There are very few adequately controlled trials of alternative teaching strategies to guide the planning of the education of these children.

The more precise analysis of the deficit entailed in the poor attention and learning difficulties of hyperactive children will be essential to guide appropriate education and remedial training (Schachar & Logan, 1990*a*,*b*; Sonuga-Barke, Taylor & Heptinstall, 1992). For example, O'Neill and Douglas (1991) studied boys with attention deficit disorder with hyperactivity (ADD-H), non-ADD-H reading-disabled and normal boys. The groups were matched for age and verbal IQ. On a story recall task, ADD-H boys did not differ from normals whereas reading disabled boys did less well than the other two groups. The ADD-H boys had less good study skills than the normal boys; they spent less time studying, expended less effort, and employed more superficial strategies.

To summarise this section on intervention for educational aspects of hyperactivity, there has been a reluctance in the UK to use stimulant treatments for problems associated with hyperactivity. In part, this is a result of the confused literature on its effectiveness and because of a reluctance by parents, teachers and doctors alike to medicalise what is seen to be a behavioural or educational difficulty. There are also doubts about the long-term benefits of stimulant treatment on school performance or behaviour problems in these children (Jacobvitz *et al.*, 1990). Interestingly studies in the USA where such treatments are more widely available have shown a similar reluctance on behalf of parents to accept stimulant treatment. However, Liu *et al.* (1991) found that, once parents knew more about methylphenidate treatment they were more accepting of it as the treatment of choice.

It is very unlikely that the complex educational difficulties of hyperactive children are going to be solved by one treatment procedure. A programme that combines medication with behavioural or cognitive–behavioural techniques is the most prudent approach. It should be recognised that the evidence reviewed earlier indicates that, for some children at least, it is possible that their hyperactivity is a secondary consequence of their primary reading deficit. The most effective treatment for this subgroup of children is one that attempts to remediate their deficits in phonological processing such as that of Bryant and Bradley (1984).

CONCLUSIONS

A few years ago it was suggested that there need to be more studies which explicitly contrast the characteristics of putative disorders to provide better validation of existing distinctions (Quay, Routh & Shapiro, 1987). This need to provide the crucial evidence for validity of types of disorder by studying children with pure types of disorder has yet to be met. Even those well-conducted epidemiological studies that avoid referral bias and that adopt well defined operational criteria have failed to resolve the disagreements over the major influences on hyperactivity, reading disability and conduct disorder. The next stage of identifying whether co-morbid cases have unique characteristics has only recently started to address questions of their validity as a separate diagnostic category. It has been suggested that a whole range of distinctive co-morbid conditions could be found linking ADHD with a conduct disorder, anxiety disorders, and so on (Biederman & Steingard, 1989; Biederman, Newcorn & Sprich, 1991). Each might have their own particular set of correlates or causes and may thereby require different approaches to treatment.

The links between hyperactivity and reading disability should be placed in the context of the lifespan development of children experiencing these difficulties. It has been well established that children diagnosed with hyperactivity experience continuing difficulties in social functioning in adulthood (Thorley, 1984). It was suggested by Lie (1992) that as many as one-third of children with ADHD continue to show these characteristics in their early adult years. Furthermore, Keller *et al.* (1992) found that ADD had an average duration over twice as long as that of conduct disorder. However, Klein and Mannuzza (1991) point out that although as adults children with ADHD remain academically 'compromised', on testing there is at best equivocal evidence of continuing cognitive deficits.

Despite the reservations mentioned above over the need for more focused studies on the characteristics of children with hyperactivity, conduct disorder and reading disability, there are a number of conclusions that can be drawn about the relationship between these conditions. First, hyperactivity and reading disability have distinctive cognitive deficits associated with each of them. Secondly, there is evidence that the cognitive deficits in hyperactivity and reading disability are influenced by genetic factors but the relationship between the genetic factors influencing them is as yet unresolved. Thirdly, there is no evidence for a cognitive deficit underlying conduct disorder nor for a genetic effect on conduct disorder. Fourthly, hyperactivity, reading disability and conduct disorder are associated via a number of mechanisms linking family and social influences. Of these, maternal depression or disrupted parenting seem to play a crucial and distinctive role. Finally, as far as management is concerned, there are guidelines available on classroom organisation and behavioural management by teachers and there is a consensus on the value of stimulant treatments for at least short changes in behaviour which show associated gains in the classroom in terms of behaviour and learning.

ACKNOWLEDGEMENTS

I would like to thank Philip Graham and David Skuse for their helpful comments on an early draft. Thalia Eley gave valuable assistance with bibliographic research during the initial stage of preparing this chapter.

REFERENCES

Abikoff, H. (1987). An evaluation of cognitive behaviour therapy for hyperactive children. In *Advances in clinical child psychology*, eds. B.B.Lahey & A.E.Kazdin, Vol.10, pp.171–216. New York: Plenum Press.

Abikoff, H. & Klein, R.G. (1992). Attention-deficit hyperactivity and conduct disorder: co-morbidity and its implications for treatment. *Journal of Consulting and Clinical Psychology*, **60**, 881–92.

Achenbach, T.M. & Edelbrock, C. (1986). *Manual for the Teacher Report and Teacher Version of the Child Behavior Profile*. Burlington, VT: University of Vermont, Department of Psychiatry.

Ackerman, P.T., Dykman, R.A. & Gardner, M.Y. (1990). ADD students with and without dyslexia differ in sensitivity to rhyme and alliteration. *Journal of Learning Disabilities*, **25**, 279–83.

Altepeter, T.S. & Breen, M.J. (1992). Situational variation in problem behaviour at home and school in attention deficit disorder with hyperactivity: a factor analytic study. *Journal of Child Psychology and Psychiatry*, **33**, 741–8.

American Psychiatric Association (1987). *Diagnostic and Statistical Manual of Mental Disorders*, ed.3–R. Washington, DC. American Psychiatric Association.

Atkins, M.S. & Pelham, W.E. (1991). School-based assessment of attention deficit-hyperactivity disorder. *Journal of Learning Disabilities,* **24**, 197–204, 255.

August, G.J. & Garfinkel, B.D. (1993). The nosology of attention-deficit hyperactivity disorder. *Journal of the American Academy of Child and Adolescent Psychiatry,* **32**, 155–65.

August, G.J. & Stewart, M.A. (1982). Is there a syndrome of pure hyperactivity? *British Journal of Psychiatry,* **140**, 305–11.

August, G.J. & Garfinkel, B.D. (1989). Behavioural and cognitive subtypes of ADHD. *Journal of the American Academy of Child & Adolescent Psychiatry,* **28**, 739–48.

August, G.J. & Garfinkel, B.D. (1990). Co-morbidity of ADHD and reading disability among clinic-referred children. *Journal of Abnormal Child Psychology,* **18**, 29–45.

Baddeley, A. (1992). Working memory. *Science,* **255**, 556–9.

Baer, R.A. & Nietzel, M.T. (1991). Cognitive and behavioral treatment of impulsivity in children: a meta-analytic review of the outcome literature. *Journal of Clinical Child Psychology,* **20**, 400–12.

Balthazor, M.J., Wagner, R.K & Pelham, W.E. (1991). The specificity of the effects of stimulant medication on classroom learning-related measures of cognitive processing for attention deficit disorder children. *Journal of Abnormal Child Psychology,* **19**, 35–52.

Barkley, R.A. (1988). The effects of methylphenidate on the interactions of preschool ADHD children with their mothers. *Journal of the American Academy of Child and Adolescent Psychiatry,* **27**, 336–41.

Barkley, R.A., Anastopoulos, A.D., Guevremont, D.C. & Fletcher, K.E. (1991). Adolescents with ADHD: patterns of behavioral adjustment, academic functioning, and treatment utilization. *Journal of the American Academy of Child and Adolescent Psychiatry,* **30**, 752–61.

Barkley, R.A., DuPaul, G.J. & McMurray, M.B. (1991). Attention deficit disorder with and without hyperactivity: clinical response to three dose levels of methylphenidate. *Pediatrics,* **87**, 519–31.

Barkley, R.A., Grodzinsky, G. & DuPaul, G.J. (1992). Frontal lobe functions in attention deficit disorder with and without hyperactivity: a review and research report. *Journal of Abnormal Child Psychology,* **20**, 163–88.

Barkley, R.A., Guevremont, D.C., Anastopoulos, A.D. & Fletcher, K.E. (1992). A comparison of three family therapy programs for treating family conflicts in adolescents with attention-deficit hyperactivity disorder. *Journal of Consulting and Clinical Psychology,* **60**, 450–62.

Bauermeister, J.J., Alegria, M., Bird, H.R., Rubio-Stipec, M. & Canino, G. (1992). Are attentional-hyperactivity deficits unidimensional or multi-dimensional syndromes? Empirical findings from a community survey. *Journal of the American Academy of Child and Adolescent Psychiatry,* **31**, 423–31.

Beck, S.J.,Young, G.H. & Tarnowski, K.J. (1990). Maternal characteristics and perceptions of pervasive and situational hyperactives and normal controls. *Journal of the American Academy of Child and Adolescent Psychiatry,* **29**, 558–65.

Beitchman, J.H., Hood, J., Rochon, J. & Peterson, M. (1989). Empirical classification of speech/language impairment in children: II: Behavioral characteristics. *Journal of the American Academy of Child and Adolescent Psychiatry,* **28**, 118–23.

Berry, C.A., Shaywitz, S.E. & Shaywitz, B.A. (1985). Girls with attention deficit disorder: a silent majority? A report on behavioral and cognitive characteristics. *Pediatrics,* **76**, 801–9.

Biederman, J. & Steingard, R. (1989). Attention-deficit hyperactivity disorder in adolescents. *Psychiatric Annals,* **19**, 587–96.

Biederman, J., Newcorn, J. & Sprich, S. (1991). Co-morbidity of attention deficit hyperactivity disorder with conduct, depressive, anxiety, and other disorders. *American Journal of Psychiatry,* **148**, 564–77.

Bishop, D.V.M. & Adams, C. (1990). A prospective study of the relationship between specific language impairment, phonological disorders and reading retardation. *Journal of Child Psychology and Psychiatry,* **31**, 1027–50.

Blouin, A.G., Conners, C.K., Seidel, W.T. & Blouin, J. (1989). The independence of hyperactivity from conduct disorder: methodological considerations. *Canadian Journal of Psychiatry,* **34**, 279–82.

Bradley, L. (1984). *Assessing Reading Difficulties: A Diagnostic and Remedial Approach*, 2nd edn. London: Macmillan.

Bradley, L. & Bryant, P. (1985). *Rhyme and Reason in Reading and Spelling*. Ann Arbor: University of Michigan Press.

Breen, M.J. (1989). Cognitive and behavioural differences in ADHD boys and girls. *Journal of Child Psychology and Psychiatry,* **30**, 711–16.

Breen, M.J. & Altepeter, T.S. (1990). Situational variability in boys and girls identified as ADHD. *Journal of Clinical Psychology,* **46**, 486–90.

Breznitz, Z. & Friedman, S.L. (1988). Toddlers' concentration: does maternal depression make a difference? *Journal of Child Psychology and Psychiatry,* **29**, 267–80.

Brown, R.T., Madan-Swain, A. & Baldwin, K. (1991). Gender differences in a clinic-referred sample of attention-deficit-disordered children. *Child Psychiatry and Human Development,* **22**, 111–28.

Bryant, P. & Bradley, L. (1984). *Childrens' Reading Problems*. Oxford: Blackwell.

Cadoret, R.J. & Stewart, M.A. (1991). An adoption study of attention deficit/hyperactivity/aggression and their relationship to adult antisocial personality. *Comprehensive Psychiatry,* **32**, 73–82.

Campbell, S.B. & Ewing, L.J. (1990). Follow-up of hard-to-manage preschoolers: adjustment at age 9 and predictors of continuing symptoms. *Journal of Child Psychology and Psychiatry,* **31**, 871–89.

Cantwell, D.P. & Baker, L. (1991). Association between attention deficit-hyperactivity disorder and learning disorders. *Journal of Learning Disabilities,* **24**, 88–95.

Cantwell, D.P. & Baker, L.(1992). Attention deficit disorder with and without hyperactivity: a review and comparison of matched groups. *Journal of the American Academy of Child and Adolescent Psychiatry,* **31**, 432–8.

Carey, W.B. (1992). Temperament issues in the school-aged child. *Pediatric Clinics of North America,* **39**, 569–84.

Caron, C. & Rutter, M. (1991). Co-morbidity in child psychopathology: concepts, issues and research strategies. *Journal of Child Psychology and Psychiatry,* **32**, 1063–80.

Caspi, A., Lynam, D., Moffitt, T.E. & Silva, P.A. (1993). Unravelling girl's delinquency: biological, dispositional and contextual contributions to adolescent misbehavior. *Developmental Psychology,* **29**, 19–30.

Coie, J.D. & Krebbiel, G. (1984). Effects of academic tutoring on the social status of low-achieving, socially rejected children. *Child Development,* **55**, 1465–78.

Costello, E.J., Loeber, R. & Stouthamer-Loeber, M. (1991). Pervasive and situational hyperactivity–confounding effect of informant: a research note. *Journal of Child Psychology and Psychiatry,* **32**, 367–76.

DeFries, J.C. & Fulker, D.W. (1985). Multiple regression analysis of twin data. *Behavior Genetics,* **15**, 467–73.

De Fries, J.C. & Fulker, D.W. (1988). Multiple regression of twin data: Etiology of deviant scores versus individual differences. *Acta Geneticae Medicae et Gemellologiae*, **37**, 1–13.

DeFries, J.C., Fulker, D.W. & LaBuda, M.C. (1987). Evidence for a genetic aetiology in reading disability in twins. *Nature, (London)* **329**, 537–539.

de Sonneville, L.M., Njiokiktjien, C. & Hilhorst, R.C. (1991). Methylphenidate-induced changes in ADDH information processors. *Journal of Child Psychology and Psychiatry,* **32**, 285–95.

Douglas, V.I., Barr, R.G., O'Neill, M.E. & Britton, B.G. (1986). Short-term effects of methylphenidate on the cognitive, learning and academic performance of children with attention deficit disorder in the laboratory and the classroom. *Journal of Child Psychology and Psychiatry,* **27**, 191–211.

Douglas, V.I. & Benezra, E. (1990). Supraspan verbal memory in attention deficit disorder with hyperactivity normal and reading-disabled boys. *Journal of Abnormal Child Psychology,* **18**, 617–38.

Duffy, F.H. & McAnulty, G. (1990). Neurophysiological heterogeneity and the definition of dyslexia: preliminary evidence for plasticity. *Neuropsychologia,* **28**, 555–71.

Duncan, C.C., Rumsey, J.M., Denckla, M.B., Hmaburger, S.D. & Odoupotkin, M. (1994) Developmental dyslexia and attention dysfunction in adults – brain potential indices of information processing. *Psychophysiology,* **31**, 386–401.

DuPaul, G.J. & Barkley, R.A. (1992). Situational variability of attention problems: Psychometric properties of the revised home and school situations questionnaires. *Journal of Clinical Child Psychology,* **21**, 178–88.

DuPaul, G.J. (1991). Parent and teacher ratings of ADHD symptoms: psychometric properties in a community-based sample. *Journal of Clinical Child Psychology,* **20**, 245–53.

Dykman, R.A. & Ackerman, P.T. (1991). Attention deficit disorder and specific reading disability: separate but often overlapping disorders. *Journal of Learning Disabilities,* **24**, 96–103.

Estrada, P., Arsenio, W.F., Hess, R.D. & Holloway, S.D. (1987). Affective quality of the mother–child relationship: longitudinal consequences for children's school-relevant cognitive functioning. *Developmental Psychology,* **23**, 210–15.

Evans, S.W. & Short, E.J. (1991). A qualitative and serial analysis of social problem solving in aggressive boys. *Journal of Abnormal Child Psychology,* **19**, 331–40.

Evans, S.W. & Pelham, W.E. (1991). Psychostimulant effects on academic and behavioral measures for ADHD junior high school students in a lecture format classroom. *Journal Abnormal Child Psychology,* **19**, 537–52.

Faraone, S.V., Biederman, J, Keenan, K., Tsuang, M.T. + ??(1991). Separation of DSM-III attention deficit disorder and conduct disorder: evidence from a family-genetic study of American child psychiatric patients. *Psychological Medicine,* **21**, 109–21.

Felton, R.H., Wood, F.B., Brown, I.B., Campbell, S.K. & Harter, M.R. (1987). Separate verbal memory and naming deficits in attention deficit disorder and reading disability. *Brain and Language,* **31**, 171–84.

Felton, R.H. & Wood, F.B. (1989). Cognitive deficits in reading disability and attention deficit disorder. *Journal of Learning Disabilities,* **22**, 3–22.

Fergusson, D.M. & Horwood, L.J. (1992). Attention deficit and reading achievement. *Journal of Child Psychology and Psychiatry,* **33**, 375–85.

Fergusson, D.M. & Horwood, L.J. (1987). The trait and method components of ratings of conduct disorder-Part 1. Maternal and teacher evaluations of conduct disorder in young children. *Journal of Child Psychology and Psychiatry,* **28**, 249–60.

Fergusson, D.M., Fergusson, J.E., Horwood, C.J. & Kinzett, N.G. (1988*a*). A Longitudinal Study of dentine lead levels, intelligence, school performance and behaviour. Part I. Dentine lead levels and exposure to environmental risk factors. *Journal of Child Psychology and Psychiatry,* **29**, 781–92.

Fergusson, D.M., Fergusson, J.E., Horwood, L.J. & Kinzett, N.G. (1988*b*). A longitudinal study of dentine lead levels, intelligence, school performance and behaviour. Part III. dentine lead levels and attention/activity. *Journal of Child Psychology and Psychiatry,* **29**, 811–24.

Flicek, M. (1992). Social status of boys with both academic problems and attention-deficit hyperactivity disorder. *Journal of Abnormal Child Psychology,* **20**, 353–66.

Forness, S.R., Cantwell, D.P., Swanson, J.M., Hanna, G.L. & Youpa, D. (1991). Differential effects of stimulant medication on reading performance of boys with hyperactivity with and without conduct disorder. *Journal of Learning Disabilities,* **24**, 304–10.

Forness, S.R., Swanson, J.M., Cantwell, D.P., Youpa, D. & Hanna, G.L. (1992*a*). Stimulant medication and reading performance: follow-up on sustained dose in ADHD boys with and without conduct disorders. *Journal of Learning Disabilities,* **25**, 115–23.

Forness, S.R., Youpa, D., Hanna, G.L., Cantwell, D.P. *et al.* (1992*b*). Classroom instructional characteristics in attention deficit hyperactivity disorder: comparison of pure and mixed subgroups. *Behavioral Disorders,* **17**, 115–25.

Frick, P.J., Lahey,B.B., Christ, M.A., Loeber, R. & Green, S. (1991). History of childhood behavior problems in biological relatives of boys with attention-deficit hyperactivity disorder and conduct disorder. *Journal of Clinical Child Psychology,* **20**, 445–51.

Gadow, K.D., Nolan, E.E., Sverd, J., Sprafkin, J. & Paolicelli, L. (1990). Methylphenidate in aggressive-hyperactive boys: I. Effects on peer aggression in public school settings. *Journal of the American Academy of Child and Adolescent Psychiatry,* **29**, 710–18.

Gadow, K.D., Nolan, E.E. & Sverd, J. (1992). Methylphenidate in hyperactive boys with comorbid tic disorder: II.Short-term behavioral effects in school settings. *Journal of the American Academy of Child and Adolescent Psychiatry,* **31**, 462–71.

Gilger, J.W., Pennington, B.F. & DeFries, J.C. (1992). A twin study of the etiology of comorbidity: attention-deficit hyperactivity disorder and dyslexia. *Journal of the American Academy of Child and Adolescent Psychiatry,* **31**, 343–8.

Gillis, J.J., Gilger, J.W., Pennington, B.F. & DeFries, J.C. (1992). Attention deficit disorder in reading-disabled twins: evidence for a genetic etiology. *Journal of Abnormal Child Psychology,* **20**, 303–15.

Goodman, R. & Stevenson, J. (1989*a*). A twin study of hyperactivity-I. An examination of hyperactivity scores and categories derived from Rutter teacher and parent questionnaires. *Journal of Child Psychology and Psychiatry,* **30**, 671–89.

Goodman, R. & Stevenson, J. (1989*b*). A twin study of hyperactivity-II. The aetiological role of genes, family relationships and perinatal adversity. *Journal of Child Psychology and Psychiatry,* **30**, 691–709.

Haddad, P.M. & Garralda, M.E. (1992). Hyperkinetic syndrome and disruptive early experiences. *British Journal of Psychiatry,* **161**, 700–3.

Harter,M.R., Diering,S. & Wood,F.B. (1988) Separate brain potential characteristics in children with reading disability and attention deficit disorder: I. Relevance-independent effects. *Brain and Cognition,* **7**, 54–86.

Hinshaw, S.P. (1987). On the distinction between attention deficit/hyperactivity and conduct/aggression in child psychopathology. *Psychological Bulletin,* **101**, 443–63.

Hinshaw, S.P. (1992*a*). Academic underachievement, attention deficits and aggression: comorbidity and implications for treatment. *Journal of Consulting and Clinical Psychology,* **60**, 893–903.

Hinshaw, S.P. (1992*b*). Externalizing behaviour problems and academic underachievement in childhood and adolescence: causal relationships and underlying mechanisms. *Psychological Bulletin,* **111**, 127–55.

Hinshaw, S.P., Morrison, D.C., Carte, E.T. & Cornsweet, C. (1987). Factorial dimensions of the revised behavior problem checklist: replication and validation within a kindergarten sample. *Journal of Abnormal Child Psychology,* **15**, 309–27.

Hodges, J. & Tizard, B. (1989). IQ and behavioural adjustment of ex-institutional adolescents. *Journal of Child Psychology and Psychiatry,* **30**, 55–76.

Hogan, A.E. & Quay, H.C. (1984). Cognition in child and adolescent behaviour disorders. in *Advances in Clinical Child Psychology*, eds. B.B.Lahey & A.E.Kazdin, Vol.7, pp.1–34. New York: Plenum Press.

Huesmann, L.R., Eron, L.D. & Yarmel, P.W. (1987). Intellectual functioning and aggression. *Journal of Personality and Social Psychology,* **52**, 232–40.

Hynd, G.W., Lorys, A.R., Semrud-Clikeman, M., Nieves, N., Huettner, M.I. & Lahey, B.B. (1991). Attention deficit disorder without hyperactivity: a distinct behavioral and neurocognitive syndrome. *Journal of Child Neurology,* 6 Suppl, S37–43.

Isaac, G. (1992). Misdiagnosed bipolar disorder in adolescents in a special educational school and treatment program. *Journal of Clinical Psychiatry,* **53**, 133–6.

Jacobvitz, D., Sroufe, L.A., Stewart, M. & Leffert, N. (1990). Treatment of attentional and hyperactivity problems in children with sympathomimetic drugs: a comprehensive review. *Journal of the American Academy of Child and Adolescent Psychiatry,* **29**, 677–88.

James, A. & Taylor, E. (1990). Sex differences in the hyperkinetic syndrome of childhood. *Journal of Child Psychology and Psychiatry,* **31**, 437–46.

Jorm, A.F., Share, D.L., Matthews, R & MacLean, R. (1986). Behaviour problems in specific reading retardation and general reading backward children: a longitudinal study. *Journal of Child Psychology and Psychiatry,* **27**, 33–43.

Kasten, E.F., Coury, D.L. & Heron, T.E. (1992). Educators' knowledge and attitudes regarding stimulants in the treatment of attention deficit hyperactivity disorder. *Journal of Developmental Behavioral Pediatrics,* **13**, 215–19.

Keller, M.B., Lavori, P.W., Beardslee, W.R. & Wunder, J. (1992). The disruptive behavioral disorder in children and adolescents: Co-morbidity and clinical course. *Journal of the American Academy of Child and Adolescent Psychiatry,* **31**, 204–9.

Klein, R.G. & Mannuzza, S. (1991). Long-term outcome of hyperactive children: a review. *Journal of the American Academy of Child and Adolescent Psychiatry,* **30**, 383–7.

Korkman, M. & Peltomaa, K. (1991). A pattern of test findings predicting attention problems at school. *Journal of Abnormal Child Psychology,* **19**, 451–67.

Kupietz, S.S. (1990). Sustained attention in normal and in reading-disabled youngsters with and without ADDH. *Journal of Abnormal Child Psychology,* **18**, 357–72.

Lahey, B.B., Russo, M.F., Walker, J.L. & Piacentini, J.C. (1989). Personality characteristics of the mothers of children with disruptive behavior disorders. *Journal of Consulting and Clinical Psychology,* **57**, 512–15.

Lahey, B.B., Piacentini, J.C., McBurnett, K., Stone, P. *et al.* (1988). Psychopathology in the parents of children with conduct disorder and hyperactivity. *Journal of the American Academy of Child and Adolescent Psychiatry,* **27**, 163–70.

Levy, F. & Hobbes, G. (1989). Reading, spelling, and vigilance in attention deficit and conduct disorder. *Journal of Abnormal Child Psychology,* **17**, 291–8.

Levy, H.B., Harper, C.R. & Weinberg, W.A. (1992). A practical approach to children failing in school. *Pediatric Clinics of North America,* **39**, 895–928.

Lie, N. (1992). Follow-ups of children with attention deficit hyperactivity disorder (ADHD).Review of literature. *Acta Psychiatrica Scandinavica Supplement,* **368**, 1–40.

Liu, C., Robin, A.L., Brenner, S. & Eastman, J. (1991). Social acceptability of methylphenidate and behaviour modification for treating attention deficit hyperactivity disorder. *Pediatrics,* **88**, 560–5.

Livingston, R.L., Dykman, R.A. & Ackerman, P.T. (1991). The frequency and significance of additional self-reported psychiatric diagnoses in children with attention deficit disorder. *Journal of Abnormal Child Psychology,* **18**, 465–78.

Loehlin, J. (1987). *Latent Variable Analysis: An Introduction to Factor, Path and Structural Analysis.* Hillsdale, NJ: Lawrence Erlbaum Associates.

Luk, S.L., Leung, P.W., Bacon-Shone, J. & Lieh-Mak, F. (1991). The structure and prevalence of behavioral problems in Hong Kong preschool children. *Journal of Abnormal Child Psychology,* **19**, 219–32.

McBurnett, K. & Pfiffner, L.J. (1991). 'Attention deficit-hyperactivity disorder: is it a learning disability or a related disorder?': Comment. *Journal of Learning Disabilities,* **24**, 258–9.

McGee, R. & Share, D.L. (1988). Attention deficit disorder-hyperactivity and academic failure: which comes first and what should be treated? *Journal of the American Academy of Child and Adolescent Psychiatry,* **27**, 318–25.

McGee, R., Williams, S., Share, D.I., Anderson, J. & Silva, P. (1986). The relationship between specific reading retardation, general reading backwardness and behaviour problems in a large sample of Dunedin boys: a longitudinal study from five to eleven years. *Journal of Child Psychology and Psychiatry*, **27**, 597–610.

McGee, R., Williams, S & Silva, P.A. (1987). A Comparison of girls and boys with teacher-identified problems of attention. *Journal of the American Academy of Child and Adolescent Psychiatry,* **26**, 711–17.

McGee, R., Williams, S., Moffitt, T. & Anderson, J. (1989). A comparison of 13-year old boys with attention deficit and/or reading disorder on neuropsychological measures. *Journal of Abnormal Child Psychology,* **17**, 37–53.

McGee, R., Partridge, F., Williams, S. & Silva, P.A. (1991). A twelve-year follow-up of preschool hyperactive children. *Journal of the American Academy of Child and Adolescent Psychiatry,* **30**, 224–32.

McGee, R., Williams,S. & Feehan, M. (1992). Attention deficit disorder and age of onset of problem behaviors. *Journal of Abnormal Psychology,* **20**, 487–502.

McGuire, J. & Richman, N. (1986). Screening for behavior problems in nurseries: the reliability and validity of the Preschool Behavior Checklist. *Journal of Child Psychology and Psychiatry*, **27**, 7–32.

Madan-Swain, A. & Zentall, S.S. (1990). Behavioural comparisons of liked and disliked hyperactive children in play contexts and the behavioural accommodations by their classmates. *Journal of Consulting and Clinical Psychology,* **58**, 197–209.

Maughan, B., Gray, G. & Rutter, M. (1985). Reading retardation and antisocial behviour: a follow up into employment. *Journal of Child Psychology and Psychiatry*, **26**, 741–59.

Miller, N.B., Cowan, P.A., Cowan, C.P., Hetherington, E.M. & Clingempeel, W.G. (1993). Externalising in preschoolers and early adolescents: a cross-study replication of a family model. *Developmental Psychology,* **29**, 3–18.

Moffitt, T.E. (1990). Juvenile delinquency and attention deficit disorder: boys' developmental trajectories from age 3 to age 15. *Child Development,* **61**, 893–910.

Murphy, V. & Hicks-Stewart, K. (1991). Learning disabilities and attention deficit–hyperactivity disorder: an interactional perspective. *Journal of Learning Disabilities,* **24**, 386–88.

Olson, R., Wise, B., Conners, F., Rack, J. & Fulker, D. (1989). Specific deficits in component reading and writing skills: genetic and environmental differences. *Reading and Writing,* **22**, 339–48.

Olweus, D. (1983). Low school achievement and aggressive behavior in adolescent boys. In *Human Development: An Interactionist Perspective*, ed. D.Magnusson, pp. 353–365. San Diego, CA: Academic Press.

O'Neill, M.E. & Douglas, V.I. (1991). Study strategies and story recall in attention deficit disorder and reading disability. *Journal of Abnormal Child Psychology,* **19**, 671–92.

Patterson, G.R., DeBaryshe, B.D. & Ramsey, E. (1989). A developmental perspective on antisocial behaviour. *American Psychologist,* **44**, 329–35.

Pelham, W.E. & Bender, M.E. (1982). Peer relationships in hyperactive children. In

Advances in Learning and Behavioral Disabilities, eds. K. Gadow & I. Bialer, pp. 365–436, Greenwich, CT: JAI Press.

Pennington, B.F. & Smith, S.D. (1988). Genetic influences on learning disabilities: an update. *Journal of Consulting and Clinical Psychology,* **56**, 817–23.

Pennington, B.F., Grossier, D. & Welsh, M.C. (1993). Contrasting neuropsychological deficits in attention deficit hyperactivity disorder versus reading disability. *Developmental Psychology*, **29**, 511–23.

Pisterman, S., McGrath, P., Firestone, P., Goodman, J.T., Webster, I. & Mallory, R. (1989). Outcome of parent-mediated treatment of preschoolers with attention deficit disorder with hyperactivity. *Journal of Consulting and Clinical Psychology*, **57**, 628–35.

Quay, H.C., Routh, D.K. & Shapiro, S.K. (1987). Psychopathology of childhood: from description to validation. *Annual Review of Psychology,* **38**, 491–532.

Reich, W., Weiner, Z., Taibelson, C & Kram, L. (1987). *The Diagnostic Interview for Children and Adolescents* – Revised – Parent. St Louis. Washington University.

Richman, N., Stevenson, J. & Graham, P. (1982). *Preschool to School:A Behavioural Study*. London: Academic Press.

Robins, P.M. (1992). A comparison of behavioural and attentional functioning in children diagnosed as hyperactive or learning-disabled. *Journal of Abnormal Child Psychology,* **20**, 65–82.

Rowe, K.J, & Rowe, K.S. (1992*a*). The relationship between inattentiveness in the classroom and reading achievement (Part A): methodological issues. *Journal of the American Academy of Child Adolescent Psychiatry,* **31**, 349–56.

Rowe, K.J. & Rowe, K.S. (1992*b*). The relationship between inattentiveness in the classroom and reading achievement (Part B): an explanatory study. *Journal of the American Academy of Child and Adolescent Psychiatry,* **31**, 357–68.

Rutter, M. (1984). Behavioural Studies: Questions and findings on the concept of a distinctive syndrome. In *Developmental Neuropsychiatry*, ed. M. Rutter, pp. 259–79. Edinburgh: Churchill Livingstone.

Rutter, M. (1987). The role of cognition in child development and disorder. *British Journal of Medical Psychology,* **60**, 1–16.

Rutter, M. & Yule, W. (1975). The concept of specific reading retardation. *Journal of Child Psychology and Psychiatry*, **16**, 181–97.

Rutter, M., Tizard, J. & Whitmore, K. (1970). *Education, Health and Behaviour*. London: Longmans.

Rutter, M., Bolton, P., Harrington, R., Le Couteur, A., Macdonald, H. & Simonoff, E. (1990). Genetic factors in child psychiatric disorder. II. Empirical findings. *Journal of Child Psychology and Psychiatry,* **31**, 39–84.

Sandberg, S.T., Wieselberg, M. & Shaffer, D. (1980). Hyperkinetic and conduct problem children in a primary school population: some epidemiological considerations. *Journal of Child Psychology and Psychiatry,* **21**, 293–311.

Scarborough, H.S. (1991). Antecedents to reading disability: preschool language development and literacy experiences of children from dyslexic families. *Reading and Writing,* **3**, 219–33.

Schachar, R. (1991). Childhood hyperactivity. *Journal of Child Psychology and Psychiatry,* **32**, 155–91.

Schachar, R. & Logan, G. (1990*a*). Are hyperactive children deficient in attentional capacity? *Journal of Abnormal Child Psychology,* **18**, 493–513.

Schachar, R. & Logan, G.D. (1990*b*). Impulsivity and inhibitory control in normal development and childhood psychopathology. *Developmental Psychology,* **26**, 710–20.

Schachar, R.J. & Wachsmuth,R. (1991). Family dysfunction and psychosocial adversity: Comparison of attention deficit disorder, conduct disorder, normal and clinical controls. *Canadian Journal of Behavioral Science,* **23**, 332–48.

Schaughency, E.A., Vannatta, K., Langhinrichsen, J., Lally, C. & Seeley, J. (1992). Correlates of sociometric status in school children in Buenos Aires. *Journal of Abnormal Child Psychology,* **20**, 317–26.

Semrud-Clikeman, M., Biederman, J., Sprich-Buckminster, S., Krifcher Lehan, B., Faraone, S.V. & Norman, D. (1992). Co-morbidity between ADDH and learning disability: A review and report in a clinically referred sample. *Journal of the American Academy of Child and Adolescent Psychiatry,* **31**, 439–48.

Sergeant, J.A. & Scholten, C.A. (1985). On resource strategy limitations in hyperactivity: cognitive impulsivity reconsidered. *Journal of Child Psychology and Psychiatry,* **26**, 97–109.

Share, D.L. (1988). Comment on Tarnowski, Prinz and Nay (1986) No evidence for differential diagnostic validity of attention deficit disorder with hyperactivity. *Journal of Abnormal Psychology*, **97**, 374–5.

Shaywitz, B,A. & Shaywitz, S.E. (1991). Co-morbidity: a critical issue in attention deficit disorder. *Journal of Child Neurology,* **6** (Suppl), S13–22.

Shonfeld, I.S., Shaffer, D., O'Connor, P. & Portnoy, S. (1988). Conduct disorder and cognitive functioning: testing three causal hypotheses. *Child Development,* **59**, 993–1007.

Silver, L.B. (1990). Attention deficit-hyperactivity disorder: is it a learning disability or a related disorder? *Journal of Learning Disabilities,* **23**, 394–7.

Silver, L.B. (1992). *Attention-Deficit Hyperactivity Disorder*. Washington, DC: American Psychiatric Press.

Sonuga-Barke, E.J., Taylor, E. & Heptinstall, E. (1992). Hyperactivity and delay aversion: II. The effect of self versus externally imposed stimulus presentation periods on memory. *Journal of Child Psychology and Psychiatry,* 33, 399–409.

Stevenson, J. (1991). Which aspects of processing text mediate genetic effects? *Reading and Writing,* **3**, 249–69.

Stevenson, J. (1992). Evidence for a genetic etiology in hyperactivity in children. *Behavior Genetics,* **22**, 337–44.

Stevenson, J. & Fredman, G. (1990). The social environmental correlates of reading ability. *Journal of Child Psychology and Psychiatry,* **31**, 681–98.

Stevenson, J. & Graham, P. (1993). Antisocial behaviour and spelling disability in a population sample of 13 year old twins. *European Journal of Child and Adolescent Psychiatry* , **2**, 179–91.

Stevenson, J., Richman, N & Graham, P. (1985). Behaviour problems and language abilities at three years and behavioural deviance at eight years. *Journal of Child Psychology and Psychiatry,* **26**, 215–30.

Stevenson, J., Pennington, B., Gilger, J.W., DeFries, J.C. & Gillis, J.J. (1993). Hyperactivity and spelling disability: testing for shared genetic aetiology. *Journal of Child Psychology and Psychiatry* , **34**, 1137–52.

Stolzenberg, J. & Cherkes-Julkowski, M. (1991). 'Attention deficit–hyperactivity disorder: is it a learning disability or a related disorder?': Comment. *Journal of Learning Disabilities,* **24**, 194–5.

Sturge, C. (1982). Reading Retardation and Antisocial Behaviour. *Journal of Child Psychology and Psychiatry,* **23**, 21–31.

Szatmari, P., Reitsma-Street, M. & Offord, D.R. (1986). Pregnancy and birth complications in antisocial adolescents and their siblings. Special Issue: Canadian Academy of Child Psychiatry: A Canadian perspective. *Canadian Journal of Psychiatry,* **31**, 513–16.

Szatmari, P., Offord, D.R. & Boyle , M.H. (1989a). Ontario child health study: prevalence of attention deficit disorder with hyperactivity. *Journal of Child Psychology and Psychiatry,* **30**, 219–30.

Szatmari, P., Offord, D.R. & Boyle, M.H. (1989b). Correlates, associated impairments & patterns of service utilization of children with attention deficit disorder: findings from the Ontario child health study. *Journal of Child Psychology and Psychiatry,* **30**, 205–17.

Szatmari, P., Offord, D.R., Siegel, L.S., Finlayson, M.A. & Tuff, L. (1990). The clinical significance of neurocognitive impairments among children with psychiatric disorders: diagnosis and situational specificity. *Journal of Child Psychology and Psychiatry,* **31**, 287–99.

Tarnowski, K.J., Prinz, R.J. & Nay, S.M. (1988). Additional considerations for children's attentional performance: reply to share. *Journal of Abnormal Psychology,* **97**, 376–77.

Tarnowski, K.J., Prinz, R.J. & Nay, S.M. (1986). Comparative analysis of attentional deficits in hyperactive and learning-disabled children. *Journal of Abnormal Psychology,* **95**, 341–5.

Taylor, E.A. (1986*a*). The causes and development of hyperactive behaviour. In *The Overactive Child*, ed. E.A. Taylor, pp. 118–60. Oxford: Blackwells.

Taylor, E.A. (1986*b*). Childhood hyperactivity. *British Journal Psychiatry,* **149**, 562–73.

Taylor, E., Sandberg, S., Thorley, G. & Giles, S. (1991). *The Epidemiology of Childhood Hyperactivity. Maudsley Monographs No. 33*. Oxford: Oxford University Press.

Taylor, E. (1987). Cultural differences in hyperactivity. *Advances in Developmental and Behavioral Pediatrics,* **8**, 125–50.

Taylor, E. & Sandberg, S. (1984). Hyperactive behaviour in English schoolchildren: a questionnaire survey. *Journal of Abnormal Child Psychology,* **12**, 143–56.

Taylor, E., Schachar, R., Thorley, G. & Wieselberg, M. (1986). Conduct disorder & hyperactivity: I. Separation of hyperactivity and antisocial conduct in British child Psychiatric patients. *British Journal of Psychiatry,* **149**, 760–7.

Thorley, G. (1984). Review of follow-up and follow-back studies of childhood hyperactivity. *Psychological Bulletin,* **96**, 116–32.

Tizard, B. & Hodges, J. (1978). The effects of early institutional rearing on the development of eight year old children. *Journal of Child Psychology and Psychiatry,* **19**, 99–118.

van der Meere, J. & Sergeant, J.A. (1988). Acquisition of attention skill in pervasively hyperactive children. *Journal of Child Psychology and Psychiatry,* **29**, 301–10.

van der Meere, J., Van Baal, M. & Sergeant, J. (1989). The additive factor method: a differential diagnostic tool in hyperactivity and learning disability. *Journal of Abnormal Child Psychology,* **17**, 409–22.

van der Meere, J., Wekking, E. & Sergeant, J. (1991). Sustained attention and pervasive hyperactivity. *Journal of Child Psychology and Psychiatry,* **32**, 275–84.

Verhulst, F.C., Althaus, M. & Versluis-den Bieman, H.J. (1990). Problem behaviour in international adoptees: I. An epidemiological study. *Journal of the American Academy of Child and Adolescent Psychiatry,* **29**, 94–103.

Victor, J., Halverson, C. & Montague, R. (1985). The relationship between reflection-impulsivity and behavioural impulsivity in preschool children. *Developmental Psychology*, **21**, 141–8.

Wagner, R.K. & Torgesen, J.K. (1987). The nature of phonological processing and its casual role in the acquisition of reading skills. *Psychological Bulletin,* **101**, 192–212.

Walker, J.L., Lahey, B.B., Hynd, G.W., Frame, C.L. (1987). Comparison of specific patterns of antisocial behavior in children with conduct disorder with or without coexisting hyperactivity. *Journal of Consulting and Clinical Psychology,* **55**, 910–13.

Werry, J.S., Elkind, G.S. & Reeves, J.C. (1987). Attention deficit, conduct, oppositional, and anxiety disorders in children: III. Laboratory differences. *Journal of Abnormal Child Psychology,* **15**, 409–28.

Willerman, L. (1973). Activity level and hyperactivity in twins. *Child Development,* **44**, 288–93.

World Health Organisation (1988). International Classification of Diseases (10th Edition). 1988 Draft Chapter V. Categories F00–F99. Mental, behavioural and developmental disorders. Geneva: World Health Organisation Division of Mental Health.

Yule, W. (1986). Behavioural methods. In *The Overactive Child*, ed. E. Taylor. Oxford: Blackwell/ MacKeith Press.

Ziegler,R. & Holden, L. (1988). Family therapy for learning disabled and attention-deficit disordered children. *American Journal of Orthopsychiatry,* **58**, 196–210.

Zoccolillo, M., Pickles, A., Quinton, D. & Rutter, M. (1992). The outcome of childhood conduct disorder: implications for defining adult personality disorder and conduct disorder. *Psychological Medicine,* **22**, 971–86.

12

Treatment

Russell Schachar, Rosemary Tannock and Charles Cunningham

INTRODUCTION

Childhood hyperactivity, currently known as attention deficit hyperactivity disorder in North America (ADHD, American Psychiatric Association, 1994) and hyperkinetic disorder internationally (HD; World Health Organisation, 1994), results in considerable impairment and suffering for affected children, their families, schools, and communities and places substantial burden on health care systems (Szatmari, Offord & Boyle, 1989*b*).

In this chapter we present a review of existing evidence for the efficacy of psychopharmacological and behavioural treatments for hyperactivity and emphasise the recent advances in the field. Since stimulants, in particular methylphenidate, are the most extensively investigated and widely prescribed treatment for childhood hyperactivity, we place greatest emphasis on the range of clinical benefits and limitations of this treatment. Behavioural interventions, on the other hand, have focused on a wider range of specific modalities for both hyperactive children and their families, in a variety of treatment settings. But fewer methodologically sound studies of behavioural interventions are available for evaluation. We also describe the limitations of pharmacological and behavioural treatments, in particular, the absence of clear evidence for the generalisation of treatment effects across settings and over time. Although the research covered is relevant to clinical practice, this chapter is not intended as a practitioner's guide to clinical management.

OVERVIEW OF DIFFICULTIES

Childhood hyperactivity has diverse clinical manifestations involving *core symptoms* such as overactivity, inattention, impulsiveness, and *associated symptoms* such as aggressiveness, defiance and academic underachievement. To facilitate discussion of treatment effects, we describe each manifestation of childhood hyperactivity briefly before discussing the effects of various treatments on these symptoms. The behavioural manifestations of childhood hyperactivity receive greater attention in Chapter 3: Chemical aspects.

Hyperactive children are more active, inattentive and impulsive than their non-hyperactive peers (for review see Campbell & Werry, 1986). In particular, these symptoms are evident in structured situations that demand social interaction with peers or adults, sustained attention to tasks or academic effort (e.g. Cunningham & Siegel, 1987). The core behavioural manifestations of hyperactive children are believed to reflect a fundamental and multifaceted cognitive deficit (for review see Douglas, 1988; Chapter 4: The role of attention). Consistent with this hypothesis, hyperactive children in comparison with non-hyperactive children, perform poorly on a range of cognitive tasks that measure inhibitory control, sustained attention and selective attention.

Academic underachievement and learning disabilities commonly complicate childhood hyperactivity. Hyperactive children tend to leave school sooner and with a poorer scholastic record than their non-hyperactive peers (Campbell & Werry, 1986); approximately 20 % of hyperactive children meet criteria for learning disability (e.g. Hinshaw, 1992; Lambert & Sandoval, 1980; McGee & Share, 1988).

Disruptive and aggressive behaviour in social situations is a frequent and problematic associated feature of childhood hyperactivity (Campbell & Werry, 1986). Hyperactive children interrupt others, act inappropriately and abruptly, tease, criticise and annoy other children, and are less attentive to their peers and to the social activities in which they are participating. They communicate less efficiently with their peers, request less feedback, disagree more often, and learn less from social experience (Whalen et al., 1979; Cunningham & Siegel, 1987). They appear to have a deficit in social cognition and lack control over anger and aggressive impulses (Pelham & Bender, 1982). The hyperactive child has an immediate and negative impact on the behaviour and achievement of normal peers with whom they come in contact (Cunningham & Siegel, 1987; Whalen, Henker & Dotemoto, 1981). Not surprisingly, they are less liked by their peers and by their teachers (Milich & Landau, 1982; Johnston, Pelham & Murphy, 1985).

The hyperactive child's difficulties with activity level, sustained attention, impulse control and self-regulation adversely affect social relationships with family members (Cunningham & Barkley, 1979; Mash & Johnston, 1982). With parents, for example, hyperactive children are less compliant and less likely to sustain attention to tasks. Parents report that their hyperactive children have difficulties in a wide variety of tasks, routines and social activities (Cunningham & Barkley, 1979; Mash & Johnston, 1982).

All core and associated manifestations of the disorder may be evident in a particular child. More typically, the hyperactive child has a subset of these difficulties. For example, a pattern of inattentiveness and impulsiveness without gross motor overactivity is common (Lahey & Carlson, 1991; Barkley, DuPaul & McMurray, 1990a). DSM-IV distinguishes three ADHD subtypes; primarily inattentiveness, primarily hyperactivity and impulsiveness and a pattern of all three symptom clusters (APA, 1994). In other children, the pattern of associated symptoms is so pronounced that the children are diagnosed as having an additional or co-morbid disorder. Co-morbid conduct disorder is evident in approximately 50% of hyperactive children and co-morbid emotional disorder in 25% of children (Szatmari *et al.*, 1989*b*).

The prognosis of childhood hyperactivity is more serious than previously believed (Gittelman *et al.*, 1985; Klein & Mannuzza, 1991; Chapter 13). Although activity level tends to diminish, social, interpersonal and academic problems either persist or develop with the passage of time (Klein & Mannuzza, 1991; Fisher *et al.*, 1989).

PREVALENCE OF VARIOUS TREATMENTS

In the United States, medication, particularly methylphenidate, is the most common treatment for childhood hyperactivity. Recent estimates indicate that as many as 5% of all children (Safer & Krager, 1988) and 75% of children with a clinical diagnosis of hyperactivity are treated with stimulants (Barkley *et al.*, 1990*b*; Copeland *et al.*, 1987; Wolraich *et al.*, 1990). Safer & Krager (1988) reported higher rates among children enrolled in special education classes (20%), among those living in low-income areas and in males. They found that rates of stimulant medication use in the United States have been increasing over the last decade, especially among females and adolescents. The vast majority of children are prescribed medication by paediatricians or by family practitioners (Safer & Krager, 1988); in most cases, medication is the sole treatment received (Sandoval, Lambert & Yandell, 1979; Copeland *et al.*, 1987; Wolraich *et al.*, 1990). Once instituted, pharmacological treatment tends to continue for three or more years (Safer & Krager, 1984; Barkley et al., 1990*b*). Only 5% of children receiving stimulants are treated with dextroamphetamine and only 2% receive pemoline (Safer & Krager, 1984). Tricyclic antidepressants are the most common alternative to the stimulants, but they have been prescribed and investigated less frequently.

Behavioural treatments are recommended and applied less often than medication in the United States (Copeland *et al.*, 1987: Wolraich *et al.*, 1990; Barkley *et al.*, 1990*b*). The typical psychosocial treatment is a combination of physician's advice about the child's management, diet and school placement. As well, special education may be provided through the child's school. Systematic programmes of behavioural therapy such as training in child management skills for parents or self–control training for the child are not commonly part of the treatment (Copeland *et al.*, 1987; Wolraich *et al.*, 1990; Barkley *et al.*, 1990*b*). Hyperactive children are not considered good candidates for psychotherapy (O'Malley & Eisenberg, 1973).

Medication is prescribed less frequently in Canada (0.3%, Szatmari, Offord & Boyle *et al.*, 1989*c*) and is rarely used in Britain and Europe. In these countries psychological interventions, particularly therapy aimed at altering parenting strategies, are the preferred therapy for hyperactive children. European clinicians seem to focus on the conduct disturbance and the educational problems of hyperactive children (Prendergast *et al.*, 1988) and direct therapy toward mitigating deficient parenting practices, disturbance in family functioning and the psycho-educational deficits of the children (Taylor *et al.*, 1991).

PHARMACOLOGICAL TREATMENTS

Methylphenidate: short-term effects

Core symptoms

Overt behaviour Treatment with methylphenidate consistently results in an improvement in the core behavioural symptoms of childhood hyperactivity. Activity level decreases, overt attention to tasks and activities increases and behavioural impulsiveness diminishes with treatment in most studies and in most subjects (e.g. Porrino *et al.*, 1983*a*). With medication, children are more consistent in their behaviour and are judged to be putting forth greater effort (Douglas *et al.*, 1989; Pelham *et al.*, 1990*b*). These effects are more obvious in structured settings such as in the classroom, but they are also evident in less structured situations (Whalen *et al.*, 1978; 1987). The major limitations of the effect of methylphenidate on core behavioural manifestations are the rapid reoccurrence of symptoms upon discontinuation of treatment (e.g. Brown et al., 1986) and a rebound increase in symptoms in some children as the medication wears off towards the end of the day (Porrino *et al.*, 1983*b*; Johnston *et al.*, 1988).

Cognition Methylphenidate improves a hyperactive child's performance on a variety of tasks believed to measure specific cognitive processes such as inhibitory control in addition to non-specific effects such as speed of information processing. For example, methylphenidate facilitates inhibition of discrete motor responses (Tannock *et al.*, 1989*a*; Trommer, Hoeppner & Zecker; 1991, Klorman *et al.*, 1991; Douglas *et al.*, 1986). In contrast, the drug's effect on the processes affecting correct choice in certain situations such as measured with the Matching Familiar Figures Task, has been inconsistent (e.g. Rapport *et al.*, 1985; Sebrechts *et al.*, 1986; Douglas *et al.*, 1986).

There is clear evidence that stimulants improve sustained attention; for example, hyperactive children taking stimulants make fewer errors of omission (Rapport *et al.*, 1987; Klorman *et al.*, 1991; de Sonneville, Njiokiktjien & Hilhorst, 1991), and their performance on the Continuous Performance Task deteriorates less over time (e.g. Peloquin & Klorman, 1986; Klorman *et al.*, 1991). However, only limited data about the effects of stimulants on selective attention are available. Earlier studies (Sebrechts *et al.*, 1986; Campbell *et al.*, 1971; Taylor *et al.*, 1987) that involved tasks such as the Embedded Figures Task, Colour Distraction Task and the selective listening task found no evidence of beneficial effects. Recent studies (de Sonneville *et al.*, 1991; Klorman *et al.*, 1991; Tannock, Schachar & Logan, 1993) involving reaction-time paradigms derived from information-processing theory report preliminary evidence of specific effects on processes involved in selective aspects of attention such as target search, stimulus evaluation and focused attention. None the less, these effects are often subtle compared to the more salient non-specific effects of generalized improvement in speed and accuracy of performance. In summary, methylphenidate facilitates a range of specific cognitive functions although some effects are not as robust as others.

Associated symptoms

Academic achievement The beneficial effects of methylphenidate on the classroom behaviour of hyperactive children are well established. Treatment results in decreased restlessness and increased attentiveness to schoolwork

(Abikoff & Gittelman, 1985). By comparison, methylphenidate's effect on academic achievement is equivocal. Earlier influential reviews of the literature (Barkley & Cunningham, 1978) concluded that there was little beneficial effect of stimulants on academic performance. These reviews recommended that stimulants be used only when the goal of treatment was improved manageability in the classroom. However, methodological limitations of earlier studies may account for some negative findings (Pelham, 1983). For example, the standardised achievement tests that were used in these investigations were relatively insensitive to change over short periods of time, dose of medication and compliance had been uncontrolled, medication was not combined with non–pharmacological interventions in a systematic fashion, and subjects were not assigned randomly to treatment conditions.

More recent research has incorporated improved methods. These studies indicate that methylphenidate results in substantial improvement in the performance of hyperactive children on tasks designed to resemble classroom assignments such as timed arithmetic problems, speed of reading short passages and reading comprehension (Pelham *et al.*, 1985; Douglas *et al.*, 1986; Douglas, 1988; Rapport *et al.*, 1985, 1986; Tannock *et al.*, 1989b), on experimental academic tasks (Douglas *et al.*, 1986; 1989), and on regular classroom work (Rapport *et al.*, 1986; Vyse & Rapport, 1989; Gadow *et al.*, 1990). The effect is comparable across setting (laboratory versus classroom; Douglas *et al.*, 1989) and across type of measure (experimental versus regular classroom work). The magnitude of improvement is variable but is apparently greater and more consistent for reading than for mathematics or spelling (Pelham *et al.*, 1989). These short-term studies provide strong evidence that stimulant treatment enhances academic productivity (i.e. children complete more of their assigned work); it remains to be determined whether these immediate improvements in productivity can be translated into gains in academic achievement with prolonged treatment.

Social interaction The effects of methylphenidate on the social behaviour of hyperactive children are immediate, often dramatic and quite consistent across numerous studies. The quality of social interaction with parents, teachers and peers improves; disruptive, non-compliant and aggressive social interactions decrease in frequency and in intensity; and fewer negative verbalisations occur (Gadow *et al.*, 1990; Pelham *et al.*, 1987; Barkley *et al.*, 1985; Hinshaw, Buhrmester & Heller, 1989*a*; Schachar *et al.*, 1987; Whalen & Henker, 1991*a*). When taking medication, the hyperactive child is rated by peers as more co–operative, greater fun to be with, and more often a best friend (Pelham & Bender, 1982; Whalen *et al.*, 1989*a*).

Despite these salutary effects, medication is far from a cure for the interpersonal ills of these children. Medication may not enhance the hyperactive child's social judgement, eliminate their negative perceptions of their peers (Whalen, Henker & Granger, 1989*b*, 1990), or normalize social behaviour of most of these children (Abikoff & Gittelman, 1985; Hinshaw *et al.*, 1989*a, b*; Whalen *et al.*, 1989*a*). A longer period of treatment may be required to counteract the negative reputation of a hyperactive child or to eliminate social deficits. Moreover, methylphenidate has been noted to decrease the frequency of aggressive social interaction without increasing the rate of pro–social behaviour (cf Pelham *et al.*, 1987; Hinshaw *et al.*, 1989*b*). Finally, although parents behave in a less intrusive, less controlling and more positive way with their medicated hyperactive children (e.g. Barkley *et al.*, 1984), they do not automatically adopt more effective parenting practices in response to drug-induced improvement in child behaviour (Schachar *et al.*, 1987).

Age, dose and subtype effects

Age and response Little is known about the relationship among age, dose, diagnostic subtype and response to methylphenidate. We know least about the effect of methylphenidate on preschoolers. Available studies (Schleifer *et al.*, 1975; Barkley, 1988; Conners, 1975; Cunningham, Siegel & Offord, 1985) point to its considerable beneficial effect on core behavioural symptoms and social interaction but also to the greater frequency of adverse effects in this age group (Schleifer *et al.*, 1975; Barkley, 1988; Cunningham *et al.*, 1985).

Primary school-aged children and adolescents consistently show reduction in core behavioural symptoms (e.g. Barkley *et al.*, 1985; Evans & Pelham, 1991) impulsiveness, and improved sustained attention (Tannock et al., 1989a; Peloquin & Klorman, 1986), academic performance (Douglas *et al.*, 1986, 1988) and social interaction (e.g. Cunningham, et al., 1985; Taylor *et al.*, 1987; cf Hinshaw *et al.*, 1989*a, b*; Klorman *et al.*, 1990). Behavioural (Klorman *et al.*, 1990) and cognitive (Klorman *et al.*, 1991) improvement, however, may be less consistent and extensive among adolescents than among primary school-aged children. For example, 40% of adolescents describe the effect of methylphenidate as unimpressive (Klorman *et al.*, 1991). In summary, methylphenidate is effective across a wide range of ages, although, in preschoolers, the benefit may not be as great and adverse effects may be more frequent.

Dose and response The series of reports from the laboratory of Sprague and colleagues (Sprague & Sleator, 1977; Brown & Sleator, 1979; Brown, Slimmer & Wynne, 1984) that examine the relationship between dose of and response to methylphenidate have been important and provocative. These reports demonstrate a decrease in performance on cognitive tasks with high dose (1 mg/kg) of methylphenidate. Sprague & Sleator (1977) concluded that behavioural and cognitive changes have different dose–response relationships and postulated that high doses of stimulant medication may impair learning and academic achievement. If substantiated, this hypothesis could have major implications for clinical practice: typically dose is increased according to parent or teacher report of child behaviour. Because the emphasis when dose level is determined is on reduction of overt activity and other disruptive behaviours, many children could receive doses that are detrimental to cognitive function and academic achievement.

The monotonic relationship between dose and core behavioural symptoms has been convincingly demonstrated in a large number of well–controlled studies (e.g. Pelham *et al.*, 1985; Rapport *et al.*, 1988; Douglas *et al.*, 1989). The relationship between dose and cognitive function, however, is unclear. The majority of studies of stimulant effects on cognition have examined effects using a single dose only. Consequently, they do not clarify the nature of the dose–response relationship for cognition. Most of the studies that have examined the effects at several levels of methylphenidate have described linear dose–response functions for a range of academic and cognitive tasks such that higher doses result in greater improvement (Douglas, 1988; Pelham *et al.*, 1985; Rapport *et al.*, 1985). However, the range of doses in these studies did not cover the range of doses used in typical clinical practice (e.g. up to 1.0 mg/kg in a single dose).

None the less, a few investigators (Peeke *et al.*, 1984; Rapport *et al.*, 1986; Douglas *et al.*, 1989; Elia *et al.*, 1991) have reported a pattern of results that is consistent with the hypothesis that cognitive performance is improved by low doses but not by moderate or high doses of methylphenidate. There also have been two reports of stimulant-induced cognitive perseveration and behavioural stereotypy in children, suggesting that high doses may result in rigidity of thought and action (Dyme *et al.*, 1982; Tannock & Schachar, 1992). However, in most of the studies reporting decrement at high doses, the changes have been subtle (Douglas, 1988), transient (Tannock & Schachar, 1992), based on a very small sample (Dyme *et al.*, 1982; Peeke *et al.*, 1984), and unconfirmed by statistical analysis (Dyme *et al.*, 1982). Adverse effects of psychostimulants on cognition are only suggested but not proven in these studies.

Diagnostic subtype and drug response Although the data are preliminary, several interesting relationships have emerged between clinical characteristics and response to methylphenidate. The response of hyperactive children with and without co-morbid conduct disorder has been researched most often. To date, the evidence points to a similar pattern of behavioural (Taylor *et al.*, 1987; Whalen *et al.*, 1987; Klorman *et al.*, 1988; Hinshaw *et al.*, 1989*b*; Barkley *et al.*, 1989; Cunningham, Siegal & Offord, 1991; cf Pelham & Bender, 1982) and cognitive response in the two subgroups (e.g. Klorman *et al.*, 1988; Barkley *et al.*, 1989; Matier *et al.*, 1992).

Nevertheless, the presence and severity of co-morbid hyperactivity and the presence of co-morbid emotional disturbance do predict response to methylphenidate. Barkley, DuPaul & McMurray (1991) reported that children with attention deficit disorder associated with hyperactivity were more likely than those without associated hyperactivity to be recommended for treatment with methylphenidate, despite equivalent clinical response during a systematic trial. Similarly, Taylor *et al.* (1987) reported that a more favourable clinical response was predicted when subjects had high pretreatment levels of hyperactivity. Both Taylor *et al.* (1987) and Pliszka (1989) reported less favourable clinical response in children with co-morbid emotional disturbance (i.e. anxiety, fearfulness).

Methylphenidate: longer-term effects In clinical practice, treatment typically continues for several years (Barkley *et al.*, 1990*b*). Yet, there have been few methodologically sound studies of methylphenidate administered for more than 3 months that permit judgement of the efficacy of the medication. Eighteen studies of methylphenidate with active treatment longer than 3 months have been conducted (for review see Schachar & Tannock, 1993). Seven of these studies (Weiss *et al.*, 1975; Hechtman, Weiss & Perlman, 1984; Blouin, Bornstein & Trites, 1978; Charles & Schain, 1981; Riddle & Rapoport, 1976; Satterfield, Satterfield & Cantwell, 1981; Sleator, von Neumann & Sprague,1974) employed a variety of quasi-experimental designs whose major flaw was their inability to ensure the pre-treatment equivalence of comparison groups. They did not preclude initial differences in factors that can bias outcome such as severity of hyperactivity (Blouin *et al.*, 1978; Weiss *et al.*, 1975) or family dysfunction (Weiss *et al.*, 1975). Comparisons based on the duration of treatment (Riddle & Rapoport, 1976; Charles & Schain, 1981; Satterfield *et al.*, 1981; Firestone *et al.*, 1986) were flawed by a tendency for the most severely disturbed children to receive the longest treatment whereas studies using historical control groups (Weiss *et al.*, 1975; Hechtman *et al.*, 1984) were confounded by uncontrollable changes in diagnostic and therapeutic practice.

Eleven of the 18 extended treatment studies involving methylphenidate were randomized control trials (one involved dextroamphetamine; Conrad *et al.*, 1971). Although randomized control trials are required to control for pre-treatment differences between comparison groups, these studies have not been without their methodological problems including small sample size (Brown *et al.*, 1986; Kupietz *et al.*, 1988), variability in sample characteristics (pervasiveness of hyperactivity, presence of co-morbid conduct disorder and co-morbid emotional disorder), high or unspecified rates of subject attrition, a tendency for premature discontinuation of medication (Brown *et al.*, 1987; Firestone *et al.*, 1986; Schain & Reynard, 1975; Rie, Rie & Stewart, 1976*a*; Rie *et al.*, 1976*b*), absence of an accepted method for establishing optimal dose of medication, and, finally, failure to specify the nature and extent of adjunctive therapy or the medication status of subjects at the time of their assessments after treatment. As a result of these limitations, any conclusions based on this body of research are tentative.

Collectively, the 11 available randomised control trials indicate that methylphenidate is more effective in ameliorating the core features of hyperactivity – at least over a period of 3 to 7 months – than placebo (Conrad *et al.*, 1971; Horn *et al.*, 1991), thioridazine (Gittelman-Klein *et al.*, 1976*b*), non-pharmacological therapy (Brown, Wynne & Medenis, 1985; Conrad *et al.*, 1971), or no treatment (Brown *et al.*, 1985). There is, however, no evidence that the beneficial effects of methylphenidate are greater than those derived from treatment with the tricyclic antidepressant imipramine (Quinn & Rapoport, 1975), nor are they potentiated by adjunctive pharmacological (thioridazine; Gittelman-Klein *et al.*, 1976*b*) or non-pharmacological therapy such as cognitive training (Brown *et al.*, 1985) or educational tutoring (Conrad *et al.*, 1971). Despite significant clinical improvement, few children make sufficient progress to be symptom- or diagnosis-free at the end of the trial of medication (Conrad *et al.*, 1971).

Favourable longer-term effects of stimulants on core behaviours have been obtained with doses of 0.3 mg/kg (Brown *et al.*, 1985), as well as with doses up to 1.5 mg/kg (Gittelman-Klein *et al.*, 1976*b*). Behavioural improvement seems to increase linearly with dose in long–term as well as in short-term studies (Horn *et al.*, 1991; Kupietz *et al.*, 1988). Longer-term benefit dissipates rapidly when treatment is terminated (Brown et al., 1987). Moreover, the beneficial effect of methylphenidate may diminish over a 6-month course of treatment, even with regular administration of medication (Kupietz *et al.*, 1988). The extent to which this reflects the development of tolerance is unclear (Winsberg *et al.*, 1987; Bertrand *et al.*, 1987). Studies of the effect of many years of methylphenidate treatment on cognition have not been conducted.

In contrast to this moderately optimistic picture of drug effects on core symptoms, little benefit on associated symptoms has been noted from the effect of prolonged methylphenidate treatment (Gittelman-Klein & Klein, 1976). Logic dictates that longer treatment would maximise the obvious immediate improvement in social interaction and peer perceptions that results from short-term treatment. Yet, there is only minimal evidence that stimulants reduce the incidence of conduct disturbance and improve the quality of peer relationships or self-esteem when administered for prolonged periods (Kupietz *et al.*, 1988; Gittelman-Klein *et al.*, 1976*b*). The clearest example of improvement in associated symptoms was obtained at a moderate dose (0.7 mg/kg) and the effect diminished between 3 and 6 months of treatment (Kupietz *et al.*, 1988). Similarly, improvement in academic attainment with longer term treatment would be predicted from the immediate increase in academic performance derived from methylphenidate. However, randomised controlled trials of longer-term effects yield only equivocal evidence of improvement in reading (e.g. Kupietz *et al.*, 1988) and no improvement in mathematics, with the single exception of the study of Gittelman-Klein *et al.* (1976*b*). It is likely that improvement in the associated features of hyperactivity requires longer-treatment than that investigated in existing studies or combinations of pharmacological and non-pharmacological treatments.

Methylphenidate: side effects

Somatic complaints

Although a number of physical and behavioural complaints have been identified as side effects of stimulant therapy, many of these complaints are common in unmedicated hyperactive children and may actually occur less frequently with treatment (Barkley *et al.*, 1990*c*). Only decreased appetite, insomnia and stomach-aches are more common with methylphenidate than with placebo therapy (Barkley *et al.*, 1990*a*). These treatment-emergent side effects are generally mild, are of questionable or unknown functional significance, and can usually be eliminated with adjustment of the drug's dose or schedule of administration. Of the children who have had a systematic trial of medication, most have minimal somatic side effects and are recommended for treatment. In general, the incidence of somatic side effects increases with dose (Tannock *et al.*, 1989*b*; Barkley *et al.*, 1990*a*): as many as 40% of children cannot tolerate doses greater than 0.9 mg/kg twice daily (Elia *et al.*, 1991).

Side effects necessitating discontinuation of medication are more common in preschoolers than in older children. In the case of the Schleifer *et al.* (1975)

study, all but 3 of 28 children discontinued medication after the trial because of side effects such as irritability, clinging, decrease in sociability, poor appetite and insomnia. One-third of parents in the Barkley (1988) preschool sample decided to discontinue their child's medication. In contrast to the Schleifer *et al.* (1975) sample, these children discontinued their medication because of the lack of benefit: few children experienced side effects warranting discontinuation. Older preschool age children (5 or 6 years of age) experience fewer side effects (Barkley *et al.*, 1985; Cunningham *et al.*, 1985). Available evidence indicates that the incidence of physical side effects and sombreness may increase with long-term treatment (e.g. Schain & Reynard *et al.*, 1975; Gittelman-Klein *et al.*, 1976*b*).

Dysphoria

Dysphoria associated with methylphenidate treatment appears to be common, occurring in almost half of treated children. This effect is characterized by a decrease in talkativeness and an increase in anxiety, euphoria, irritability, sadness and staring (Barkley *et al.*, 1990*b*; Whalen *et al.*, 1989*a*, *b*; Buhrmester *et al.*, 1992). The functional significance of this dysphoria is unknown. It is more common among hyperactive children who present with co-morbid emotional disorder, is serious enough to warrant discontinuation of methylphenidate in approximately 25% of children, and is more likely to occur as dose increases (Tannock & Schachar, 1992; Ickowicz *et al.*, 1992).

Abnormal movements, perseveration and over-focusing

Movement abnormalities and perseverative or compulsive symptoms are surprisingly frequent side effects of stimulant medication even in the absence of any history of tic disorders or obsessive compulsive disorder (Barkley *et al.*, 1990*a*, *b*; Borcherding *et al.*, 1990; Denckla, Bemporad & MacKay *et al.*, 1976; Ickowicz *et al.*, 1992). Motor and vocal tics and stereotyped movements have been observed in 30–70% of hyperactive children receiving stimulant treatment compared to 20% receiving placebo; persevering or obsessive–compulsive symptoms, such as persevering thought and rigidity in behaviour that resembles obsessive compulsive disorder, occur in 30–50% of these children (Borcherding *et al.*, 1990; Ickowicz *et al.*, 1992; Tannock & Schachar, 1992). Obsessive–compulsive behaviour, but not movement abnormalities, have been found to be related to dose (Borcherding *et al.*, 1990; Ickowicz *et al.*, 1992). Moreover, obsessive–compulsive symptoms hav been found to occur more frequently with dextroamphetamine than methylphenidate (Borcherding *et al.*, 1990).

In spite of the high rate of these treatment-emergent symptoms, their clinical significance is not known. None the less, some clinical implications do emerge. These side effects are best determined by direct observation during the active period of pharmacological action of the medication by individuals who have been trained and sensitised to these possible effects (Borcherding *et al.*, 1990; Ickowicz *et al.*, 1992). The movement abnormalities and obsessive–compulsive symptoms are often subtle, transient, and virtually always disappear when the dose is lowered or another stimulant is used (Borcherding *et al.*, 1990). Close monitoring of the child is crucial, however, because the causative or precipitative role of stimulants in Tourette's Syndrome has not been resolved (Borcherding *et al.*, 1990; Comings & Comings, 1987; Gadow & Sverd, 1990; Sverd *et al.*, 1988).

Growth retardation

There has not been a randomised control trial to examine the effect of methylphenidate on the growth of hyperactive children. However, several studies with less rigorous designs indicate that some degree of growth suppression occurs with methylphenidate treatment. Length and consistency of treatment as well as dose are crucial determinants of the extent of growth suppression and could explain the absence of the effect in some samples (Mattes & Gittelman, 1983). No evidence has been found that the ultimate height of hyperactive children is suppressed, even in patients whose growth rate was adversely affected during active treatment (Klein *et al.*, 1988; cf Vincent, Varley & Leger, 1990). The results of these studies indicate that the occurrence of a compensatory growth rebound must occur following discontinuation of medication. Interruption of methylphenidate during summer months results in significantly greater height and weight than continuous treatment (Klein *et al.*, 1988). The magnitude of growth suppression is small and of questionable clinical significance, but may be a concern for some children who are short before treatment. The mechanism of this growth suppression is unclear (Greenhill, 1981).

Self-confidence

Clinicians and researchers have proposed that medication may undermine a child's sense of personal responsibility for their successes and failures (Henker

& Whalen, 1989; Whalen & Henker, 1991*b*). If true, medicated children might become less persistent in the face of new challenges and less responsible for their own actions both while on and off medication. In general, investigators (Milich *et al.*, 1989, 1991) have observed that methylphenidate engenders improvement in the attributions that children make about their competence and enhances the correspondence between self-evaluations and objective performance levels. Moreover, in the only study to examine the question (Horn *et al.*, 1991), longer-term treatment (6 months) did not engender an external locus of control.

Other stimulants

Dextroamphetamine

Although there have been few direct comparisons and despite somewhat different neurochemical effects, in general, dextroamphetamine and methylphenidate are believed to have equivalent effects. Elia *et al.* (1991) studied the overall clinical and cognitive effects of relatively high doses of these two drugs. By and large, the therapeutic and adverse effects of the two stimulants were similar (Borcherding *et al.*, 1990). Of 48 hyperactive children, the vast majority responded well to both medications. However, four responded to methylphenidate but not to dextroamphetamine, eight responded to dextroamphetamine but not to methylphenidate. Only two failed to respond to either medication. This finding indicates that poor response to one stimulant does not necessarily predict a similarly poor response to an alternative stimulant.

Longer-acting stimulants

Longer-acting stimulants (pemoline, dextroamphetamine spansules, ritalin slow-release) have the advantage of less frequent dosing that makes them an attractive alternative to regular acting preparations for situations at school in which medication cannot be taken or those in whom compliance is low. In general, all long-acting preparations have effects on core and associated symptoms that are equally as beneficial as those of the short-acting preparation of methylphenidate and have an equivalent time-course (from 1 to 9 hours after ingestion for long-acting preparations and for regular methylphenidate administered twice a day) (Pelham *et al.*, 1987; 1990*a*). However, some aspects of some children's behaviour or performance are more improved by one preparation than another. Selection of the optimal preparation requires investigation of various preparations within a particular child (Pelham *et al.*, 1990*a*). However, it is not yet clear whether there are clinically important differences between long-acting and short-acting stimulants. Longer-acting preparations are more likely to cause insomnia and loss of appetite than regular-acting preparations (Pelham *et al.*, 1990*a*). On the other hand, longer-acting preparations might yield greater consistency in performance during the day and from day to day than other preparations (Pelham *et al.*, 1990*a*). Pemoline may cause liver toxicity (Greenhill, 1992) and choreoathetotic movements, which occur later in the course of treatment (Sallee *et al.*, 1989). Contrary to earlier belief, pemoline exerts its effect within several days (Pelham *et al.*, 1990*a*).

Tricyclic antidepressants

Tricyclic antidepressants have been used to treat childhood hyperactivity but few direct comparisons of antidepressants and stimulants have been conducted to evaluate the relative merit of the two classes of medication. Tricyclic antidepressants are an alternative to stimulants for those few children who fail to respond to stimulants; for those who have a response that is considered clinically inadequate; or for those who experience side effects, such as dysphoria, tics or insomnia, that necessitate discontinuation of methylphenidate. Tricyclic antidepressants have the additional advantage of requiring less frequent administration. They are longer-acting and have low abuse potential. They are thought to enhance the functional availability of noradrenaline – a neurochemical mechanism that is quite different from the dopaminergic action of stimulants.

Tricyclic antidepressants reduce activity level, but have demonstrated little effect on cognitive task performance (Gualtieri, Keenan & Chandler, 1991; Biederman *et al.*, 1989; Donnelly *et al.*, 1986), although Gualtieri *et al.*, 1991 argue for a drug-related improvement in memory. Improvement in symptoms of dysphoria has not been observed consistently (Biederman *et al.*, 1989; Gualtieri, *et al.*, 1991), and some evidence of impairment in motor performance has been detected (Gualtieri *et al.*, 1991).

The potential for adverse effects poses a major limitation on the clinical application of tricyclic medications. Twenty to 30% of hyperactive children treated with these medications experience dry mouth, decreased appetite, headache, abdominal discomfort, tiredness, dizziness or insomnia (Biederman *et al.*, 1989). Perhaps more seriously, tricyclics are associated with statistically significant although minimal increase in pulse, diastolic blood pressure, and frequency of cardiac conduction defects. The clinical significance of these effects is unclear and hotly debated especially since several children have died suddenly while being treated with tricyclic medication. Careful monitoring of the child's electrocardiogram before and after treatment, as well as blood levels of medication, are recommended (Biederman 1991). Tricyclics are best avoided in patients with heart disease or a history of heart disease. The frequency of side effects increases with serum level of drug, but the relationship of serum level and oral dose is unclear.

The risk and expense of monitoring tricyclics render their role in the clinical management of hyperactivity unclear. There is little to recommend these medications as a first choice in the pharmacological management of hyperactivity. Further study of the role of tricyclics for those who fail to derive sufficient benefit from any stimulant, those who present with co-morbid emotional disorder or those who experience debilitating dysphoria on stimulants is required.

Summary of pharmacological therapy

Stimulant treatment provides considerable benefit for hyperactive children. Core symptoms are reduced in intensity (e.g. Porrino *et al.*, 1983*a*), performance on cognitive tasks improves (e.g. Tannock *et al.*, 1989*a*), academic productivity and possibly learning improves (Douglas *et al.*, 1989) and children become less defiant, disobedient and aggressive (Whalen & Henker, 1991*a*). Nevertheless, several factors limit their clinical utility. Some children do not seem to benefit from stimulants. Others experience side effects necessitating withdrawal from medication (Barkley *et al.*, 1990*a*). A significant number of children discontinue their treatment for unknown reasons and without consultation with their doctor suggesting that the treatment might be unhelpful or undesirable for other reasons (Firestone *et al.*, 1986). Few children with favourable response to stimulants are considered free of difficulties in behaviour or social interaction following treatment. The possibility remains that some children receive a dose of methylphenidate which optimises their behaviour but which impedes academic or intellectual functioning.

Symptoms reoccur rapidly upon termination of treatment (Brown *et al.*, 1986) and there is little evidence that medicated children use the period during which their symptoms are suppressed by methylphenidate to acquire new, more permanent social, academic or self-regulatory skills. Logistical problems in the administration of medication may compromise the effectiveness of stimulants. Older children and adolescents may refuse to take medication, schools may be reluctant to administer noontime doses, or parents may be unable to comply with the pharmacological regimen. Some parents disagree on philosophical or religious grounds with pharmacological approaches to child management. Finally, as the time course of stimulant medication generally limits their effectiveness to the school day, parents may continue to experience difficulties during early morning and evening periods when chores, homework, meal-–times, peer interactions, and important family activities occur. Thus behavioural approaches to the management of the hyperactive child represent either an alternative or an adjunct to stimulant medication.

BEHAVIOURAL INTERVENTIONS

By comparison to trials of medication, the complexity of behavioural interventions makes comparisons of outcome studies difficult. For example, the target of behavioural interventions might include core symptoms, associated conduct problems, academic difficulties, social relationships with peers, parenting skills, or family functioning. Secondly, the mediator responsible for implementing behavioural interventions might include the child's parents, a teacher, or a professional therapist. Thirdly, behavioural interventions might involve a manipulation of the situational variables controlling problem behaviours, a shift in reinforcement contingencies for positive or negative behaviours, cognitive-behavioural strategies designed to improve the child's planning and self-regulatory skills, social learning interventions designed to teach new skills via modelling and observational learning, or combinations of these models. Within each of these approaches, the duration and frequency of training sessions, and the strength of the procedures used may vary considerably. Finally, the setting in which behavioural interventions are conducted might include the school, playground, home, community or mental health clinic. Difficulties establishing the relative efficacy of behavioural interventions is compounded by the inclusion of several components whose individual integrity has not been established.

The efficacy of behavioural interventions will be described according to the main target of intervention. Also, the organisation of the review of behavioural treatments will reflect differences related to mediator, type of intervention and setting. Age, dose and subtype issues as well as the effects of combined treatments will be recounted separately.

Behavioural interventions: short–term effects

Core and associated symptoms

Interventions implemented by teachers Interventions that are conducted by teachers who reinforce the positive behaviour and academic accomplishments of individual hyperactive children (Allyon, Layman & Kandel, 1975; Friedling & O'Leary, 1979; Robinson, Newby & Ganzell, 1981) or incorporate reinforcement procedures into specially designed classrooms (Barkley, Copeland & Sivage, 1980; Carlson *et al.*, 1992; Pfiffner, Rosen & O'Leary, 1985; Wolraich *et al.*, 1978) yield short-term improvements in both cores symptoms and academic performance. The effectiveness of reinforcing positive behaviour appears to be enhanced by the inclusion of negative consequences for disruptive behaviour. Thus, response–cost procedures (e.g. deducting points), loss of privileges, reprimands or time-out procedures may contribute to reductions in disruptive and aggressive behaviour (Acker & O'Leary, 1987; Rapport, Murphy & Bailey 1982; Rosen *et al.*, 1984; Pfiffner & Barkley, 1990; Sullivan & O'Leary, 1989). While the short-term effects of reward versus response–cost procedures appear comparable, response–cost procedures may improve maintenance when treatments are subsequently faded (Sullivan & O'Leary, 1989). Although most studies reveal a positive linear relationship between reinforcement magnitude and behavioural improvement, some studies suggest that quiet, private, "prudent" negative consequences yield more favourable outcomes than more intensive public consequences (Rosen *et al.*, 1984).

Under optimal conditions, the outcome of classroom-based behavioural interventions matches or exceeds (Loney, Kramer & Milich, 1979; Gittelman *et al.*, 1980; Gittelman-Klein *et al.*, 1976*a*) those of stimulant medications (Allyon *et al.*, 1975; Loney, Langhorne & Paternite, 1978; O'Leary *et al.*, 1976; Pelham *et al.*, 1980; Rapport *et al.*, 1982; Wolraich *et al.*, 1978). In addition to improving the behaviour of individual ADHD children, behavioural interventions may yield positive effects on performance (Rapport *et al.*, 1982; Wolraich *et al.*, 1978) of untargeted overactive peers (Loney *et al.*, 1979). None the less, many hyperactive children remain more problematic than peers (Abikoff & Gittelman, 1984; Pelham *et al.*, 1980). Although specially designed classroom programmes (Barkley *et al.*, 1980) may yield immediate behavioural improvements, generalisation to regular class placements is limited (Barkley *et al.*, 1980). Moreover, while some large–scale programmes executed by teachers trained in classroom management procedures have demonstrated significant improvements (O'Leary & Pelham, 1978; Pelham *et al.*,

1980), others have reported less promising results (Abikoff & Gittelman, 1984). The failure of larger-scale school-based studies to obtain the effects observed in earlier interventions suggests that teachers may not adhere to behavioural recommendations which impose an additional logistical burden, are inconsistent with prevailing educational beliefs, or disrupt classroom ecologies (Witt, 1986). Future studies, therefore, need to monitor the fidelity of behavioural interventions and explore approaches to classroom management which enhance adherence (Meichenbaum & Turk, 1987).

Community based interventions While interventions conducted by parents and teachers may yield improvements at home and school, it is unclear whether these benefits extend to after-school, early evening, weekend and vacation periods when hyperactive children spend large amounts of poorly supervised time with peers. Given the high prevalence of conduct disorders among hyperactive children (Szatmari, Boyle & Offord 1989*a*; Hinshaw, 1987), these represent high risk periods when constructive alternative activities might reduce antisocial behaviour. Extracurricular skill building programmes, for example, lower rates of antisocial behaviour and enhance the self-esteem of children in high-risk communities (Jones & Offord, 1989). While these gains did not generalise to the school setting and reversed when this programme was terminated, the magnitude of the reduction in police, fire, and vandalism expenditures offset the cost of the intervention. Although Jones and Offord (1989) did not target hyperactivc children, the possibility that programmes engaging hyperactive children in constructive activities during high-risk times may reduce the opportunity to engage in antisocial behaviour deserves careful study.

Enhancing self control

Cognitive–behavioural strategies Programmes designed to enhance self-control by teaching hyperactive children self-instructional strategies represent a potentially important approach to the hyperactive child's difficulties with self-regulation and impulsiveness (Kendal & Braswell, 1985). While early self-control studies were conducted in clinic settings, this approach is often applied in classroom settings (e.g. Barkley *et al.*, 1980). Whereas some early studies supported the efficacy of self-instructional programmes (Bornstein & Quevillon, 1976; Reid & Borkowski, 1987), later studies yielded less promising outcomes (Cohen *et al.*, 1981; Douglas *et al.*, 1976; Friedling & O'Leary, 1979). Although evidence on the incremental benefits of self-instructional strategies is limited, some studies suggest that self-evaluation procedures may enhance the effectiveness of reinforcement procedures. Moreover, although classrooms combining behavioural and self-regulatory interventions yield positive short-term outcomes (Barkley *et al.*, 1980; Barkley, 1991), generalisation of the gains accomplished via cognitive interventions is often limited (Abikoff, 1985, 1991). Despite the conceptual promise of interventions designed to improve self-control or self-regulatory strategies, their potential contribution to behavioural interventions in the classroom remains to be demonstrated (Abikoff, 1985, 1991).

Social skills training While there are some promising efforts to improve the social competence of hyperactive children (Cunningham *et al.*, 1989; Guevremont, 1990; Hinshaw, Whalen & Henker, 1984; Kendall & Braswell, 1985), skills acquired in social-skill training programmes may not generalise from the clinical settings in which training is conducted to the educational and social contexts where the hyperactive child's problems with social competence are most evident (Berler, Gross & Drabman, 1982; Abikoff, 1991). Moreover, the unpopular child's reputation may negatively bias the response of peers to improvements in social competence (Hymel, Wagner & Butler, 1992). Generalised improvements in the hyperactive child's relationships with peers may be more likely when social skills training is integrated into educational and extracurricular activities. Cunningham *et al.* (1989), for example, conducted a pre-class social skills group for hyperactive and learning disabled students which improved both prosocial behaviour and sociometric evaluations by peers. None the less, while positive interactions improved, reinforcement of non-aggressive behaviour in class was required to reduce negative interactions (Cunningham *et al.*, 1989).

Parenting skills

Parent training programmes Parent training programmes employ parents as mediators of home- and community-based behavioural interventions for their hyperactive children. While parents represent important allies in the management of hyperactive children, their child's poorly regulated behaviour often elicits controlling, less positive parenting strategies (Cunningham & Barkley, 1979; Mash & Johnston, 1982; Barkley *et al.*, 1984) which may compound the child's difficulties (Patterson, 1982). Parenting programmes, therefore, are designed to increase the frequency with which parents reinforce positive behaviour, to decrease the use of overly controlling punitive strategies, and to develop more effective responses to oppositional or aggressive behaviour (Barkley, 1989; Cunningham, 1990). The content of parent training programmes varies considerably. While many parent training studies incorporate components of the programmes described by Barkley (1981), Forehand & McMahon (1981), or Patterson (1976), the curriculum included is not consistent across studies. In addition to variations in specific child management strategies, programmes may include general information on attention deficit disorder or readings introducing social learning principles. Moreover, key dimensions of the training process may vary. These may include required participation by both parents (Gittelman-Klein *et al.*, 1976*a*), the completion of prerequisite assignments (Firestone *et al.*, 1981), combinations of group and individual sessions (Pisterman *et al.*, 1989, 1992), modelling of new skills, opportunities to role-play new strategies, in-session practice with the child, and homework projects applying new strategies at home. Other programmes address the hyperactive child's difficulties at school by teaching parents strategies for working collaboratively with teachers, developing home–school contracts, or consulting directly to teachers regarding the management of hyperactive children in the classroom.

Parent training programmes have been shown to improve child management skills (Pisterman *et al.*, 1989, 1992), enhance parental confidence, and reduce their stress (Anastopoulos *et al.*, 1993). These positive shifts in parenting are accompanied by a reduction in both primary symptoms of inattention and overactivity (Freeman, Phillips & Johnston, 1992) and secondary problems with noncompliant (Pisterman *et al.*, 1989, 1992) and aggressive behaviour (Freeman *et al.*, 1992).

Despite generally favourable outcomes, the clinical significance and specific areas in which parent training accomplishes change varies across studies. Whereas many studies report improvements in primary symptoms of inattention and overactivity (Anastopoulos *et al.*, 1993; Freeman *et al.*, 1992), others do not (Pisterman *et al.*, 1989, 1992). This heterogeneity in outcome may reflect differences in sampling frames, diagnostic procedures, drop-out rates, and the content and design of individual parent training programmes. Thus, parent training programmes are unlikely to improve classroom behaviour unless parents link school behaviour to home-based incentives (Firestone *et al.*, 1981) or teachers are trained in more effective classroom management strategies (Firestone *et al.*, 1981; Gittelman *et al.*, 1980; O'Leary & Pelham, 1978).

The effectiveness of programmes for parents of hyperactive children may be limited by several factors. First, the costs and logistical demands involved in obtaining service, arranging child care, travel, weekly sessions, readings, and homework assignments may limit attendance (Cunningham, Bremner & Secord-Gilbert, 1990). Secondly, particularly high risk families may not participate in parent training programmes. Thus, younger (Firestone & Witt, 1982), economically disadvantaged, socially isolated (Wahler, 1980), single (Webster-Stratton & Hammond, 1988*a, b*), or depressed parents (Webster-Stratton & Hammond, 1988*a*) seem most likely to discontinue participation (Firestone & Witt, 1982). Finally, the availability of parent training programs for this prevalent problem is often limited.

Books and videotapes In addition to formal training programmes for parents and teachers, a variety of books and videotapes provide suggestions regarding the management of hyperactive children (Barkley *et al.,* 1992*a*, *b*; Goldstein & Goldstein, 1987, 1990*a*, *b*; Gordon, 1991; Goldstein, 1989; Ingersoll, 1988; Parker, 1988). Whereas videotaped programmes have proven effective for parents of young conduct disordered children (Webster–Stratton, 1990), follow-up studies suggest that only programmes combining videotaped modelling with therapist led group discussion result in stable improvements (Webster-Stratton, 1990; Webster-Stratton *et al.*, 1988*b*). Although these types of programmes may prove to be useful adjuncts to more formal parent training programmes, their effectiveness with hyperactive children has not been established.

Family functioning

Several factors suggest that the management of child behaviour problems might be approached more effectively from a perspective which considers the influence of relationships within the child's family, peer group, and school (Mash & Terdal, 1988; Mash, 1989; Miller & Prinz, 1990). These include links between marital conflict and childhood behaviour problems (Emery, 1982; Grych & Finchman, 1990), the more specific association between family dysfunction and conduct disorder among hyperactive children (Szatmari *et al.*, Offord, 1989*a*; McGee, Silva & Williams, 1984) and an increased prevalence of alcohol abuse (Cunningham, Benness & Siegel, 1988; Owings-West & Prinz, 1987) and parental psychopathology (Barkley *et al.*, 1992*a*; Cunninghamet *al.*, 1988; Schachar & Wachsmuth, 1990; Lahey *et al.*, 1988) among the families of hyperactive children.

Despite the promise of a family system's perspective, simply including fathers in parent training programmes typically attended by mothers does not appear to enhance outcome (Adesso & Lipson, 1981; Firestone, Kelly & Fike, 1980; Martin, 1977). Moreover, family therapy interventions may not outperform standard parent training programmes (Barkley *et al.*, 1991). None the less, parent training programmes which target problem solving, communication, and conflict resolution skills appear to improve outcome for discordant families (Dadds, Schwartz & Sanders, 1987). Moreover, the improvements in management skill, parental confidence and child behaviour accomplished in parent training programmes may be associated with collateral improvement in marital functioning (Anastopoulos *et al.*, 1993).

Social networks

Families of hyperactive children move frequently (Barkley *et al.*, 1990*b*), consider relationships with relatives to be disruptive, and have fewer contacts with extended family members (Cunningham et al., 1988) who may be an important source of direct assistance, child rearing information, and personal support (Cochran & Brassard, 1979; Crnic & Greenberg, 1990). For boys, moves themselves may be associated with fewer peer contacts, less intimate friendships, and an increase in social rejection (Vernberg, 1990). For adults social isolation may adversely influence child management (Dumas, 1986) and limit the effectiveness of parent training programmes (Wahler, 1980). Interventions enhancing the effectiveness of personal networks represent promising, though unstudied directions (Miller & Prinz, 1990).

Age, dose and subtype effects – age and response

School-based interventions While single case studies have demonstrated the efficacy of classroom-based behavioural interventions for preschoolers and trials of kindergarten programmes designed specifically for hyperactive children are in progress (Barkley *et al.*, 1992*a*, *b*), little is known regarding the efficacy of behavioural procedures in preschool settings. Although the efficacy of classroom-based behavioural interventions for school-aged hyperactive children is well established (Carlson *et al.*, 1992), the outcome of behavioural interventions at the secondary level where rotating schedules, multiple teachers, and large classes might compromise adherence, requires study.

Parent training The relative efficacy of a single programme of parent training at different age levels has not been investiagted. Moreover, differences in sampling frames, inclusion criteria, and treatment programmes make comparisons across studies difficult. Nonetheless, studies of different age groups suggest that existing parenting programmes may be more effective with preschool and school-aged children than with adolescents. While trials with preschoolers and school-aged children report a decrease in parent reported problems, improvements in parenting skill, and a reduction in child management problems (Pisterman *et al.*, 1989; Dubey, O'Leary & Kaufman, 1983; Pollard, Ward & Barkley, 1983), the single adolescent study (Barkley *et al.*, 1992*a*), found few clinically meaningful improvements among adolescent hyperactive children randomly assigned to eight to ten session interventions designed to improve either child management skills, communication and problem solving skills, or family functioning.

Dose and response

Behavioural interventions, like pharmacological interventions, can vary in dose. The concept of dose in a behavioural intervention reflects factors such as length of intervention, intensity in terms of the number of sessions per week or the density of reinforcement contingencies. While the relationships between dose and response has not been investigated for school-based contingency management procedures with hyperactive children, programmes which deliver powerful consequences more contingently and frequently across situations and activities should yield more favourable outcomes than less consistently administered programmes. Accordingly, interventions conducted by highly trained mediators administering individualised consequences (Allyon *et al.*, 1975), enriched reinforcement contingencies (Pfiffner *et al.*, 1985), or specially designed classrooms (Barkley *et al.*, 1980; Wolraich *et al.*, 1978), appear to yield more pronounced short-term results than programmes introduced by consultants, implemented by teachers, in regular classroom placements (Abikoff & Gittleman, 1984).

In contrast to studies of stimulant medications, parent training studies have not examined the relationship between programme length, session duration, session frequency, and outcome. Moreover, little is known regarding the relative contribution of the various components of the training process, or the different skills introduced via parenting programmes. Those few studies addressing this issue have yielded conflicting results. Thus, while some investigators find little relationship between attendance, homework completion and outcome (Pisterman *et al.*, 1992), others suggest that increasing the length of parent training may yield more favourable follow-ups (Horn *et al.*, 1991).

Diagnostic subtype and response

As parent training reduces non-compliance and aggressive behaviour in both hyperactive and conduct disordered children (Bank *et al.*, 1991; Forehand & McMahon, 1981; Patterson, 1982; Kazdin, 1987; Webster-Stratton, Kolpacoff & Hollinsworth, 1988; Webster-Stratton, 1990), parent training may be particularly useful with the considerable percentage of hyperactive children presenting, or at risk for, oppositional or conduct disorders (Szatmari *et al.*, 1989*a*; Hinshaw, 1987).

Behavioural treatments: Longer–term effects

Follow-up studies have consistently demonstrated that the gains established in parent training programmes are maintained over short periods of time. These include 6-week (Freeman *et al.*, 1992), 2-month (Anastopoulos *et al.*, 1992), 3-month (Pisterman *et al.*, 1989), and 6-month (Dubey *et al.*, 1983) follow-up intervals. Studies examining the longer term impact of parent training programs for this population are unavailable. One study measuring longer-term outcomes suggested that short-term gains may dissipate over time (Abikoff, 1985). Longer-term follow-up studies are clearly needed.

COMBINED INTERVENTIONS

Combining behavioural approaches

Individual hyperactive children present a situationally variable pattern of problems in home, school, and extracurricular contexts (Whalen & Henker, 1991*b*). As the beneficial results of behaviour interventions introduced in one setting may not generalise to another (Forehand & Atkeson, 1978; Pelham & Hinshaw, in press), combining interventions which target different settings or behaviours may yield more comprehensive outcomes for children with pervasive difficulties.

Available evidence supports benefit of combining interventions. Gittelman *et al.* (1980) found limited evidence that parent training and classroom-based behavioural intervention yielded greater effects on activity level and inattention that either intervention alone. Abikoff & Gittelman (1984) found that, although a combined parent training and classroom management programme normalised levels of aggressive behaviour in hyperactive children, other measures did not shift significantly. Horn *et al.* (1991) found that combining parent training and self-instructional training for school–aged hyperactive children yielded more positive outcomes at follow-up than either programme in isolation.

Combining behavioural and pharmacological interventions

Uncontrolled cohort studies have suggested that multimodal interventions combining behavioural and pharmacological treatments might enhance outcome (Satterfield *et al.*, 1981). Indeed, there are a variety of mechanisms by which a combination of behavioural and pharmacological interventions might prove more effective than either form of therapy in isolation. First, combined interventions might yield greater effects on individual target behaviours than individually administered treatments. Pelham *et al.* (1980), for example, reported that methylphenidate (MPH) plus an intervention combining parent training and classroom behaviour management yielded greater effects on teacher ratings and direct observations of on task behaviour than behavioural interventions alone. Moreover, the effects of methylphenidate appeared to be greater after 13 weeks of behavioural intervention. In a later study, Pelham *et al.* (1988) found that a combination of methylphenidate and classroom behaviour therapy yielded greater reductions in teacher ratings of inattentive overactive behaviour than behaviour therapy alone. Pelham, Milich & Walker (1986), reported that a combination of methylphenidate and reinforcement of correct responses yielded a greater effect on a nonsense word spelling task than either intervention individually. Similarly, Richardson *et al.* (1988) reported that ADHD children who responded favourably to methylphenidate showed greater gains in reading grade equivalents during a remedial programme than those children evidencing a less favourable response to methylphenidate.

Alternatively, the addition of behavioural interventions to pharmacological treatments might allow the use of lower doses of medication. Thus, while Horn *et al.* (1991) concluded that the combination of parent training and methylphenidate was no better than drug alone, this study provided weak but suggestive evidence that a combined behavioural intervention consisting of parent training and social skills training plus a low dose of methylphenidate yielded improvements in teacher reports matching those of high dose methylphenidate conditions. Carlson *et al.* (1992) presented a more convincing demonstration that a combination of classroom behaviour therapy and 0.3mg/kg of MPH yielded behavioural improvements comparable to those observed at 0.6mg/kg of MPH alone.

Secondly, MPH's effects on sustained attention and self-regulation might allow children to participate more effectively and derive more benefit from behavioural or educational interventions. Thus, Hinshaw *et al.* (1984) found that methylphenidate increased the accuracy of ADHD children's self-evaluations in a cognitive–behavioural intervention in which accurate self-evaluation resulted in more point reinforcers than inaccurate self-evaluations. Moreover, only interventions combining methylphenidate and reinforced self-evaluation (versus medication, reinforced self-evaluation, or reinforcement alone) reduced negative behaviour to a level below that of normal peers (Hinshaw *et al.*, 1984). Abikoff and Gittelman (1985), in contrast, found that a 16-week cognitive training programme designed to improve social problem-solving skills did not enhance the effects of stimulant medication on academic, behavioural, and cognitive measures.

Thirdly, it is possible that behavioural and pharmacological interventions might affect different target responses in the same situation. For example, while behaviourally orientated social skills training programmes enhance positive interactions between ADHD and their peers, negative behaviour may not be affected (Cunningham *et al.*, 1989). Stimulant medications, in contrast, reduce negative peer interactions but do not increase positive interactions (Cunningham *et al.*, 1985, 1991). A combination of these interventions, therefore, might yield a more comprehensive influence on both positive and negative social interactions. Similarly, Wolraich *et al.* (1978) found that classroom-based behavioural intervention during group activities decreased non-attending, out-of-seat behaviour, inappropriate vocalisations, and disruptive peer interactions, whereas stimulant medication effected a different response, fidgeting.

Fourthly, combining treatments with different daily time courses might yield effects across a wider range of situations than either treatment individually. Wolraich *et al.* (1978), reported that a classroom-based behaviour management programme appeared most effective during group work scheduled early in the school day, whereas methylphenidate exerted a greater effect on later individual activities. Similarly, while parent training might be expected to improve parenting skill, parent–child relationships, and child behaviour at home, its effects may not generalise to problems at school (Forehand & Atkeson, 1978). Stimulants, whose time course coincides with the school day, on the other hand, might be expected to influence behaviour and performance in classroom contexts.

In addition to potentially positive effects, combining behavioural and pharmacological interventions might yield negative effects. Firestone *et al.* (1986), for example, reported a negative interaction with combined methylphenidate and parent training inferior to methylphenidate alone on teacher ratings of hyperactivity and (to some extent) measures of academic ability.

Assessing the combined effects of behavioural and pharmacological interventions places complex demands on subject selection, experimental design, and the selection of dependent measures. The outcome of those studies conducted to date, consequently, have yielded a pattern of results which is difficult to interpret. Few studies comparing the combined versus individual effects of methylphenidate and behavioural interventions with ADHD children, for example, begin with sample sizes providing the power needed to detect the incremental benefits of combined versus individual treatments. Thus, it is doubtful whether studies reporting main effects for methylphenidate and behavioural interventions had the statistical power needed to detect interactions between these interventions (Wolraich *et al.*, 1978; Pelham *et al.*, 1988).

Secondly, detecting the combined effects of behavioural and pharmacological interventions on an individual behaviour within a single situation (e.g. aggressive peer interactions at school) which is likely to show treatment related declines in frequency requires measures with 'floors' low enough to detect combined effects. If the effects of either intervention approach the floor of a given measure, it is unlikely that combined effects will be detected. Horn *et al.* (1991), for example, suggested that the absence of an incremental effect when methylphenidate and parent training were combined was attributable to relatively low pretest conduct disorder scores. Detecting effects on behaviour which increase in frequency (math problems completed correctly), in contrast, require measures with ceilings capable of detecting combined versus individual effects. Thus Abikoff and Gittelman (1985) questioned (but rejected) whether ceiling effects prevented the detection of the incremental effects of an intervention combining methylphenidate and cognitive training.

Studies comparing the effects of combined interventions on different target behaviours in a given situation must employ equally sensitive measures of each behaviour. Detecting potential cross-situational effects of combined interventions on a single measure, moreover, requires equally sensitive measurement of the same construct in each situation (e.g. aggressive behaviour at home and at school).

In addition to symmetry in the design and selection of dependent measures, studies comparing treatments must ensure the integrity (Moncher & Prinz,

1991) and potency of individual interventions. While it is relatively easy to ensure pharmacological interventions are titrated carefully and administered reliably, the complexity of behavioural interventions makes the evaluation of treatment integrity, therapist/experimenter commitment, and potency more complex. It is not surprising, therefore, that with the exception of one single case study (Horn, Chatoor & Conners, 1983) cognitive interventions, whose benefits are questionable (Abikoff, 1985, 1991), have not been shown to enhance the efficacy of methylphenidate (Abikoff & Gittelman, 1985; Brown *et al.*, 1985, 1986; Cohen *et al.*, 1981).

As well as assessing immediate response to alternative treatments, studies need to include follow-up measures designed to detect the longer term course of children treated with combined versus individual interventions. While stimulants yield relatively immediate effects, their positive effects on classroom behaviour and performance are lost when treatment is discontinued (Pelham *et al.*, 1988). The effects of behavioural interventions, in contrast, should emerge more gradually as parents or teachers acquire more effective behaviour management skills and introduce these at home or school. Moreover, longer-term follow-ups show that, in contrast to methylphenidate, the effects of parent training are generally maintained at 1 to 6-month follow-ups (Anastropoulos et al., 1992; Dubey *et al.*, 1983; Freeman *et al.*, 1992; Pisterman *et al.*, 1989). Thus, short-term studies with observations completed immediately after treatment may show an advantage of stimulant drug effects, whereas longer follow-up periods might favour behavioural interventions.

Summary of behavioural interventions

Behavioural interventions appear to be effective although they do not constitute a complete treatment for childhood hyperactivity. In particular, teacher-mediated behavioural interventions can benefit core and academic symptoms and parent training improves parenting skills, parents' sense of competence and child behaviour. As is the case for pharmacological therapy, longer-term benefits have been inadequately studied and are, as a result, unestablished. Behavioural interventions for hyperactive adolescents have been studied little but seem less effective than similar interventions for preschoolers and school-age hyperactive children. The major limitation of these therapies is their poor generalisation across situations, for example, classroom-based interventions do not generalise to home or community.

DIRECTIONS FOR FUTURE RESEARCH

Future studies of psychostimulants and other medications for childhood hyperactivity must delineate possible adverse effects such as cognitive impairment and dysphoria. These adverse effects could account for the apparently poor showing of medication in longer-term trials. More careful attention must be paid to methods of establishing optimal doses of medication which are practical in typical clinical settings. Randomised control trials of extended treatment are urgently required. Careful attention should be paid to differential responsiveness of various subgroup of hyperactive children. In particular, those with symptoms of emotional disturbance might respond to psychostimulants in an unique fashion and might be good candidates for a trial of another medication.

Several issues need to be addressed in future studies of behavioural interventions with hyperactive children. First, the transfer of positive effects across situations and maintenance of gains over time need to be explored. In the absence of generalisation, integrated interventions addressing problems in home, school, and extracurricular settings need to be evaluated.

Secondly, future studies must pay more careful attention to the magnitude of treatment effects and the relative effects sizes of different interventions. Utilisation of more conservative recovery statistics which consider both the test–retest reliability of dependent measures and the effect size needed to obtain a clinically meaningful yield of more modest outcomes for behavioural interventions (Jacobson & Truax, 1991).

Thirdly, little is known regarding the effects of behavioural interventions on different subtypes of hyperactive children. For example, as families of hyperactive children with conduct problems may be more dysfunctional, for example, differential outcome might be expected. Fourthly, given the evidence that parents and teachers fail to implement behavioural interventions, studies examining variables influencing adherence are indicated. Fifthly, programmes such as self-control training that have strong theoretical rationale with this poorly regulated group of children (Kendal & Braswell, 1985) but do not yield effects in short-term trials (Abikoff, 1985; 1991) may need to be conducted on a class-wide basis in the context of ongoing curriculum, activities, and peer groups.

Finally, high prevalence, limited professional resources, and evidence that a significant number of children do not receive or utilise existing treatments (Szatmari *et al.*, 1989*c*), emphasises the importance of developing accessible, cost-effective service delivery models. Although the needs of individual children often appear unique, it is generally possible to deliver services such as parent (Cunningham *et al.*, 1990) or social skills training (Cunningham, *et al.*, 1989) in more cost–effective groups or class–wide contexts.

CLINICAL IMPLICATIONS AND CONCLUSIONS

This chapter is not intended to provide details about clinical management of hyperactive children. Nevertheless, several of the issues that have been discussed bear on clinical management in a direct fashion. This review supports the opinion that stimulants are beneficial in treating hyperactive children. The immediate benefit in both core and several associated symptoms of hyperactivity typically noted by parents, peers and teachers is substantial and helpful. Nevertheless, medication has significant limitations as a complete treatment for such a multifaceted disorder as hyperactivity. Stimulants are not a cure for the social and academic problems of these children. Stimulants do not appear to improve a child's academic or social abilities, nor do they improve parenting knowledge or competence. It is possible that adequately designed studies of drug effects over longer periods of time would demonstrate normalization of many symptoms. For the moment, however, long–term treatment with methylphenidate appears to be associated with poor compliance, limited effectiveness and possibly with tolerance. Perhaps it is best to view drugs as providing a window of opportunity for other interventions. Behavioural interventions require much further study but appear beneficial in the short term. Combinations of behavioural therapies and medication are a logical choice for long-term combined treatment.

REFERENCES

Abikoff, H. (1985). Efficacy of congitive training interventions in hyperactive children: A critical review. *Clinical Psychology Review* **5**, 479–512.

Abikoff, H. (1991). Cognitive training in ADHD children: less to it than meets the eye. *Journal of Learning Disabilities*, **24**, 205–9.

Abikoff, H. & Gittelman, R. (1984). Does behaviour therapy normalize the classroom behaviour of hyperactive children? *Archives of General Psychiatry,* 41, 449–54.

Abikoff, H. & Gittelman, R. (1985). Hyperactive children treated with stimulants: Is cognitive training a useful adjunct? *Archives of General Psychiatry,* **42**, 953–61.

Acker, M. M. & O'Leary, S.G. (1987). Effects of reprimands and praise on appropriate behavior in the classroom. *Journal of Abnormal Child Psychology,* **15**, 549–57.

Adesso, V. J. & Lipson, J. W. (1981). Group training of parents as therapists for their children. *Behavior Therapy,* **12**, 625–33.

Allyon, T., Layman, D. & Kandel, H. (1975). A behavioral educational alternative to drug control of hyperactive children. *Journal of Applied Behavior Analysis,* **8**, 137–46.

Bank, L., Marlow, H., Reid, J.B., Patterson, G.R., & Weinrott, M.R. (1991). A comparative evaluation of parent-training interventions for families of chronic delinquents. *Journal of Abnormal Child Psychology,* **19**, 15–33.

American Academy of Pediatrics, Committee on Children with Disabilities, Committee on Drugs (1987). Medication for children with an attention deficit disorder. *Pediatrics,* **80**, 758–60.

American Psychiatric Association. (1987). *Diagnostic and Statistical Manual of Mental Disorders, rev. 3rd edn.* Washington, DC.

American Psychiatric Association. (1994). *Diagnostic and Statistical Manual of Mental Disorders.* 4th edn. Washington, DC.

Anastopoulos, A. D., Shelton, T. L., DuPaul, G. J. & Guevremont, D.C. (1993). Parent training for attention deficit hyperactivity disorder: its impact on child and parent functioning. *Journal of Abnormal Child Psychology*, **21**, 581–96.

Barkley, R. A. (1981). *Hyperactive children. A Handbook for Diagnosis and Treatment.* New York: Guilford Press.

Barkley, R.A. (1988). The effects of methylphenidate on the interactions of preschool ADHD children with their mothers. *Journal of the American Academy of Child and Adolescent Psychiatry,* **27**, 336–41.

Barkley, R. A. (1989). The ecological validity of laboratory and analogue assessments of ADHD symptoms. In *Proceedings of the Second International Symposium on ADHD*, eds. J. Sargeant & A. Kalverboer. Oxford: Pergamon Press.

Barkley, R.A. (1990). *Attention Deficit Hyperactivity Disorder: A Handbook for Diagnosis and Treatment,* New York: Guilford Press.

Barkley, R.A. & Cunningham, C.E. (1978). Do stimulant drugs improve the academic performance of hyperkinetic children?: A review of outcome studies. *Clinical Pediatrics,* **17**, 85–92.

Barkley, R.A., Copeland, A.P. & Sivage, C. (1980). A self–control classroom for hyperactive children. *Journal of Autism and Developmental Disorders,* **10**, 75–89.

Barkley, R.A., Karlsson, J., Strzelecki, E. & Murphy, J.V. (1984). Effects of age and ritalin dosage on the mother–child interactions of hyperactive children. *Journal of Consulting and Clinical Psychology,* **52**, 750–58.

Barkley, R.A., Karlson, J., Pollard, S. & Murphy, J.V. (1985). Developmental changes in the mother–child interactions of hyperactive boys: effects of two dose levels of Ritalin. *Journal of Child Psychology and Psychiatry*, **26**, 705–15.

Barkley, R.A., McMurray, M.B., Edelbrock, C.S. & Robbins, K. (1989). The response of aggressive and nonaggressive ADHD children to two doses of methylphenidate. *Journal of the American Academy of Child and Adolescent Psychiatry,* **28**, 873–81.

Barkley, R.A., DuPaul, G.J. & McMurray, M.B. (1990a). Comprehensive evaluation of attention deficit disorder with or without hyperactivity as defined by research criteria. *Journal of Consulting and Clinical Psychology,* **58**, 775–89.

Barkley, R.A., Fischer, M., Edelbrock, C.S. & Smallish, L. (1990b). The adolescent outcome of hyperactive children diagnosed by research criteria: I. An 8–year prospective follow–up study. *Journal of the American Academy of Child and Adolescent Psychiatry,* **29**, 546–57.

Barkley, R.A., McMurray, M.B., Edelbrock, C.S. & Robbins, K. (1990c). Side effects of methylphenidate in children with attention deficit hyperactivity disorder: systemic, placebo-controlled evaluation. *Pediatrics,* **86**, 184–92.

Barkley, R.A., DuPaul, G.J. & McMurray, M.B. (1991). Attention deficit disorder with and without hyperactivity: clinical response to three dose levels of methylphenidate. *Pediatrics*, **87**, 519–31.

Barkley, R. A., Anastopoulos, A.D., Guevremont, D.C. & Fletcher, K.E. (1992*a*). Adolescents with attention deficit hyperactivity disorder: mother–adolescent interactions, family beliefs and conflicts, and maternal psychopathology. *Journal of Abnormal Child Psychology*, **20**, 263–88.

Barkley, R. A., Guevremont, D. C., Anastopoulos, A. D. & Fletcher, K. F. (1992b). A comparison of three family therapy programs for treating family conflicts in adolescents with ADHD. *Journal of Consulting and Clinical Psychology,* **60**, 450–62.

Berler, E. S., Gross, A. M. & Drabman, R. S. (1982). Social skills training with children: Proceed with caution. *Journal of Applied Behavior Analysis*, **15**, 41–53.

Bertrand, W., Matinsky, S., Kupietz, S. & Richardson, E. (1987). Is there dose-dependent tolerance associated with chronic methylphenidate therapy in hyperactive children?: oral dose and plasma considerations. *Psychopharmacology Bulletin*, **23**, 107–10.

Biederman, J., (1991). Sudden death in children treated with a tricyclic antidepressant. *Journal of the American Academy of Child and Adolescent Psychiatry,* **30**, 495–8.

Biederman, J., Baldessarini, R. J., Wright, V., Knee, D., Harmatz, J. S. & Goldblatt, A. (1989). A double-blind placebo controlled study of desipramine in the treatment of ADD: II. Serum drug levels and cardiovascular findings. *Journal of the American Academy of Child and Adolescent Psychiatry*, **28**, 903–11.

Blouin, A. G. A., Bornstein, R. A. & Trites, R. L. (1978). Teenage alcohol use among hyperactive children: a five-year follow-up study. *Journal of Pediatric Psychology,* **3**, 188–94.

Borcherding, B.G., Keysor, C.S., Rapoport, J.L., Elia, J. & Amass, J. (1990). Motor/vocal tics and compulsive behaviors on stimulant drugs: is there a common vulnerability? *Psychiatry Research*, **33**, 83–94.

Bornstein, P. H. & Quevillon, R. P. (1976). The effects of a self-instructional package on overactive preschool boys. *Journal of Applied Behavior Analysis,* **9**, 179–88.

Brown, R.T. & Sleater, E.K. (1979). Methylphenidate in hyperkinetic children: differences in dose effects on impulsive behaviour. *Pediatrics*, **64**, 408–11.

Brown, R.J., Slimmer, L.W. & Wynne, M.E. (1984). How much stimulant medication is appropriate for hyperactive school children? *JOSH*, **54**, 128–30.

Brown, R.T., Wynne, M.E. & Medenis, R. (1985). Methylphenidate and cognitive therapy: a comparison of treatment approaches with hyperactive boys. *Journal of Abnormal Child Psychology,* **13**, 69–87.

Brown, R.J., Borden, K.A., Wynne, M.E., Schleser, R. & Clingerman, S.R. (1986). Methylphenidate and cognitive therapy with ADD children: a methodological reconsideration. *Journal of Abnormal Child Psychology,* **14**, 481–97.

Brown, R.T., Borden, K.A., Wynne, M.E., Spunt, A.L. & Clingerman, S.R. (1987). Compliance with pharmacological and cognitive treatments for attention deficit disorder. *Journal of the American Academy of Child and Adolescent Psychiatry,* **26**, 521–6.

Buhrmester, D., Whalen, C.K., Henker, B., MacDonald, V. & Hinshaw, S.P. (1992). Prosocial behavior in hyperactive boys: effects of stimulant medication and comparison with normal boys. *Journal of Abnormal Child Psychology,* **20**, 103–21.

Campbell, S.B., Douglas, V.I. & Morgenstern, G. (1971). Cognitive styles in hyperactive children and the effect of methylphenidate. *Child Psychology and Psychiatry,* **12**, 55–67.

Campbell, S.B. & Werry, J.S. (1986). Attention deficit disorder (hyperactivity). In *Psychopathological Disorders of Childhood,* eds. H.C. Quay & J.S. Werry, *3rd edn.* New York, NY: John Wiley & Sons.

Carlson, C.L., Pelham, W.E. Jr., Milich, R. & Dixon, J. (1992). Single and combined effects of methylphenidate and behaviour therapy on the classroom performance of children with attention deficit hyperactivity disorder. *Journal of Abnormal Child Psychology*, **20**, 213–32.

Charles, L. & Schain, R. (1981). A four-year follow-up study of the effects of methylphenidate on the behaviour and academic achievement of hyperactive children. *Journal of Abnormal Child Psychology*, **9**, 495–505.

Cochran, M. & Brassard, J.A., (1979). Child development and personal social networks. *Child Development*, **50**, 601–15.

Cohen, N. J., Sullivan, J., Minde, K., Novak, C. & Helwig, C. (1981). Evaluation of the relative effectiveness of methylphenidate and cognitive behavior modification in the treatment of kindergarten-aged hyperactive children. *Journal of Abnormal Child Psychology*, **9**, 43–54.

Comings, D.E. & Comings, B.G. (1987). A controlled study of Tourette syndrome. I. Attention-deficit disorder, learning disorders, and school problems. *American Journal of Human Genetics*, **4**, 701–41.

Conners, C.K., (1975). Controlled trial of methylphenidate in preschool children with minimal brain dysfunction. *Advances in Child Psychopharmacology*, New York, Human Sciences Press, 65–78.

Conrad, W. G., Dworkin, E. S., Shai, A. & Tobiessen, J. E. (1971). Effects of amphetamine therapy and prescriptive tutoring on the behavior and achievement of lower class hyperactive children. *Journal of Learning Disabilities*, **4**, 45–53.

Copeland, L., Wolraich, M., Lindgren, S., Milich, R. & Woolson, R. (1987). Pediatricians' reported practices in the assessment and treatment of attention deficit disorders. *Journal of Developmental and Behavioral Pediatrics*, **8**, 191–7.

Crnic, K.A. & Greenburg, M.T. (1990). Minor parenting stresses with young children. *Child Development*, 61, 1628–37.

Cunningham, C.E. (1990). A family-system-oriented training program for parents of language delayed children with behavior problems. In *Handbook of Parent Training: Parents as Co-Therapists for Children's Behavior Problems*, eds. C.E. Schaefer & J.M. Breismeister, pp. 133–76. New York: Wiley.

Cunningham, C. E. & Barkley, R. A. (1979). The interactions of normal and hyperactive children with their mothers in free play and structured tasks. *Child Development*, **50**, 217–24.

Cunningham, C.E., Siegel, C.S. & Offord, D.R. (1985). A developmental dose response analysis of the effects of methylphenidate on the peer interactions of attention deficit disordered boys. *Journal of Child Psychology and Psychiatry*, **26**, 955–71.

Cunningham, C.E. & Siegel, L.S. (1987). Peer interactions of normal and attention-deficit-disabled boys during free-play, cooperative task, and simulated classroom situations. *Journal of Abnormal Child Psychology*, **15**, 247–68.

Cunningham, C.E., Benness, B.B. & Siegel, L.S. (1988). Family functioning, time allocation, and parental depression in the families of normal and ADDH children. *Journal of Clinical Child Psychology*, **17**, 169–77.

Cunningham, C. E., Clark, M. L., Heaven, R., Durrant, J. & Cunningham, L. J. (1989). The effects of coping modelling, problem solving and contingency management procedures on the positive and negative interactions of learning disabled and attention deficit disordered boys with an autistic peer. *Child and Family Behavior Therapy*, **11**, 89–106.

Cunningham, C.E., Bremner, B. & Secord–Gilbert, M. (1990). A family and community-systems-oriented-course for parents of ADHD children. *Chadder*, **4**, 10–11, 26.

Cunningham, C.E., Siegel, L.S. & Offord, D.R. (1991). A dose–response analysis of the effects of methylphenidate on the peer interactions and simulated classroom performance of ADD children with and without conduct problems. *Journal of Child Psychology and Psychiatry*, **32**, 439–52.

Dadds, M. R., Schwartz, S. & Sanders, M. R. (1987). Marital discord and treatment outcome in behavioral treatment of child conduct disorders. *Journal of Consulting and Clinical Psychology*, **55**, 396–403.

Denckla, M.B., Bemporad, J.R. & MacKay, M.D. (1976). Tics following methylphenidate administration. *Journal of the American Medical Association*, **235**, 1349–51.

de Sonneville, L.M.J., Njiokiktjien, C. & Hilhorst, R.C. (1991). Methylphenidate-induced changes in ADDH information processors. *Journal of Child Psychology and Psychiatry*, **32**, 285–95.

Donnelly, M., Zametkin, A.J., Rapoport, J., Ismond, D., Weingartner, H. *et al.* (1986). Treatment of childhood hyperactivity with desipramine: plasma drug concentration, cardiovascular effects, plasma and urinary catecholamine levels and clinical response. *Clinical Pharmacology and Therapics*, **39**, 72–81.

Douglas,V.I. (1988). Cognitive deficits in children with attention deficit disorder with hyperactivity. In *Attention Deficit Disorder: Criteria, Cognition, Intervention*, eds. L.M. Bloomingdale & J.A. Sergeant, pp. 65–81. Oxford: Pergamon Press.

Douglas, V. I., Parry, P., Marton, P. & Garson, C. (1976). Assessment of a cognitive training program for hyperactive children. *Journal of Abnormal Child Psychology*, **4**, 389–410.

Douglas, V.I., Barr, R.G., O'Neill, M.E. & Britton, B.G. (1986). Short term effects of methylphenidate on the cognitive, learning and academic performance of children with attention deficit disorder in the laboratory and the classroom. *Journal of Child Psychology and Psychiatry*, **27**, 191–211.

Douglas, V.I., Barr, R.G., Amin, K., O'Neill, M.E. & Britton, B.G. (1989). Dosage effects and individual responsivity to methylphenidate in attention deficit disorder. *Journal of Child Psychology and Psychiatry*, **29**, 453–75.

Dubey, D.R., O'Leary, S. & Kaufman, K.F. (1983). Training parents of hyperactive children in child management: a comparative outcome study. *Journal of Abnormal Child Psychology*, **11**, 229–46.

Dumas, J. E. (1986). Indirect influence of maternal social contacts on mother–child interactions: a setting event analysis. *Journal of Abnormal Child Psychology*, **14**, 203–16.

Dyme, I.Z., Sahakian, B.J., Golinko, B.E. & Rabe, E.F. (1982). Perseveration induced by methylphenidate in children: preliminary findings. *Progress in Neuro-Psychopharmacology and Biological Psychiatry*, **6**, 269–73.

Elia, J., Borcherding, B.G., Rapoport, J.L. & Keysor, C.S. (1991). Methylphenidate and dextroamphetamine treatments of hyperactivity: are there true nonresponders? *Psychiatry Research*, **36**, 141–55.

Emery, R.E. (1982). Interparental conflict and the children of discord and divorce. *Psychological Bulletin*, **92**, 310–30.

Evans, S.W. & Pelham W.E. (1991). Psychostimulant effects on academic and behavioral measures for ADHD junior high school students in a lecture format classroom. *Journal of Abnormal Child Psychology*, **19**, 537–52.

Firestone, P., Kelly, M. J. & Fike, S. (1980). Are fathers necessary in parent training groups? *Journal of Clinical Psychology*, **10**, 44–7.

Firestone, P., Kelly, M.J., Goodman, J. & Davey, J. (1981). Differential effects of parent training and stimulant medication with hyperactive children. *Journal of the American Academy of Child Psychiatry*, **20**, 135–47.

Firestone, P. & Witt, J.E. (1982). Characteristics of families completing and prematurely discontinuing a behavioral parent-training program. *Journal of Pediatric Psychology*, **7**, 209–22.

Firestone, P., Crowe, D., Goodman, J.T. & McGrath, P. (1986). Vicissitudes of follow–up studies: Differential effects of parent training and stimulant medication with hyperactives. *American Journal of Orthopsychiatry*, **56**, 184–94.

Fisher, M., Barkley, R.A., Edelbrock, C.S. & Smallish, L. (1989). The adolescent outcome of hyperactive children diagnosed by research criteria: II. Academic, attentional, and neuropsychological status. *Journal of Consulting and Clinical Psychology*, **58**, 580–8.

Forehand, R. & Atkeson, B. (1978). Parents' behavioural training for problem children: An examination of studies using multiple outcome measures. *Journal of Abnormal Child Psychology*, **8**, 449–60.

Forehand, R. & McMahon, R. (1981). *Helping the Noncompliant Child: A Clinician's Guide to Parent Training.* New York: Guilford Press.

Forness, S.R., Cantwell, D.P., Swanson, J.M., Hanna, G.L. & Youpa, D. (1991). Differential effects of stimulant medication on reading performance of boys with hyperactivity with and without conduct disorder. *Journal of Learning Disabilities*, **24**, 304–10.

Freeman, W., Phillips, J. & Johnston, C. (1992). Treatment effects on hyperactive and aggressive behaviours in ADHD children. *Paper presented at the meeting of the Canadian Psychological Association, Quebec City, June, 1992.*

Friedling, C. & O'Leary, S.G. (1979). Effects of self-instructional training on second- and third-grade hyperactive children: a failure to replicate. *Journal of Applied Behavior Analysis*, **12**, 211–19.

Gadow, K.D. (1983). Effects of stimulant drugs on academic performance in hyperactive and learning disabled children. *Journal of Learning Disabilities*, **16**, 290–9.

Gadow, K.D., Nolan, E.E., Sverd, J. Sprafkin, J., & Paolicelli, L. (1990). Methylphenidate in aggressive-hyperactive boys: I. Effects on peer aggression in public school settings. *Journal of the American Academy of Child and Adolescent Psychiatry*, **29**, 710.

Gadow, K.D. & Sverd, J., (1990). Stimulants for ADHD in child patients with Tourette's Syndrome: The issue of relative risk. *Developmental and Behavioral Pediatrics,* **11**, 269–71.

Gittelman–Klein, R. & Klein, D.F. (1976). Methylphenidate effects in learning disabilities. Psychometric changes. *Archives of General Psychiatry*, **33**, 655–64.

Gittelman–Klein, R., Klein, D. F., Abikoff, H., Katz, S., Gloisten, C. & Kates, W. (1976*a*). Relative efficacy of methylphenidate and behavior modification in hyperkinetic children: An interim report. *Journal of Abnormal Child Psychology*, **4**, 361–79.

Gittelman–Klein, R., Klein, D.F., Katz, S., Saraf, K. & Pollack, E. (1976b). Comparative effects of methylphenidate and thioridazine in hyperkinetic children. I. Clinical results. *Archives of General Psychiatry*, **33**, 1217–31.

Gittelman, R., Abikoff, H., Pollack, E., Klein, D.F., Katz, S. & Mattes, J. (1980). A controlled trial of behavior modification and methylphenidate in hyperactive children. In *Hyperactive Children*: *The Social Ecology of Identification and Treatment,* eds. C.K. Whalen & C. Henker, pp. 221–43. New York: Academic Press.

Gittelman, R., Mannuzza, S., Shenker, R. & Bonagura, N. (1985). Hyperactive boys almost grown up. I. Psychiatic status. *Archives of General Psychiatry*, **42**, 937–47.

Gittelman, R. & Mannuzza, S. (1988). Hyperactive boys almost grown up. III. Methylphenidate effects on ultimate height. *Archives of General Psychiatry*, **45**, 1131–4.

Goldstein, S.(1989). Why won't my child pay attention?: *A Video Guide for Parents of Hyperactive and Inattentive Children.* Salt Lake City, Utah: Neurology, Learning & Behavior Center.

Goldstein, S. & Goldstein, M. (1987). *A Teacher's Guide: Attention–deficit Hyperactivity Disorder in Children.* Salt Lake City, Utah: Neurology, Learning & Behavior Center.

Goldstein, S. & Goldstein, M. (1989). *A Parent's Guide: Attention–deficit Hyperactivity Disorder in Children.* Salt Lake City, Utah: Neurology, Learning & Behavior Center.

Goldstein, S. & Goldstein, M. (1990*a*). *Educating Inattentive Children: A Guide for the Classroom.* Salt Lake City, Utah: Neurology, Learning & Behavior Center.

Goldstein, S. & Goldstein, M. (1990*b*). *Managing Attention Disorders In Children.* John Wiley & Sons, Inc. Salt Lake City, Utah: Neurology, Learning & Behavior Center.

Gordon, M.F. (1991). *ADHD/hyperactivity: A Consumer's Guide.* Dewitt: GSI Publications.

Greenhill, L.L. (1981). Stimulant–related growth inhibition in children: a review. *In Strategic Interventions for Hyperactive Children.* ed. M.G. Helman, pp 39–63. M.E. Sharpe, Armonk, NY.

Greenhill, L.L., Puig–Antich, J., Novacenko, H., et al. (1984). Prolactin, growth hormone and growth responses in boys with attention deficit disorder and hyperactivity treated with methylphenidate. *Journal of the American Academy of Child and Adolescent Psychiatry*, **23**, 58–67.

Greenhill, L.L. (1992). Pharmacological treatment of attention deficit hyperactivity disorder. In *Pediatric Psychopharmacology, Psychiatric Clinics of North America*, ed. D. Shaffer vol. 15, pp. 1–27. Philadelphia: Saunders.

Grych, J.H. & Finchman, F.D. (1990). Marital conflict and children's adjustment: a cognitive-contextual framework. *Psychological Bulletin*, **108**, 276–90.

Gualtieri, C. T., Keenan, P.A. & Chandler, M. (1991). Clinical and neuropsychological effects of desipramine in children with attention deficit hyperactivity disorder. *Journal of Clinical Psychopharmacology*, **II**, 155–9.

Guevremont, D. (1990). Social skills and peer relationship training. In *Attention–Deficit Hyperactivity Disorder: A Handbook for Diagnosis and Treatment,* ed. R.A. Barkley, pp. 540–572. New York: Guilford Press.

Hechtman, L., Weiss, G. & Perlman, T. (1984). Young adult outcome of hyperactive children who received long-term stimulant treatment. *Journal of the American Academy of Child and Adolescent Psychiatry*, **23**, 261–9.

Henker, B. & Whalen, C.K. (1989). Hyperactivity and attention deficits. *American Psychologist,* 44**,** 216–23.

Hinshaw, S.P. (1987). On the distinction between attentional deficit/hyperactivity and conduct problems/aggression in child psychopathology. *Psychological Review*, **101**, 443–63.

Hinshaw, S.P. (1992). Externalizing behavior problems and academic underachievement in childhood and adolescence: causal relationships and underlying mechanisms. *Psychological Bulletin*, **111**, 127–55.

Hinshaw, S.P., Whalen, C.K. & Henker, B. (1984). Cognitive-behavioural and pharmacological interventions for hyperactive boys: comparative and combined effects. *Journal of Consulting and Clinical Psychology*, **52**, 739–49.

Hinshaw, S.P., Buhrmester, D. & Heller, T. (1989*a*). Anger control in response to verbal provocation: effects of stimulant medication for boys with ADHD. *Journal of Abnormal Child Psychology*, **17**, 393–408.

Hinshaw, S.P., Henker B., Whalen, C.K., Erhardt, D. & Dunnington, R.E. (1989*b*). Aggressive, prosocial, and nonsocial behavior in hyperactive boys: dose effects of methylphenidate in naturalistic settings. *Journal of Consulting and Clinical Psychology*, **57**, 636–43.

Horn, W. F., Chatoor, I. & Conners, C. K. (1983). Additive effects of Dexedrine and self-control training. *Behavior Modification*, **7**, 383–402.

Horn, W.F., Ialongo, N., Greenberg, G., Packard, T. & Smith-Winberry, C. (1990). Additive effects of behavioral parent training and self-control therapy with attention-deficit hyperactivity disordered children. *Journal of Clinical Child Psychology*, **19**, 98–110.

Horn, W. F., Ialongo, N. S., Pascoe, J. J., Greenberg, G., Packard, T., Lopez, M., Wagner, A. & Puttler, L. (1991). Additive effects of psychostimulants, parent training, and self-control therapy with ADHD children. *Journal of the American Academy of Child and Adolescent Psychiatry*, **30**, 233–40.

Horn, W.F., Ialongo, N., Popovich, S., & Peradotto, D. (1987). Behavioral parent training and cognitive-behavioral self control therapy with ADDH children: Comparative and combined effects. *Journal of Clinical Child Psychology*, **16**, 57–68.

Hymel, S., Wagner, E. & Butler, L.J. (1992). Reputational bias: View from the peer group. In *Peer Rejection in Childhood.* eds. S.R Asher & J.D. Coie. Cambridge: Cambridge University Press.

Ickowicz, A., Tannock, R., Fulford, P., Purvis, K. & Schachar, R. (1992). Transient tics and compulsive behavior following methylphenidate: evidence from a placebo controlled double blind clinical trial. Presented at the 39th Annual meeting of the American Academy of Child and Adolescent Psychiatry, Washington DC (published abstract).

Ingersoll, B. (1988). *Your Hyperactive Child: A Parent's Guide to Coping with Attention Deficit Disorder.* Doubleday, New York.

Jacobson, N. S. & Truax, P. (1991). Clinical significance: A statistical approach to defining meaningful change in psychotherapy research. *Journal of Consulting and Clinical Psychology*, **59**, 12–9.

Johnston, C., Pelham, W.E. & Murphy A.H. (1985). Peer relationships in ADDH and normal children: a developmental analysis of peer and teacher ratings. *Journal of Abnormal Child Psychology*, **13**, 89–100.

Johnston, C., Pelham, W.E., Hoza, J. & Sturges, J. (1988). Psychostimulant rebound in attention deficit disordered boys. *Journal of the American Academy of Child and Adolescent Psychiatry*, 27, 806–10.

Jones, M.B. & Offord, D.R. (1989). Reduction of antisocial behavior in poor children by non–school skill development. *Journal of Child Psychology and Psychiatry,* **30**, 737–50.

Kazdin, A.E. (1987). Treatment of antisocial behavior in children: current status and future directions. *Psychological Bulletin*, **102**, 187–203.

Kendall, P. & Braswell, L. (1985). *Cognitive-Behavioral Therapy for Impulsive Children.* New York: Guilford Press.

Klein, R.G., Landa, B., Mattes, J.A. & Klein, D.F. (1988). Methylphenidate and growth in hyperactive children: a controlled withdrawal study. *Archives of General Psychiatry*, **45**, 1127–30.

Klein, R G. & Mannuzza, S. (1991). Long-term outcome of hyperactive children: a review. *Journal of the American Academy of Child and Adolescent Psychiatry*, **30**, 383–7.

Klorman, R., Brumaghim, J.T., Salzman, L.F., Strauss, J., Borgstedt, A.D., McBride, M.C. & Loeb, S. (1988). Effects of methylphenidate on attention-deficit hyperactivity disorder with and without aggressive/noncompliant features. *Journal of Abnormal Psychology*, **97**, 413–22.

Klorman, R., Brugmaghim, J.T., Fitzpatrick, P.A. & Borgstedt, A.D. (1990). Clinical effects of a controlled trial of methylphenidate on adolescents with attention deficit disorder. *Journal of the American Academy of Child and Adolescent Psychiatry*, **29**, 702–9.

Klorman, R., Brugmaghim, J.T., Fitzpatrick, P.A. Borgstedt, A.D. (1991). Methylphenidate speeds evaluation processes of attention deficit disorder adolescents during a continuous performance test. *Journal of Abnormal Child Psychology*, **19**, 263–83.

Kupietz, S.S., Winsberg, B.G., Richardson, E., Maitinsky, S. & Mendell, N. (1988). Effects of methylphenidate dosage in hyperactive reading-disabled children: I. Behavior and cognitive performance effects. *Journal of the American Academy of Child and Adolescent Psychiatry*, **27**, 70–7.

Lahey, B.B., Piacentini, J.C., McBurnett, K., Stone, P., Hartdagen, S. & Hynd, G. (1988). Psychopathology in the parents of children with conduct disorder and hyperactivity. *Journal of the American Academy of Child and Adolescent Psychiatry*, **27**, 163–70.

Lahey, B.B. & Carlson, C.L. (1991). Validity of the diagnostic category of attention deficit disorder without hyperactivity: A review of the literature. *Journal of Learning Disabilities*, **24**, 110–20.

Lambert, N. & Sandoval, J. (1980). Prevalence of learning disabilities in a sample of children considered hyperactive. *Journal of Abnormal Child Psychology*, **8**, 33–50.

Laufer, M.W., Denhoff, E. & Riverside, R.I. (1957). Hyperactice syndrome in children. *Journal of Pediatrics*, **50**, 463–74.

Loney, J., Kramer, J. & Milich, R. (1979). The hyperkinetic child grows up: Predictors of symptoms, delinquency, and achievement at follow-up. Paper presented at the meeting of the American Association for the Advancement of Science.

Loney, J., Langhorne, J. & Paternite, C. (1978). An empirical basis for subgrouping the hyperkinetic/minimal brain dysfunction syndrome. *Journal of Abnormal Psychology*, **87**, 431–41.

Lowe, T.L., Cohen, D.J., Detlor, J., Kremenitzer, M.W. & Shaywitz, B.A. (1982). Stimulant medications precipitate Tourette's disorder. *Journal of the American Medical Association,* **247**, 1168–9.

McGee, R., Silva, P.A. & Williams, S. (1984). Behaviour problems in a population of seven-year-old children: prevalence, stability and types of disorder – A research report. *Journal of Child Psychology and Psychiatry*, **25**, 251–9.

McGee, R. & Share, D.L. (1988). Attention deficit disorder – hyperactivity and academic failure: Which comes first and what should be treated? *Journal of the American Academy of Child and Adolescent Psychiatry*, **27**, 318–25.

Mattes, J.A. & Gittelman, R. (1983). Growth of hyperactive children on maintenance regimen of methylphenidate. *Archives of General Psychiatry*, **40**, 317–21.

Martin, B. (1977). Brief family intervention: The effectiveness and importance of including the father. *Journal of Consulting and Clinical Psychology*, **45**, 1002–10.

Mash, E.J. (1989). Treatment of child and family disturbance: A behavioral-systems perspective. In *Treatment of Childhood Disorders,* eds. E. J. Mash & R.A. Barkley, pp. 3–36. New York: Guilford Press.

Mash, E.J. & Johnston, C. (1982). A comparison of the mother–child interactions of younger and older hyperactive and normal children. *Child Development*, **53**, 1371–81.

Mash, E.J. & Terdal, L.G.(1988) *Behavioral Assessment of Childhood Disorders* (2nd ed.). New York: Guilford Press.

Matier, K., Halperin, J.M., Sharma, V., Newcorn, J.H. & Sathaye, N. (1992). Methylphenidate response in aggressive and non–aggressive ADHD children: distinctions on laboratory measures of symptoms. *Journal of the American Academy of Child and Adolescent Psychiatry*, **31**, 219–25.

Meichenbaum, D. & Turk, D. C. (1987). *Facilitating Treatment Adherence*: *A Practitioner's Guidebook.* New York: Plenum Press.

Milich, R. & Landau, S. (1982). Socialization and peer relations in hyperactive children. In *Advances in Learning and Behavioral Disabilities,* eds. K.D. Gadow & I. Bialer, Vol. 1, pp. 283–339. Greenwich, CT: JAI Press.

Milich, R., Licht, B.G., Murphy, D.A. & Pelham, W.E., (1989). Attention–deficit hyperactivity disordered boys' evaluations of and attributions for task performance on medication versus placebo. *Journal of Abnormal Psychology*, **98**, 280–4.

Milich, R., Carlson, C.L., Pelham W.E. Jr. & Licht, B.G., (1991). Effects of methylphenidate on the persistence of ADHD boys following failure experiences. *Journal of Abnormal Child Psychology*, **19**, 519–36.

Miller, G. E. & Prinz, R. J. (1990). Enhancement of social learning family interventions for childhood conduct disorder. *Psychological Bulletin*, **108**, 291–307.

Moncher, F. J. & Prinz R. J. (1991). Treatment fidelity in outcome studies. *Clinical Psychology Review*, **11**, 247–66.

O'Leary, K. D., Pelham, W. E., Rosenbaum, A. & Price, G. H. (1976). Behavioral treatment of hyperkinetic children: an experimental evaluation of its usefulness. *Clinical Pediatrics*, **15**, 510–15.

O'Leary, S.G. & Pelham, W.E. (1978). Behavior therapy and withdrawal of stimulant reduction with hyperactive children. *Pediatrics*, **61**, 211–17.

O'Malley, J.E. & Eisenberg, L. (1973). The hyperkinetic syndrome. *Seminars in Psychiatry*, **5**, 95–103.

Owings-West, N. & Prinz, R.J. (1987). Parental alcoholism and childhood psychopathology. *Psychological Bulletin*, **102**, 204–18.

Parker, H. (1988). *The ADD Hyperactivity Workbook for Parents, Teachers and Kids.* Plantation, Florida: Impact Publications.

Patterson, G. R. (1976). The aggressive child: victim and architect of a coercive system. In *Behavior Modification and Families*, eds. E. Mash, L. Hamerlynck & L. Handy, pp. 267–316. New York: Brunner/Mazel.

Patterson, G. R. (1982). *Coercive Family Process*. Eugene, OR: Castalia.

Peeke, S., Halliday, R., Callaway, E., Prael, R. & Reus, V. (1984). Effects of two doses of methylphenidate on verbal information processing in hyperactive children. *Journal of Clinical Psychopharmacology*, **4**, 82–8.

Pelham, W.E. (1983). The effects of psychostimulants on academic achievement in hyperactive and learning disabled children. *Thalamus*, **3**, 1–47.

Pelham, W.E., Schnedler, R.W., Bologna, N. & Contreras, A. (1980). Behavioural and stimulant treatment of hyperactive children: a therapy study with methylphenidate probes in a within-subject design. *Journal of Applied Behaviour Analysis*, **13**, 221–36.

Pelham, W.E. & Bender, M.E. (1982). Peer relationships in hyperactive children: Description and treatment. In *Advances in Learning and Behavioral Disabilities*, eds. K.D. Gadow & I. Bialer, Vol 1, pp. 365–436, Greenwich, CT: JAI Press.

Pelham, W.E., Bender, M.E., Caddell, J., Booth, S. & Moorer, S.H. (1985). Methylphenidate and children with attention deficit disorder. Dose effects on classroom academic and social behavior. *Archives of General Psychiatry*, **42**, 948–52.

Pelham, W.E., Milich, R. & Walker, J. (1986). The effects on continuous and partial reinforcement and methylphenidate on learning in children with attention deficit disorder. *Journal of Abnormal Psychology*, **95**, 319–25.

Pelham, W.E., Sturges, J., Hoza, J., Schmidt, C., Bijlsma, J.J., Milich, R. & Moorer, S. (1987). Sustained release and standard methylphenidate effects on cognitive and social behavior in children with attention deficit disorder. *Pediatrics*, **80**, 491–501.

Pelham, W.E., Schnedler, R.W., Bender, M.E., Nilsson, D.E., Miller, J., Budrow, M.S., Ronnei, M., Paluchowski, C. & Marks, D.A. (1988). The combination of behaviour therapy and methylphenidate in the treatment of attention deficit disorders: A therapy outcome study. *Journal of Attention Deficit Disorder*, **3**, 29–48.

Pelham, W.E., Walker, J.L., Sturges, J. *et al.* (1989). Comparative effects of methylphenidate on ADD girls and boys. *Journal of the American Academy of Child and Adolescent Psychiatry*, **28**, 773–6.

Pelham, W.E., Greenslade, K.E., Vodde–Hamilton, M., Murphy, D.A., Greenstein, J.J., Gnagy, E.M., Guthrie, K.J., Hoover, M.D. & Dahl, R.E. (1990*a*). Relative efficacy of long-acting stimulants on children with attention deficit-hyperactivity disorder: a comparison of standard methylphenidate, sustained-release methylphenidate, sustained-release dextroamphetamine, and pemoline. *Pediatrics*, **86**, 226–37.

Pelham, W.E., Harper, G.W., McBurnett, K., Milich, R., Murphy D.A., Clinton, J. & Thiele, C. (1990*b*). Methylphenidate and baseball playing in ADHD children: Who's on first? *Journal of Consulting and Clinical Psychology*, **58**, 130–3.

Pelham, W.E. & Hinshaw, S.P. (in press). Behavioral intervention for attention deficit-hyperactivity disorder. In *Handbook of Clinical Behavior Therapy*. eds. S. Turner, K. Calhoun, & H. Adams, New York: Wiley & Sons.

Peloquin, L.J. & Klorman, R (1986). Effects of methylphenidate on normal children's mood, event-related potentials, and performance in memory scanning and vigilance. *Journal of Abnormal Psychology*, **95**, 88–9.

Pfiffner, L.J. & Barkley, R.A. (1990). Educational placement and classroom management. In *Attention–Deficit Hyperactivity Disorder: A Handbook For Diagnosis and Treatment,* ed. R.A. Barkley, pp. 498–539. New York: Guilford Press.

Pfiffner, L.J., Rosen, L.A. & O'Leary, S.G. (1985). The efficacy of an all–positive approach to classroom management. *Journal of Applied Behavior Analysis*, **18**, 257–61.

Pisterman, S., McGrath, P.J., Firestone, P., Goodman, J.T., Webster, I. & Mallory, R. (1989). Outcome of parent-mediated treatment of preschoolers with attention deficit disorder with hyperactivity. *Journal of Consulting and Clinical Psychology*, **57**, 628–35.

Pisterman, S., McGrath, P., Firestone, P., Goodman, J.T., Webster, I., Mallory, R. & Goffin, B. (1992). The effects of parent training on parental stress and parenting sense of competence. *Canadian Journal of Behavioral Science*, **24**, 41–58.

Pliszka, S.R. (1989). Effect of anxiety on cognition, behaviour, and stimulant resopnse in ADHD. *Journal of the American Academy of Child and Adolescent Psychiatry*, **28**, 882–7.

Pollard, S., Ward, E.M. & Barkley, R.A. (1983). The effects of parent training and Ritalin on the parent–child interactions of hyperactive boys. *Child and Family Therapy*, **5**, 51–69.

Porrino, L.J., Rapoport, J.L., Behar, D., Ismond, D.R. & Bunney, W.E. Jr. (1983a). A naturalistic assessment of the motor activity of hyperactive boys. II. Stimulant drug effects. *Archives of General Psychiatry*, **40**, 688–93.

Porrino, L.J., Rapoport, J.L., Behar, D., Sceery, W., Ismond, D.R. & Bunney, W.E. (1983b). A naturalistic assessment of the motor activity of hyperactive boys. I. Comparison with normal controls. *Archives of General Psychiatry*, **40**, 681–7.

Prendergast, M., Taylor, E., Rapoport, J.L., Bartko, J., Donnelly, M., Zametkin, A., Ahearn, M.B., Dunn, G. & Weiselberg, H.M. (1988). The diagnosis of childhood hyperactivity. A US–UK cross-national study of DSM-III and ICD-9. *Journal of Child Psychology and Psychiatry*, **29**, 289–300.

Quinn, P.O. & Rapoport, J.L. (1975). One-year follow-up of hyperactive boys treated with imipramine or methylphenidate. *American Journal of Psychiatry*, **132**, 241–5.

Rapport, M.D., Murphy, H.A. & Bailey, J.S. (1982). Ritalin vs. response cost in the control of hyperactive children: a within-subject comparison. *Journal of Applied Behavior Analysis*, **15**, 205–16.

Rapport, M.D., Stoner, G., DuPaul, G.J., Birmingham, B.K. & Tucker, S. (1985). Methylphenidate in hyperactive children: differential effects of dose on academic learning, and social behavior. *Journal of Abnormal Child Psychology*, **13**, 227–43.

Rapport, M.D., DuPaul, G.J., Stoner, G. & Jones, J.T. (1986). Comparing classroom and clinic measures of attention deficit disorder: differential, idiosyncratic, and dose–response effects of methylphenidate. *Journal of Consulting and Clinical Psychology*, **54**, 334–41.

Rapport, M.D., Jones, J.T., DePaul, G.J., *et al.* (1987). Attention deficit disorder and methylphenidate: Group and single–subject analyses of dose effects on attention in clinic and classroom settings. *Journal of Clinical Child Psychology*, **16**, 329–38.

Rapport, M.D., Stoner, G., DuPaul G.J., Kelly, KL., Tucker, S.B. & Schoeler, T. (1988). Attention deficit disorder and methylphenidate; a multilevel analysis of dose–response effects on children's inpulsivity across settings. *Journal of the American Academy of Child and Adolescent Psychiatry*, **27**, 60–9.

Reid, M. K. & Borkowski, J. G. (1987). Causal attributions of hyperactive children: Implication for teaching strategies and self–control. *Journal of Education Psychology*, **79**, 296–307.

Richardson, E., Kupietz, S.S., Winsberg, B.G. Maitinsky, S. & Mendell, N. (1988). Effects of methylphenidate dosage in hyperactive reading disabled children: II. Reading achievement. *Journal of the American Academy of Child and Adolescent Psychiatry*, **27**, 78–87.

Riddle, K.D. & Rapoport, J.L. (1976). A two-year follow-up of 72 hyperactive boys. Classroom behaviour and peer acceptance. *The Journal of Nervous and Mental Disease*, **162**, 126–34.

Rie, H.E., Rie, E.D. & Stewart, S. (1976*a*). Effects of methylphenidate on underachieving children. *Journal of Consulting and Clinical Psychology*, **44**, 250–60.

Rie, H.E., Rie, E.D., Stewart, S. & Ambuel, J.P. (1976*b*). Effects of Ritalin on underachieving children: a replication. *American Journal of Orthopsychiatry*, **46**, 313–22.

Robbins, T.W. & Sahakian, B.J. (1979). 'Paradoxical' effects of psychomotor stimulant drugs in hyperactive children from the standpoint of behavioural pharmacology. *Neuropharmacology*, **18**, 931–50.

Robinson, P.W., Newby, T.J. & Ganzell, S.L. (1981). A token system for a class of underachieving children. *Journal of Applied Behavior Analysis*, **14**, 307–35.

Rosen, L.A., O'Leary, S.G., Joyce, S.A., Conway, G. & Pfiffner, L.J. (1984). The importance of prudent negative consequences for maintaining the appropriate behavior of hyperactive students. *Journal of Abnormal Child Psychology*, **12**, 581–604.

Safer, D.J. & Krager,J.M. (1984). Trends in medication treatment of hyperactive school children. In *Advances in Learning and Behavioral Disabilities*, **3**, 125–49, ed. K.D. Gadow. Greenwich, CT: JAI Press.

Safer, D.J. & Krager, J.M. (1988). A survey of medication treatment for hyperactive–inattentive students. *Journal of the American Medical Association,* **260**, 2256–8.

Sallee, F.R., Stiller, R.L., Perel, J.M. & Everett, G. (1989). Pemoline–induced abnormal involuntary movements (see comments). *Journal of Clinical Psychopharmacology*, **9**, 125–9.

Sandoval, J., Lambert, N.M. & Yandell, W. (1979). Current medical practice and hyperactive children. In *Behavior Therapy with Hyperactive and Learning Disabled Children*, ed. B.B. Lahey, pp. 120–9. New York: Oxford University Press.

Satterfield, J.H., Satterfield, B. & Cantwell, D.P. (1981). Three-year multimodality treatment study of 100 hyperactive boys. *Journal of Pediatrics*, **98**, 650–5.

Schachar, R., Taylor, E., Wieselberg, M., Thorley,G. & Rutter, M. (1987). Changes in family function and relationships in children who respond to methylphenidate. *Journal of the American Academy of Child and Adolescent Psychiatry*, **26**, 728–32.

Schachar, R. & Logan, G.D. (1990). Impulsivity and inhibitory control in normal development and childhood psychopathology. *Developmental Psychology*, **26**, 710–20.

Schachar, R. & Wachsmuth, R. (1990). Hyperactivity and parental psychopathology. *Journal of Child Psychology and Psychiatry*, **31**, 381–92.

Schachar, R. & Tannock, R. (1993). Childhood hyperactivity and psychostimulants: a review of extended treatment studies. *Journal of Child and Adolescent Psychopharmacology*, **3**, 81–97.

Schain, R.J. & Reynard, C.L. (1975). Observations on effects of a central stimulant drug (methylphenidate) in children with hyperactive behaviour. *Pediatrics*, **55**, 709–16.

Schleifer, M., Weiss, G., Cohen, N., Elman, M., Cvejic, H. & Kruger, E. (1975). Hyperactivity in preschoolers and the effect of methylphenidate. *American Journal of Orthopsychiatry*, **45**, 38–50.

Sebrechts, M.M., Shaywitz, S.E., Shaywitz, B.A., Jatlow, P., Anderson, G.M. & Cohen, D.J. (1986). Components of attention, methylphenidate dosage, and blood levels in children with attention deficit disorder. *Pediatrics*, **77**, 222–8.

Sleator, E.K., von Neumann, A. & Sprague, R.L. (1974). Hyperactive children. A continuous long-term placebo-controlled follow-up. *Journal of the American Medical Association*, **229**, 316–17.

Sprague, R.L. & Sleator, E.K. (1977). Methylphenidate in hyperkinetic children: differences in dose effects on learning and social behaviour. *Science,* **198**, 1274–6.

Sullivan, M.A. & O'Leary, S.G. (1989). Differential maintenance following reward and cost token programs with children. *Behavior Therapy,* **21**, 139–51.

Sverd, J., Curley, A.D., Jandorf, L. et al, (1988). Behavior disorder and attention deficits in boys with Tourette syndrome. *Journal of the American Academy of Child and Adolescent Psychiatry,* **27**, 413–7.

Sykes, D.H., Douglas, V.I. & Morgenstern, G. (1973). Sustained attention in hyperactive children. *Journal of Child Psychology and Psychiatry*, **14**, 213–20.

Szatmari, P., Boyle, M. & Offord, D.R. (1989*a*). ADDH and conduct disorder: degree of diagnostic overlap and differences among correlates. *Journal of the American Academy of Child and Adolescent Psychiatry*, **28**, 865–72.

Szatmari, P., Offord, D.R. & Boyle, M.H. (1989*b*). Ontario child Health Study: prevalence of attention deficit disorder with hyperactivity. *Journal of Child Psychology and Psychiatry*, **30**, 205–17.

Szatmari, P., Offord, D.R. & Boyle, M.H. (1989*c*). Correlates, associated impairments and patterns of service utilization of children with attention deficit disorder: Findings from the Ontario child health study. *Journal of Child Psychology and Psychiatry*, **30**, 205–17.

Tannock, R. & Schachar, R. (1992). Is ADHD with co-morbid overanxious disorder different from ADHD? Symposium on Comorbidity of ADHD: Discriminating features and methodological problems, at the 39th Annual meeting of the American Academy of Child and Adolescent Psychiatry, Washington DC (published abstract).

Tannock, R., Schachar, R.J., Carr, R.P., Chajczyk, D. & Logan G.D. (1989*a*). Effects of methylphenidate on inhibitory control in hyperactive children. *Journal of Abnormal Child Psychology*, **17**, 473–91.

Tannock, R., Schachar, R.J., Carr, R.P. & Logan, G.D. (1989*b*). Dose–response effects of methylphenidate on academic performance and overt behavior in hyperactive children. *Pediatrics*, 84, 648–57.

Tannock, R. & Schachar, R. (1992). Methylphenidate and cognitive perseveration in hyperactive children. *Journal of Child Psychology and Psychiatry*, **33**, 1217–28.

Tannock, R., Schachar,R. & Logan, G. (1993). Does methylphenidate induce overfocusing in hyperactive children? *Journal of Clinical Child Psychology*, **22**, 28–41.

Taylor, E.,Schachar, R., Thorley, G., Wieselberg, H.M., Everitt, B. & Rutter, M. (1987). Which boys respond to stimulant medication? A controlled trial of methylphenidate in boys with disruptive behaviour. *Psychological Medicine*, **17**, 121–43.

Taylor, E., Sandberg, S., Thorley, G. & Giles, S. (1991). *The Epidemiology of Childhood Hyperactivity. Institute of Psychiatry Maudsley Monographs.* London: Oxford University Press.

Trommer, B.L., Hoeppner, J.A. & Zecker, S.G. (1991). The go–no go test in attention deficit disorder is sensitive to methylphenidate. *Journal of Child Neurology*, **6**, 128–31.

Vernberg, E.M. (1990). Experiences with peers following relocation during early adolescence. *American Journal of Orthopsychiatry*, **60**, 466–72.

Vyse, S.A. & Rapport, M.D. (1989). The effects of methylphenidate on learning in children with ADDH: the stimulus equivalence paradigm. *Journal of Consulting and Clinical Psychology*, **57**, 425–35.

Vincent, J., Varley, C.K. & Leger, P. (1990). Effects of methylphenidate on early adolescent growth. *American Journal of Psychiatry*, **147**, 501–2.

Wahler, R.G. (1980). The insular mother: her problems in parent–child treatment. *Journal of Applied Behavior Analysis*, **13**, 207–19.

Webster-Stratton, C. (1990). Enhancing the effectiveness of self-administered videotape parent training for families with conduct-problem children. *Journal of Abnormal Child Psychology*, **18**, 479–92.

Webster-Stratton C. & Hammond, M. (1988*a*). Maternal depression and its relationship to life stress, perceptions of child behavior problems, parenting behaviours, and child conduct problems. *Journal of Abnormal Child Psychology*, **16,** 299–315.

Webster-Stratton, C., Kolpacoff, M. & Hollinsworth, T. (1988*b*). Self-administered videotape therapy for families with conduct-problem children: comparison with two cost-effective treatments and a control group. *Journal of Consulting and Clinical Psychology*, **56,** 558–66.

Weiss, G., Kruger, E., Danielson, U. & Elman, M. (1975). Effect of long-term treatment of hyperactive children with methylphenidate. *Canadian Medical Association Journal*, **112**, 159–65.

Whalen, C.K., Collins, B.E., Henker, B., Alkus, S.R., Adams, D. & Stapp, J. (1978). Behavior observations of hyperactive children and methylphenidate (Ritalin) effects in systematically structured classroom environments: Now you see them, now you don't. *Journal of Pediatric Psychology*, **3**, 177–87.

Whalen, C.K., Henker, B., Collins, B.E., McAuliffe, S., & Vaux, A. (1979). Peer interaction in a structured communication task: comparisons of normal and hyperactive boys and of methylphenidate (Ritalin) and placebo effects. *Child Development*, **50**, 388–401.

Whalen, C.K., Henker, B. & Dotemoto, S. (1981). Teacher response to the methylphenidate (Ritalin) versus placebo status of hyperactive boys in the classroom. *Child Development*, **52**, 1005–14.

Whalen, C.K., Henker, B., Swanson, J.M., Granger, D., Kliewer, W., Spenser, J. (1987). Natural social behaviors in hyperactive children: dose effects of methylphenidate. *Journal of Consulting and Clinical Psychology*, **55**, 187–93.

Whalen, C.K., Henker, B., Buhrmester, D., Hinshaw, S.P., Huber, A. & Laski, K. (1989*a*). Does stimulant medication improve the peer status of hyperactive children? *Journal of Consulting and Clinical Psychology*, **57**, 545–9.

Whalen, C.K., Henker, B. & Granger, D.A. (1989b). Ratings of medication effects in hyperactive children: Viable or vulnerable? *Behavioral Assessment*, **111**, 179–99.

Whalen, C.K., Henker, B. & Granger D.A. (1990). Social judgment processes in hyperactive boys: effects of methylphenidate and comparisons with normal peers. *Journal of Abnormal Child Psychology*, **18**, 297–316.

Whalen, C. K. & Henker, B. (1991a). Therapies for hyperactive children: comparisons, combinations, and compromises. *Journal of Consulting and Clinical Psychology*, **59**, 126–37.

Whalen, C. K. & Henker, B. (1991b). Social impact of stimulant treatment for hyperactive children. *Journal of Learning Disabilities*, **24**, 231–41.

Winsberg, B., Matinsky, S., Kupietz, S. & Richardson, E. (1987). Is there dose–dependent tolerance associated with chronic methylphenidate therapy in hyperactive children: oral dose and plasma considerations. *Psychopharmacology Bulletin*, **23**, 107–10.

Witt, J.C. (1986). Teachers' resistance to the use of school-based interventions. *Journal of School Psychology*, **24,** 37–64

Wolraich, M., Drummond, T., Salomon, M.K., O'Brien, M.L. & Sivage, C. (1978). Effects of methylphenidate alone and in combination with behaviour modification procedures on the behaviour and academic performance of hyperactive children. *Journal of Abnormal Child Psychology*, **6,** 149–61.

Wolraich, M.L., Lindgren, S., Strömquist, A., Milich, R., Davis, C. & Watson, D. (1990). Stimulant medication use by primary care physicians in the treatment of attention deficit hyperactivity disorder. *Pediatrics*, **86**, 95–101.

World Health Organisation. (1994). *International Classification of Diseases* 10th edn. Geneva.

13

Outcome

Christopher Gillberg and Lars Hellgren

INTRODUCTION

The study of the long-term outcome of disorders associated with attention deficits has been hampered by a number of problems. First, the definition of attention deficit has varied from one study to another. Secondly, attention deficits are often associated with other disorders making it difficult to tease out the specific contribution of attention problems to ultimate outcome. Thirdly, very few studies have referred to population based samples with appropriate comparison groups rendering generalised conclusions impossible. Fourthly, the numbers included in each study have tended to be small and this too has rendered generalisation hazardous – at least when results have been equivocal and not appropriate for pooling with those of other studies. Fifthly, prospective longitudinal studies are needed, but only a handful of studies have used this design and included a reasonable time span for follow-up. Sixthly, the study of the natural history of attention deficits has been problematic because many children have received treatment of various kinds, most notably with central nervous system stimulants, which are known to effectively reduce attention problem, at least in the short term. Finally, a number of other methodological problems, including non-blindness of diagnosticians, pertain to virtually all studies of outcome in so-called attention deficit hyperactivity disorder (ADHD) (APA ,1987), attention deficit disorder (ADD) (APA, 1980), and hyperkinetic disorder (WHO, 1980).

This chapter aims to review the evidence concerning the natural outcome of childhood onset disorders of attention. The term 'disorders of attention' will be used throughout as an umbrella concept. There is no clear consensus in the field as to which overriding concept to use. ADD suffers from its inherent tautology: it is either 'deficit' or 'disorder', hardly both. ADHD excludes children who are not hyperactive, which is inappropriate (Shaywitz & Shaywitz, 1988). Hyperkinetic disorder seems to be the least convincing term of all, considering that most authors seem to agree that extremes of hyperactivity are not usually present in so-called hyperkinetic syndromes. Most children with severe and pervasive attention deficits have additional problems of motor control and perception (Landgren, Petterson, Kjellman & Gillberg, 1996). The term DAMP (deficits in attention, motor control and perception) has been suggested (Gillberg, Gillberg & Groth, 1989). At least half of all children with DAMP also meet criteria for ADHD and all have considerable problems attending to tasks even if full criteria for ADHD are not met (Landgren *et al.*, 1995). However, because of controversy in the field, and because it is yet not clear what proportion (if any) of children with severe attention deficits does not exhibit motor–perceptual problems, the most neutral term, namely disorders of attention will be used. It needs emphasising, however, that not even this term is neutral enough in that it has not been unequivocally demonstrated that children who receive a clinical diagnosis of attention deficit actually have a core dysfunction in the field of basic attentional processes. (The issues of measurement and classification are more fully discussed in Chapters 2, 4 and 6.)

The following areas will be covered:
(i) In the present review the long-term outcome studies up until the early 1980s, (ii) recent long-term follow-up studies of disorders of attention making use of appropriate comparison groups, (iii) recent controlled follow-up studies of problems often associated with disorders of attention, (iv) treatment related to outcome, (v) neurophysiological aspects in relation to outcome, (vi) follow-back studies, and cross sectional studies shedding light on certain outcome aspects, and (vii) case studies of potential clinical importance for the understanding of specific outcome issues.

OLDER LONG-TERM OUTCOME STUDIES

Thorley (1984) and Weiss (1985) reviewed outcome studies in the field of 'hyperactivity'/disorders of attention up until the early 1980s.

Thorley found 17 prospective and 7 retrospective studies. He concluded, on the basis of his review that 'hyperactives have a worse outcome than normal children'. Persistent conduct problems and antisocial behaviour tended to be the most common type of problem encountered in teenage and early adult life. However, the inadequacy of many of the studies reviewed, both in terms of small patient cohorts, selected rather than representative patient groups, atypically high boy:girl ratios as compared with attention disordered cases drawn from the general population, and the failure to include other psychiatric problem cases for contrast led Thorley to the view that the clinical validity (concurrent validity) of a specific hyperkinetic syndrome of childhood was largely unsupported. Instead, he asked whether the presence of marked hyperactivity in a whole range of children with various kinds of disorders (irrespective of clinical diagnosis and including those with autism and mental retardation) could signal a generally worse outcome in terms of social adjustment and personal well-being. He did not consider that – at the time of his review – the evidence was there to suggest such a dimensional approach to the whole issue of hyperkinetic disorder, and that the elucidation of it in future follow-up studies would contribute towards a valuable answer.

Weiss (1985), on the other hand, although equally critical of the quality of most of the outcome studies in the field, arrived at, superficially, rather different conclusions. She highlighted the fact that, although the majority of children with disorders of attention grow up without serious psychopathology, about half continue to show one or more symptoms of the original syndrome in adolescence and young adulthood. She further stated that 10–50% of sufferers of childhood hyperactivity developed antisocial behaviour and that other adult psychiatric problems (except alcoholism, schizophrenia and major depression) might be a common outcome also.

Both Thorley and Weiss acknowledge a host of methodological problems that render generalised conclusions impossible. However, they do not strongly emphasise the most serious drawback of all, namely that virtually all of the published studies pertained to potentially heavily biased samples recruited in various clinical settings. Such samples, no matter how sophisticated the methodology used, will tell us little, if anything, about the outcome of disorders of attention in the general population. Knowledge about the outcome of clinic patients is not necessarily useful, given the enormous cultural (and even intracultural) differences in respect of service availability and organisation and different levels of 'tolerance' of attention deficits in one place as compared to another. One recent example of the extreme bias that clinic referral can introduce was provided by the total population study of anorexia nervosa performed by Råstam, Gillberg & Garton (1989). Anorexia nervosa, of course, is not generally associated with attention deficits, but the same general rules apply when discussing various types of selection bias. In the Råstam *et al.* (1989) study, every single child in the Göteborg population born in 1970 was examined without clothes on in 1985. All cases of anorexia nervosa in the population were traced by this procedure. The total population prevalence was 0.47%. Only

15% (3 out of 20) of these anorexia cases had attended child and adolescent psychiatric clinics. On follow-up several years later, only a few more cases had attended any type of clinic for eating disorders, and only 25% of the total population could be said to have received treatment. Among those who had not attended a clinic between age 15 and 22 years were some of the most emaciated and severely disturbed cases. If outcome studies in anorexia nervosa are based only on clinic referred populations, it is quite likely that the conclusions drawn may be seriously misleading. The follow-up at age 22 years of the anorexia and control cases in the Råstam *et al.* study suggested that some cases seen in clinics are different from those who never attend clinics and that, in some respects, the latter group may be even more disturbed and with poorer outcome. The same line of reasoning might well prove to be relevant in the study of attention disorders. The truth of the matter is that we still know very little about the long-term prognosis of attention disorders in the general population.

RECENT LONG-TERM FOLLOW-UP STUDIES

Six sets of studies of outcome in disorders of attention have been published since the mid-1980s (Table 13.1). Four of these (Gittelman *et al.*, 1985; Howell, Huessy & Hassuk, 1985; Lambert *et al.*, 1987; Fischer *et al.*, 1990) originated in the United States, one in Canada (Hechtman & Weiss, 1986) and one in Sweden (Gillberg & Gillberg, 1989*a*). Only the Swedish study was clearly population based. The New York and Milwaukee follow-up groups may have been biased towards heavily selected samples because they only involved cases that had been referred to a specialised 'hyperactivity centre' specifically for treatment of hyperactivity. Only the Canadian and Swedish studies included personal interview by a trained psychiatrist both at initial assessment and follow-up. Only the Swedish study concerned children who did not receive any kind of specific treatment.

The diagnostic criteria used have been different in all the published studies. Only the Gittelman and Gillberg studies included groups with pervasive attention deficits according to defined measures, even though it is likely that several of the other studies referred to behaviourally similar groups. The Gillberg study included children who had the combination of pervasive 'ADD' and motor control/ perceptual problems. Many of the ADD/hyperactivity cases in the other studies also showed such problems, but it had not been a requirement for entry into the study. On the other hand, the Gillberg study from Sweden and the study by the Huessy group from Vermont, USA, were the only two which did not require that the children included in the study had a perceived major behaviour problem.

The attrition rates for follow-up numbers compared with numbers of cases on entry into study ranged from 0–42%. Taken together, these differences across studies detract from the possibility of drawing firm conclusions. In spite of all the major shortcomings of research in the field so far, a few cautious conclusions appear to be warranted.

First of all, it appears that at psychiatric examination or interview by research assistants using standardised instruments, a substantial proportion of children with disorders of attention are indistinguishable from normal contrast groups in teenage/early adult life (Gittelman *et al.,* 1985; Hechtman & Weiss, 1986; Mannuzza *et al.*, 1991). It is yet too early to determine just how large this proportion is. According to Gillberg *et al.* (1989) and Hellgren *et al.* (1994), it is no more than 16% in early teenage and 36% in later teens. The New York group found that 48–52% of childhood onset attention disorders had no DSM-III-R diagnosis in late teenage/early adult life. These cases (without a DSM-III-R diagnosis in teenage/early adult life) were strikingly similar to normal 'controls'. The Montreal group reported a generally good outcome in the mid-20s, but acknowledged the high rate of problems in teenage.

Secondly, a relatively large group continue to show attention deficit problems in teenage/adult life. All the follow-up studies that have reported specifically on the persistence/disappearance of attention deficits, have agreed that at least 40% (peaking at 72% in the Barkley *et al.*, 1990 study) meet criteria for ADD, ADHD or pervasive hyperactivity at age 13–23 years. According to the Milwaukee study findings (Fischer *et al.*, 1990) direct observational measures suggest that the vast majority of childhood 'hyperactives' continue to show attention deficits in teenage. This would imply that the old notion of a maturational lag with gradual amelioration of attention problems might be mistaken. There is also the possibility that there might exist a subgroup of cases with attention disorders which are of a developmental character with slow disappearance of deficits over time, and another subgroup for which the prognosis should be considerably more guarded. If such subgroups do exist, the evidence for subdividing in early childhood (something that clinicians, parents and teachers often hope for and even demand) is scanty. The onset of hyperactivity symptoms during the first few years of life could be an indicator of poor outcome (Sandberg, Rutter & Taylor, 1978), but, even in this respect, the evidence is not clearly convincing: one of the few population studies in the field (Gillberg & Gillberg 1988) confirmed the presence of a 'pervasive hyperkinesis' syndrome with a less positive outlook for early teenage, but there appeared to be a fairly large subgroup even within this group, which showed a much better prognosis.

Table 13.1 *Attention disorders. Outcome studies.*

Study	N (male:female)	Approximate attrition compared with original study %	Source	Diagnosis	Contrast group (age-matched)	Specific treatment	Age at diagnosis (yrs)	Age at follow-up (yrs)	Outcome at follow-up
USA									
New York									
1. Gittelman *et al.*, 1985	101 (101:0)	2%	Referred to clinic for stimulant treatment	DSM-II hyperkinetic +questionnaire cross-situational attention deficit (Conners)	Male. Non-psychiatric clinic patients recruited at follow-up	Stimulant	6–12	16–23	40% ADD (DSM-III) 16% drugs other than alcohol 27% conduct/antisocial
2. Mannuzza & Gittelman, 1984	12 (0:12)	0%				Stimulant?	6–12	16–18	20% had multiple convictions according to official arrest records 25% ADD (DSM-III)
3. Mannuzza *et al.*, 1989 and Mannuzza *et al.*, 1991	94 (94:0)	10%	Referred to clinic for stimulant/behaviour treatment			Stimulant+ behaviour therapy	5–11	16–21	43% ADD (DSM-III) 10% drugs other than alcohol 32% conduct/antisocial
Milwaukee									
4. Fischer *et al.*, 1990 and Barkley *et al.*, 1990	123 (111:12)	22%	Consecutive referrals to clinic specialised in treatment of hyperactives	Parent-rated hyperactivity (Conners) +'teacher complaints' (DSM-III-R?)	Normal children of friends of parents in index group (approximately sexmatched)	Many treated with stimulants up until 48 hrs before study	4–12	12–20	72% ADHD (DSM-III-R) 60% conduct/oppositional/ defiant disorder 15-17% (DSM-III-R) marijuana use Academic failure in many
California									
5. Lambert *et al.*, 1987	59 (59:0)	?	Mixed medically identified and epidemiological survey cases	DSM-II hyperkinetic	Male random from same grade and school	Stimulant	9.9 (mean)	14.3 (mean) (>12)	43% reported to be still treated for hyperactivity
Vermont									
6. Howell *et al.*, 1985	49 (?:?)	29%	Rural epidemiological sample	>80th percentile on Huessy scale (similar to Conners)	80th percentile on Huessy scale	?	7(?)	22(?)	More antisocial acts and learning problems in high than low scorers (IQ 91 versus 105)

Table 13.1 (*cont.*)

Study	N (male:female)	Approximate attrition compared with original study %	Source	Diagnosis	Contrast group (age-matched)	Specific treatment	Age at diagnosis (yrs)	Age at follow-up (yrs)	Outcome at follow-up
Canada Montreal									
7. Hechtman & Weiss, 1986*	61	42%	Referred to Child Psychiatry Clinic for sustained hyperactivity at home and at school	Clinically based judgement – often in combination with learning disability, behavioural problems or neurotic problems	Normal high-school class mates (approximately sex-matched)	No 'sustained' stimulants Other 'acute' drug trials	6–12	21–23	Generally good outcome except in small subgroup 23% 'clinically' antisocial Better result could be due to this group having been followed into adult age. Many had had severe problems in adolescence
Sweden Göteborg									
8. Gillberg & Gillberg, 1988*	15 (11:4)	17%	Urban population screening	Extreme overactivity in 3 different settings. Cross-situational	Population groups with moderate over-activity and no overactivity	None	7	13	40%pervasivce overactivity 27% Conduct problem 70%School achievement problems 18% Asperger syndrome
9. Gillberg & Gillberg, 1989a* and Gillberg *et al.*, 1989*	42 (33:9)	0–11%	Urban population screening	ADD (DSM-III) in combination with mild/ moderate motor–perceptual problems	Population group without ADD	None	7	13	49% Attention deficit 40% Conduct disorder 60% School achievement problems 7% Asperger syndrome High rates of accidents and fractures
10. Hellgren *et al.*, 1993	42 (33:9)	0-8%	Urban population screening	ADD (DSM-III) in combination with mild/ moderate motor-perceptual problems	Population group without ADD	None	7	13	36% Overall motor clumsiness 13% Substance abuse 53% Delayed visual reaction time Even higher rates of accidents and fractures than at age 13

* included comprehensive assessment by psychiatrist both at entry and follow-up.

Thirdly, about a fourth to a third of hyperactive children show severe conduct problems/antisocial acts in teenage (Gittelman *et al.*, 1985; Hechtman & Weiss 1986; Gillberg *et al.*, 1989; Mannuzza *et al.*, 1991). In the Montreal study, there appeared to be a trend towards conduct/antisocial problems subsiding with increasing age (Hechtman & Weiss 1986). According to the New York studies, a large subgroup of 'hyperactives' have been involved in criminal activities, and a full 20% (compared with 2% in the normal contrast group) had had multiple convictions for criminal offences.

Related to the issue of antisocial activity outcome is the question of whether or not it would be possible to separate at an earlier stage those hyperactive children with a fair prognosis from those with a poor prognosis. In the New York study, the association between arrest history and childhood disorders of attention was mediated almost entirely by the occurrence of antisocial disorders in late adolescence and young adulthood (Mannuzza *et al.*, 1989). Continuing attention deficit disorder with hyperactivity at follow-up, by itself, was not associated with arrest history.

Fourthly, the incidence of drug use (other than alcohol) appears to be much higher in those with childhood hyperactivity than in those without. The rate of such drug use has been surprisingly stable in the US studies, ranging from 10–17% in teenage/early adult life in the hyperactive groups and 1–5% in the normal contrast groups. However, Hechtman and Weiss (1986) found no clear evidence of higher rates of illicit drug use in former hyperactives by the age of about 25 years. In the Swedish study, between 10 and 13% in the various groups with deficits in attention, motor control and perception, compared with 2% in the group without such problems, had substance abuse disorder at age 16.5 years. Only half of this proportion was accounted for by drugs other than alcohol (Hellgren *et al.*, 1993). As with antisocial behaviour, drug use in teenage/early adult life among those who had shown disorders of attention in childhood was strongly related to the occurrence of a conduct disorder by early teenage (Gittelman *et al.*, 1985; Barkley *et al.*, 1990; Mannuzza *et al.*, 1991).

The fifth conclusion is that, although there has been a great degree of variability across studies in respect to type of data reported, it appears that school achievement problems and academic failure may be one very important type of outcome in a large minority (perhaps even a majority) of those with childhood hyperactivity. The Swedish studies suggest that childhood disorders of attention predispose to reading disorders during the early and middle school years (Gillberg & Gillberg, 1989*a*) and that reading problems in the early teens reflect childhood attention disorders in at least 40% of the cases (Gillberg, 1987).

Finally, all the above conclusions pertain to boys only. Several of the cited studies have included only boys, and in those few that studied both sexes, the number of girls was too small for any generalised statements to be appropriate. There have been a very limited number of reports specifically geared to the study of outcome in girls with hyperactivity. Mannuzza and Gittelman (1984) reported on the adolescent outcome of 12 girls diagnosed hyperactive in childhood, and compared it to that of hyperactive boys and male control subjects. No differences emerged in respect of rate of mental disorder between hyperactive females and males. However, subjects were matched for age and social class and all cases had an IQ above 85, and these as well as other selection factors (the sample was not epidemiologically based) might have biased conclusions. James and Taylor (1990), in a clinical cross-sectional study, found clear differences between boys and girls with ICD-9 hyperkinetic syndrome: the girls had significantly higher rates of language disorders, neurological disorders and mental handicap. Unlike the New York group, the London group included a sample in which the majority of cases had IQs under 85.

A few other interesting hypotheses have emerged from the follow-up studies published so far. A subgroup of patients diagnosed as suffering from ADD or ADHD in early childhood may turn out to meet current criteria for Asperger syndrome (Gillberg & Gillberg, 1989*b*; Hellgren *et al.*, 1994). Children with Asperger syndrome often have 'concentration difficulties' and 'motor control problems' (Asperger, 1944; Wing, 1981), both of which are common features in attention disorders. Conversely, a number of children who have been given a 'primary' diagnosis of attention deficit disorder (in combination with motor control problems) show symptoms from Lorna Wing's 'triad' of social, communicative and behavioural impairments (Wing, 1991) or 'autistic features/psychotic behaviour' (Gillberg, 1983). The diagnosis of Asperger syndrome is not in widespread use in the US (although it has now been included in the DSM-IV (APA, 1994)), but is increasingly recognised as a useful clinical concept in Europe. It is generally believed that genetic factors play a major role in the pathogenetic chain of events in this syndrome and that there is a major risk that symptoms of the disorder will persist throughout childhood and adolescence well into adult life (Frith, 1991). The finding of a link between attention disorder and Asperger syndrome in some cases, if upheld by other studies, could indicate that there is a certain degree of overlap between so called 'autism spectrum disorders' and attention disorders (Gillberg, 1992).

Not highlighted in the studies reviewed here, but certainly evident in the literature on Tourette syndrome, is the link between attention disorders and tics (Comings, 1990). Virtually all studies of Tourette syndrome (currently believed to exist in at least 0.1% of all school-age children (Ehlers & Gillberg, 1993) acknowledge the presence of attentional problems in young people with tics.

However, tics have not generally received much attention in the study of hyperactivity syndromes or attention deficits. Nevertheless, it appears that attention problems are almost part and parcel of the full-blown Tourette syndrome (Shapiro *et al.,* 1988). Recently, there has been mention of a possible link between the Tourette and Asperger syndromes (Realmuto & Main, 1982; Burd *et al.,* 1987; Ritvo *et al.,* 1990; Gillberg 1992; Ehlers and Gillberg, 1993). It is quite conceivable that those young people with attention deficits who also meet criteria for Tourette and/or Asperger syndrome might represent a specific subgroup, genetically different from the other attention disorders. A clinical impression gained over the years by the present authors is that the attention deficits associated with the Tourette and Asperger syndromes are of a different quality than those encountered in the larger group of attention disorders generally. Whereas, in an unselected group of children and adolescents with attention deficits, these are often associated with hyperactivity and inability to sit still (observed restlessness), in the Tourette and Asperger syndromes the attention deficits encountered are often associated with a feeling of restlessness but no, or only mildly, reduced ability to be still. Impulsivity may more often be a feature of Tourette syndrome (Landgren *et al.,* 1996), but more rarely so of other disorders comprising attention deficits. To be sure, there are cases with Asperger syndrome and Tourette syndrome who resemble those with attention disorders generally and who have clear problems controlling their activity level, but, by and large, there appear to be qualitative differences between these and the other cases with attention disorders.

The interrelationships between attention disorders, tics, Tourette syndrome and Asperger syndrome suggest that 'ADHD' covers a heterogeneous group of disorders in which attention problems or hyperactivity may be important features but not necessarily the only key problem.

Another finding, suggested by at least two of the follow-up studies reviewed in this section (Howell *et al.,* 1985; Gillberg & Gillberg, 1989*b*) – and supported by findings from cross-sectional studies (Taylor *et al.,* 1986) and follow-up studies of ADD-related problems (e.g. Astbury *et al.,* 1990) – is that children with disorders of attention may be considerably more 'accident prone' and more likely to suffer fractures than matched comparison children. The association of attention dificit disorder with accidents (such as ingestion of washing-up detergent and bicycle accidents) could be due to attention problems, impulsivity, motor control problems, perceptual difficulties or associated behaviour problems and risks related to these – or any combination of problems of this kind. In the Swedish study, there was a four-fold increase in the number of accidents requiring hospital admission sustained by the DAMP group as compared with the non-DAMP group already at age 13 years (24% and 6%, respectively, $p<.05$) and the difference was even more pronounced at age 16 and 22 years (Hellgren *et al.,* 1993; Gillberg, personal communication).

The Swedish studies suggest that an associated major psychiatric disorder other than ADD/ADHD is common (Gillberg, 1983). Asperger syndrome and other autistic-type features appear to be relatively common in the most severely affected cases, whereas conduct disorders and depressive syndromes abound in the mildly to moderately attention disordered groups. Conduct and depressive disorders were particularly evident around age 10 years. At age 13 and 16 years, psychiatric/behavioural/emotional problems were still present in more than half of all cases having received a DAMP-diagnosis at age 7 years, but the clinical picture was more varied. Nevertheless, at age 16.5 years, DSM-III-R affective and anxiety disorders were common relative to the comparison group without DAMP. Personality disorders involving restriction of social interaction (paranoid, schizotypal, schizoid, avoidant or obsessive–compulsive) were much more common in the DAMP group, affecting about one in three, compared to fewer than one in ten in the non-DAMP comparison group. Off all individuals in the DAMP group (0% in the comparison group) 10% had suffered at least one episode of mania (Hellgren *et al.*, 1994). Also, some clinical follow-up studies suggest that a subgroup of young children with ADHD go on to develop tics and Tourette syndrome around age 10 years and then to affective disorders (including mania) at a later age (teenage) (Biedermann *et al.,* 1994).

Furthermore, motor control problems seem to abate with time in many, but not all cases (Gillberg *et al.,* 1989). Whereas a vast majority of children with severe cross-situational attention deficit show motor control problems during the early school years (Rasmussen *et al.,* 1983), only 55% still do so at age 10 years, and 30% continue to show such problems (as compared with a contrast group of children without motor–perceptual and attentional deficits) at age 16 years. Finally, some studies (Hechtman & Weiss, 1986; Gillberg, 1987; Barkley *et al.,* 1990) indicate that the family status changed (parental divorce, father changes jobs, moves etc) much more often during the course of the follow-up studies in children with hyperactivity than in normal children.

Some of the particular problems and assets of the longitudinal follow-up studies reviewed will be briefly highlighted here. The New York studies (Gittelman *et al.,* 1985; Mannuzza & Gittelman, 1984; Mannuzza *et al.,* 1989; 1991) are among the best with regard to reliability and validity aspects of the follow-up measures used. They also have included large enough numbers to allow reasonable statistical comparisons and they have tried specifically to address the special (if any) problems encountered by females with childhood hyperactivity. On the other hand, the original material is likely to have been biased by the fact that all cases had been referred to a specialised clinic for

Table 13.2. *Outcome in DAMP (deficits in attention, motor control and perception) diagnosed at age 7 years. Follow-up findings at age 10,13 and 16 years. Percentage showing problem at follow-up age.* (Figures in brackets refer to findings in non-DAMP age-matched controls examined blind as to group status).

Outcome variable	7	10	13	16 years
Attention deficits	100 (0)	60	50	45
Motor control problems	100 (0)	55	30	36
Learning disorder/ perceptual deficits*	67 (0)	80	67	n.e.
Psychiatric disorder/ behaviour problem	64 (64)	80	67	64
Accidents	5	10	25	32
Psychiatric treatment (cumulative)	40	42	55	68

* all cases had IQ>70.
n.e. = not evaluated.
Based on findings from studies reported in Gillberg *et al.*, 1985, Gillberg *et al.*, 1989, and Hellgren *et al.*, 1994.

some kind of treatment. Furthermore, a majority of the cases received stimulant treatment. It is also unclear whether the comparison group can be seen as representative of the general population.

The Milwaukee studies (Fischer *et al.*, 1990; Barkley *et al.*, 1990) show roughly the same type of strengths and weaknesses. The fact that the parents of hyperactive children were actively involved in selecting the comparison group of children could have introduced further bias and skewing of results.

The California study (Lambert *et al.*, 1987) is too sketchily described to allow detailed evaluation of assets and drawbacks. Also, as in the New York and Milwaukee studies, stimulant treatment of the index group was the rule rather than the exception.

The Vermont sample (Howell *et al.*, 1985) has the advantage of being a (rural) population group, but the level of clinical investigation both at the time of entry into the study and at the time of follow-up was rather low.

The Montreal studies (Hechtman & Weiss, 1986) appear to have been 'in-depth', performed on a reasonably large group and including an acceptable comparison group. Also, sustained stimulant treatment was not used. However, the attrition was large (42% lost to follow-up), and the original sample may have been biased because of referral selection bias.

The Göteborg studies (e.g. Gillberg *et al.*, 1989) have the advantage of being the only clearly population-based 'in depth' study in the field. Longitudinal follow-up (by psychiatrists blind to original group status), after original screening at age 6, has been performed at age 7, 10, 13, and 16 years (Hellgren *et al.,* 1994) (and follow-up at age 21 years is on-going). These studies are the only ones which have included detailed neurodevelopmental examination at all follow-up ages. None of the cases has received specific treatments (Table 13.2).

The main problem with this set of studies is the fact that motor–perceptual dysfunction (MPD), as well as cross-situational attention deficit, were required for entry into the study. (The combination of ADD and MPD has been labelled DAMP (deficits in attention, motor control and perception) by the Swedish group). Even though it seems reasonable to assume that minor/moderate motor–perceptual problems have been present in hyperactive subjects of most other follow-up studies also, there is currently no way of finding out how comparable the subjects in the Swedish studies are to those of the US and Canadian groups. Also, the number of cases included is rather small.

Brief mention of the interesting longitudinal study of criminal development in a low social class population sample performed by David Farrington and his group is warranted. Farrington recently reanalysed his data to provide some clues as to the contribution of childhood inattention to later criminal outcome (Farrington, Loeber & van Kammen, 1990). It needs emphasising that Farrington did not delineate a clinical syndrome of hyperactivity/inattention, but used prospectively gathered information obtained from teachers, parents, children and peers retrospectively to assign indices of hyperactivity/inattention, on the one hand, and conduct problems on the other. The 411 males originally included in the study were derived from a working class area in London. The probands were followed up at ages 8, 10, 14, 16, 18, 21 and 25 years using various measures and with varying degree of comprehensiveness. The main object of the study was to identify precursors of later criminal behaviour. It was established that the measure of inattention/hyperactivity predicted later criminality partly independently of the measure of conduct problems. Inattention/hyperactivity was particularly predictive of early conviction (but not adult conviction) and contributed strongly to the development of chronic offending (more than six convictions before age 25 years), which, in turn, occurred only in a small subgroup of the general population sample. Inattention/hyperactivity and conduct problems were partly correlated with different sets of background factors. This and other aspects of the findings (such as the association of inattention/hyperactivity with learning problems) led the authors to conclude that hyperactivity and conduct problems 'are distinctly different disorders'. Their results convincingly demonstrate that inattention and conduct problems may represent two, at least partly, discrete – but partly overlapping – dimensions of behaviour, but not that they are different disorders. As the authors themselves note, no measures were used which had been specifically designed for the study of disorders with modern criteria in mind. Also, their inclusion of 'daring' behaviour as a sign of inattention and not of conduct problem appears slightly confusing. Nevertheless, the Farrington studies add to the evidence that inattention/hyperactivity can be usefully separated from conduct problems and that while both types of behaviour may predict similar outcomes, they may do so along partly different pathways and on the basis of partly different mechanisms.

Finally, the studies of Schaughency and colleagues in New Zealand warrant some discussion. A whole birth cohort of Dunedin children born in the early 1970s was studied. Out of 943 children examined at age 15 years, only 4 (0.4%) met full DSM-III criteria for ADD. Several more met the criteria for operationally defined attention dysfunction, but only a minority of these were reported both by the 15 year-olds and their parents. About half the group with attention dysfunction had a history of ADD, whereas the other half had 'late onset' ADD symptoms. Both groups received more comorbid diagnoses, and had experienced more adverse educational and social outcomes at both age 15 and 18 years than those with 'non-ADD' (Schaughency *et al.,* 1994). This is an excellent study, but the number of clearly clinically significant cases of ADD is much too small for generalised conclusions to be drawn.

RECENT CONTROLLED FOLLOW-UP STUDIES OF PROBLEMS WHICH ARE OFTEN ASSOCIATED WITH DISORDERS OF ATTENTION

The follow-up and follow-back studies of language delayed and behaviourally impaired children merit brief mention here because of the strong association of attention disorders with language delay and behaviour problems. At least 40% of children who exhibit DAMP at age 7 years have shown clearly delayed language development according to maternal report as compared with 2% of children who do not exhibit DAMP (Rasmussen & Gillberg, 1983). Significant language impairment – clinically significant language or speech impairment (not mild dysarticulation) leading to referral for speech therapy – was present in 46% of the DAMP children but in none of the children without DAMP at age 7 years (Rasmussen *et al.,* 1983). Almost 90% of the DAMP group compared to 10% of those without DAMP had some (mild, moderate or severe) language or speech impairment (including mild dysarticulation). In a recent selective review of studies of early language delay as a predictor of later reading failure Stevenson (1988) concluded that 50–75% of children showing approximately

9 months' language delay at age 3 years (which applies to 3–4.9% of the general population according to Fundudis, Kolvin & Garside (1979), Stevenson and Graham (1982), and Silva, McGee & Williams (1983)), experience either IQ under 85, reading problems or behaviour problems at age 8 years. 'Behaviour problems' were not specifically defined in the relevant studies but were measured by the Rutter teacher or parent scales (Rutter, 1967; Rutter, Tizard & Whitmore, 1970). This scale includes several items reflecting problems associated with attention disorders.

It is quite clear that disorders of speech and language (now often referred to as 'specific language impairment' (SLI) in spite of the lack of specificity of this broad concept) are rarely isolated phenomena but rather represent one group of several co-morbid problems, including attention deficits, unspecific behaviour problems, motor control problems, reading problems and 'perceptual' abnormalities of various kinds. 'Auditory perceptual impairments' are strongly associated with SLI (Tallal *et al.,* 1981), but it is unclear to what extent such impairments also underlie/covary with 'attention deficit' and the complex web of problems associated with it (Bishop, 1992). The association of attention problems with SLI brings out the important issue as to which of these diagnoses should be considered 'more important'. Even if one decides that the evidence is not there to suggest that one is more basic than the other, the clinical problem of choosing the most appropriate screening device (if screening is considered important) cannot be overlooked. Also, the literature in both fields (language and attention/behaviour oriented) tends to – largely – disregard the existence of the other. This has left us in a situation in which language specialists diagnose SLI and child psychiatrists diagnose ADHD or psychiatric disorder in general (and developmental paediatricians diagnose delayed motor development and teachers diagnose reading problems) in groups of children with a developmental disorder affecting many different aspects of functioning and presenting with variable clinical symptoms depending on such factors as age, sex and social–educational circumstances, to mention but a few. By pretending that attention disorders is one class of disorder and language disorder a very different one we are creating parallel paths of scientific development which may be counterproductive in the process of trying to develop appropriate clinical intervention strategies.

Motor control problems in childhood are common associated problems in disorders of attention. Losse *et al.* (1991) studied outcome from mean age of 6 years to 16 years in a group of 17 'clumsy' and 17 'non-clumsy' London children (sex ratio 14:3 in both groups). At age 6 years there had been non-significant trends towards lower verbal and performance IQs in the 'clumsy' group, but both groups were well within normal IQ ranges. At follow-up verbal

IQ was significantly lower in the 'clumsy' group. The 'clumsy' group remained clumsy on a number of motor measures. They also showed more emotional and behaviour problems including social interaction problems and attention deficits (more than half of the 'clumsy' group showed persisting problems of this type). These findings are in accord with the Göteborg studies reported in the previous section: many children with attention deficits and motor control problems show persistent clumsiness, attention problems and social interaction problems throughout teenage (Gillberg & Gillberg 1988). The results also corroborate those of Roussonis and Gaussen (1987) in Leeds (UK) who found motor clumsiness (even though less pronounced) to persist from age 5 1/2 years through age 7 1/2 years (17 clumsy and 17 'control' cases, sex ratios 11:6 in both groups). Furthermore, the clumsy children showed impaired educational attainment and they were more fidgety and showed poorer conduct than control cases.

Very low birthweight (VLBW) survivors have been followed from birth to pre-school and school age in a number of studies. Several children in such follow-up studies show 'ADD'. Astbury *et al.* (1990) followed 57 Melbourne VLBW children through age 2 and 5 years. DSM-III-ADD was diagnosed in 23 (40%) at age 2 years. Of these, 18 still showed ADD at age 5 years. At least two further children not diagnosed as ADD at age 2 years, received this diagnosis at age 5 years. The ADD group had significantly more motor control problems, lower IQ, more conduct problems, 'minor surgery' and 'hospital admissions' than the non-ADD group. Thus, within a sample of VLBW children (< 1500 g), the risk of developing ADD during the pre-school years appears to be increased manifold as compared with the general population. The presence of ADD also predicts clumsiness, cognitive/learning problems and accident proneness to a considerable extent. Children with even lower birthweights appear to have an even higher risk of developing attention disorders and learning problems (Hack *et al.*, 1994).

Behaviour and school achievement, at the age of nine years were studied in singletons without (*n*=230), with minimally (*n*=205) and moderately (*n*=133) abnormal results on neurological examination in the newborn period (Hadders-Algra *et al.,* 1988). Overtly handicapped children were excluded. School failure was predicted by moderately abnormal neurological status in the newborn period and by social class. The neurological status and male sex also contributed to the development of ADD type problems and to motor clumsiness at age 9 years.

In a study from Pittsburgh, Campbell and Elwing (1990) followed 'hard-to-manage' pre-schoolers from age 3 to 4, 6, and 9 years. They found that, of the 15 children who showed persistent behaviour problems by age 6 years, 10

(67%) still showed an externalising disorder (mostly 'ADDH') at age 9 years. Among those 14 children who had improved by age 6 years, 4 (29%) were given a diagnosis of an externalising disorder at age 9 years. This was true also of 4 of the 24 (16%) original 'not-hard-to-manage' pre-schoolers. This study adds to the evidence that disorders of attention often show as unspecific behaviour problems in infancy and early childhood (Richman, Stevenson & Graham, 1982) and that, once recognised as belonging in the ADDH – ADHD – DAMP class of disorders, show a high degree of stability across time.

STUDIES OF OUTCOME IN RELATION TO TREATMENT

No long-term follow-up studies of the effects of stimulant treatment of childhood hyperactivity have been able to answer the critical question whether or not medication predicts overall long-term behavioural improvement (see Jacobvitz *et al.* (1990) for a recent overview). That there are certain short-term benefits, such as improved attention, behaviour (including reduction of negativistic, 'conduct disordered' behaviours), social interaction, family interaction and performance (accurate school-work completed) cannot be in doubt (Gadow, 1992), but the extent to which benefits are also there in a 'several years perspective' is not known.

Even though long-term beneficial effects of stimulant treatment of attention disorders have not been adequately demonstrated, there is considerable evidence that long-term adverse effects are not a major problem. Teachers rating the behaviour of hyperactive children in the classroom actually report more side-effects if children are on placebo than if they are on stimulant treatment. During the 50-year history of stimulant treatment of hyperactive disorders, concern has been expressed that growth could be stunted and depression, tic disorder, psychosis and drug abuse provoked. Ultimate height is not significantly reduced in most cases after chronic stimulant drug therapy (Roche *et al.*, 1979; Klein & Mannuzza, 1988), but there may be temporary reductions of growth in height in mid-adolescence (Gittelman-Klein *et al.*, 1988). Depressive symptoms appear to be ameliorated rather than provoked, at least in the short-term perspective (Barkley *et al.*, 1990; Klorman *et al.*, 1990). Tic disorders are probably not provoked *de novo* in hyperactive children receiving stimulant treatment, but could possibly sometimes be exacerbated when present as a co-morbid problem already at the start of therapy (for a review, see Gadow, 1992). There is some evidence that stimulant treatment may be a safe and effective form of intervention in children with attention disorders and tics

(Konkol, Fischer & Newby, 1990). Development of psychosis or drug abuse are not important risks in the overall panorama of effects and side-effects in stimulant treatment of attention disorders. However, depending on the type of underlying aetiology, the possibility of differential outcomes in this respect has to be acknowledged (Jacobvitz *et al.*, 1990). Stimulant treatment has, almost 'by tradition' been banned from the treatment of children with autism because it was believed that 'psychotic symptoms' might be triggered. However, there is no good empirical evidence to suggest any connection of this kind. However, there is some evidence that overfocused obsessive/compulsive behaviours are fairly common features in attention disordered children who receive stimulant medication (Borcherding *et al.,* 1990). Dosage adjustment and the selection of a different type of stimulant drug can sometimes help alleviate such problems. Severe self-injury can occasionally occur in children treated with stimulants (Sokol *et al.,* 1987).

What is needed now are longer-term studies of the effects of stimulant treatment compared with other types of intervention. The issues relating to the widely discrepant levels of stimulant prescription in the US (very frequent), and in Europe (rare or very rare), should be addressed.

A recent study comparing the effects of information to parents and teachers with those of individual psychotherapy to the child for a school year, motor training for a school year, and no intervention around the time of school entry in a group of 6 year-old children with DAMP (= ADD + motor, perceptual dysfunction)/recruited after general population screening, indicated that outcome at age 10 years was better in the group of children who, together with parents and teachers received information about the diagnosis as such but then had no further specific intervention (Gillberg, Winnergård & Gillberg, 1993). However, the conclusions of that study have to be very cautious, because of the small number of children included (n=25) and several methodological problems in assessing the outcome status of the patients.

NEUROPHYSIOLOGICAL/NEURODEVELOPMENTAL ASPECTS IN RELATION TO OUTCOME

Satterfield *et al.* (1990) examined 15 boys with ADDH (DSM-III) – who also met ADHD (DSM-III-R) criteria – and 15 normal boys at age 6 years and again at age 7 years 8 months. They recorded auditory and visual event-related potentials (ERP) in these boys. The degree of abnormality in the so called P3b responses to target stimuli in ADHD boys (lower than normal boys) was found to increase with age. The P3b is one of several endogenous-evoked brain waves elicited by selectively attending to stimuli from the environment. It is generally believed to reflect cognitive processing after discrimination and decision to act (automatically) on a stimulus has occurred. Its appearance and amplitude could signal revision, updating of memory and 'intrachannel stimulus selection'. The authors suggested that an insufficient noradrenergic drive from the locus coeruleus might be partly responsible for the abnormally low P3b response. Thus, noradrenaline could be involved in the learning and attentional processes by augmenting neural responsivity to novel or important events or by habituating the brain's responses to repetitious or unimportant events. Hypothetically, improved attention with central stimulant treatment could be linked to the effect of such treatment on the locus coeruleus.

In another study, Satterfield, Schell & Backs (1987) found abnormal auditory ERP maturational changes in 25 children with hyperactivity who had not developed delinquent behaviour 8 years after the initial evaluation (at age 6–12 years). Nine 'hyperactives' with delinquent behaviour showed the same type of maturational change as did the 34 non-delinquent normal children. The findings suggested that, from the neurophysiological point of view, delinquent and non-delinquent ADDH cases may represent different clinical entities. Neither subgroup could be considered to represent a 'maturational lag' theory: the non-delinquents were clearly abnormal and the delinquents normal. The authors suggested that those ADDH boys without CNS dysfunction who later become delinquent have their disorder as consequence of social/environmental factors, whereas the non-delinquent ADDH boys show hyperactivity/attention deficit because of underlying neuronal impairment.

In one study, not specifically addressing attention deficits, underarousal of the central and autonomic nervous systems at age 15 years (as measured electrodermally and by monitoring heart rate and power spectral density EEG) correctly classified 75% of cases of criminality at age 24 years (Raine, Venables & Williams, 1990). Underarousal has been proposed by several groups to be an important background factor in attention disorders and hyperactivity (Hastings & Barkley, 1978). (See also Chapter 7 for a full review of neurophysiological studies.)

The Göteborg longitudinal studies of DAMP (= ADD + motor/perception dysfunction) showed that behavioural and school achievement problems tended to persist, even in those many cases showing gradual amelioration of motor control problems. The implication was that children with ADHD examined in teenage might have no obvious motor–perception difficulties even in cases with such problems prominent at age 6–7 years (Gillberg *et al.,* 1989). There was also a clear tendency for a subgroup of attention deficient children (about one in four of the whole original group diagnosed at age 6–7 years) to show persistent motor control problems throughout teenage (Hellgren *et al.*, 1993). Whether or not this group has a better or worse prognosis from the point of view of delinquency (cf. the Satterfield study referred to in the previous section) has yet to be determined.

FOLLOW-BACK AND CROSS-SECTIONAL STUDIES

In a study of 56 adults (48 males, 8 females) (aged 19–65 years) who presented with adult ADHD, psychiatric co-morbidity was found to be at a very high level (Shekim *et al.*, 1990). Generalised anxiety disorder was found in 53%, alcohol abuse in 34%, drug abuse in 30%, dysthymic disorder in 25% and cyclothymic disorder in 25%. Only 13% received no other DSM-III-R diagnosis than ADHD.

The findings differ markedly from those of the longitudinal follow-up studies, in particular as regards generalised anxiety disorder. Of the 194 probands in the New York studies, not a single one met criteria for generalised anxiety disorder.

Selection factors are likely to contribute to atypical findings in follow-back studies of this kind. The sample as such is probably biased towards cases with psychiatric/emotional problems causing personal rather than 'external' suffering. In other words, anxiety disorders, even if – hypothetically – extremely rare in ADHD generally, might be a common companion of attention problems in those patients who suffer themselves and therefore apply for psychiatric help. This is only one of the reasons why follow-back studies cannot contribute to the understanding of the relative scope of problems associated with disorders of attention during the course of development.

In an epidemiological study of teenage psychosis, DAMP (deficits in attention, motor control and perception) was found to be an extremely common associated factor according to 'prospectively blind' data in school health reports (Hellgren, Gillberg & Enerskog, 1987).

A study employing both a cross-sectional design and longitudinal and follow-back data was performed by Moffitt (1990). In the Dunedin longitudinal follow-up study, four groups of boys were identified at age 13 years: (i) ADD (DSM-III criteria) without delinquency (*n*= 16); (ii) ADD with delinquency (*n*= 19); (iii) delinquents without ADD (*n*= 52); and (iv) non-disordered (*n*= 348). The boys in group (i) had normal IQ and reading scores and had normal family relationships. They showed mild and transient conduct problems in middle childhood. Those in group (ii) had low verbal IQ and reading scores and poor family conditions. Their conduct problems dated from before school entry and persisted into adolescence. Group (iii) did not show major early risk factors and remained relatively free of conduct problems, until at age 13 years they initiated delinquency. This study is interesting not only because of the original design but also because it adds considerable strength to the notion that it is the combination of ADD and conduct/antisocial/delinquency problems which predicts a poor outcome.

CASE STUDIES

The follow-up studies seem to agree that major affective illness and schizophrenia are no more common outcomes in groups of children with disorders of attention than in groups without such problems. However, since ADHD (counting in many per cent) is very common and schizophrenia with onset under age 20 years very rare (amounting to no more than 0.2% of the population in that age range), a connection might exist which would not show up in follow-up studies of ADHD unless very large numbers of cases were included. The case for a possible connection was highlighted in the teenage psychosis study by Hellgren *et al.* (1987).

A recent publication (Schmidt & Freidson, 1990) described two cases of 'psychotic' breakdown at age 13 years in boys with ADHD diagnosed during the early school years who had initially responded well to stimulant medication. One boy had signs suggestive of schizophrenia and the other of bipolar affective disorder. The authors acknowledge that these may be atypical outcomes. However, the longitudinal follow-up studies which have been published to this date have not gone into 'developmental' detail in this respect. There is a need in future follow-up studies of attention deficit disorder to look in more detail for signs and symptoms suggestive of 'psychosis' disturbance.

The value of careful individual case studies as a complement to large scale controlled studies should not be underestimated. Case studies can often be the starting point for generating new hypotheses for testing in controlled systematic studies. They also serve the purpose of bridging the gap between clinicians and researchers by highlighting in a concentrated format issues relating to treatment and follow-up, which might not immediately present themselves in the findings of a larger-scale study.

CONCLUSIONS

In conclusion, there is still a great need for population-based controlled longitudinal follow-up studies of children who show early onset disorders of attention. The few studies that exist in the field are hampered by many deficiencies and even some of the most consistent findings remain open to some doubt. Nevertheless, it seems safe to assume that (i) many children continue to show persistent attentional problems well into adolescence and early adult life, (ii) a subgroup develop severe conduct/antisocial problems, (iii) this subgroup has a poor prognosis with regard to continued conduct/antisocial problems and – to some extent with regard to illicit drug use also, (iv) many, perhaps the majority, face school achievement problems, (v) associated disorders, other than conduct problems, are common and include learning disorders, motor control problems and minor injuries/fractures, (vi) some grow out of attentional problems and do well by early adult age.

The effects of treatment on the long-term outcome are poorly understood and prospective controlled (placebo or otherwise) intervention studies are much in need. Future outcome studies need to consider disorders of attention in a broader perspective, acknowledging the comparative lack of 'pure' cases, the overlap with conduct and 'empathy' disorders and the relationship with various measures of neurodevelopmental dysfunction. Population samples are needed to study the natural history of the disorder. Clinic referred samples can be helpful in a given cultural setting but results derived on the basis of such samples do not necessarily generalise to other populations of children in other countries, or even in other cities. The number of population studies in the field of attention deficit disorders is so small that there is considerable scope for doubting many of the rather poorly underpinned conclusions. In particular, the evidence for a distinct syndrome of hyperactivity, clearly delineated *vis-à-vis* other child psychiatric disorders, and motor–perceptual–language disorders, is scant. However, this is true of a number of other so called child psychiatric disorders as well, including conduct disorder.

There is still good reason to consider Thorley´s proposition that attention deficits and hyperactivity may best be regarded as dimensional problems that cut across other diagnostic entities, and that, as such, they may have considerable prognostic impact even if they do not qualify for the status of true 'disorder'. In this respect, problems of inattention and activity regulation might best be conceptualised along lines familiar to researchers in the field of mental retardation: intellectual deficiency is not a syndrome or disorder, but a very important feature, which is shared by a number of syndromes and disorders, and which is often a better prognostic instrument than the diagnosis of the disorder as such. For instance, attentional problems are very common in Tourette syndrome; perhaps the overall outcome in that disorder is better predicted by the presence or absence of attention deficits than by the presence or absence of Tourette syndrome as such. Severe attention problems are also common in autism (Gillberg, 1989) and epilepsy (Ounsted, Lindsay & Richards, 1987) and it is possible that attention problems contribute to poor outcome in these 'disorders' also. Therefore, so long as we do not have specific biological or psychological 'markers' for attention deficits, it is prudent (and probably wise) to consider attentional functions as dimensional rather than the matrix for a simple dichotomous distinction between normality and disorder.

REFERENCES

American Psychiatric Association (1980). *Diagnostic and Statistical Manual of Mental Disorders*, Third Edition. Washington, DC: APA.

American Psychiatric Association (1987). *Diagnostic and Statistical Manual of Mental Disorders*, (3rd edn. – revised). Washington, DC: APA.

American Psychiatric Association (1994). *Diagnostic and Statistical Manual of Mental Disorders*, (4th edn). Washington, DC: APA.

Asperger, H. (1944). Die autistischen Psychopathen im Kindesalter. *Archiv für Psychiatrie und Nervenkrankheiten*, **117,** 76–136.

Astbury, J., Orgill, A. A., Bajuk, B. & Yu, V. Y. (1990). Neurodevelopmental outcome, growth and health of extremely low-birthweight survivors: how soon can we tell? *Developmental Medicine and Child Neurology*, **32**, 582–9.

Barkley, R. A., Fischer, M., Edelbrock, C. S. & Smallish, L. (1990). The adolescent outcome of hyperactive children diagnosed by research criteria. I. An 8 year prospective follow-up study. *Journal of the American Academy of Child and Adolescent Psychiatry*, **29**, 546–57.

Biederman, J., Spencer, T., Wilens, T. & Wozniak, J. (1994). *Current Concepts in Psychotherapy and Pharmacotherapy and Issues in Co-morbidity and the Treatment of ADHD in Children and Adolescents.* Paper presented at the CHADD Conference on Attention Deficit Disorders. A Global Perspective (October 13–15, 1994), New York.

Bishop, D. (1992). The underlying nature of specific language impairment. *Journal of Child Psychology and Psychiatry*, **33**, 3–66.

Borcherding, B. G., Keysor, C. S., Rapoport, J. L., Elia, J. & Amass, J. (1990). Motor/vocal tics and compulsive behaviors on stimulant drugs: is there a common vulnerability? *Psychiatry Research*, **33**, 83–94.

Burd, L., Fisher, W.W., Kerbeshiam, J. & Arnold, M.E. (1987). Is development of Tourette disorder a marker for improvement in patients with autism and other pervasive developmental disorders? *Journal of the American Academy of Child and Adolescent Psychiatry*, **26**, 162–5.

Campbell, S. B. & Ewing, L. (1990). Follow-up of hard-to-manage preschoolers: adjustment at age 9 and predictors of continuing symptoms. *Journal of Child Psychology and Psychiatry*, **31**, 871–89.

Comings, D. (1990). *Tourette Syndrome and Human Behavior*. Duarte, CA: Hope Press.

Ehlers, S. & Gillberg, C. (1993). The epidemiology of Asperger syndrome. A total population study. *Journal of Child Psychology and Psychiatry*, **34**, 1327–50.

Farrington, D. P., Loeber, R. & van Kammen, W. B. (1990). Long-term criminal outcomes of hyperactivity-impulsivity-attention deficit and conduct problems in childhood. In *Straight and Devious Pathways from Childhood and Adulthood*, eds. L. Robins & M. Rutter, pp. 72–73. Cambridge: Cambridge University Press.

Fischer, M., Barkley, R. A., Edelbrock, C. S. & Smallish, L. (1990). The adolescent outcome of hyperactive children diagnosed by research criteria: II. Academic, attentional, and neuropsychological status. *Journal of Consulting and Clinical Psychology*, **58,** 580–8.

Frith, U. (ed.) (1991). *Autism and Asperger Syndrome*. Cambridge: Cambridge University Press.

Fundudis, T., Kolvin, I. & Garside, R. F. (1979). *Speech Retarded and Deaf Children: Their Psychological Development*. London: Academic Press.

Gadow, K. D. (1992). Pediatric psychopharmacotherapy: a review of recent research. *Journal of Child Psychology and Psychiatry*, **33**, 153–95.

Gillberg, C. (1983). Psychotic behaviour in children and young adults in a mental handicap hostel. *Acta Psychiatrica Scandinavica*, **68**, 351–8.

Gillberg, C. (1989). Autism: neurobiological correlates. *Current Opinion in Psychiatry*, **2**, 93–7.

Gillberg, C. (1992). The Emanuel Miller Memorial Lecture 1991: Autism and autistic-like conditions: subclasses among disorders of empathy. *Journal of Child Psychology and Psychiatry*, **33**, 813–42.

Gillberg, C. & Gillberg, I. C. (1988). Children with deficits in attention, motor control and perception (DAMP): need for specialist treatment. *Acta Paediatrica Scandinavica*, **77**, 450–1.

Gillberg, C., Gillberg, I. C. & Rasmussen, P. (1985). Minimal brain dysfunction. In *Risks of Labour*, ed. J. W. Crawford, pp. 147–55. New York: Wiley.

Gillberg, I. C. (1987). *Deficits in Attention, Motor Control and Perception: Follow-up from Pre-School to Early Teens*. MD Thesis, University of Uppsala.

Gillberg, I. C. & Gillberg, C. (1989*a*). Children with preschool minor neurodevelopmental disorders. IV: Behaviour and school achievement at age 13. *Developmental Medicine and Child Neurology*, **31**, 3–13.

Gillberg, I. C. & Gillberg, C. (1989*b*). Asperger syndrome – some epidemiological considerations: a research note. *Journal of Child Psychology and Psychiatry*, **30**, 631–8.

Gillberg, I. C., Gillberg, C. & Groth, J. (1989). Children with preschool minor neurodevelopmental disorders. V: Neurodevelopmental profiles at age 13. *Developmental Medicine and Child Neurology*, **31**, 14–24.

Gillberg, I. C., Winnergård, I. & Gillberg, C. (1993). Screening methods, epidemiology and evaluation of intervention in DAMP in preschool children. *European Child and Adolescent Psychiatry*, **2**, 121–35.

Gittelman, R., Mannuzza, S., Shenker, R. & Bonagura, N. (1985). Hyperactive boys almost grown up: I. Psychiatric status. *Archives of General Psychiatry*, **42**, 937–47.

Gittelman-Klein, R., Landa, B., Mattes, J. A. & Klein, D. F. (1988). Methylphenidate and growth in hyperactive children. *Archives of General Psychiatry*, **45**, 1127–30.

Hack, M., Taylor, H. G., Klein, N., Eiben, R., Schatschneider, C. & Mercuri-Minich, N. (1994). School-age outcomes in children with birth weights under 750 g. *New England Journal of Medicine*, **331**, 802–3.

Hadders-Algra, M., Huisjes, H. J. & Touwen, B. C. L. (1988). Perinatal risk factors and minor neurological dysfunction: significance for behaviour and school achievement at nine years. *Developmental Medicine and Child Neurology*, **30**, 482–91.

Hastings, J. E. & Barkley, R. A. (1978). A review of psychophysiological research with hyperkinetic children. *Journal of Abnormal Child Psychology*, **6**, 413–48.

Hechtman, L. & Weiss, G. (1986). Controlled prospective fifteen year follow-up of hyperactives as adults: non-medical drug and alcohol use and anti-social behaviour. *Canadian Journal of Psychiatry*, **31**, 557–67.

Hellgren, L., Gillberg, C. & Enerskog, I. (1987). Antecedents of adolescent psychoses: a population-based study of school health problems in children who develop psychosis in adolescence. *Journal of the American Academy of Child and Adolescent Psychiatry*, **26**, 351–5.

Hellgren, L., Gillberg, C., Gillberg, I. C. & Enerskog, I. (1993). Children with deficits in attention, motor control and perception (DAMP) almost grown up. General health at age 16 years. *Developmental Medicine and Child Neurology*, **35**, 881–92.

Hellgren, L., Gillberg, I. C., Bågenholm, A. & Gillberg, C. (1994). Children with Deficits in Attention, Motor control and Perception (DAMP) almost grown up: psychiatric and personality disorders at age 16 years. *Journal of Child Psychology and Psychiatry*, **35**, 1255–71.

Howell, D. C., Huessy, H. R. & Hassuk, B. (1985). Fifteen-year follow-up of a behavioral history of attention deficit disorder. *Pediatrics*, **76**, 185–90.

Jacobvitz, D., Sroufe, L. A., Stewart, M. & Leffert, N. (1990). Treatment of additional and hyperactivity problems in children with sympathomimetric drugs: a comprehensive review. *Journal of the American Academy of Child and Adolescent Psychiatry*, **29**, 677–88.

James, A. & Taylor, E. (1990). Sex differences in the hyperkinetic syndrome of childhood. *Journal of Child Psychology and Psychiatry*, **31**, 437–46.

Klein, R. G. & Mannuzza, S. (1988). Hyperactive boys almost grown up. III. Methylphenidate effects on ultimate height. *Archives of General Psychiatry*, **45**, 1131–4.

Klorman, R., Brumaghim, J. T., Fitzpatrick, P.A. & Borgstedt. A. D. (1990). Clinical effects of a controlled trial of methylphenidate on adolescents with attention deficit disorder: see comments in: 1992 Jan; *Journal of the American Academy of Child and Adolescent Psychiatry*, **31**, 171–2, **29**, 702–9.

Konkol, R. J., Fischer, M. & Newby, R. F. (1990). Double-blind placebo-controlled stimulant trial in children with Tourette syndrome and attention deficit hyperactivity disorder. Meeting abstract. *Annals of Neurology*, **28**(3), 424.

Lambert, N. M., Hartsough, C. S., Sassone, D. & Sandoval, J. (1987). Persistence of hyperactivity symptoms from childhood to adolescence and associated outcomes. *American Journal of Orthopsychiatry*, **57**, 22–32.

Landgren, M., Petterson, R., Kjellman, B. & Gillberg, C. (1996). ADHD, DAMP and other neurodevelopmental neuropsychiatric disorders in 6 year-olds. *Developmental Medicine and Child Neurology* (In Press).

Losse, A., Henderson, S. E., Elliman, D., Hall, D., Knight, E. & Jongmans, M. (1991). Clumsiness in children–do they grow out of it? A 10-year follow-up study. *Developmental Medicine and Child Neurology*, **33**, 55–68.

Mannuzza, S. & Gittelman, R. (1984). The adolescent outcome of hyperactive girls. *Psychiatry Research*, **13**, 19–29.

Mannuzza, S., Klein, R. G., Konig, P. H. & Ciampino, T. L. (1989). Hyperactive boys almost grown up. IV. Criminality and its relationship to psychiatric status. *Archives of General Psychiatry*, **46**, 1073–9.

Mannuzza, S., Klein, R. G., Bonagura, N., Malloy, P., Giampino, T. L. & Addalli, K. A. (1991). Hyperactive boys almost grown up. V. Replication of psychiatric status. *Archives of General Psychiatry*, **48**, 77–83.

Moffitt, T. E. (1990). Juvenile delinquency and attention deficit disorder: boys' developmental trajectories from age 3 to age 15. *Child Development*, **61**, 893–910.

Ounsted, C., Lindsay, J. & Richards, P. (1987). *Temporal Lobe Epilepsy. A Biographical Study 1948–1986 (Clinics in Developmental Medicine No 103)*. Oxford: MacKeith Press.

Raine, A., Venables, P.H. & Williams, M. (1990). Relationships between central and autonomic measures of arousal at age 15 years and criminality at age 24 years. *Archives of General Psychiatry*, **47**, 1003–7.

Rasmussen, P. & Gillberg, C. (1983). Perceptual, motor and attentional deficits in seven-year-old children. Paediatric aspects. *Acta Paediatrica Scandinavica*, **72**, 125–30.

Rasmussen, P., Gillberg, C., Waldenström, E. & Svenson, B. (1983). Perceptual, motor and attentional deficits in seven-year-old children: neurological and neurodevelopmental aspects. *Developmental Medicine and Child Neurology*, **25**, 315–33.

Råstam, M., Gillberg, C. & Garton, M. (1989). Anorexia nervosa in a Swedish urban region. A population-based study. *British Journal of Psychiatry*, **155**, 642–6.

Realmuto, G. M. & Main, B. (1982). Coincidence of Tourette's disorder and infantile autism. *Journal of Autism and Developmental Disorder*, **12**, 367–72.

Richman, N., Stevenson, J. & Graham, P. (1982). *Pre-School to School: A Behavioural Study*. London: Academic Press.

Ritvo, E. R., Mason-Brothers, A., Freeman, B. J., Pingree, C., Jenson, W. R., McMahon, W. M., Petersen, P. B., Jorde, L. B., Mo, A. & Ritvo, A. (1990). The UCLA-University of Utah epidemiologic survey of autism: the etiologic role of rare diseases. *American Journal of Psychiatry*, **147**, 1614–21.

Roche, A. F., Lipman, R. S., Overall, J. E. & Hung, W. (1979). Effects of stimulant medication on the growth of hyperkinetic children. *Pediatrics*, **5**, 847–50.

Roussounis, S. H. & Gaussen, T. H. (1987). Measurement of attention in severely motor impaired infants: a clinical evaluation of a new approach. *Child Care Health Development*, **13**, 257–68.

Rutter, M. (1967). A children's behaviour questionnaire for completion by teachers: preliminary findings. *Journal of Child Psychology and Psychiatry*, **8**, 1–11.

Rutter, M., Tizard, J. & Whitmore, K. (1970). *Education, Health and Behaviour*. London: Longmans.

Sandberg, S. T., Rutter, M. & Taylor, E. (1978). Hyperkinetic disorder in psychiatric clinic attenders. *Developmental Medicine and Child Neurology*, **20**, 279–99.

Satterfield, J. H., Schell, A. M. & Backs, R. W. (1987). Longitudinal study of AERPs in hyperactive and normal children: relationship to antisocial behavior. *Electroencephalography and Clinical Neurophysiology*, **67**, 531–6.

Satterfield, J. H., Schell, A. M., Nicholas, T. W. & Satterfield, B. T. (1990). Ontogeny of selective attention effects on event-related potentials in attention-deficit hyperactivity disorder and normal boys. *Biological Psychiatry*, **28**, 879–903.

Schaughency, E., McGee, R., Raja, S. N., Feehan, M. & Silva, P. A. (1994). Self-reported inattention, impulsivity, and hyperactivity at ages 15 and 18 years in the general population. *Journal of the American Academy of Child and Adolescent Psychiatry*, **33**, 173–84.

Schmidt, K. & Freidson, S. (1990). Atypical outcome in attention deficit hyperactivity disorder. *Journal of the American Academy of Child and Adolescent Psychiatry*, **29**, 566–70.

Shapiro, A. K., Shapiro, E. S., Young, J. G. & Feinberg, T. E. (eds.) (1988). *Gilles de la Tourette Syndrome*. New York: Raven Press.

Shaywitz, S.E. & Shaywitz, B. A. (1988). Increased medication use in attention-deficit hyperactivity disorder: regressive or appropriate? *Journal of the America Medical Association*, 21; **260**, 2270–2.

Shekim, W. O., Asarnow, R. F., Hess, E., Zaucha, K. & Wheeler, N. (1990). A clinical and demographic profile of a sample of adults with attention deficit hyperactivity disorder, residual state. *Comprehensive Psychiatry*, **31**, 416–25.

Silva, P. A., McGee, R. & Williams, S. M. (1983). Developmental language delay from three to seven years and its significance for low intelligence and reading difficulties at age seven. *Developmental Medicine and Child Neurology*, **25**, 783–93.

Sokol, M. S., Campbell, M., Goldstein, M. & Kriechman, A. M. (1987). Attention deficit disorder with hyperactivity and the dopamine hypothesis: case presentations with theoretical background (clinical conference). *Journal of the American Academy of Child and Adolescent Psychiatry*, **26**, 428–33.

Stevenson, J. (1988). Which aspects of reading ability show a 'hump' in their distribution? *Applied Cognitive Psychology*, **2**, 77–85.

Stevenson, J. & Graham, P. (1982). Temperament: a consideration of concepts and methods. *Ciba Foundation Symposium*, **89**, 36–50.

Tallal, P., Stark, R., Kallman, C. & Mellits, D. (1981). A reexamination of some nonverbal perceptual abilities of language-impaired and normal children as a function of age and sensory modality. *Journal of Speech and Hearing Research*, **24**, 351–7.

Taylor, E., Schachar, R., Thorley, G. & Wieselberg, M. (1986). Conduct disorder and hyperactivity: I. Separation of hyperactivity and antisocial conduct in British child psychiatric patients. *British Journal of Psychiatry*, **149**, 760–7.

Thorley, G. (1984). Review of follow-up and follow-back studies of childhood hyperactivity. *Psychological Bulletin*, **96**, 116–32.

Weiss, G. (1985). Hyperactivity. Overview and new directions. *Psychiatric Clinics of North America*, **8**, 737–53.

WHO (1980). *International Classification of Diseases and Disorders (ICD-9)*. (9th edn). Geneva: Author.

Wing, L. (1981). Asperger's syndrome: a clinical account. *Psychological Medicine*, **11**, 115–29.

Wing, L. (1991). The relationship between Asperger's syndrome and Kanner's autism. In *Autism and Asperger Syndrome*, ed. U. Frith, pp. 93–121. Cambridge: Cambridge University Press.

Index

The terms *attention deficit disorder*, *attention deficit disorder with or without hyperactivity*, *attention deficit hyperactivity disorder (ADHD)*, *hyperkinetic disorder*, *hyperlinetic syndrome*, *hyperactivity*, occur throughout the book. The index has included a number of references to page numbers under these headings (except for hyperactivity which is included under ADHD) but references cannot be exhaustive and other more specific entries can be found throughout the index. The same applies to *diagnosis*, *differential diagnosis*, *terminology*, *clinical aspects* and *clinical assessment*.

Index